Antioxidants

Edited by Emad Shalaby

Published in London, United Kingdom

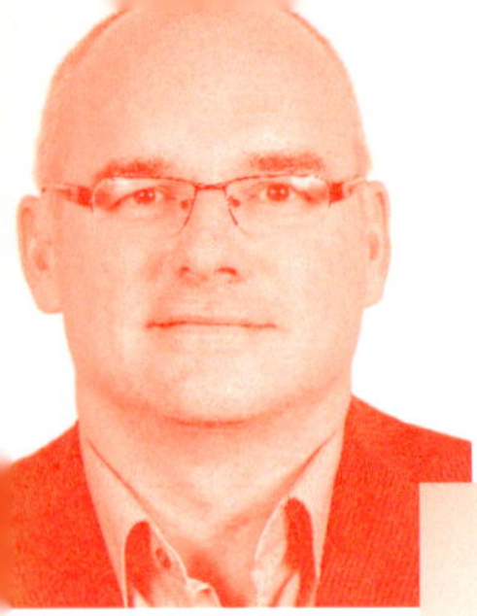
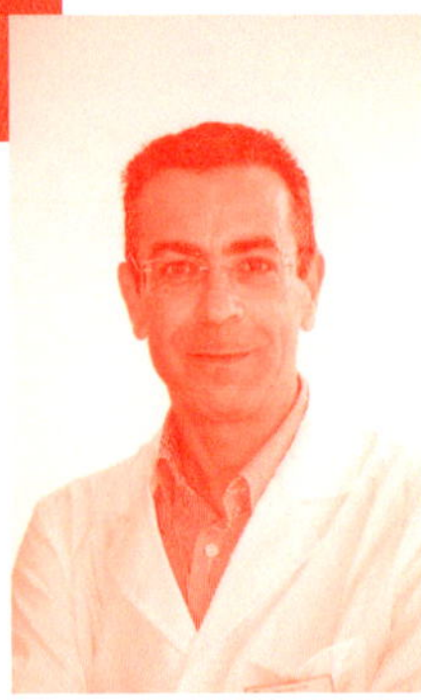
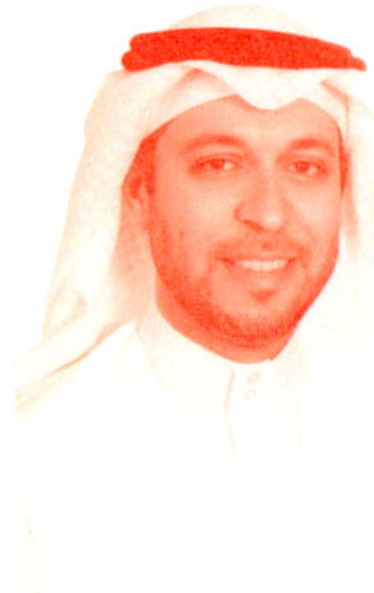
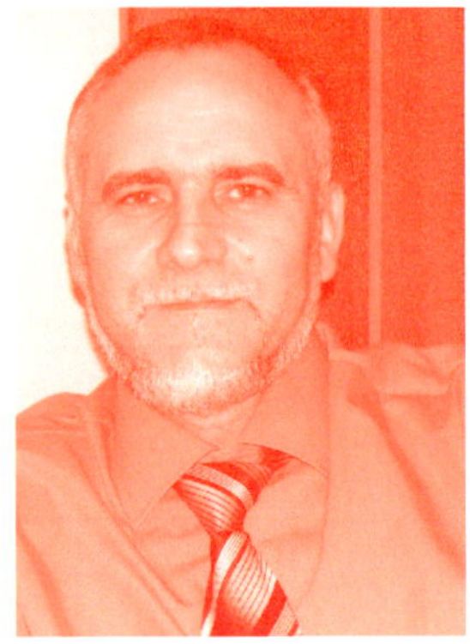
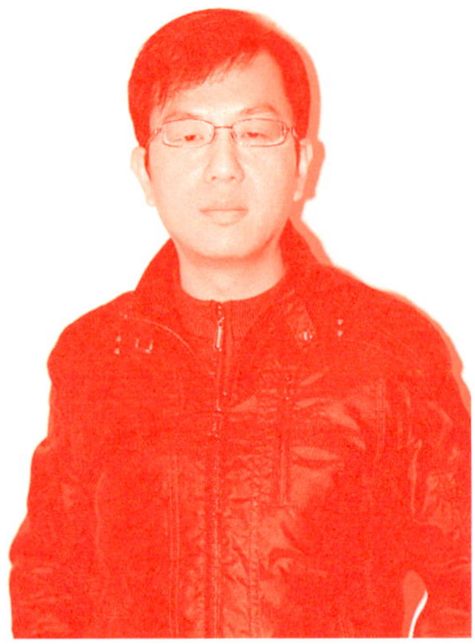
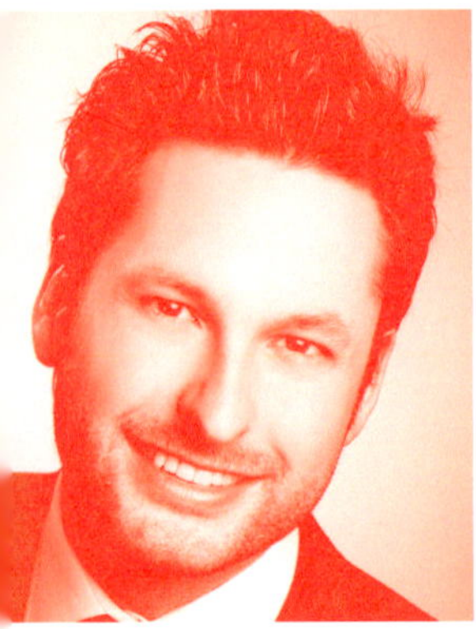
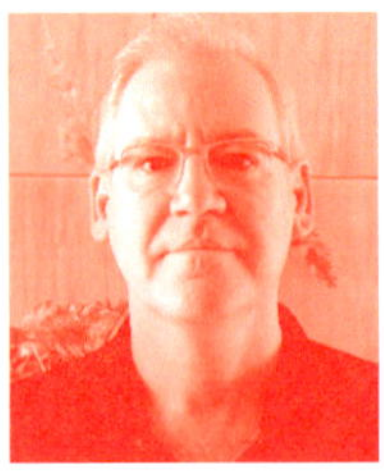

IntechOpen

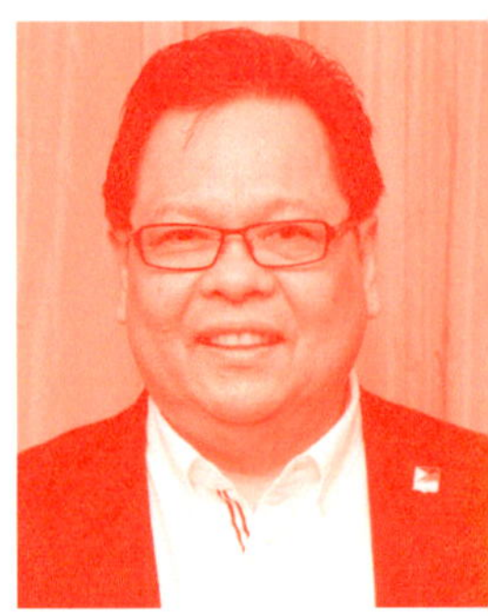
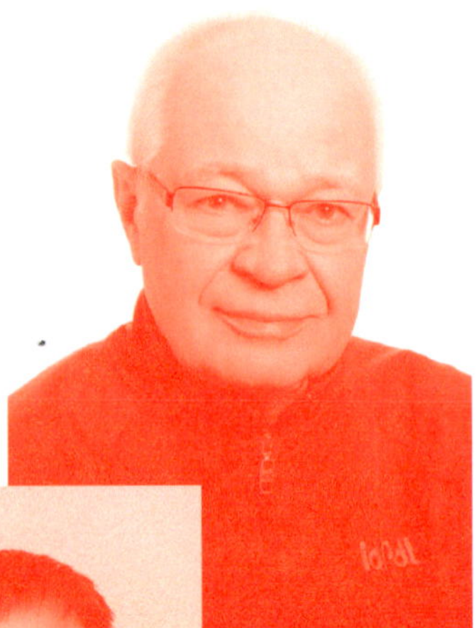
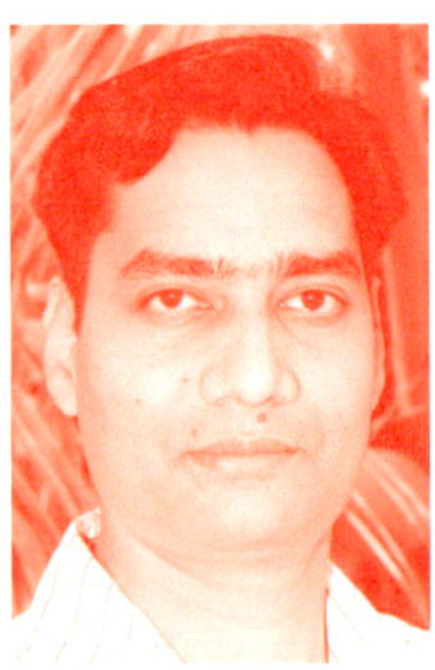
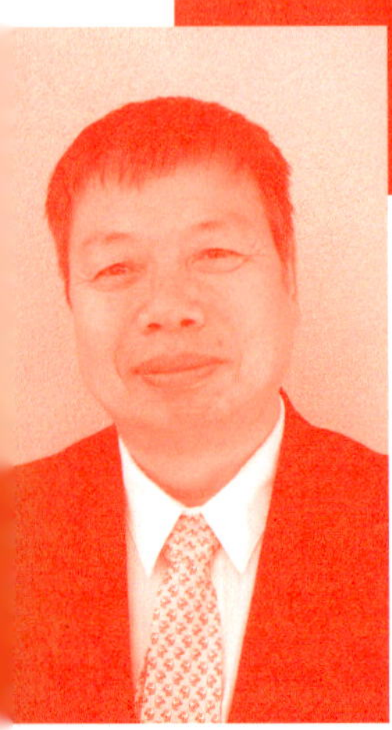
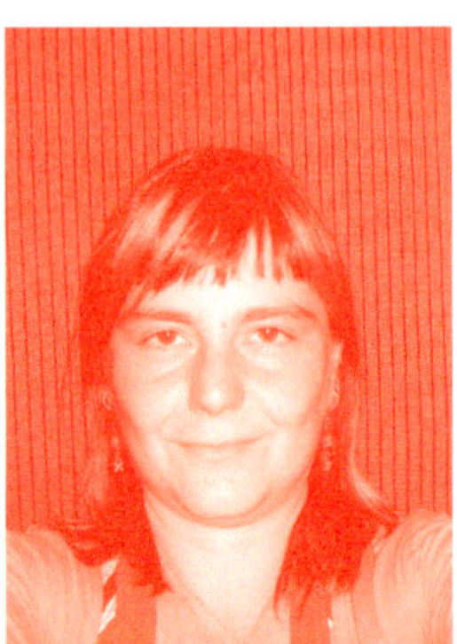
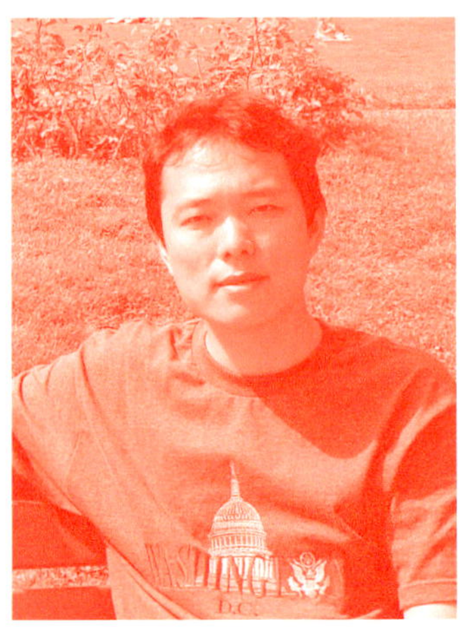

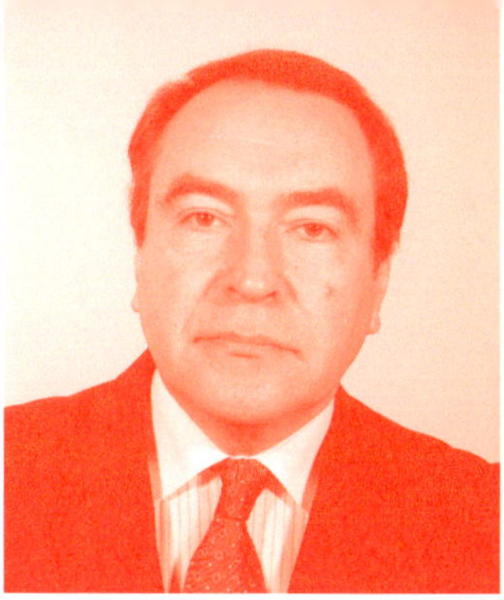
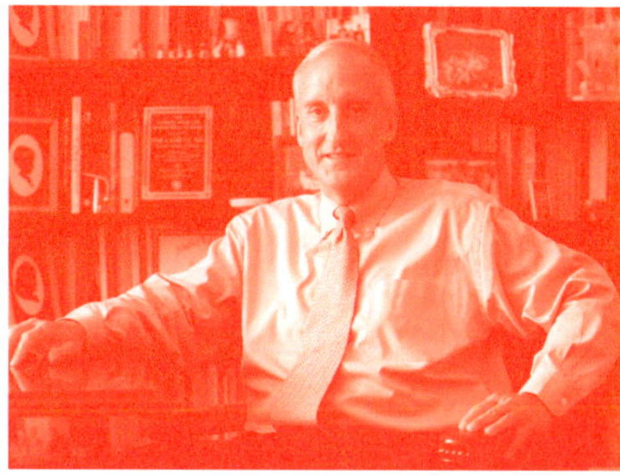
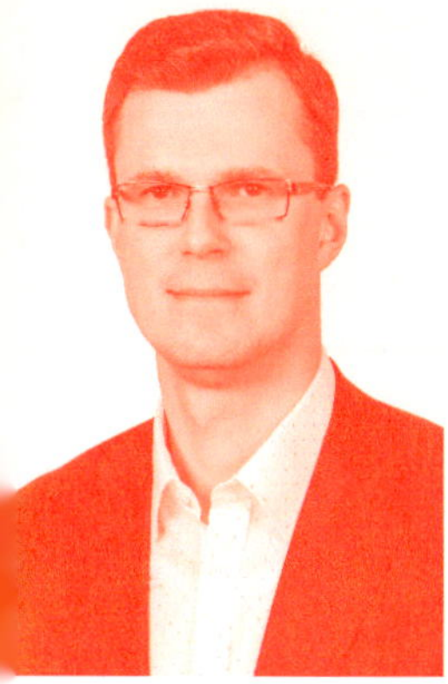
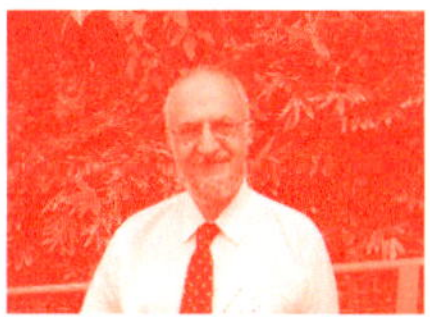
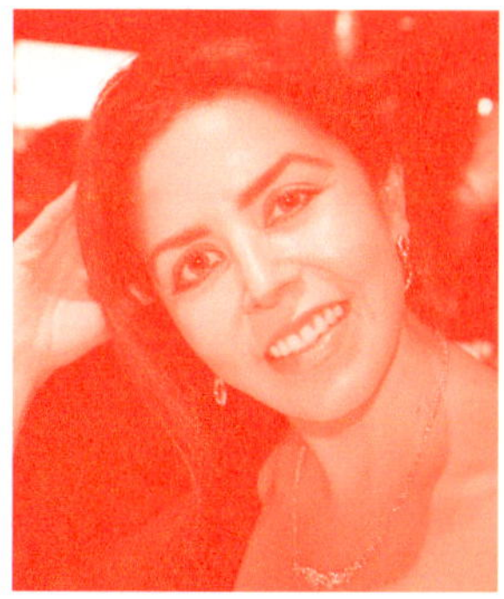

Supporting open minds since 2005

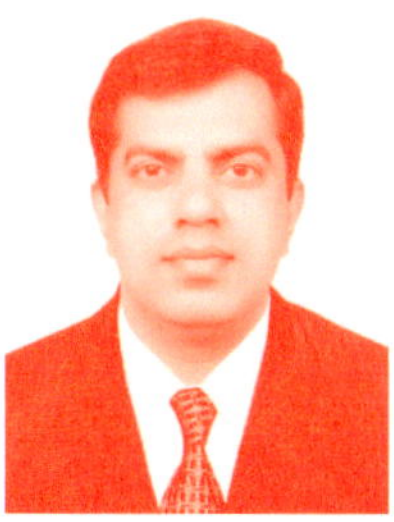
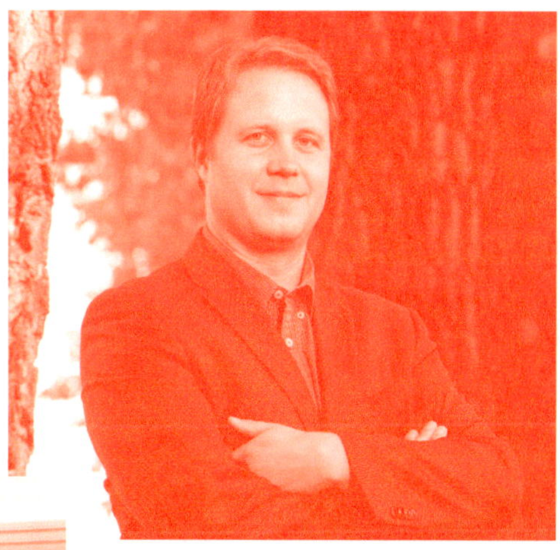
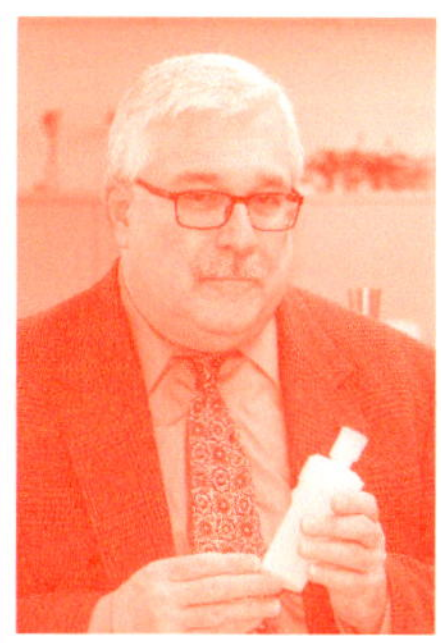
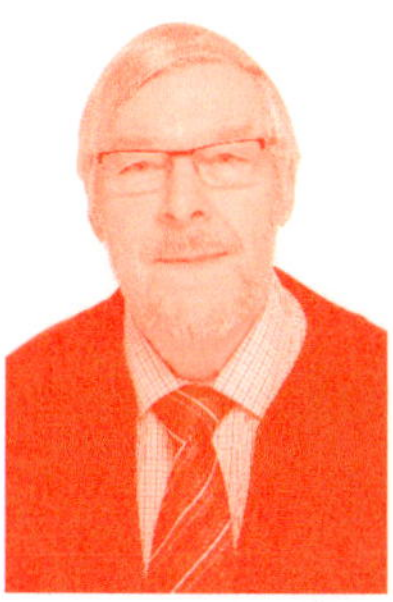
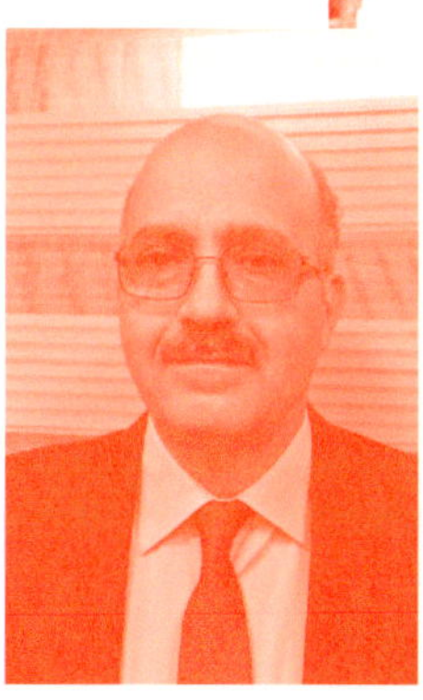
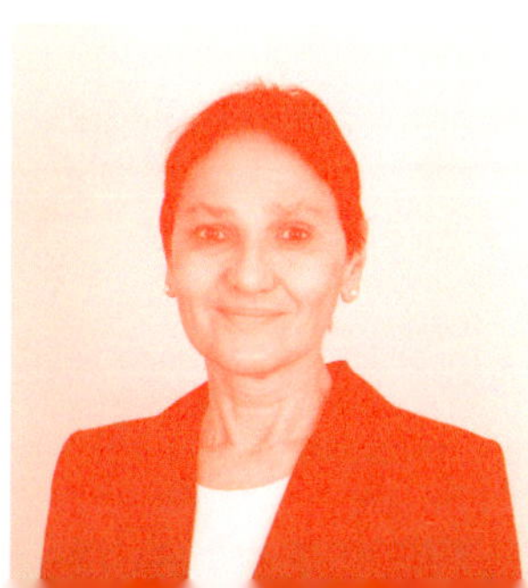
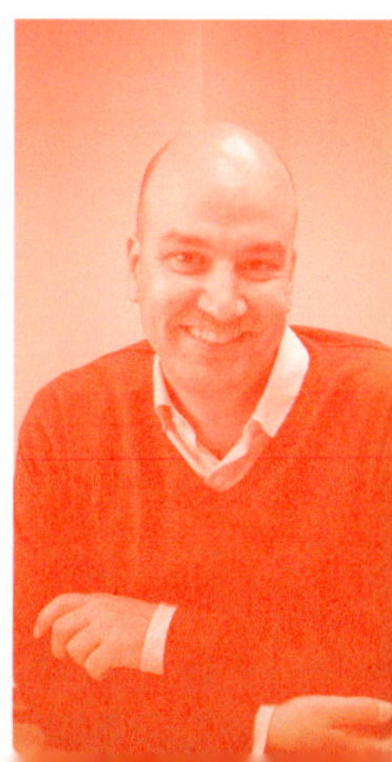

Antioxidants
http://dx.doi.org/10.5772/intechopen.77838
Edited by Emad Shalaby

Part of IntechOpen Book Series: Physiology, Volume 5
Book Series Editor: Angel Catala

Contributors
Melinda Matyas, Gabriela Zaharie, Narendra Maddu, Alejandra Guillermina Miranda-Diaz, Julio Alejandro Gutiérrez-Prieto, Javier Soto-Vargas, Renato Parra-Michel, Andrés García-Sánchez, Leonardo Pazarín-Villaseñor, Norma Francenia Santos-Sánchez, Raúl Salas-Coronado, Beatriz Hernández-Carlos, Claudia Villanueva-Cañongo, Marielba De Los Angeles Rodriguez Salazar, Glides Rafael Olivo Urbina, Priscila do Nascimento Bezerra, Vânia Maria Borges Cunha, Marcilene Paiva Da Silva, Flávia Cristina Seabra Pires, Ana Paula de Souza e Silva, Sérgio Henrique Brabo De Sousa, Raul Nunes de Carvalho Jr, Yapo Guillaume Aboua, Omolola Rebecca Oyenihi, Claudine Manirafasha, Nicole Lisa Brooks, Stefan S. Du Plessis, Manal Azat Aziz, Abdulkareem Shehab Diab, Abeer Abdulrazak Mohammed, Darryl R. Peterson, Ernest J. Sukowski, Syed Ali Raza Naqvi, Sana Nadeem, Sana Komal, Muhammad Samee Mubarik, Muhammad Zahid, Ali Abbas, Syed Ali Asad Naqvi, Sajid Yaqub Qureshi, Naeem-Ul-Haq Khan, Nosheen Aslam, Shahzad Ahmad, Syed Shujat Raza, Daniel Martin Márquez López, Sergio O. Flores-Valle, Tomás A. Fregoso-Aguilar, Jorge A. Mendoza-Pérez, Abdulameer Allaith, Andriy Zagayko, Anna Kravchenko, Victoria Fylymonenko, Tatiana Briukhanova, Dmytro Lytkin, Biljana Kaurinovic, Djendji Vastag, Katarína Bauerova, Vladimir Jakus, Jarmila Kucharska, Jana Muchova, Silvester Ponist, Lukas Slovak, Karol Svik, Paula Cecilia Guadarrama-Mendoza, Mehmet Bozkurt, Percin Karakol, Melihcan Sezgic, Can Uslu, Tevfik Balikci, Danuta Zielińska, Vadim A. Kosolapov, Alexander A. Spasov, Vera A. Anisimova, Olga N. Zhukovskaya, Eva María Molina-Trinidad, Marco Antonio Becerril Flores, José Luis Imbert Palafox, Laura Vargas Servín, Donovan McGrowder, Dwayne Tucker, Melisa Anderson, Lennox Anderson-Jackson, Fabian Miller, Kurt Vaz, Majid Asadi-Samani, Najmeh Kafash Farkhad, Mohammad Reza Mahmoudian-Sani, Hedayatollah Shirzad

First published in London, United Kingdom, 2019 by IntechOpen
IntechOpen is the global imprint of INTECHOPEN LIMITED, registered in England and Wales, registration number: 11086078, 7th floor, 10 Lower Thames Street, London,
EC3R 6AF, United Kingdom
Printed in Croatia

British Library Cataloguing-in-Publication Data
A catalogue record for this book is available from the British Library

Additional hard and PDF copies can be obtained from orders@intechopen.com

Antioxidants
Edited by Emad Shalaby
p. cm.
Print ISBN 978-1-78923-919-5
Online ISBN 978-1-78923-920-1
eBook (PDF) ISBN 978-1-83962-725-5
ISSN 2631-8261

For EU product safety concerns:
IN TECH d.o.o., Prolaz Marije Krucifikse Kozulić 3, 51000 Rijeka, Croatia,
info@intechopen.com or visit our website at intechopen.com.

IntechOpen Book Series

Physiology

Volume 5

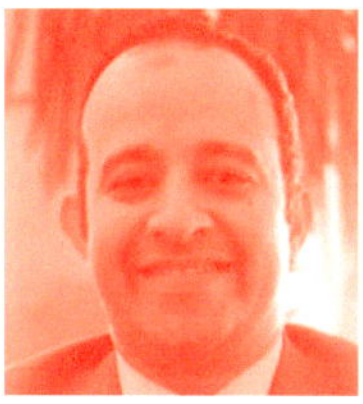

Dr. Emad Shalaby is a professor of biochemistry on the Biochemistry Department Faculty of Agriculture, Cairo University. He received a short-term scholarship to carry out his post-doctoral studies abroad, from Japan International Cooperation Agency (JICA), in coordination with the Egyptian government. Dr. Shalaby speaks fluent English and his native Arabic. He has 77 internationally published research papers, has attended 15 international conferences, and has contributed to 18 international books and chapters. Dr. Shalaby works as a reviewer on over one hundred international journals and is on the editorial board of more than twenty-five international journals. He is a member of seven international specialized scientific societies, besides his local one, and he has won seven prizes.

Editor of Volume 5: Emad Shalaby
Biochemistry Department, Faculty of Agriculture
Cairo University, Giza, Egypt

Book Series Editor: Angel Catala
National University of La Plata, Argentina

Scope of the Series

Modern physiology requires a comprehensive understanding of the integration of tissues and organs throughout the mammalian body, including the expression, structure, and function of molecular and cellular components. While a daunting task, learning is facilitated by our identification of common, effective signaling pathways employed by nature to sustain life. As a main example, the cellular interplay between intracellular Ca2 increases and changes in plasma membrane potential is integral to coordinating blood flow, governing the exocytosis of neurotransmitters and modulating genetic expression. Further, in this manner, understanding the systemic interplay between the cardiovascular and nervous systems has now become more important than ever as human populations age and mechanisms of cellular oxidative signaling are utilized for sustaining life. Altogether, physiological research enables our identification of clear and precise points of transition from health to development of multi-morbidity during the inevitable aging process (e.g., diabetes, hypertension, chronic kidney disease, heart failure, age-related macular degeneration; cancer). With consideration of all organ systems (e.g., brain, heart, lung, liver; gut, kidney, eye) and the interactions thereof, this Physiology Series will address aims of resolve (1) Aging physiology and progress of chronic diseases (2) Examination of key cellular pathways as they relate to calcium, oxidative stress, and electrical signaling & (3) how changes in plasma membrane produced by lipid peroxidation products affects aging physiology

Contents

Preface

Damage in biological compounds such as nucleic acid, protein, lipids, etc. occurs when the free radical encounters another molecule and seeks to find another electron to pair its unpaired electron. Free radicals can cause mutations in different biological compounds and lead to various diseases (cancer, cardiovascular disease, aging, etc.). Antioxidants are chemical substances that protect different human cells from free radical damage that can occur from exposure to certain chemicals, smoking, pollution, radiation, and as a by-product of normal metabolism. Most antioxidants come from natural sources, which include wild plants, herbs and spices, fruits and vegetables, aquatic organisms, and microorganisms, and from antioxidant compounds, including vitamins A, C, and E, carotenoids such as beta-carotene, minerals, phenolic compounds, and other natural chemicals with antioxidant properties. There is developing interest in the utilization of natural antioxidants for the preservation of different kinds of foods and in the management of a number of diseases and conditions. The implication of oxidative stress in the etiology and progression of several acute and chronic clinical diseases has led to the suggestion that antioxidant compounds can have health benefits as prophylactic agents. Several studies have consistently shown an inverse association between consumption of natural products (as fruits, vegetables, herbs, algae etc.), the risk of cardiovascular diseases, and certain kinds of cancer. Although the protective effects have been primarily attributed to well-known antioxidants, such as vitamins A, C and E and beta-carotene, plant phenolic compounds may also play a significant role. Moreover, restrictions on the consumption of synthetic antioxidants such as Butylated hydroxyl anisole and Butylated hydroxyl toluene in food further strengthen the concept of using naturally occurring compounds as antioxidants.

The aim of this book is to illustrate the definition of oxidative stress and antioxidant in addition to identifying antioxidant sources, mechanisms, its applications in different fields, and the relation between antioxidant compounds and their preventive effect against several diseases such as cancer, cardiovascular disease, inflammation, diabetes, atherosclerosis, etc.

The current book will be of interest to students, researchers, and scientists in the field of biological science and applications.

I would like to thank all the contributing authors for their time and great efforts in the careful construction of the chapters and for making this project realizable.

I am grateful to Ms. Sandra Maljavac (Author Service Manager) for her great efforts, encouragement, and guidance during the preparation of this book.

Finally, I would like to express my deepest gratitude towards my parents, my wife (Ghada M. Azzam), and my daughters (Hana, Farida, and Zaina) for their kind cooperation and encouragement, which helped me in completing this book.

Dr. Emad Shalaby
Professor of Biochemistry,
Biochemistry Department,
Faculty of Agriculture,
Cairo University,
Giza, Egypt

Section 1

Antioxidants: Sources and Modes of Actions

Chapter 1

Antioxidant Categories and Mode of Action

Manal Azat Aziz, Abdulkareem Shehab Diab and Abeer Abdulrazak Mohammed

Abstract

Oxidative stress has received a considerable scientific attention as a mediator in the etiology of many human diseases. Oxidative stress is the result of an imbalance between free radicals and antioxidants. Cells can be damaged by free radicals that are considered to play a main role in the aging process and diseases development. Antioxidants are the first line of defense against the detrimental effects of free radical damage, and it is essential to maintain optimal health via different mechanisms of action. Types of antioxidants range from those generated endogenously by the body cells, to exogenous agents such as dietary supplements. Antioxidant insufficiency can be developed as a result of decreased antioxidant intake, synthesis of endogenous enzymes, or increased antioxidant utilization. To maintain optimal body function, antioxidant supplementation has become an increasingly popular practice through improving free radical protection. In this chapter, we first elucidate the oxidative stress, and then define the antioxidant and its categories. Finally, introduce the antioxidants mode of actions for cell protection from free radicals.

Keywords: oxidative stress, antioxidants, reactive oxygen species, antioxidant enzymes, free radicals, antioxidant mechanisms

1. Introduction

Oxidative stress refers to the imbalance between oxidants and antioxidants within the body due to antioxidant deficiency or increased reactive oxygen species (ROS), reactive nitrogen species (RNA), and reactive sulfur species (RSS) production, which lead to potential cellular damage [1, 2]. ROS is a collective term that encompasses all highly reactive forms of oxygen, including free radicals. ROS categories include hydroxyl radical ($OH^{\bullet}$), perhydroxyl radical ($HO_2^{\bullet}$), hypochlorous acid (HOCl), superoxide anion radical ($O_2^{\bullet-}$), hydrogen peroxide (H_2O_2), singlet oxygen ($^1O_2$), nitric oxide radical ($NO^{\bullet}$), hypochlorite radical ($OCl^{\bullet}$), peroxynitrite (ONOO), and different lipid peroxides. RNS are derived from nitric oxide by the reaction with $O_2^{\bullet-}$ to form $ONOO^-$, while RSS are easily produced from thiols through a reaction with ROS [3, 4].

Due to unpaired electrons of free radicals, these free radicals show high activity to react with other molecules in order to be neutralized. The free radicals have important functions in cell signaling, apoptosis, ion transportation, and gene expression [4]. Chemical reactivity of inactivated free radicals can damage all cellular macromolecules including carbohydrates, proteins, lipids, and nucleic acids. In general, cells are able to protect themselves against ROS damage via intracellular enzymatic reactions, metal

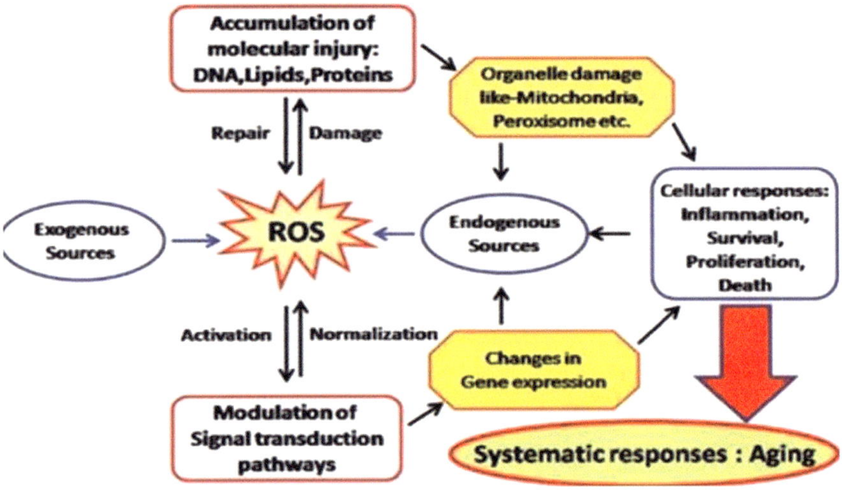

Figure 1.
Reactive oxygen species (ROS) generation by endogenous and exogenous sources can lead to oxidative damage and accumulation of proteins, lipids and DNA, when defensive (repair) mechanisms of the body become weak. These ROS also modulate the signal transduction pathways, which result in organelle damage, and changes in gene expression followed by altered responses of the cells, which finally results into aging. Adapted from Pandey and Rizvi [5].

chelating, and free radical scavenging actions to keep the ROS homeostasis at a low level. In addition, dietary antioxidants can assist to keep an adequate antioxidant status in the body. Nevertheless, during environmental stress and cell dysfunction, levels of ROS can increase dramatically and cause significant cellular damage in the body. Consequently, oxidative stress significantly contributes to the pathogenesis of different diseases, such as heart disease, inflammatory disease, cancer, diabetes mellitus, Alzheimer's disease, autism, and to the aging process (**Figure 1**) [3–5]. The chapter clarifies oxidative stress. Then classify the antioxidants and their applications. Finally, we describe antioxidants' mode of action and how they prevent the cell damage.

2. Oxidative stress

2.1 Oxidative damage to proteins

Protein oxidation can lead to amino acid modification, fragmentation of the peptide chain, aggregation of cross-linked reaction products, and increased electrical charges. Oxidized proteins are more susceptible to proteolysis, and a raise in oxidized proteins may be responsible for the loss of selected physiological and biochemical roles. Free radical damage to proteins may play a role in the causation of cataracts and aging (**Figure 2**) [1, 6].

2.2 Oxidative damage to lipids

Lipids have an important structural and functional role in cell membranes. After cell death, membrane lipids are susceptible to peroxidation and this process can cause misinterpretation of some lipid peroxidation assays. In particular, polyunsaturated fatty acids are susceptible targets for ROS attack. The important reactive moiety and initiator for ROS chain reaction and lipoperoxidation of polyunsaturated is $OH^{\bullet}$ [7]. Because of lipid peroxidation, several compounds are produced, such as alkanes, malondialdehyde, and isoprostanes. These compounds are utilized

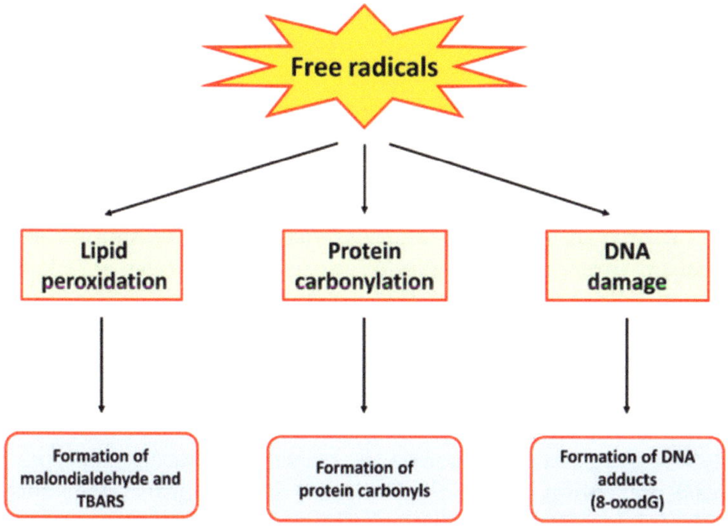

Figure 2.
A schematic diagram illustrating the detrimental effects of free radicals on biomolecules. Adapted from Law et al. [1].

as indicators in lipid peroxidation assay, and have been confirmed in diseases including neurogenerative diseases, heart disease, and diabetes (**Figure 2**) [1, 8].

2.3 Oxidative damage to DNA

Activated oxygen and agents that produce oxygen-free radicals, for example, ionizing radiations, promote damage in DNA that leads to deletion, mutations, and other fatal genetic effects. Through this DNA damage, both sugar and base moieties are susceptible to oxidation, leading to base degradation, single-strand breakage, and cross links to proteins. Free radical damage to DNA is associated in the causation of cancer and accelerated aging (**Figure 2**) [1, 5, 9].

2.4 Oxidative damage to carbohydrates

According to carbohydrates, the production of oxygen-free radicals during early glycation could contribute to glycoxidative damage. Through the primary stages of nonenzymatic glycosylation, fragmentation of sugar forms short-chain species like glycoaldehyde whose chain is too short to cyclize and is thus prone to autoxidation, producing the superoxide radical that can lead to the formation of β-dicarbonyls, which are well-known mutagens [10]. Carbohydrates free radical oxidation mechanisms are comparable to those of lipids. Low molecular carbohydrates, such as glucose, mannitol, and deoxyribose, are well known to interact with $HO^{\bullet}$, forming oxidized intermediates, which does not affect food quality [11].

3. Antioxidants

Antioxidants are inhibitors of oxidation, even at small concentrations; therefore, antioxidants have different physiological functions in the body. In addition, antioxidants act as free radical scavengers, by reacting with the reactive radicals and demolishing them to become less active, less dangerous, and long-lived substance than those radicals that have been neutralized. Antioxidants may be able to neutralize free radicals via accepting or donating electron(s) to remove the unpaired status of the radical [4]. Also, antioxidants can be defined as compounds able to inhibit oxygen-mediated oxidation of different substances from simple molecule to polymer and complicated bio-system [8].

The US Food and Drug Administration (FDA) defined antioxidants as substances utilized to preserve food by retarding deterioration, rancidity, or discoloration owing to oxidation. Whereas antioxidants are important to the food industry to prevent rancidity, antioxidants are also important to biologists and clinicians as they may assist to protect the human body against diseases from ROS danger by regulating ROS-related enzymes [8]. Cellular level of free radicals may be decreased by antioxidants either via inhibiting the activities or expression of free radical generating enzymes such as NAD(P)H oxidase and xanthine oxidase (XO), or by promoting the activities and expression of antioxidant enzymes such as superoxide dismutase (SOD), catalase (CAT), and glutathione peroxidase (GPx) [12–14].

Since 1990s, antioxidant research has increased dramatically due to its potential role in disease prevention and health promotion. In biological systems such as animal models and clinical trials, the antioxidant action of pure compounds, foods, and dietary supplements has been extensively examined [4, 15, 16]. Numerous study models have been determined in chemical and/or biological systems to examine the mechanism of action of antioxidants, as well as the identification and recognition of new antioxidants, particularly from natural substances. Further research in animal models and cell cultures has provided critical information on the bioavailability, metabolism, and toxicity issues of antioxidants, suggesting probable clinical applications of these substances. Nevertheless, animal models and human research are expensive and not suitable for early antioxidant screening of foods and dietary supplements. Therefore, cell culture models have been utilized for early screening and study proceeding to animal research and human clinical trials [4].

Antioxidants can protect the cells and organs of the body against the harmful effect of the oxidative stress through various defense mechanisms by both enzymatic and nonenzymatic reactions, which work synergistically and together with each other. To prevent lipid peroxidation in food, nonenzymatic antioxidants are often added. The use of antioxidants for food and therapeutic purposes must be characterized carefully, because several lipid antioxidants can exert a prooxidant effect to other molecules under particular circumstances [5, 7].

The feature of a perfect antioxidant is that it should be readily absorbed, eliminate free radicals, and chelate redox metals at physiologically suitable levels. In addition, it should work in both aqueous and membrane domains, and have a positive effect on gene expression [7].

4. Antioxidant categories

Antioxidants can be classified in several ways [17, 18].

1. Based on their activity, they can be classified as enzymatic and nonenzymatic antioxidants. Dangerous oxidative products can be converted to H_2O_2 and then to water by enzymatic antioxidants that are able to break down and get rid of free radicals in a multistep process in the presence of cofactors such as copper (Cu), zinc (Zn), manganese (Mn), selenium (Se), and iron (Fe).

2. Vitamin C, vitamin E, plant polyphenol, carotenoids, and glutathione are nonenzymatic antioxidants, which act by interrupting free radicals chain reactions.

3. Based on solubility, antioxidants can be classified as water-soluble or lipid-soluble antioxidants. Vitamin C is a type of water-soluble vitamin found in cellular fluids such as cytosol or cytoplasmic matrix.

4. According to size, antioxidants can be categorized as small or large-molecule antioxidants. The small molecule antioxidants neutralize the ROS in a process named radicals scavenging and carry them away. Vitamin C, vitamin E, carotenoids, and glutathione (GSH) are the main antioxidants in this category. Large molecule antioxidants include enzymes (SOD, CAT, and GPx) and sacrificial proteins (albumin) that absorb ROS and prevent them from attacking other essential proteins.

5. Kinetically antioxidants can be categorized as below:

    a. Antioxidants that are able to break chains through reacting with peroxyl radicals containing weak O–H or N–H bonds, phenol, naphthol, hydroquinone, aromatic amines, and aminophenols.

    b. Antioxidants with a capability to break chains by reacting with alkyl radicals: quinines, nitrones, and iminoquinones.

    c. Antioxidants that terminate cyclic chain such as aromatic amines, nitroxyl radicals, and variable valence metal compounds.

    d. Hydroperoxide decomposing antioxidants such as sulfide, phosphide, and thiophosphate.

    e. Metal-deactivating antioxidants include diamines, hydroxyl acids, and bifunctional compounds.

    f. Synergism action of a number of antioxidants including phenol sulfide in which the phenolic group reacts with the peroxylradical's sulfide group with hydroperoxide.

6. Based on their occurrence, antioxidants are categorized as natural or synthetic [19, 20].

    a. Natural antioxidants

They are classified as chain-breaking antioxidants, which react with radicals and convert them into more stable products. Generally, antioxidants of this group are phenolic in structure and include the following:

1. Antioxidant minerals: these are antioxidant enzymes cofactors like selenium, copper, iron, zinc, and manganese. Absence of the cofactors will definitely enhance many macromolecules metabolism such as carbohydrates.

2. Antioxidant vitamins: these are important and required for most body metabolism functions such as, vitamin C, E, and B.

3. Phytochemicals: these are phenolic compounds derivatives that are neither vitamins nor minerals. Examples include flavonoids, catechins, carotenoids, carotene, lycopene, and herbs and spices such as diterpene, rosmariquinone, thyme, nutmeg, clove, black pepper, ginger, garlic, curcumin, and derivatives.

b. Synthetic antioxidants

These are phenolic compounds that carry out the role of capturing free radicals and stopping the chain reaction. These compounds include butylated hydroxyl anisole (BHA), butylated hydroxyltoluene (BHT), propyl gallate (PG), metal chelating agent (EDTA), tertiary butyl hydroquinone (TBHQ), and nordihydroguaiaretic acid (NDGA).

4.1 Antioxidant enzymes

There are several enzymes that catalyze reactions to neutralize free radicals and ROS. These enzymes form the body's endogenous defense mechanisms from free radicals to protect the cell. The enzyme antioxidants GPx, CAT, and SOD are the best-known substances of the antioxidant protection system, and they are responsible for the free radical change [21]. Enzymes are important components of the protection and defense mechanisms, by decreasing ROS generation via removing potential oxidants/transferring ROS/RNS into relatively stable compounds [5]. For optimum catalytic activity, these enzymes require micronutrient cofactors such as Se, Fe, Cu, Zn, and Mn [21].

4.1.1 Superoxide dismutase (SOD)

Irwin Fridovitch of Duke University and Joe McCord discovered antioxidant enzyme (SOD) (EC 1.15.1.1) in 1967, which belongs to the group of oxidoreductases. SOD is an important cellular defense against free radical damage. Therefore, medical scientists have begun to look seriously at free radicals [3]. SOD antioxidant enzymes are metal-containing proteins that catalyze the dismutation of the highly reactive superoxide anion to O_2 and to the less reactive species H_2O_2 (Eq. (1)). The result is that peroxide can be destroyed by reaction of CAT or GPX [22, 23].

$$O_2^{-} + O_2^{-} + 2H^{+} \xrightarrow{SOD} H_2O_2 + O_2 \tag{1}$$

In mammals, there are three forms of SOD; the active site of the enzyme contains one or two different atoms of a transition metal in a certain oxidation state. SODs are categorized by their metal cofactors into known forms: cytosolic SOD, extracellular SOD [CuZnSOD], and mitochondrial SOD [MnSOD]. Each form is produced by distinct genes and distinct subcellular localization, but catalyzes the same reaction. This distinct subcellular localization of the three SOD forms is especially significant for compartmentalized redox signaling [24].

CuZnSOD enzymes have two identical subunits of about 32 kDa, though a monomeric structure is found in a high concentration of protein from *E. coli*. Each subunit includes a metal cluster, an active site, and a Cu and a Zn atom bridged By a histamine residue. The Cu and Zn which are important for SOD enzymatic activity. Zn contributes in appropriate protein folding and stability. Cu is not replaceable with another metal, while Zn is replaceable with cobalt and Cu, and it is not essential for enzyme action at low pH. CuZnSOD plays a major function in the first line of antioxidant defense [25].

MnSOD is a homotetramer 96 kDa; each subunit contains one Mn atom, those cycles from Mn^{3+} to Mn^{2+} and back to Mn^{3+} during the two-step dismutation of superoxide. In mitochondria, the main source of oxygen radicals is the respiratory chain. It was shown that this enzyme is greatly stimulated and decreased by cytokines, while oxidants moderately influenced it [26–28].

Extracellular SOD (ECSOD) is a tetrameric protein, containing Cu and Zn having a high affinity for certain glycosaminoglycans such as heparin and heparin sulfate [7]. ECSOD is found primarily in the extracellular membrane and to a lesser extent, in the extracellular fluids. It protects against the inactivation of NO liberating from the endothelium by $O_2^{\bullet-}$ through diffusion to smooth muscle, thus preserving endothelial function. Studies have shown that ECSOD plays an essential role in various oxidative stress-dependent pathophysiologies, such as hypertension, ischemia reperfusion injury, and lung injury. In addition, a number of lines of research propose a role for ECSOD in aging. ECSOD plasma levels decrease with aging, and in old rats, gene transfer of ECSOD improves endothelial function. However, it is still unknown whether ECSOD expression or activity in blood vessels is adjusted by aging and whether endogenous ECSOD is engaged in regulation of vascular functions during aging [29].

4.1.1.1 Application

SOD enzymes enhance the rejuvenation and cellular repair, while decreasing the damage caused by free radicals. SOD is necessary to generate sufficient amounts of skin building cells named fibroblasts and plays an essential role in preventing the progress of amyotrophic lateral sclerosis (ALS), which causes death if it affects the nerve cells in the spinal cord and brain. In addition, this enzyme is also utilized for inflammatory diseases treatment, burn injuries, prostate problems, corneal ulcer, arthritis, and reversing the long-term consequences of radiation and smoke exposure. Furthermore, it prevents wrinkle formation if the skin lotion contains this enzyme. Also, it enhances wound healing, reduces scars, and lightens skin pigmentation caused by UV rays.

Moreover, SOD facilitates nitric oxide moving into hair follicles. This is beneficial for people with a genetic predisposition or free radicals for premature hair loss. SOD is a very potent antioxidant, in that it combats the effect of free radicals on the hair follicles. Because of nitric oxide's ability as a blood vessel relaxant, allowing more blood to reach the hair follicle, and SOD ability to remove free radicals, hair loss can be prevented or reversed. Maintaining overall well-being and health, as well as free radical protection, can be achieved by taking dietary supplement that provides an adequate supply of SOD [3].

4.1.2 Catalase (CAT)

Catalase (EC 1.11.1.6) is an enzyme responsible for H_2O_2 degradation that is generated by oxidases involved in β-oxidation of fatty acids, respiration, and purine catabolism [3]. It is present in nearly all animal cells as a protective enzyme. The highest levels of CAT activity are measured in the liver, kidney, and red blood cells.

Human CAT composes four identical subunits of 62 kDa, each subunit containing four distinct domains and one prosthetic heme group, and has a molecular mass of about 240 kDa [30]. CAT enzyme reacts with H_2O_2 to form water and molecular oxygen and with H donors such as methanol, ethanol, formic acid, or phenols with peroxidase activity. CAT protects cells from H_2O_2 generated within them. Therefore, it has an essential role in the acquisition of tolerance to oxidative stress in the adaptive response of cells. Various disease conditions and abnormalities are associated with the deficiency or mutation of CAT enzyme [30, 31].

4.1.2.1 Application

In the food industry, CAT enzyme is used to remove H_2O_2 from milk prior to cheese production, and to prevent food from oxidizing in food wrappers. In addition,

CAT enzyme is used in the textile industry for H_2O_2 removal from fabrics, to make sure the material is peroxide free. Recently, esthetics industries have begun to use CAT enzyme in facial masks, as the combination of CAT enzyme with H_2O_2 on the face can be used to increase cellular oxygenation in the upper layers of the epidermis [3].

4.1.3 Glutathione perioxidases (GPx)

Glutathione peroxidase (EC 1.11.1.9) contains a single selenocysteine residue in each of the four identical subunits, which is important for enzyme activity. GPx (80 kDa) is an imperative intracellular enzyme that catalyzes H_2O_2 to water and lipid peroxides to their corresponding alcohols mainly in the mitochondria and sometimes in the cytosol. In mammals, there are five GPx isoenzymes. Though their expression is ubiquitous, the level of each isoform differs depending on their tissue type. Mitochondrial and cytosolic glutathione peroxidase (GPx1 or cGPx) reduces fatty acid hydroperoxides and H_2O_2 at the expense of glutathione [32].

GPx1 is the main ubiquitous selenoperoxidase present in most cells; found in the cytosolic, mitochondrial, and peroxisomal compartments. It is an important antioxidant enzyme required in the detoxification of H_2O_2 and lipid hydroperoxides and preventing DNA, protein and lipids damage by harmful accumulation of intracellular H_2O_2 [33]. GPx1 uses GHS as an obligate co-substrate in the reduction of H_2O_2 to water [32]. Phospholipid hydroperoxidase glutathione (PHGPX) is found in most tissues and can directly reduce the phospholipid hydroperoxides, fatty acid hydroperoxides, and cholesterol hydroperoxides that are produced in peroxidized membranes and oxidized lipoproteins [30].

GPx4 is found in both the cytosol and the membrane fraction, and is highly expressed in renal epithelial cells and tests. Cytosolic GPx2 or extracellular GPx3 is inadequately found in nearly all tissues except for the gastrointestinal tract and kidney. In recent, GPx5, a new kind, expressed particularly in mouse epididymis, is selenium independent [34].

Several studies underlined the clinical importance of GPx. In addition, GPx, especially GPx1, have been implicated in the progression and prevention of many frequent and complex diseases, including cancer and cardiovascular disease [34, 35].

4.1.3.1 Application

GPx is an important antioxidant enzyme in the body. Glutathione (GHS), the master antioxidant, is important for GPx levels due to the closely linked relationship; GHS is a tripeptide that protects the cells against the negative effects of pollution and functions as the body's immune system booster. GHS plays an essential role in red blood cells to remain intact and protects white blood cells, which are responsible for the immune system. An antioxidant's role is specifically essential for the brain because it is sensitive to the presence of free radicals. To increase the body's protection from free radicals, it is imperative to combine certain antioxidants such as glutathione, vitamin C and E, Se, and GPx [3].

4.2 Nonenzymatic antioxidants

In previous decades, there has been increasing evidence that large amounts of antioxidants present in our diet contribute to the antioxidant defense system by preventing oxidative stress and specific human diseases. Phytochemicals, the plant-derived compounds, are one of the classes of the dietary factors, which play an essential role in functions of the body. Food materials contain a number of natural compounds reported to have antioxidant characteristics due to the presence of hydroxyl groups in their structure. Synthetic and natural antioxidants prevent the oxidative damage to the most important macromolecules such as lipids, proteins, and nucleic acids found in human body through scavenging the free radicals formed in different biochemical processes [36]. These antioxidants consist of small molecules including vitamin C, E, and β-carotene or natural antioxidants such as flavonoids, tannins, coumarins, phenolics, and terpenoids [37]. Because of oxidative stress, the free radicals that have been produced react with lipids, proteins and nucleic acids and lead to stimulation of apoptosis, which causes various neurological, cardiovascular, and physiological disorders [38].

In addition to phytochemical antioxidants, which can protect the body from oxidative damage, there are other antioxidants for example polyphenols, lycopene, and lutein [39]. Even though there has been a considerable concentration on antioxidant function of phytochemicals for several years, it is distinguished that phytochemicals have nonantioxidant effects important for health such as cell signaling and gene expression [40].

4.2.1 Glutathione

Glutathione (γ-glutamyl-cysteinyl-glycine; GSH) is a tripeptide and is the most abundant intracellular antioxidant protecting normal cells from oxidative injury due to its role as a substrate of ROS scavenging enzymes. Glutathione is primarily present in its reduced form (GSH) in normal conditions, with only a small amount being found in the fully oxidized state (GSSG) [41]. Glutathione functions as a nonenzymatic antioxidant through free radical scavenging in cells and serves as a cofactor for several enzymes, include GPx, glutathione reductase (GR), and glutathione transferase (GST) [42, 43].

4.2.1.1 Application

Recently, there is a new era of therapeutic applications of glutathione through the association of decreased GSH levels with the common features of aging and a wide range of pathological conditions, including neurodegenerative disorders. Remarkably, depletion and alterations of GSH in its metabolism appear to be crucial in the onset of Parkinson's disease [44].

4.2.2 Vitamin E

Vitamin E, C, and β-carotene are the main antioxidant vitamins for tissues against free radical damage. Vitamin E, a major lipid soluble antioxidant, functions as the most important membrane-bound antioxidant, neutralizing free radicals, and preventing oxidation of lipids within membranes [45]. Vitamin E is the free radical scavenger in the prevention of chronic diseases [46]. α-Tocopherol is the main form of vitamin E with antioxidant and immune functions. α-tocopherol has been revealed to be a more effective inhibitor of peroxynitrite-induced lipid peroxidation and inflammatory reactions [47]. *In vitro* tocotrienols have excellent antioxidant activity and have been proposed to restrain ROS more effectively than tocopherols [48].

4.2.2.1 Application

The main function of vitamin E is to protect against lipid peroxidation through evidence suggesting that α-tocopherol and vitamin C function together in a cyclic type of process. It has been reported that vitamin E supplementation in hypercholesterolemic patients has shown to increase autoantibody levels against oxidized LDL, and prevent ischemic heart disease [49].

4.2.3 Vitamin C

In extracellular fluids, vitamin C, a water-soluble vitamin, is the most important antioxidant and can protect biomembranes against lipid peroxidation injury through eliminating peroxyl radicals in the aqueous phase before peroxidation initiation. Vitamin C is an effective antioxidant located in the aqueous phase of cells; it simply loses electrons to give stability to reactive species such as ROS [45]. In addition to vitamin C's biological functions as a superoxide and hydroxyl radicals' scavenger, it also functions as an enzyme cofactor [42].

4.2.3.1 Application

Vitamin C plays an essential function in the defense against oxidative damage particularly in leukocytes, as well as the possible effect it may have on the treatment of chronic degenerative diseases, autoimmune diseases, and cancer [42, 45].

4.2.4 Carotenoids

Carotenoids are structurally and functionally different natural pigments found in many fruits and vegetables. A combination of carotenoids and tocopherols antioxidants in the lipid phase of biological membranes may enhance better antioxidant protection than tocopherols alone. Antioxidant characteristics of carotenoids include scavenging single oxygen and peroxyl radicals, thiyl, sulfonyl, sulfur, and NO_2 radicals and giving protection to lipids from superoxide and hydroxyl radical attack [49].

4.2.4.1 Application

Carotenoids and some of their metabolites are proposed to play a protective function in several ROS-mediated disorders, include cardiovascular, cancer, and myocardial infarction among smokers. Carotenoid-rich food and supplementation decrease morbidity in nonsmokers and reduce the risk of prostate cancer [42].

4.2.5 Vitamin A

Vitamin A, a lipid soluble vitamin, is important for human health and has free radicals scavenging features that aid it to act as a physiological antioxidant in protecting a number of chronic diseases such as cardiovascular disease and cancer. All transretinol, the parent compound, are the most abundant dietary form of vitamin A that occurs naturally in the form of fatty acid esters such as retinyl palmitate, while retinal and retinoic acid are the minor natural dietary components of vitamin A [45]. Vitamin A was first labeled as an inhibitor of the effect of linoleic acid on the oxidation processes. At present, vitamin A and carotenoids are known for their antioxidant actions depending on their capability to interact with radicals and prohibit cell lipid peroxidation [9].

4.2.5.1 Application

Vitamin A is important for life in mammals; it cannot be synthesized in body and has to be supplied by food. Due to its role as antioxidant, vitamin A has a new role in preventive nutrition against neurodegenerative diseases. Recently, vitamin A has increased the interest in supplementation via food [50].

4.2.6 Uric acid

Uric acid, hyperuricemia, is a potent free radical scavenger and estimated ~60% of free radical scavenging capacity in plasma [51]. Uric acid is a physiological antioxidant and an effective preventer of the production of ROS species during the action of xanthine oxidase (XO) in catalysis reaction of xanthine and hypoxanthine [42]. A study illustrated the urate ability to scavenge oxygen radicals and protect the erythrocyte membrane from lipid oxidation, characterized further by Ames et al. through the effect of uric acid in protection of cells from oxidants, which related to a variety of physiological situation [51]. Nevertheless, it is probable that the increase in serum level of uric acid is a response to protect against the detrimental effects of extreme free radicals and oxidative stress [52].

4.2.6.1 Application

Studies showed that serum uric acid levels are highly predictive of mortality in patients with coronary artery disease, heart failure, or diabetes. In addition, high uric acid level is associated with deleterious effect on vascular function. Recently, it has been found that patients with high serum uric acid level had impaired flow-mediated dilation, which was normalized by therapy for 3 months with the xo inhibitor allopurinol [53].

4.2.7 Lipoic acid

Lipoic acid is a strong antioxidant, and it reveals a great capability of antioxidant when given natural or as a synthetic drug. Lipoic acid is a short-chain fatty acid, composed of sulfur in their structure that is known for its contribution in the reaction that catalyzes the oxidation decarboxylation of α-keto acids, for example pyruvate and α-ketoglutarate, in the citric acid cycle. Lipoic acid and its reduced form, dihydrolipoic acid (DHLA), are capable of quenching free radicals in both lipid and aqueous domains. Lipoic acid and DHLA have been revealed to have antioxidant, cardiovascular, antiaging, detoxifying, anti-inflammatory, anticancer, and neuroprotective pharmacological properties [40, 54].

4.2.7.1 Application

Regarding the pathology of diabetes, there are many potential applications for lipoic acid. In type I diabetes, destruction of pancreatic β-cells leads to loss secretion of insulin, while the major problem in type II diabetes is insulin resistance of peripheral tissues. Lipoic acid has potential preventive or ameliorative effect in both type I and type II diabetes [54].

4.2.8 Flavonoids

Flavonoids are low in molecular weight and are the main type of phenolic compounds in plants. They are structured by 15 carbon atoms, organized in a C6-C3-C6 configuration. Due to their high redox potential, flavonoids are, in particular, important antioxidants that allow them to function as reducing agents, hydrogen donors, and singlet oxygen quenchers. In addition, they include a metal chelating potential [55].

4.2.8.1 Application

Flavonoids are generally found in many fruits and vegetables. When human increasingly consumed it, flavonoids have been linked with a decrease in the incidence of diseases such as prostate [56, 57] or breast cancer [58, 59].

4.2.9 Tannins

Tannins are relatively high-molecular compounds, which comprise the third essential group of phenolics and can be divided into condensed and hydrolysable tannins. Condensed tannins are produced by the polymerization of flavonoid units. The mainly studied condensed tannins are based on flavan-3-ols: (−)-epicatechin and (+)-catechin. Hydrolysable tannins are heterogeneous polymers containing phenolic acids, in particular, gallic acid (3,4,5 trihydroxyl benzoic acid) and simple sugar [42, 55].

4.2.9.1 Application

Because of tannin features, such as being the potential metal ion chelators, protein-precipitating agents, and biological antioxidants, tannins have different effects on biological systems. As a consequence of the diverse tannins biological roles and structural variation, it has been difficult to modify models that would let a precise prediction of their effects in any system. Therefore, the tannin structure modification and activity relationship are important to predict their biological effect [42].

5. Antioxidants: mechanisms of action

Generally, the antioxidants defend against free-radicals-induced oxidative damage by various mechanisms as discussed in below sections.

5.1 Preventive antioxidants

ROS such as H_2O_2, $O_2^{\bullet}$, and $OH^{\bullet}$ are produced irreversibly during metabolism. Therefore, methods have been extensively studied to reduce the damage enhanced by oxidative stress. Intracellular antioxidant enzymes produced in the cell are an essential protective mechanism against free radicals formation. SOD, CAT, GPx, GR, GST, thioredoxin reductase, and hemeoxygenase are the most important antioxidants enzymes. SODs convert $O_2^{\bullet}$ into H_2O_2, which is then converted into water by CAT, GPx, and Fenton reaction. Thus, two toxic species are converted into a harmless product (**Figure 3**) [5].

During metabolism, peroxides are formed and then eliminated via both GST and GPX. GRd regulates the equivalent of GSH and oxidized glutathione (GSSG), and the ratio of GSH/GSSG is a known index of oxidative stress [60]. The action of GRd plays an imperative role in increasing GSH concentration, which maintains the oxido-redox condition in the organism [14]. Consequently, the oxidative stress role has been reported in the progress and clinical symptom of autism. Recently, a comparison study between autism and control individuals showed decrease in GSH/GSSG ratio and increase in free radical generation in autism compared to control cells [60]. In addition, GPx is presented throughout the cell, while CAT is frequently limited to peroxisomes. In the brain, which is very sensitive to free radical damage, it has seven times more GPx activity than CAT activity. Moreover, CAT's highest levels are found in the liver, kidney, and erythrocytes, where it decomposes the most of H_2O_2 [61].

5.2 Free radical scavengers

5.2.1 Scavenging superoxide and other ROS

Superoxide ($O_2^{\bullet -}$), a predominant cellular free radical, is contributed in a huge number of deleterious alterations often linked to a low concentration of antioxidants

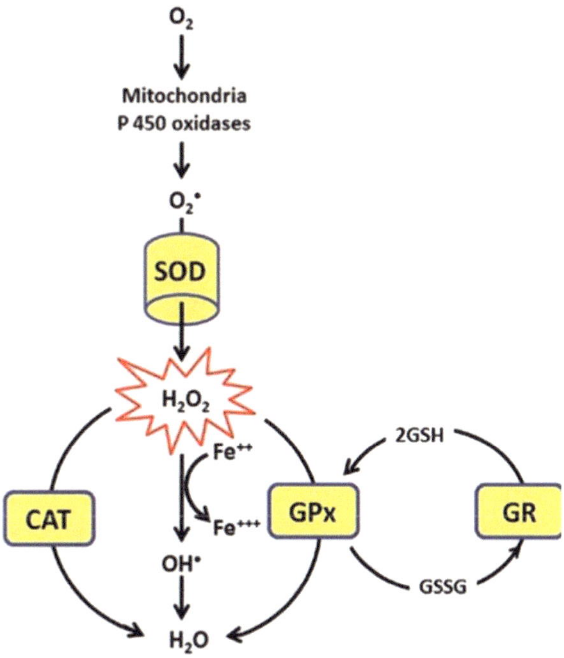

Figure 3.
Antioxidant enzyme system, $O_2^{\bullet}$, is dismutaed toH_2O_2 by SOD enzyme. The resulted H_2O_2 is converted into water by CAT and GPx. In this way, two toxic species, $O_2^{\bullet}$ and H_2O_2, are converted into the harmless product water. GPx neutralized H_2O_2 via taking hydrogen from two GSH molecules forming two molecules of water and GSSG. GR then regenerates GSH from GSSG. CAT, the essential part of enzymatic defense, neutralizes H_2O_2 into water. By Fenton reaction, H_2O_2 is also converted to the highly reactive $OH^{\bullet}$ and then to water through oxidation of Fe^{2+} to Fe^{3+}. Adapted from Pandey and Rizvi [5].

and associated with a raise in peroxidative processes. Though $O_2^{\bullet-}$ itself is not reactive to biomolecules, it assists in production of stronger $OH^{\bullet}$' and $ONOO^-$.$O_2^{\bullet-}$ is formed in large quantities, in phagocytes via NADPH oxidase enzyme during pathogen-killing process. In addition, it is a byproduct of mitochondrial respiration [3].

5.2.2 Scavenging hydroxyl radical and other ROS

Hydroxyl radical ($OH^{\bullet}$) is an extremely active and more toxic radical on biologic molecules such as DNA, lipids, and proteins than other radical species. In general, $OH^{\bullet}$ is considered to be formed from the Fe^{2+} or Cu^+/H_2O_2 Fenton reaction system, through incubation $FeSO_4$ and H_2O_2 in aqueous solution. Therefore, antioxidants activity as $OH^{\bullet}$ scavenger can be accomplished by direct scavenging or prohibiting of $OH^{\bullet}$ generation by the chelation of free metal ions or altering H_2O_2 to other nontoxic compounds [3].

5.2.3 Metal ion (Fe^{2+}, Fe^{3+}, Cu^{2+}, and Cu^+) chelating

Even though trace minerals are essential dietary components, they can function as prooxidants (through enhancing formation of free radicals). Fe^{2+} and Cu^+ react with H_2O_2, which is a product produced by the dismutation of the $O_2^{\bullet-}$ via SOD, to form extremely reactive $OH^{\bullet}$ (Eq. (2)). Dissimilarly, iron and copper's reaction with H_2O_2 forms more singlet oxygen than $OH^{\bullet}$. Fe^{2+} and Cu^+ are oxidized to Fe^{3+} and Cu^{2+}, respectively. Cellular reductant such as NADH and oxidized metal ions Fe^{3+}, and Cu^{2+} are reduced and permit the recycling to react with another molecule of H_2O_2 to produce $OH^{\bullet}$ radical in the presence of vitamin C (Eq. (3)). $OH^{\bullet}$ is strongly reactive and can directly react with proteins and lipids to produce carbonyls (aldehydes and ketones), cross linking, and lipid peroxidation. Chelating metal ions are able to decrease their action, thus reducing the ROS formation.

$$Fe^{2+}\ (\text{or } Cu^{+}) + H_2O_2\ Fe^{3+}\ (\text{or } Cu^{2+}) + OH^{\bullet} + OH^{-} \tag{2}$$

$$Fe^{3+}\ (\text{or } Cu^{2+}) + \text{vit C H}^{-}\ Fe^{2+}\ (\text{or } Cu^{+}) + \text{vitamin C}^{-\bullet} + H^{+} \tag{3}$$

Studies showed that Se antioxidant is able to chelate Cu^{+} (formed in situ with Cu^{2+}/ascorbic acid) extremely efficiently and prevent the damage of DNA by $OH^{\bullet}$ radical (formed via Cu^{+}/H_2O_2) [3].

5.3 Free radical generating enzyme inhibitors

It has been reported that the main sources of free radicals in different physiological and pathological conditions is associated with a number of enzymes. NADPH oxidases are a type of plasma membrane linked enzymes that have an ability to transfer one electron from the cytosolic donor NADPH to a molecule of extracellular oxygen, forming $O_2^{\bullet-}$ [62]. Uric acid is formed by xanthin oxidase enzyme through catalyzing the oxidation of hypoxanthine and xanthin to uric acid yielding $O_2^{\bullet-}$ and H_2O_2 and increase the oxidation level in an organism [63]. In addition, $O_2^{\bullet-}$ is also formed as a by-product of mitochondrial respiration as well as several other enzymes, for example NADH oxidase, monooxygenases and cyclooxygenases. $O_2^{\bullet-}$ is biologically quite toxic and is produced in significant amounts by the enzyme NADPH oxidase to be used in oxygen dependent killing mechanisms for invading pathogens. During the respiratory burst, it is an important control of reactive oxygen derivatives production for the defense of an organism against invading microorganisms, without causing an important loss of tissue functions [3]. Nonetheless, excessive ROS enhance oxidative stress such as low density lipoprotein (LDL) oxidation. A direct link between elevated phagocytic NADPH oxidase activities and increased circulating oxidized LDL in metabolic syndrome patients has been found. As a result, both modulation of NADPH oxidase to prohibit ROS overproduction and antioxidants supplementation have been reported as active strategies to prevent the deleterious effect of oxidative stress in hemodialysis patients [64]. In recent years, many natural antioxidants have revealed potential to inhibit enzymes that promote $O_2^{\bullet-}$ generation as well as the development of new therapeutic agents for oxidative stress-related diseases [3].

5.4 Prevention of lipid peroxidation

Lipid peroxidation is defined as oxidative deterioration of lipids composed of C-C double bonds such as unsaturated fatty acids, glycolipids, cholesterol, cholesterol ester, phospholipids. ROS damage the unsaturated fatty acids, which include numerous double bonds and the methylene-CH2-groups with particularly reactive hydrogen atoms, and begin the radical peroxidation chain reactions [65]. Antioxidants are able to directly react and quench peroxide radicals to stop the chain reaction. Lipid peroxidation and DNA damage are related to different chronic diseases, such as cancer, and atherosclerosis. Antioxidants can scavenge ROS and peroxide radicals, therefore prohibiting or treating certain pathogenic situations. Scientific attention has been concentrated in lipid peroxidation for recognizing natural antioxidants and studying their mechanism of action. Researches on antioxidants such as vitamins, polyphenols and flavones against free radical enhanced lipid peroxidation have been assumed in many systems such as lipid, red blood cells and LDL. The antioxidant activity of these polyphenols depends considerably on molecules structure, the initiation conditions and the microenvironment of the reaction medium [3].

5.5 Prevention of DNA damage

In vivo, the $OH^•$ and $ONOO^-$ radicals produced from nitric oxide and $O_2^{•-}$ are able to react directly with plasmid DNA macromolecules to cleave one DNA strand, leading to oxidative DNA damage. Cell death and mutation as a result of DNA damage are associated with neurodegenerative and heart diseases, cancer and aging. Consequently, DNA or plasmid damage has received attention and been utilized as models for the study and identification of antioxidants [66]. A study has been progressed include DNA damage caused by Cu^+ induced $OH^•$, through metal-free plasmid DNA mixed with Cu^{2+}, ascorbic acid and H_2O_2 at pH 7. The reaction includes reduction of Cu^{2+} to Cu^+ in situ with ascorbic acid. The $OH^•$ radical formed via Cu^+/H_2O_2 cleaves one DNA strand, causing the ordinarily supercoiled plasmid DNA to unwind [3].

5.6 Prevention of protein modification

Besides lipid peroxidation and DNA damage, protein modification through nitration or chloration of amino acids also is caused by ROS. *In vivo*, peroxynitrite, $O{=}N{-}O{-}O^-$, is a powerful oxidant and nitrating agent formed through the reaction of $O_2^{•-}$ with free radical nitric oxide via a diffusion-controlled reaction. In cells, $ONOO^-$ is a much stronger oxidizing agent than $O_2^{•-}$ and is able to damage a wide range of different molecules such as DNA and proteins. $ONOO^-$ and its protonated form peroxynitrous acids (ONOOH) are capable of exerting direct oxidative modifications during one or two electron oxidation processes [67]. *In vivo*, $ONOO^-$ reacts nucleophically with CO_2 to produce nitrosoperoxy carbonate, which is the predominant pathway for $ONOO^-$. These modifications often cause the alteration of protein function or structure, in addition to enzyme activities inhibition. Proteins containing nitrotyrosine residues have been detected in various pathogenic conditions, such as diabetes, hypertension, and atherosclerosis, all linked with promoted oxidative stress, including increased formation of $ONOO^-$. Antioxidants and antioxidant enzyme are utilized to prevent the protein modification of $ONOO^-$. Antioxidants or enzyme such as CAT is able to remove H_2O_2 and also inhibit HOCl formation; similarly, SOD or antioxidants, like polyphenols, may scavenge $O_2^{•-}$ and inhibit $ONOO^-$ formation [3].

6. Conclusion

This chapter briefly summarized types of antioxidants, and their mode of action. The harmful products formed during normal cellular functions are oxygen radical derivatives that are the most important free radical in the biological system. For normal physiological functioning, it is important to maintain a tolerated antioxidant status by increasing intake of natural antioxidants. Studies have shown that different types of antioxidants, including natural and synthetic antioxidants, can help in disease prevention. The antioxidant compounds may directly react with the reactive radicals to destroy them via accepting or donating electron(s) to directly remove the unpaired status of the radical. Moreover, they may indirectly reduce the production of free radicals by inhibiting the efficacy or expressions of free radical creating enzymes or by stimulating the activities and expressions of other antioxidant enzymes. Thus, it is essential to know the antioxidant mechanisms of action with the free radicals.

Conflict of interest

The authors declare they have no financial or other conflict of interests related to this chapter.

Author details

Manal Azat Aziz[1*], Abdulkareem Shehab Diab[2] and Abeer Abdulrazak Mohammed[3]

1 Department of Medical Laboratories, Al Mansour Institute of Medical Technology, Middle Technical University, Baghdad, Iraq

2 Department of Physiotherapy, College of Health and Medical Technology, Middle Technical University, Baghdad, Iraq

3 Department of Chemistry, College of Sciences, University of Mustanseriya, Baghdad, Iraq

*Address all correspondence to: manalbazaz@yahoo.com

References

[1] Law BMH, Waye MMY, So WKW, Chair SY. Hypotheses on the potential of rice bran intake to prevent gastrointestinal cancer through the modulation of oxidative stress. International Journal of Molecular Sciences. 2017;**18**:1-20

[2] Aziz MA, Ghanim HM, Diab KS, Al-Tamimi RJ. The association of oxidant-antioxidant status in patients with chronic renal failure. Renal Failure. 2016;**38**(1):20-26

[3] Krishnamurthy P, Wadhwani A. Antioxidant enzymes and human health. In: El-Missiry MA, editor. Antioxidant Enzyme. Croatia: In Tech; 2012. pp. 3-18. DOI: 10.3109/0886022X.2015.1103654

[4] Lü JM, Lin PH, Yao Q, Chen C. Chemical and molecular mechanisms of antioxidants: Experimental approaches and model systems. Journal of Cellular and Molecular Medicine. 2009;**14**(4):840-860

[5] Pandey KB, Rizvi SI. Markers of oxidative stress in erythrocytes and plasma during aging in humans. Oxidative Medicine and Cellular Longevity. 2010;**3**(1):2-12

[6] Kumar S. Free radicals and antioxidants: Human and food system. Advanced in Applied Science Research. 2011;**2**(1):129-135

[7] KurutasEB. The importance of antioxidants which play the role in cellular response against oxidative/nitrosative stress: Current state. Kurutas Nutrition Journal. 2016;**15**:71-93

[8] Bagchi K, Puri S. Free radicals and antioxidants in health and disease: A review. Eastern Mediterranean Health Journal. 1998;**4**(2):350-360

[9] Zadák Z et al. Antioxidants and vitamins in clinical conditions. Physiological Research. 2009;**58**(1): S13-S17

[10] Benov L, Beema AF. Superoxide-dependence of the short chain sugars-induced mutagenesis. Free Radical Biology and Medicine. 2003;**34**:429-433

[11] Polumbryk M, Ivanov S, Polumbryk O. Antioxidants in food systems. Mechanism of action. Ukrainian Journal of Food Science. 2013;**1**(1):15-40

[12] Shebis Y et al. Natural antioxidants: Function and sources. Food and Nutrition Sciences. 2013;**4**:643-649

[13] Panchatcharam M et al. Curcumin improves wound healing by modulating collagen and decreasing reactive oxygen species. Molecular and Cellular Biochemistry. 2006;**290**:87-96

[14] Shih PH, Yeh CT, Yen GC. Anthocyanins induce the activation of phase II enzymes through the antioxidant response element pathway against oxidative stress-induced apoptosis. Journal of Agricultural and Food Chemistry. 2007;**55**:9427-9435

[15] Williamson G, Manach C. Bioavailability and bioefficacy of polyphenols in humans. II. Review of 93 intervention studies. American Journal of Clinical Nutrition. 2005;**81**:243S-2255S

[16] Lotito SB, Frei B. Consumption of flavonoid-rich foods and increased plasma antioxidant capacity in humans: Cause, consequence, or epiphenomenon? Free Radical Biology and Medicine. 2006;**41**:1727-1746

[17] Shahidi F, Zhong Y. Novel antioxidants in food quality preservation and health promotion. European Journal of Lipid Science Technology. 2010;**112**:930-940

[18] Nimse SB, Pal D. Free radicals, natural antioxidants, antheir reaction mechanisms. Royal Society of Chemistry Advances. 2015;**5**:27986-28006

[19] Mathew BB, Tiwari A, Jatawa SK. Free radicals and antioxidants: A review. Journal of Pharmacy Research. 2011;**4**(12):4340-4343

[20] Hurrell RF. Influences of vegetable protein sources on trace element and mineral bioavailability. Journal of Nutrition. 2003;**133**(9):2973S-2977S

[21] Butnariu M, Grozea I. Antioxidant (antiradical) compounds. Journal of Bioequivalence and Bioavailability. 2012;**4**(6):4-6

[22] Vitale M, Di Matola T, Ďascoli F. Iodide excess induces apoptosis in thyroid cells trough a p53-independent mechanism involving oxidative stress. Endrocriology Scoeity. 2000;**141**:598-605

[23] Fernandez V, Barrientos X, Kiperos K, Valenzuela A, Videla LA. Superoxide radical generation, NADPH oxidase activity and cytochrome P-450 content of rat liver microsomal fractions in an experimental hyperthyroid state: Relation to lipid peroxidation. Endocrinology. 1985;**117**:496-501

[24] Fukai T, Ushio-Fukai M. Role in redox signaling, vascular function, and diseases. Antioxidants and Redox Signaling. 2011;**15**(6):1583-1606

[25] Ghafourifar P, Cadenas E. Mitochondrial nitric oxide synthase. Trends in Pharmacological Sciences. 2005;**26**(4):190-195

[26] Maggi-Capeyron MF, Cases J, Badia E, et al. A diet high in cholesterol and deficient in vitamin E induces lipid peroxidation but does not enhance antioxidantenzyme expression in rat liver. Journal of Nutritional Biochemistry. 2002;**13**:296-301

[27] Ighodaro OM, Akinloye OA. First line defence antioxidants-superoxide dismutase (SOD), catalase (CAT) and glutathione peroxidase (GPX): Their fundamental role in the enrire antioxidant defence grid. Alexandria Journal of Medicine. 2017;**54**(4):287-293. https://doi.org/10.1016/j.ajme.2017.09.001

[28] MacMillan-Crow LA, Crow JP, Thompson JA. Peroxynitrite-mediated inactivation of manganese superoxide dismutase involves nitration and oxidation of critical tyrosine residues. Biochemistry. 1998;**37**:1613-1622

[29] Fukai T. Extracellular SOD and aged blood vessels. American Journal of Physiology—Heart and Circulatory Physiology. 2009;**297**(1):H10-H12

[30] Buschfort C, Muller MR, Seeber S, et al. DNA excision repair profiles of normal and leukemic human lymphocytes: Functional analysis at the single cell level. Cancer Research. 1997;**57**:651-658

[31] Góth L, Rass P, Pȧy A. Catalase enzyme mutations and their association with diseases. Molecular Diagnostics. 2004;**8**:141-149

[32] Esworthy RS, Ho YS, Chu FF. The GPx1 gene encodes mitochondrial glutathione peroxidase in the mouse liver. Archives Biochemistry Biophysics. 1997;**340**:59-63

[33] JB DH et al. Lack of the antioxidant enzyme glutathione peroxidase-1 (GPx1) does not increase atherosclerosis in C57BL/J6 mice fed a high fat diet. Journal of Lipid Research. 2006;**47**(6):1157-1167

[34] Imai H, Narashima K, Arai M, Sakamoto H, Chiba N, Nakagawa Y. Suppression of leukotriene formation

in RBL-2H3 cells that overexpressed phospholipid hydroperoxide glutathione peroxidase. Journal of Biological Chemistry. 1998;**273**:1990-1997

[35] Rayman MP. Selenium in cancer prevention: A review of the evidence and mechanism of action. Proceedings of the Nutrition Scoiety. 2005;**64**:527-542

[36] Shui GH, Leong LP. Analysis of polyphenolic antioxidants in star fruit using liquid chromatography and mass spectrometry. Journal of Chromatography A. 2004;**1022**:67-75

[37] Perumalla VS, Hettiarachchy NS. Green tea and grape seed extracts potential applications in food safety and quality. Food Research International. 2011;**44**(4):827-839

[38] Uttara B, Singh AV, Zamboni P, Mahajan RT. Oxidative stress and neurodegenerative diseases: A review of upstream and downstream antioxidant therapeutic options. Current Neuropharmacology. 2009;**7**(1):65-74

[39] Moon JK, Shibamoto T. Antioxidant assays for plant and food components. Journal of Agricultural and Food Chemistry. 2009;**57**(5):1655-1666

[40] El Barky AR, Hussein SA, Mohamed TM. The potent antioxidant alpha lipoic acid. Journal of Plant Chemistry and Ecophysiology. 2017;**2**(1):1-5

[41] Pocsi I, Prade RA, Penninckx MJ. Glutathione, altruistic metabolite in fungi. Advances in Microbial Physiology. 2004;**49**:1-76

[42] Skowyra M. Antioxidant properties of extracts from selected plant materials (*Caesalpinia spinosa*, *Perilla frutescens*, *Artemisia annua* and Viola wittrockiana) in vitro and in model food systems [thesis]. Department of Chemical Engineering, Universitat Politècnica de Catalunya; 2014

[43] Sun SY. N-acetylcysteine, reactive oxygen species and beyond. Cancer Biology & Therapy. 2010;**9**(2):109-110

[44] Homma T, Fujii J. Application of glutathione as anti-oxidative and anti-aging drugs. Current Drug Metabolism. 2015;**16**(7):560-571

[45] Arredondo ML. Relationship between vitamin intake and total antioxidant capacity in elderly adults. Universitas Scientiarum. 2016;**21**(2):167-177

[46] Herrera E, Barbas C. Vitamin E: Action, metabolism and perspective. Journal of Physiology and Biochemistry. 2001;**57**:43-56

[47] McCormick CC, Parker RS. The cytotoxicity of vitamin E is both vitamer and cell specific and involves a selectable trait. Journal of Nutrition. 2004;**134**:3335

[48] Schaffer S, MullerbWE, Eckert GP. Tocotrienols: Constitutional effects in aging and disease. Journal of Nutrition.2005;**135**:151

[49] Rahman K. Studies on free eadicals, antioxidants, and co-factors. Clinical Interventions in Aging. 2007;**2**(2):219-236

[50] Sauvant P, Cansell M, Hadj A, Atgie C. Vitamin a enrichment: Caution with encapsulation strategies used for food applications. Food Research International. 2012;**46**(2):469-479

[51] Ames BN, Cathcart R, Schwiers E, Hochstein P. Uric acid provides an antioxidant defense in humans against oxidant-and radical-caused aging and cancer: A hypothesis. Proceedings of the National Academy Sciences of the United States of America. 1981;**78**:6858-6862

[52] Johnson RJ. Essential hypertension, progressive renal disease, and uric acid: A pathogenetic link?

Journal of Anerican Nephrology. 2005;**16**:1909-1919

[53] Mercuro G et al. Effect of hyperuricemia upon endothelial function in patients at increased cardiovascular risk. The American Journal of Cardiology. 2004;**94**:93293-93295

[54] Packer L, Witt EH, Tritschler HJ. Alpha lipoic acid as a biological antioxidant. Free Radical Biology and Medicine. 1995;**19**(2):227-250

[55] Walter M, Marchesan E. Phenolic compounds and antioxidant activity of rice. Brazilizn Archives of Biology and Technology. 2011;**54**(1):371-377

[56] Tsao R, Yang R. Optimization of a new mobile phase to know the complex and real polyphenolic composition: Towards a total phenolic index using high performance liquid chromatography. Journal of Chromatography. 2003;**1018**(1):29-40

[57] Jaganathan SK et al. Role of pomegranate and citrus fruit juices in colon cancer prevention. World Journal Gastroenterology. 2014;**20**(16):4618-4625

[58] Sharmila G et al. Chemopreventive effect of quercetin, a natural dietary flavonoid on prostate cancer in in vivo model. Clinical Nutrition (Edinburgh, Scotland). 2014;**33**(4):718-726

[59] Yiannakopoulou EC. Effect of green tea catechins on breast carcinogenesis: A systematic review of in-vitro and in-vivo experimental studies. European Journal of Cancer Prevention: The official Journal of the European Cancer Prevention Organisation. 2014;**23**(2):84-89

[60] James SJ, Rose S, Melnyk S, et al. Cellular and mitochondrial glutathione redox imbalance in lymphoblastoid cells derived from children with autism. Federation of American Societies For Experimental Biology Journal. 2009;**23**:237-283

[61] Marklund SL, Westman NG, Lundgren E, et al. Copper and zinc containing superoxide dismutase, catalase, and glutathione peroxidase in normal and neoplastic human cell lines and normal human tissues. Cancer Research. 1982;**42**:1955-1961

[62] Lin HC, Tsal SH, Chen CS, et al. Structure-activity relationship of coumarin derivatives on xanthine oxidase-inhibiting and free radical-scavenging activities. Biocmeical Pharmacology. 2008;**75**:1416-1425

[63] Schroder K, Vecchione C, Jung O, et al. Xanthine oxidase inhibitor tungsten prevents the development of atherosclerosis in ApoE knockout mice fed a Western-type diet. Free Radical Biology and Medicine. 2006;**41**:1353-1360

[64] Castilla P, Davalos A, Teruel JL, et al. Comparative effects of dietary supplementation with red grape juice and vitamin E on production of superoxide by circulating neutrophil NADPH oxidase in hemodialysis patients. American Journal of Clinical Nutrition. 2008;**87**:1053-1561

[65] Porter NA, Caldwell SE, Mills KA. Mechanisms of free radical oxidation of unsaturated lipids. Lipids. 1995;**30**:277-290

[66] Zhao F, Tang YZ, Liu ZQ. Protective effect of icariin on DNA against induced oxidative damage. Journal of Pharmacy and Pharmacology. 2007;**59**:1729-1732

[67] Pacher P, Beckman JB, Liaudet L. Nitric oxide and peroxynitrite in health and disease. Physiolagical Review. 2007;**87**:315-424

Chapter 2

Antioxidant Compounds and Their Antioxidant Mechanism

Norma Francenia Santos-Sánchez, Raúl Salas-Coronado, Claudia Villanueva-Cañongo and Beatriz Hernández-Carlos

Abstract

An antioxidant is a substance that at low concentrations delays or prevents oxidation of a substrate. Antioxidant compounds act through several chemical mechanisms: hydrogen atom transfer (HAT), single electron transfer (SET), and the ability to chelate transition metals. The importance of antioxidant mechanisms is to understand the biological meaning of antioxidants, their possible uses, their production by organic synthesis or biotechnological methods, or for the standardization of the determination of antioxidant activity. In general, antioxidant molecules can react either by multiple mechanisms or by a predominant mechanism. The chemical structure of the antioxidant substance allows understanding of the antioxidant reaction mechanism. This chapter reviews the *in vitro* antioxidant reaction mechanisms of organic compounds polyphenols, carotenoids, and vitamins C against free radicals (FR) and prooxidant compounds under diverse conditions, as well as the most commonly used methods to evaluate the antioxidant activity of these compounds according to the mechanism involved in the reaction with free radicals and the methods of *in vitro* antioxidant evaluation that are used frequently depending on the reaction mechanism of the antioxidant.

Keywords: antioxidants, oxidative stress, reactive oxygen species, free radical, hydrogen atom transfer, single electron transfer

1. Introduction

Oxidative stress in biological systems is a complex process that is characterized by an imbalance between the production of free radicals (FR) and the ability of the body to eliminate these reactive species through the use of endogenous and exogenous antioxidants. During the metabolic processes, a great variety of reactions take place, where the promoters are the reactive oxygen species (ROS), such as hydrogen peroxide (H_2O_2) and the superoxide radical anion ($O_2^{\bullet-}$), among others. A biological system in the presence of an excess of ROS can present different pathologies, from cardiovascular diseases to the promotion of cancer. Biological systems have antioxidant mechanisms to control damage of enzymatic and nonenzymatic natures that allow ROS to be inactivated. The endogenous antioxidants are enzymes, such as superoxide dismutase (SOD), catalase (CAT), glutathione peroxidase, or non-enzymatic compounds, such as bilirubin and albumin. When an organism is exposed to a high concentration of ROS, the endogenous antioxidant system is compromised and, consequently, it fails to guarantee complete protection of the organism. To compensate this deficit of antioxidants, the body can use exogenous antioxidants supplied through food, nutritional supplements, or pharmaceuticals. Among the most important exogenous antioxidants are phenolic compounds carotenoids and vitamins C and some minerals such as selenium and zinc.

In the study of antioxidant compounds and the mechanisms involved, it is important to distinguish between the concepts of antioxidant activity and capacity. These terms are often used interchangeably. However, antioxidant activity refers to the rate constant of a reaction between an antioxidant and an oxidant. The antioxidant capacity is a measure of the amount of a certain free radical captured by an antioxidant sample [1]. Therefore, during the selection of a method, the response parameter must be considered to evaluate the antioxidant properties of a sample, which may be a function of the concentration of the substrate or concentration and the time required to inhibit a defined concentration of the ROS.

The reaction mechanisms of the antioxidant compounds are closely related to the reactivity and chemical structure of FR as well as the environment in which these reactive species are found. Therefore, it is very important to describe the ROS and, to a lesser degree, the reactive nitrogen species (RNS), which include both precursors and free radicals.

In the literature, there are many *in vitro* methods to evaluate the effectiveness of antioxidant compounds present in a variety of matrices (plant extracts, blood serum, etc.) using lipophilic, hydrophilic, and amphiphilic media (emulsions). The *in vitro* methods can be divided into two main groups: (1) hydrogen atom transfer (HAT) reactions and (2) transfer reactions of a single electron (SET). These methods are widely used because of their high speed and sensitivity. When carrying out a study related to the antioxidant properties of a sample, more than one method is usually used to evaluate the antioxidant capacity/activity [2]. This chapter describes the methods of *in vitro* antioxidant evaluation that are used frequently depending on the reaction mechanism of the antioxidant.

2. Oxidative stress

Oxygen is associated with aerobic life conditions [3], representing the driving force for the maintenance of cell metabolism and viability and at the same time involving a potential danger due to its paramagnetic characteristics. These characteristics promote the formation of partially oxidized intermediates with a high reactivity. These compounds are known as reactive oxygen species (ROS). ROS are free radicals (FR) or radical precursors. In stable neutral molecules, the electrons are paired in their respective molecular orbitals, known as maximum natural stability. Therefore, if there are unpaired electrons in an orbital, highly reactive, molecular species are generated that tend to trap an electron from any other molecule to compensate for its electron deficiency. The oxygen triplet is the main free radical, since it has two unpaired electrons. The reaction rate of triplet oxygen in biological systems is slow. However, it can become highly toxic because it metabolically transforms into one or more highly reactive intermediates that can react with cellular components. This metabolic activation is favored in biological systems, because the reduction of O_2 to H_2O in the electron transport chain occurs by the transfer of an electron to form FR or ROS [4].

Free radicals in a biological system can be produced by exogenous factors such as solar radiation, due to the presence of ultraviolet rays. Ultraviolet radiation causes the homolytic breakdown of bonds in molecules. FR also occur during the course of a disease. In a heart attack, for example, when the supply of oxygen and glucose to the heart muscle is suspended, many FR are produced. Another exogenous factor is chemical intoxication, which promotes the formation of FR. The organism, because it requires the conversion of toxic substances to less dangerous substances, promotes the release of FR. The toxicity of many drugs is actually due to their conversion into free radicals or their effect on the formation of FR. The presence of contaminants, additives, pesticides, etc., in food can also become a source of FR.

Inflammatory processes are due to endogenous factors that promote the presence of FR in the system. These FR, present inside the cleansing cells of the immune system, have the function of killing pathogenic microorganisms. Tissue damage is caused when FR are excessive during this process. Phagocytic cells (neutrophils, monocytes, or macrophages) use the NADPH oxidase system directly generating the superoxide ion ($O_2^{\bullet-}$). $O_2^{\bullet-}$ is considered the primary ROS and when reacting with other molecules through enzymatic processes or catalyzed by metals generates secondary ROS. $O_2^{\bullet-}$ is protonated to produce H_2O_2 and $HO_2^{\bullet}$. $O_2^{\bullet-}$ is produced from the irradiation of molecular oxygen with UV rays, photolysis of water, and by exposure of O_2 to organic radicals formed in aerobic cells such as $NAD^{\bullet}$, $FpH^{\bullet}$, semiquinone radicals, cation radical pyridinium or by hemoproteins. Likewise, it is produced by phagocytic leukocytes as the initial product of the respiratory explosion when consuming O_2. The radical $O_2^{\bullet-}$ does not react directly with polypeptides, sugars, or nucleic acids.

As a defense mechanism cells generate $^{\bullet}NO$ by the action of nitric oxide-synthase on intracellular arginine. The combination of O_2 with $^{\bullet}NO$ results in the formation of $ONOO^{\bullet}$, which induces lipid peroxidation in lipoproteins. This happens in a very marked way in autoimmune diseases such as rheumatoid arthritis, systemic lupus erythematosus, primary biliary cirrhosis, type 1 diabetes, celiac disease, Graves' disease, Hashimoto's disease, inflammatory bowel disease, scleroderma, multiple sclerosis, psoriasis, and vitiligo.

FR are necessarily present during metabolic processes because many of the chemical reactions involved require these chemical species. For example, the reactions of polymerization of amino acids to form proteins or the reactions of polymerization of glucose to form glycogen involve the participation of FR. FR are also involved in the catalytic activation of various enzymes of intermediary metabolism, such as hypoxanthine, xanthine oxidase, aldehyde oxidase, monoamine oxidase, cyclooxygenase, and lipoxygenase [5]. Generally, antioxidant enzymes efficiently control these radicals.

Another generating source of ROS is the structural alteration of essential macromolecules of the cell (DNA, protein, and lipids) by irreversible chemical reactions. These reactions generate derivatives, such as malonaldehyde and hydroperoxides that propagate oxidative damage.

Additionally, there are also RNS, such as nitric oxide ($NO^{\bullet}$), nitrogen dioxide ($NO_2^{\bullet}$), as well as peroxynitrite ($ONOO^-$), nitrosoperoxycarbonate ($ONOOCO_2^-$), and nitronium ions (NO_2^+), and the neutral species, peroxynitrous acid (ONOOH) and dinitrogen trioxide (N_2O_3). These species are generated in small amounts during normal cellular processes such as cell signaling, neurotransmission, muscle relaxation, peristalsis, platelet aggregation, blood pressure modulation, immune system control, phagocytosis, production of cellular energy, and regulation of cell growth [6]. **Table 1** shows the most representative FR present during the process of energy production in aerobic biological systems.

2.1 Oxidative damage to biomolecules

There are many ROS that act as biological oxidants, but the $O_2^{\bullet-}$ is the largest oxidant; the simple addition of a proton leads to the formation of $HO_2^{\bullet}$, becoming a very active oxidizing agent. These transformations are summarized in **Figure 1**.

Specie	Source	Function
$O_2^{\bullet-}$	Enzymatic process, autoxidation reaction, and nonenzymatic electron transfer reactions	It can act as reducing agent of iron complexes such as cytochrome-c or oxidizing agent to oxidize ascorbic acid and α-tocopherol
$HO_2^{\bullet}$	Protonation of $O_2^{\bullet-}$	$HO_2^{\bullet}$ initiates fatty acid peroxidation
$HO^{\bullet}$	H_2O_2 generates $HO^{\bullet}$ through the metal-catalyzed Fenton reaction	$HO^{\bullet}$ reacts with both organic and inorganic molecules including DNA, proteins, lipids, and carbohydrates
$NO^{\bullet}$	Action of nitric oxide-synthase using arginine as a substrate and NADPH as an electron source	$NO^{\bullet}$ is an intracellular second messenger stimulates guanylate cyclase and protein kinases and helps in smooth muscle relaxation in blood vessels
$NO^{\bullet}_2$	Protonation of $ONOO^-$ or homolytic fragmentation of $ONOOCO_2^-$	This radical acts on the antioxidative mechanism decreasing ascorbate and α-tocopherol in plasma
$ONOO^{\bullet}$	Reaction of O_2 with $NO^{\bullet}$	$ONOO^{\bullet}$ is a strong oxidizing and nitrating species of methionine and tyrosine residues in proteins and oxidizes DNA to form nitroguanine
$CO_3^{\bullet-}$	The intermediate of reaction superoxide dismutase (SOD)-Cu^{2+}-$OH^{\bullet}$ react with bicarbonate to generates $CO_3^{\bullet-}$	$CO_3^{\bullet-}$ oxidizes biomolecules such as proteins and nucleic acids
$ONOOCO_2^-$	The peroxynytrite-CO_2 adduct is obtained by reaction of $ONOO^-$ with CO_2	This anion promotes nitration of tyrosine fragments of the oxyhemoglobin via FR

Table 1.
Free radicals (FR) generated in biological systems.

Free radicals produce diverse actions on the metabolism of immediate principles, which can be the origin of cell damage [7]:

1. In the polyunsaturated lipids of membranes, producing loss of fluidity and cell lysis because of lipid peroxidation (**Figure 2**).

2. In the glycosides, altering cellular functions such as those associated with the activity of interleukins and the formation of prostaglandins, hormones, and neurotransmitters (**Figure 3**) [8].

3. In proteins, producing inactivation and denaturation (**Figure 4**) [9].

4. In nucleic acids, by modifying bases (**Figure 5**) [8], producing mutagenesis and carcinogenesis.

2.2 Physiological and physiopathological processes related to free radicals (FR)

The human body responds to oxidative stress with antioxidant defense, but in certain cases, it may be insufficient, triggering different physiological and physiopathological processes. Currently, many processes are identified related to the production of free radicals. Among them are mutagenesis, cell transformation, cancer, arteriosclerosis, myocardial infarction, diabetes, inflammatory diseases, central nervous system disorders, and cell aging [10, 11].

$$O_2^{\bullet -} + HO_2^{\bullet} + H^+ \rightarrow H_2O_2 + O_2$$
$$HO_2^{\bullet} + HO_2^{\bullet} \rightarrow H_2O_2 + O_2$$
$$O_2^{\bullet -} + O_2^{\bullet -} + 2H^+ \rightarrow H_2O_2 + O_2$$

Figure 1.
Reaction mechanism of superoxide radical.

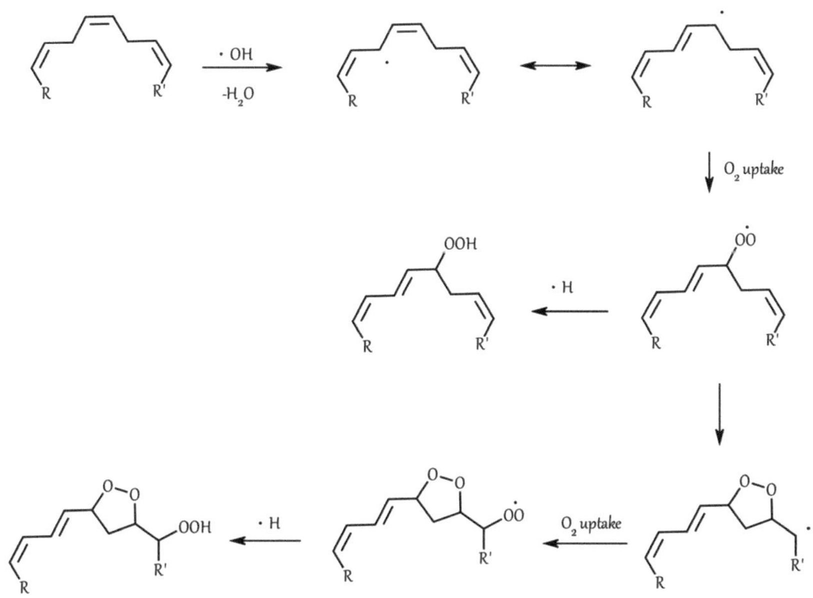

Figure 2.
Reaction of hydroxyl radical with polyunsaturated fatty acids.

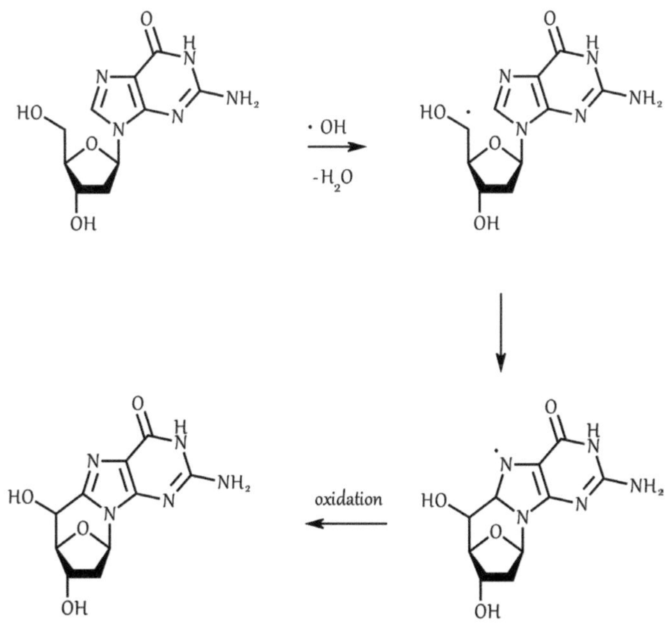

Figure 3.
Reaction of hydroxyl radical with sugar [8].

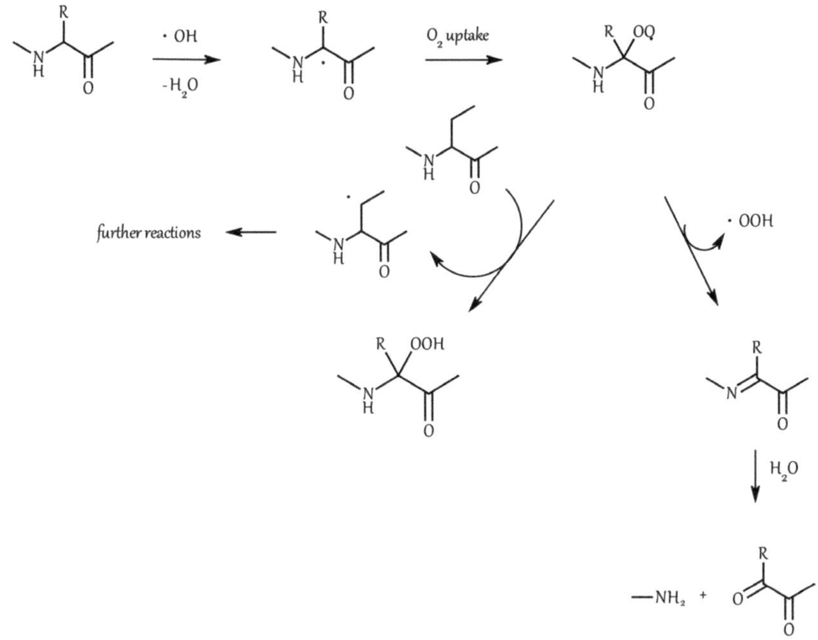

Figure 4.
Reaction of hydroxyl radical with α-aminoacids [9].

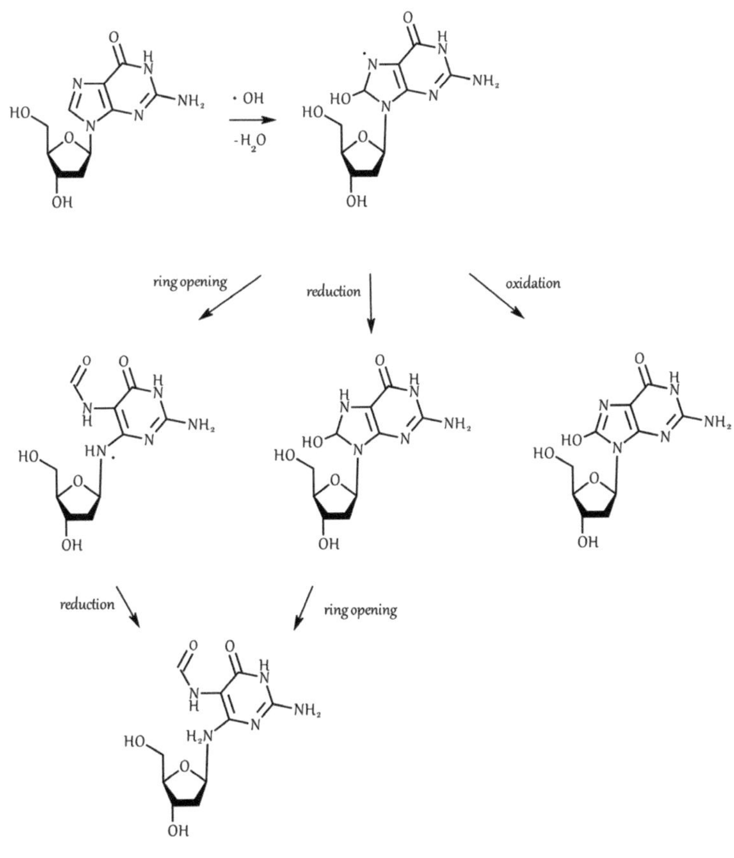

Figure 5.
Reaction of hydroxyl radical with the basepair of DNA guanosine [8].

3. Role of antioxidants

Biological systems in oxygenated environments have developed defense mechanisms, both physiological and biochemical. Among them, at the physiological level, is a microvascular system with the function of maintaining the levels of O_2 in the tissues, and at a biochemical level, the antioxidant defense can be enzymatic or nonenzymatic, as well as being a system for repairing molecules.

3.1 Primary enzymatic system

Aerobic organisms have developed antioxidant enzymes such as superoxide dismutase (SOD), catalase (CAT), glutathione peroxidase (GPx), and DT-diaphorase. SOD is responsible for the dismutation reaction of O_2 to H_2O_2, which in subsequent reactions, catalyzed by catalase or by GPx, is converted into H_2O and O_2. SOD is the most important and most powerful detoxification enzyme in the cell. SOD is a metalloenzyme and, therefore, requires a metal as a cofactor for its activity. Depending on the type of metal ion required as a cofactor by SOD, there are several forms of the enzyme [12, 13]. CAT uses iron or manganese as a cofactor and catalyzes the degradation or reduction of hydrogen peroxide (H_2O_2) to produce water and molecular oxygen, thus completing the detoxification process initiated by SOD [14, 15]. CAT is highly efficient at breaking down millions of H_2O_2 molecules in a second. CAT is mainly found in peroxisomes, and its main function is to eliminate the H_2O_2 generated during the oxidation of fatty acids. GPx is an important intracellular enzyme that breaks down H_2O_2 in water and lipid peroxides in their corresponding alcohols; this happens mainly in the mitochondria and sometimes in the cytosol [16]. The activity of GPx depends on selenium. In humans, there are at least eight enzymes GPx, GPx1–GPx8 [17]. Among glutathione peroxidases, GPx1 is the most abundant selenoperoxidase and is present in virtually all cells. The enzyme plays an important role in inhibiting the process of lipid peroxidation and, therefore, protects cells from oxidative stress [18]. Low GPx activity leads to oxidative damage of the functional proteins and the fatty acids of the cell membrane. GPx, particularly GPx1, has been implicated in the development and prevention of many diseases, such as cancer and cardiovascular diseases [19]. DT-diaphorase catalyzes the reduction of quinone to quinol and participates in the reduction of drugs of quinone structure [20]. DNA regulates the production of these enzymes in cells.

3.2 Nonenzymatic system

This system of antioxidants consists of antioxidants that trap FR. They capture FR to avoid the radical initiation reaction. Neutralize the radicals or capture them by donating electrons, and during this process, the antioxidants become free radicals, but they are less reactive than the initial FR. FR from antioxidants are easily neutralized by other antioxidants in this group. The cells use a series of antioxidant compounds or free radical scavengers such as vitamin E, vitamin C, carotenes, ferritin, ceruloplasmin, selenium, reduced glutathione (GSH), manganese, ubiquinone, zinc, flavonoids, coenzyme Q, melatonin, bilirubin, taurine, and cysteine. The flavonoids that are extracted from certain foods interact directly with the reactive species to produce stable complexes or complexes with less reactivity, while in other foods, the flavonoids perform the function of co-substrate in the catalytic action of some enzymes.

3.3 Repair system

Enzymes that repair or eliminate the biomolecules that have been damaged by ROS, such as lipids, proteins, and DNA, constitute the repair systems. Common examples include systems of DNA repair enzymes (polymerases, glycosylases, and nucleases) and proteolytic enzymes (proteinases, proteases, and peptidases) found in both the cytosol and the mitochondria of mammalian cells. Specific examples of these enzymes are GPx, glutathione reductase (GR), and methionine sulfoxide reductase (MSR). These enzymes act as intermediaries in the repair process of the oxidative damage caused by the attack of excess ROS. Any environmental factor that inhibits or modifies a regular biological activity becomes a condition that favors the appearance or reinforcement of oxidative stress.

4. Characteristics of antioxidants

The main characteristic of a compound or antioxidant system is the prevention or detection of a chain of oxidative propagation, by stabilizing the generated radical, thus helping to reduce oxidative damage in the human body [21]. Gordon [22] provided a classification of antioxidants, mentioning that characteristic. There are two main types of antioxidants, the primary (breaking the chain reaction, free radical scavengers) and the secondary or preventive. The secondary antioxidant mechanisms may include the deactivation of metals, inhibition of lipid hydroperoxides by interrupting the production of undesirable volatiles, the regeneration of primary antioxidants, and the elimination of singlet oxygen. Therefore, antioxidants can be defined as "those substances that, in low quantities, act by preventing or greatly retarding the oxidation of easily oxidizable materials such as fats" [23].

5. Mechanisms of action of antioxidants

A compound that reduces *in vitro* radicals does not necessarily behave as an antioxidant in an *in vivo* system. This is because FR diffuse and spread easily. Some have extremely short life spans, on the order of nanoseconds, so it is difficult for the antioxidant to be present at the time and place where oxidative damage is being generated. Additionally, the reactions between antioxidants and FR are second order reactions. Therefore, they not only depend on the concentration of antioxidants and free radicals but are also dependent on factors related to the chemical structure of both reagents, the medium and the reaction conditions.

5.1 Phenolic compounds

The phenolic compounds constitute a wide group of chemical substances, with diverse chemical structures and different biological activities, encompassing more than 8000 different compounds which are a significant part of the human and animal diet [24]. The phenolic compounds are important components in the mechanism of signaling and defense of plants. These compounds combat the stress brought about by pathogenic organisms and predators. The function of these compounds in plants is diverse: they are found as precursors of compounds of greater complexity or the intervention in the processes of regulation and control of plant growth, as well as the defensive medium of plants. Phenolic compounds have the capacity to act as hydrogen donors or to chelate metal ions such as iron and copper, by inhibiting the oxidation of low-density lipoproteins (LDL). These characteristics in the phenolic compounds are associated with a decrease in risks of neurodegenerative diseases, such as cardiovascular diseases [25], gastrointestinal cancers [26], colon [27], breast and ovarian cancers [28], and leukemia [29–31]. Phenolic compounds also have vasorelaxation and anti-allergenic activity [32]. The phenolic compounds inhibit the oxidation of *in vitro* LDL [33].

Phenolic compounds reduce or inhibit free radicals by transfer of a hydrogen atom, from its hydroxyl group. The reaction mechanism of a phenolic compound with a peroxyl radical ($ROO^{\bullet}$) involves a concerted transfer of the hydrogen cation from the phenol to the radical, forming a transition state of an H-O bond with one electron. The antioxidant capacity of the phenolic compounds is strongly reduced when the reaction medium consists of a solvent prone to the formation of hydrogen bonds with the phenolic compounds. For example, alcohols have a double effect on the reaction rate between the phenol and the peroxyl radical. On the one hand, the alcohols act as acceptors of hydrogen bonds. On the other hand, they favor the ionization of the phenols to anion phenoxides, which can react rapidly with the peroxyl radicals, through an electron transfer. The overall effect of the solvent on the antioxidant activity of the phenolic compounds depends to a great extent on the degree of ionization of the last compounds [34]. Leopoldini et al. [35] conducted a theoretical study to determine the dissociation energy of OH bonds and the adiabatic ionization potentials of phenolic compounds of varied structure and polarity, among them tyrosol, hydroxytyrosol, and gallic and caffeic acids. These studies were performed simulating solvated and vacuum conditions. The results showed a clear difference in the behavior of these phenolic compounds. The compounds most likely to undergo a HAT were tocopherol, followed by hydroxytyrosol, gallic acid, caffeic acid, and epicatechin (**Figure 6**), while the phenolic compounds, which were better able to SET, were kaempferol and resveratrol (**Figure 7**). This undoubtedly gives us an indication that phenolic compounds can suffer both HAT and SET and that this depends mainly on the chemical structure of the phenolic compounds.

The method based on the Folin-Ciocalteu reagent is commonly used to determine and quantify total phenols. This method evaluates the ability of phenols to react with oxidizing agents. The Folin-Ciocalteu reagent contains sodium molybdate and tungstate, which react with any type of phenol [36]. The transfer of electrons at basic pH reduces the sodium molybdate and tungstate in oxides of tungsten (W_8O_{23}) and molybdenum (Mo_8O_{23}), which have a bright blue color in solution. This color intensity is proportional to the number of hydroxyl groups of the molecule [37].

5.2 Carotenoids

Carotenoids are found in virtually all plants, animals, and microorganisms, and more than 700 carotenoids have been identified and characterized [38]. Most carotenoids have a characteristic symmetrical tetraterpene skeleton. The linear hydrocarbon skeleton is made up of 40 carbons and is susceptible to various structural modifications. These structural characteristics are related to degree of hydrogenation, *cis-trans* isomerization, presence of cycles at one or both ends of the linear skeleton, or the addition of side groups (which often contain oxygen) with their subsequent glycosylation. The most complex changes are related to the shortening or elongation of the resulting tetraterpene skeleton, to form carotenoids with chains of 50 carbons. It is also possible to find carotenoids with tetraterpene skeletons of 30 carbons, from the condensation of two units of farnesyl [39]. These compounds, in addition to conferring pigmentation on biological systems, fulfill other important functions. The most recent studies of these compounds are focused mainly on evaluating their function as antioxidants. The structural base fragment of the carotenoids is a conjugated polyunsaturated chain. This fragment is primarily responsible for the ability of these compounds to inhibit free radicals. Variations in the polyunsaturated chain from one carotenoid to another, together with the presence of hydroxyl groups, substantially modify the reactivity of the carotenoids. The reactivity of these compounds is also affected by the environmental conditions where they are

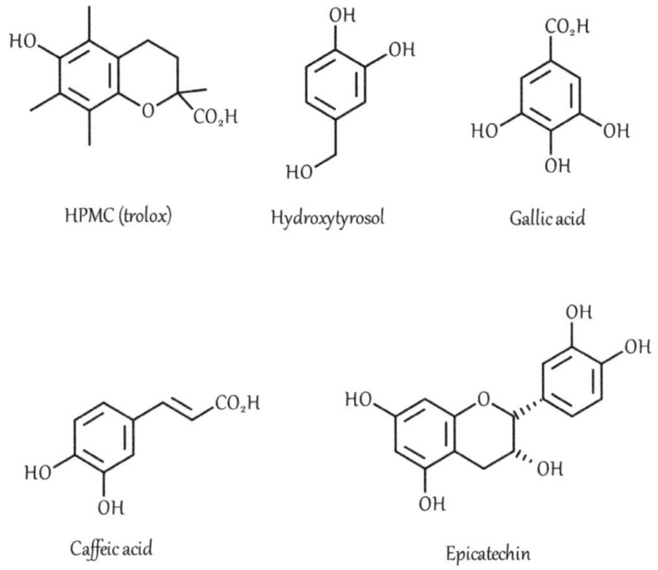

Figure 6.
Phenolic compounds with ability to HAT.

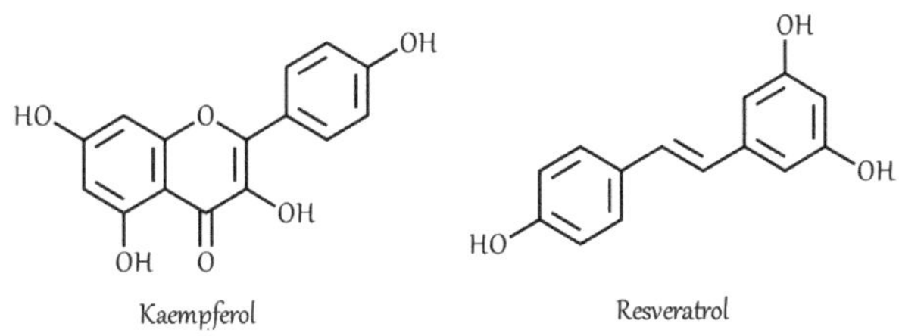

Figure 7.
Phenolic compounds with ability to SET.

found. For example, Edge and Truscott [40] found that carotenoids switch the antioxidant behavior to the prooxidant as a function of oxygen concentration. The study used a system that emulates a cell, to observe the protection effect induced by lycopene when exposing the system to high-energy radiation. Total protection is achieved in the absence of O_2, but in the presence of 100% O_2, protection is completely lost. Carotenoids are characterized as excellent peroxyl radical scavengers. The polyunsaturated chains that make up the base structure of carotenoids give these compounds a lipophilic character. Carotenoids play an important role in the protection of cell membranes and lipoproteins against peroxyl radicals.

The carotenoids react as antioxidant agents through three mechanisms: the first is the SET, the second from the formation of one adduct, and the third by HAT. In general, the antioxidant properties of carotenoids are related to their high capacity for electron donation. Everett et al. [41] found that β-carotene reacts with $NO_2^{\bullet}$ via SET. Carotenoid reactivity studies have also been carried out in the presence of the benzyl peroxyl radical, which has low reactivity, and it was concluded that in this case, the reaction mechanisms involved the formation of an adduct, while reactions by HAT are of little relevance [42].

Other studies have evaluated the effect of the chemical structure of carotenoids on the reactivity toward FR. One of these studies found that carotenoids substituted with electrons are more susceptible to oxidation than carotenoids with withdrawn electron groups. A study of carotenoid reactivity with phenoxy radicals shows the

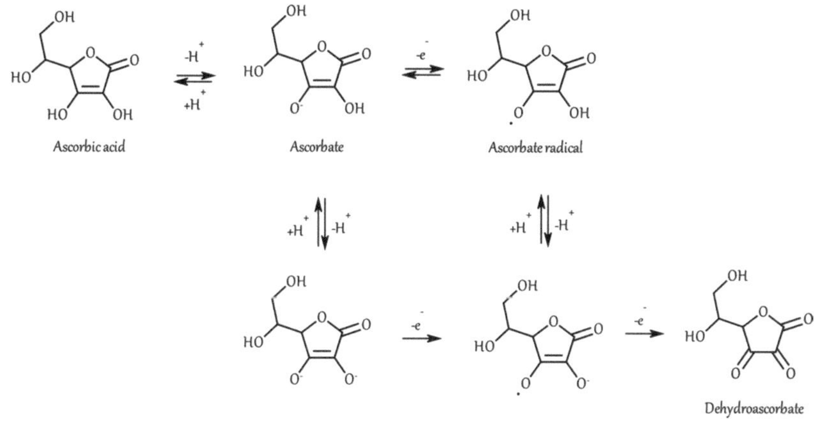

Figure 8.
Chemical species related to vitamin C.

order of reactivity to be lycopene > β-carotene > zeaxanthin > lutein > echinenone > astaxanthin [43].

The effect of the solvent on the reactivity of carotenoids in the presence of FR has also been evaluated, and it was found that in nonpolar solvents, the reactions are promoted via adduct formation; while in polar solvents, the formation of adducts takes place first and then the SET [44].

5.3 Vitamin C

Vitamin C refers to a group of ascorbic acid analogs that can be both synthetic and natural molecules. Ascorbic acid is a water-soluble ketolactone with two ionizable hydroxyl groups. Anion ascorbate is the dominant form at physiological pH (**Figure 8**). Ascorbate is a potent reducing agent and undergoes two subsequent losses of an electron, to form an ascorbate radical and dehydroascorbic acid. The ascorbate radical is relatively stable because the unpaired electron is delocalized by resonance. The ascorbate concentration in plasma of healthy humans is around 10 μg/mL. At these concentrations, the ascorbate is a co-antioxidant with vitamin E to protect LDL from peroxyl radicals [45]. The ascorbate radical is poorly reactive and can be reduced to ascorbate by reductase-dependent NADH and NADPH [46]. The ascorbate radical can alternatively undergo a disproportionation reaction that depends on pH, resulting in the formation of ascorbate and dehydroascorbic acid [47].

Vitamin C is chemically capable of reacting with most of the physiologically important ROS and acts as a hydrosoluble antioxidant. The antioxidant reaction mechanisms of vitamin C are based on the HAT to peroxyl radicals, the inactivation of singlet oxygen, and the elimination of molecular oxygen [48, 49]. For example, ascorbic acid can donate a hydrogen atom to a tocopheroxyl radical at the rate of 2×10^5 mol/s [50]. Also, it has been proven that ascorbate can produce reactions with oxidizing agents through SET [51] or a concerted transfer of electron/protons (SET/HAT) [52].

6. Methods to evaluate antioxidant activity

The antioxidant activity of a compound can be evaluated *in vitro* or *in vivo* by means of simple experiments, and at the same time, the possible prooxidant effect on different molecules can be evaluated. Antioxidant activity cannot be measured directly but is determined by the effects of the antioxidant to control the degree of oxidation. There are a variety of methods to evaluate antioxidant activity. Some methods involve a different oxidation step followed by the measurement of the response, which depends on the method used to evaluate the activity.

When the antioxidant activity of a sample is studied, it is necessary to consider the source of ROS as well as the target substrate. An antioxidant can protect lipids against oxidative damage, while, on the other hand, it can promote the oxidation of other biological molecules [53].

Most assays of antioxidant activity involve inducing accelerated oxidation in the presence of a promoter and controlling one or more variables in the test system, for example, temperature, antioxidant concentration, pH, etc. However, the oxidation mechanisms can change when modifications are carried out on some of these variables. Therefore, it is important to evaluate the intervals in which the quantification of the antioxidant activity is done to generate reliable results.

Method	Reaction mechanism	Characteristics	Reference
Total radical-trapping antioxidant parameter (TRAP)	HAT	TRAP assay involves the initiation of lipid peroxidation by generating water-soluble $ROO^{\bullet}$ and is sensitive to all known chain-breaking antioxidants	[58]
Total oxyradical scavenging capacity total assay (TOSCA)	HAT	Evaluates inhibition oxidation of α-keto-γ-methiolbutyric acid (KMBA) by ROS. The antioxidant activity is measured through ethylene concentration, generated during decomposition of KMBA, relative to a control reaction monitored by headspace gas chromatography (HS-GC)	[59]
Crocin-bleaching assays (CBAs)	HAT	CBA is based on the abstraction of hydrogen atoms and/or addition of radical to the polyene structure of crocin and results in a disruption of the conjugated system accounting for crocin bleaching	[60]
Oxygen radical absorbance capacity (ORAC)	HAT	ORAC assay is based upon the inhibition of peroxyl radical induced oxidation initiated by thermal decomposition of azo compounds such as AAPH	[61]
Inhibition of 2,2-diphenyl-1-picrylhydracyl radical ($DPPH^{\bullet}$)	SET or HAT	Colorimetric method based on the measurement of the scavenging capacity of antioxidants towards $DPPH^{\bullet}$	[62]
Inhibition of 2,2′-azino-bis-(3-ethylbenzothiazoline-6-sulphonic acid) ($ABTS^{\bullet+}$) cation radical	SET or HAT	Colorimetric method to evaluate the decay of $ABTS^{\bullet+}$ in the presence of an antioxidant agent	[63]
Total phenols assay by Folin-Ciocalteu reagent	SET	A mixture of phosphomolybdate and phosphotungstate in highly basic medium oxidized phenolic compounds	[64]
Ferric-reducing antioxidant power (FRAP)	SET	Colorimetric method that evaluates the reduction of Fe^{3+}-tripyridyltriazine complex (Fe^{3+}-TPTZ) by turning it into a ferrous form (Fe^{2+}-TPTZ)	[65]
Total antioxidant capacity (TAC)	SET	This method is used to measure the peroxide level during the initial stage of lipid oxidation. Peroxides are formed during the linoleic acid oxidation, which reacts with Fe^{2+} to form Fe^{3+} and later these ions form a complex with thiocyanate	[66]

Table 2.
Methods most commonly used to evaluate antioxidant capacity/activity in vitro.

The methods to determine the antioxidant capacity are divided into two general groups. This division is based on the reaction mechanisms involved in the RF reduction process. The first group of methods is based on the SET and the second group is based on the HAT. The result is the same: the inactivation of free radicals; however, the kinetics and secondary reactions involved in the process are different. The methods based on SET detect the capacity of a potential antioxidant for the transmission of a chemical species, including metals, carbonyls, and radicals. SET is shown through a change in color as the oxidant is reduced by antioxidant [54]. The group of methods based on HAT measures the ability of an antioxidant to inactivate FR through the donation of a hydrogen atom. HAT reactions are theoretically independent of solvent nature and pH. These reactions are rapid and occur in no more than a few minutes. The presence of other reducing agents in samples, in addition to the antioxidants under study, makes HAT testing difficult and can lead to significant errors [55]. **Table 2** shows the methods of evaluation of the antioxidant activity *in vitro*.

7. Antioxidant capacity/activity *in vitro* evaluation

The methods of evaluation of antioxidant activity must be fast, reproducible, and require small amounts of the chemical compounds to be analyzed, in addition to not being influenced by the physical properties of said compounds [56]. The results of *in vitro* assays can be used as a direct indicator of antioxidant activity *in vivo*; a compound that is ineffective *in vitro* will not be better *in vivo* [53]. These tests can also serve as warnings of possible harmful effects of chemical compounds. Because many factors can affect oxidation, including temperature, the concentration of oxygen in the reaction medium, and metal catalysts, the results may vary depending on the oxidation conditions employed. Tests that measure substrates or products can also give variable results depending on their specificity [57].

These methods are briefly described below.

7.1 Total radical-trapping antioxidant parameter (TRAP)

The TRAP is used to determine the status of a secondary antioxidant in plasma. The results (TRAP value) are expressed as μmol of $ROO^{\bullet}$ trapped per liter of plasma [58]. The test is based on the measurement of O_2 uptake during a controlled peroxidation reaction, promoted by the thermal decomposition of 2,2′-azobis-(2-amidopropane) (ABAP), which produces $ROO^{\bullet}$ at a constant rate (**Figure 9**). This starts with the addition of ABAP to human plasma; the parameter to be evaluated is the "delay time" of the O_2 absorption in plasma induced by the antioxidant compounds present in the medium. The delay time is measured from the O_2 concentration data in plasma diluted in a buffer solution monitored with an electrode. In addition to ABAP, other free radical initiators have been used, such as the ABTS [67], dichlorofluorescein diacetate [68], phycoerythrin [69], and luminol [70].

One of the main disadvantages of the TRAP method is the possibility of an error in the detection of the end point caused by the instability of the O_2 electrode, because this point can take 2 h to reach. To minimize this problem, the electrochemical detection of O_2 can be performed with a chemiluminescent detection based on the use of luminol and horseradish peroxidase [71].

7.2 Total oxyradical scavenging capacity assay (TOSCA)

This method is based on the evaluation of antioxidant activity in the gas phase, which consists of exposing α-keto-γ-methylthiobutyric acid (KMBA) to powerful oxidizing agents, such as $^{\bullet}OH$, $ROO^{\bullet}$, and $ONOO^{-}$ [59] (**Figure 10**). These oxidizing agents induce a transformation of KMBA to ethylene. To evaluate the effect of antioxidants, the ethylene formation is evaluated and compared to a control reaction by the use of headspace gas chromatography (HS-GC). The TOSCA assay is based on the inhibition of ethylene formation in the presence of antioxidant compounds that compete with KMBA for ROS.

The TOSCA method is not suitable for a high performance analysis because multiple injections of each sample are required to measure ethylene production [55]. The reaction kinetics of this method do not allow a linear relationship between the percentage of inhibition of KMBA oxidation and the concentration of antioxidants [72], which is a serious limitation.

7.3 Crocin-bleaching assay (CBA)

The crocin bleaching test (CBA) is a method originally proposed to evaluate the inhibition of alkoxyl radicals produced photolytically. This is done by measuring the protective effect exerted by antioxidant compounds on crocin, a carotenoid that presents an intense red color, under the effect of alkoxyl radicals [60] (**Figure 11**). To achieve this, reaction kinetics are carried out in a UV-Vis spectrophotometer, measuring the absorbance at a wavelength of 440 nm to obtain the relative velocity constants. These constants present a good correlation with the known antioxidant activity of reference compounds. The absolute bleaching velocity of crocin depends strongly on the type of radical that attacks the polyene structure of crocin. Crocin exhibits a high selectivity toward the alkoxyl radicals produced during the photolysis of hydroperoxides, as well as peroxyl radicals produced after the thermolysis of azo initiators. Ordoudi and Tsimidou [73] carried out a detailed evaluation of the CBA, and among the factors, they considered the crocin probe, the antioxidant compound to be evaluated, the peroxyl radical generation conditions, and the monitoring of the reaction. As a result of this, they found that any commercial saffron could be used as a source of crocin for the preparation of the probe, because it is possible to eliminate interferences, such as tocopherols. They also found that the concentration of the working solution could be adjusted and that changes in the

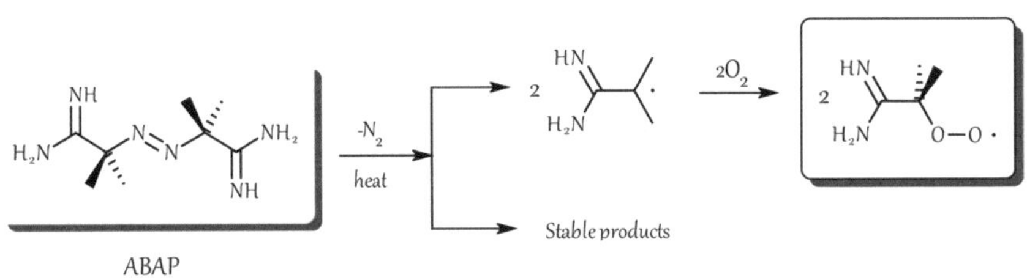

Figure 9.
Formation of peroxyl radical from ABAP.

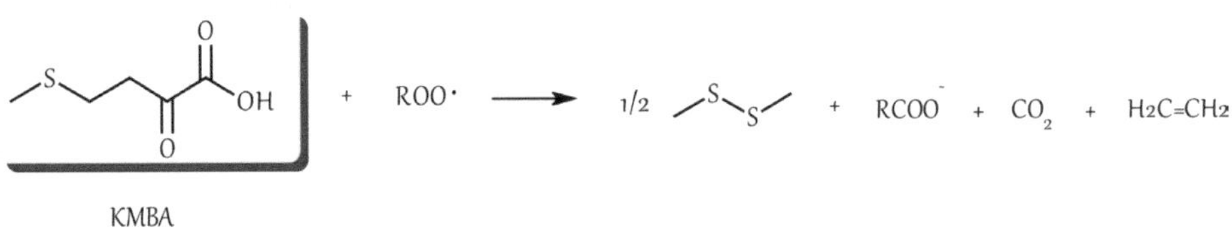

Figure 10.
Reaction between $ROO^{\bullet}$ and KMBA.

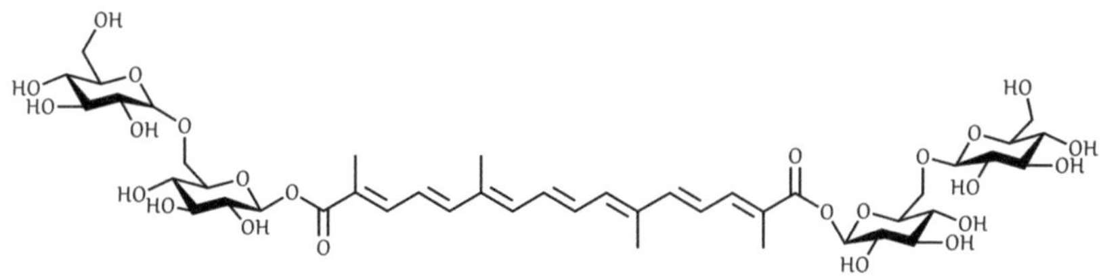

Figure 11.
Chemical structure of crocin.

stock solution of the probe can occur during storage. Ordoudi and Tsimidou [74] also evaluated a group of 39 phenolic compounds of diverse structures, including hydroxybenzoic, hydroxyphenylacetic, hydroxyphenylpropanoic, and hydroxycinnamic acids. The results of that study showed that the activity depends strongly on the position of -COOH groups in relation to the position of the -OH groups. Therefore, the CBA allows evaluation of the effect of the position of functional groups that cause antioxidant activity in a chemical compound.

7.4 Oxygen radical absorbance capacity (ORAC) method

The ORAC method is based on the inhibition of oxidation induced by peroxyl radicals and simultaneously evaluates the time effect and the inhibition degree. The ORAC test is based on hydrogen atom transfer (HAT) and uses a reaction mechanism that competes between antioxidants and a fluorescence probe (fluorescein) for a radical [61]. The test begins with the thermal decomposition of azo compounds, such as [2,2′-azobis-(2-amidino-propane)dihydrochloride (AAPH)], which is the source of free radicals that promotes the degradation of fluorescein. The antioxidant to be evaluated promotes the elimination of the peroxyl radicals, protecting the fluorescein from degradation. The decay in fluorescence due to the attack of the radicals and the protection by the antioxidants results in a curve. The antioxidant capacity is calculated from the area under the fluorescence decrease curve (AUC). This assay uses trolox as a standard; therefore, generally the antioxidant activity in this assay is expressed in terms of trolox equivalents. The ORAC method has been widely used to measure the antioxidant capacity of beverages [75], supplements [55], and vegetables and fruits [55, 76].

There are modifications to this assay that include the use of fluorescein as a probe, adaptation to a high performance format, and the ability to measure the lipophilic, hydrophilic, and total antioxidant capacity of a substance.

The ORAC assay is carried out at pH 7.4, adjusted with a phosphate buffer, in the presence of the antioxidant, AAPH, and fluorescein at a constant temperature of 37°C. Fluorescence is monitored at 1 min intervals for 35 min at an excitation wavelength of 485 nm and an emission wavelength of 520 nm [77].

The ORAC method can also be used for the detection of $^{\bullet}OH$ and other radicals by modifying the initiators. In addition, the method has been modified for the detection of lipophilic antioxidants, encapsulating these compounds in β-cyclodextrins [78].

7.5 Radical scavenging capacity DPPH$^{\bullet}$ method

The 1,1-diphenyl-2-picrylhydrazyl radical (DPPH$^{\bullet}$) (**Figure 12**) is characterized as a stable free radical because pi electrons of the aromatic systems present in the molecule can compensate for the lack of an electron. DPPH$^{\bullet}$ does not dimerize, as most other free radicals do. The delocalization of the electron also gives rise to a

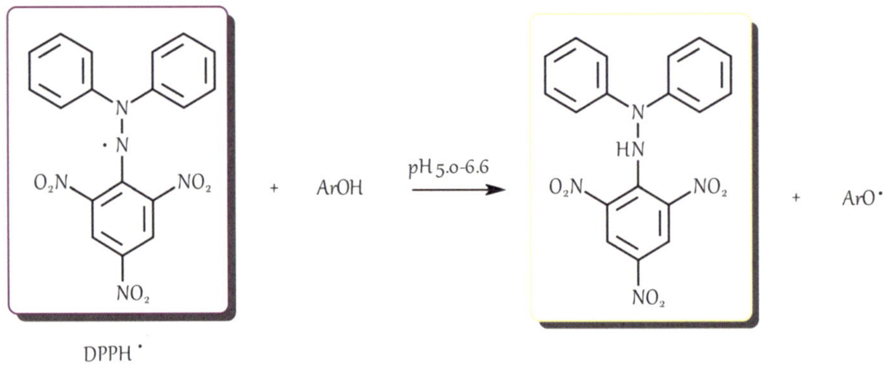

Figure 12.
DPPH• reduction by an antioxidant.

deep violet color, characterized by absorption in solution at around 517 nm. Brand-Williams et al. [62] evaluated the activity of specific compounds or extracts using DPPH• in solution. When a solution of DPPH• is in contact with a substance that can donate a hydrogen atom or with another radical (R•), the reduced form DPPH-H or DPPH-R is produced with the consequent loss of color and therefore the decrease or loss of absorbance (**Figure 8**). Consequently, the reduction of DPPH• provides an index to estimate the ability of the test compound to trap radicals. The alcoholic solutions of 0.5 mM are densely colored, and in this concentration, the law of Lambert-Beer is fulfilled in the useful absorption interval [79].

ArOH is an antioxidant that acts by donating hydrogen atoms, to obtain radicals with stable molecular structures that will stop the chain reaction. The new radical (ArO•) can interact with another radical to form stable molecules (DPPH-OAr, ArO-OAr). The reaction between DPPH• and an antioxidant compound depends on the structural conformation of the same, so quantitative comparisons are not always appropriate.

The basis of this methodology is focused on measuring the reduction of free radicals by antioxidant compounds. Different concentrations and the time of the reaction are measured (30 min or until the steady state is reached). So far, there are no reports about the existence of a mathematical kinetic model that helps to understand the behavior of antioxidants [80].

The experimental models use the percentage of DPPH• remaining to obtain the necessary quantities that are required to reduce the initial concentration to 50% (EC_{50}). In addition, kinetics is performed to determine the amount of time needed for the steady state to reach EC_{50} from the curves. EC_{50} and effective concentration 50 (TEC_{50}) are used to calculate antiradical efficiency (AE). Low values of EC_{50} and TEC_{50} show a high antioxidant strength, and a rapid decrease in absorption is observed during the reaction [81]. The antiradical efficiency can be estimated based on the scale contained in **Table 3**.

It is a fast, simple, inexpensive, and widely used method to measure the ability of compounds to act as free radical scavengers or hydrogen donors. It can also be used to quantify antioxidants in complex biological systems, for solid or liquid samples. The method is applied to measure the overall antioxidant capacity [82] and the activity of eliminating free radicals from fruit and vegetable juices [83]. It has been successfully used to investigate the antioxidant properties of wheat grain and bran, vegetables, oils, and flours in various solvents, including ethanol, aqueous acetone, methanol, and benzene [84–87].

The radical scavenging DPPH• method allows for a reaction with almost any type of antioxidant due to the stability of DPPH•. This means there is sufficient time for even weak antioxidants to react with DPPH• [82]. This method can be used with both polar and nonpolar organic solvents to evaluate hydrophilic and lipophilic antioxidants [55].

The method has some disadvantages, among which is that DPPH• can react with other radicals and consequently the time to reach the stable state is not linear to the concentration ratio of the antioxidant/DPPH• [62, 80]. The stability of DPPH• can be affected by solvents with properties of a Lewis base, as well as the presence of dissolved oxygen [88]. The absorbance of DPPH• in methanol and acetone is lower than with other solvents [89].

Because the radical scavenging DPPH• method is quite simple and used in various fields of chemistry, automated assays combined with analytical techniques have been developed (**Table 4**).

7.6 Ferric reducing/antioxidant power (FRAP) method

The FRAP analysis was introduced by [65, 96] to measure total antioxidant activity and is based on the ability of samples to reduce ferric ion Fe^{3+} to ferrous ion

Range	Antiradical efficiency classification
$AE = 1 \times 10^{-3}$	Low
$1 \times 10^{-3} < AE = 5 \times 10^{-3}$	Medium
$5 \times 10^{-3} < AE = 10 \times 10^{-3}$	High
$AE \gg 10 \times 10^{-3}$	Very high

Table 3.
Scale of antiradical efficiency (AE) against DPPH• [81].

Automation	Characteristics	References
Flow injection analysis (FIA) by high performance liquid chromatography (HPLC)	Bioassay-guided fractionation of natural products or food samples	[90]
PC-controlled sequential injection analysis (SIA)	SIA is a FIA technique modified by using a pump to continuously draw sample and reagent solutions into different lines of tubing	[91]
Electrochemical selective determination of antioxidant activity based on DPPH•/DPPH	Current intensity is proportional to the residual concentration of DPPH• after reaction with the antioxidant	[92]
Relative DPPH radical scavenging capacity (RDSC)	The RDSC uses the area under the curve, expressed as trolox equivalents. These approaches take into account both the kinetic and the thermodynamic measurements of the radical-antioxidant reactions	[93]
High performance thin layer chromatography (TLC)-DPPH•	Post-chromatographic derivatization is carried out with DPPH•. The plates are scanned before DPPH• and 30 min after DPPH derivatization in absorption-reflection mode at optimized wavelengths	[94]
Hyphenated high speed counter current chromatography (HSCCC)-DPPH•	After the HSCCC separation, the effluent is split into two streams by use of an adjustable high-pressure stream splitter. One portion is sent through the detector and the fraction collector, while the second portion is sent to a secondary coil for on-line radical-scavenging detection	[95]

Table 4.
Automated modes to evaluate radical scavenging capacity DPPH•.

Fe^{2+}, forming a blue complex. A high absorption at a wavelength of 700 nm indicates a high reduction power of the chemical compound or extract [66]. The value of FRAP has been used to determine the antioxidant activity of red wines [97]. The work of Schleisier et al. [98] was designed to determine the antioxidant activity in tea extracts and juices expressed in Fe^{2+} equivalents. The absolute initial index of the reduction of ferrylmyoglobin determined by spectroscopy in the visible region has been suggested to characterize the antioxidant activity of individual flavonoids [99]. There are several trials to evaluate FRAP; one of them is to evaluate the power of a compound or extract to reduce the complex of 2,4,6-tripyridyl-s-triazine-Fe^{2+} (TPTZ-Fe^{2+}). An antioxidant reduces the ferric ion (Fe^{3+}) to ferrous ion (Fe^{2+}) in the TPTZ complex; the latter forms a blue complex (Fe^{2+}/TPTZ), which absorbs at a wavelength of 590 nm (**Figure 13**). The reaction must be carried out under acidic conditions (pH 3.6) to preserve the solubility of Fe. The reducing power is related to the degree of hydroxylation and the conjugation in the phenols [55].

The FRAP assay has an incubation time of 4 min at 37°C for the antioxidant activity of most samples. This is done because the redox reactions, involved in the assay, occur within the incubation period. However, it has been shown that FRAP values can vary significantly, depending on the time scale of analysis [55, 96].

7.7 Method of inhibition of the (2,2′-azinobis-(3-ethylbenozothiazoline-6-sulfonate)) radical cation ($ABTS^{•+}$)

ABTS is a target molecule used to evaluate the reactivity of antioxidant samples in the presence of peroxides. The ABTS initially is subjected to an oxidation reaction with potassium permanganate, potassium persulfate or 2,2′-azo-bis (2-amidinopropane), producing the radical cation of the ABTS ($ABTS^{•+}$) with a blue greenish color that absorbs at wavelengths of 415, 645, 734, and 815 nm [100–102]. The $ABTS^{•+}$ is stable for several minutes. The $ABTS^{•+}$ is subjected to the antioxidant sample causing the reduction of $ABTS^{•+}$ and consequently the discoloration of the reaction mixture (**Figure 14**). Therefore, the degree of discoloration can be expressed as the inhibition percentage of $ABTS^{•+}$, which is determined as a function of antioxidant concentration and time. This method can be used at different pH and is useful to study the effect of pH on antioxidant activity. ABTS is soluble in both aqueous and organic solvents and consequently is useful for evaluating the antioxidant activity of samples in different media and is commonly used in solutions that simulate an ionic serum (pH 7.4) based on a phosphate buffer (PBS) containing 150 mM NaCl. When a medium of PBS is used, the samples react in a time interval of approximately 30 min, while in alcohol, they require longer reaction times [103]. The level of peroxide is determined by the absorbance at some of the above-mentioned wavelengths. The IC50 is calculated by plotting the percentage of inhibition against different

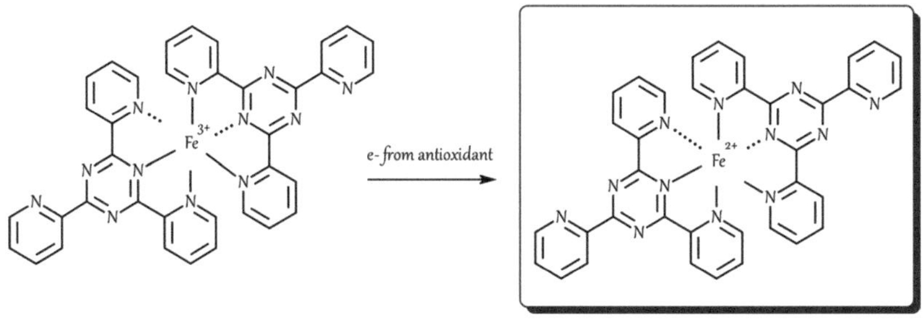

Figure 13.
Reaction mechanism for the FRAP assay in the presence of an antioxidant [55].

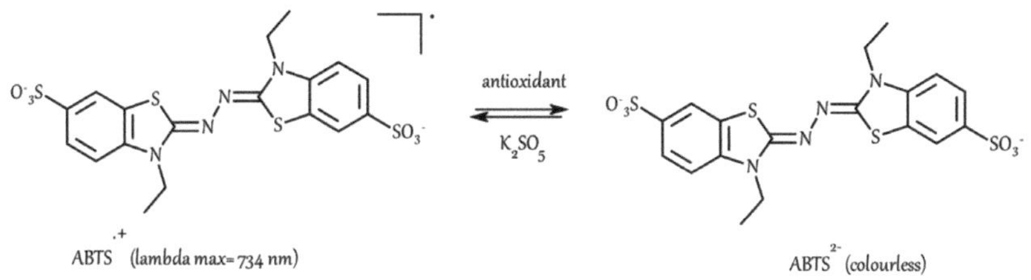

Figure 14.
Reaction of $ABTS^{\bullet +}$ with antioxidant compounds.

concentrations of the antioxidant sample [104]. The IC_{50} values indicate the sample concentration required to eliminate 50% of the $ABTS^{\bullet +}$. Low IC_{50} values indicate high radical uptake activity. The antioxidant activity against $ABTS^{\bullet +}$ can also be evaluated through the unit of antioxidant activity (TAA), which expresses the equivalents of trolox in μmol with respect to each gram of sample extract in dry base.

The inhibition of $ABTS^{\bullet +}$ activity in an antioxidant sample has a strong correlation with the radical scavenging capacity $DPPH^{\bullet}$ because both radicals have the capacity to accept electrons and $H^{\bullet}$ from the antioxidant compounds present in the samples [105, 106].

7.8 Total antioxidant capacity (TAC)

TAC is defined as the ability of a compound to inhibit the oxidative degradation of lipids [66]. Lipid peroxidation involves the oxidative deterioration of lipids with unsaturation. This peroxidation, called the initiation process, begins with the formation of conjugated dienes and trienes, known as primary oxidation products due to the abstraction of a hydrogen atom. Subsequently, a propagation process is carried out that consists of the reaction of the deprotonated species derived from the lipids with O_2, leading to the formation of peroxyl radicals ($ROO^{\bullet}$). The high energy of free radicals promotes the abstraction of hydrogen atoms from neighboring fatty acids. This leads to the formation of hydroperoxides that promotes the formation of new $R^{\bullet}$ radicals. The latter radicals react with each other to produce stable molecules of the R-R and ROOR type [107]. To encourage the antioxidant activity of a chemical compound, it is necessary to inhibit the peroxidation of a fatty acid emulsion; linoleic acid is generally used as a model. The hydroperoxides derived from linoleic acid subsequently react with Fe^{2+}, causing the oxidation of this ion to produce Fe^{3+}. The Fe^{3+} ions form a complex with thiocyanate (SCN^-), and this complex has a maximum absorbance at 500 nm [108]. This complex is used to measure the peroxide value.

The ferric thiocyanate method is used to measure the peroxide value in edible oils. To avoid errors in the determination of the peroxide value, it is important to avoid the presence of oxygen in the reaction medium and this can be achieved by bubbling nitrogen [109]. These authors found that the results of the thiocyanate assay also depend on the solvent, reducing agent and type of hydroperoxides present in the sample.

8. Conclusions

The reaction mechanisms involved in the antioxidant activity/capacity of different groups of compounds depend on several factors. Among these factors are the chemical structure of these compounds, the nature of the solvent, the temperature and pH, as well as the reactivity and chemical structure of free radicals. All these factors can also influence the reaction rate. Consequently, it is very important that, for studies of antioxidant properties, at least three evaluation methods are selected: one to exclusively evaluate the HAT, another the SET, and a combined method, HAT/SET. Also, it is important to perform reaction kinetics. In addition to this, it is essential to consider that in mixtures of antioxidant compounds, possible synergistic effects are present and can enhance the activity/capacity or even modify their reaction mechanisms.

Acknowledgements

The authors thank Carol Ann Hayenga for her English assistance in the preparation of this manuscript. Support was provided by the Technological University of the Mixteca.

Conflict of interest

The authors have no conflict of interest to declare and are responsible for the content and writing of the manuscript.

Ethical approval

This chapter does not contain any studies with human participants or animals performed by any of the authors.

Author details

Norma Francenia Santos-Sánchez*, Raúl Salas-Coronado, Claudia Villanueva-Cañongo and Beatriz Hernández-Carlos
Institute of Agroindustry, Technological University of the Mixteca, Huajuapan de León, Oaxaca, Mexico

*Address all correspondence to: nsantos@mixteco.utm.mx

References

[1] MacDonald-Wicks LK, Wood LG, Garg ML. Methodology for the determination of biological antioxidant capacity in vitro: A review. Journal of the Science of Food and Agriculture. 2006;**86**:2046-2056. DOI: 10.1002/jsfa.2603

[2] Salazar R, Pozos ME, Cordero P, Perez J, Salinas MC, Waksman N. Determination of the antioxidant activity of plants from Northeast Mexico. Pharmaceutical Biology. 2008;**46**(3):166-170. DOI: 10.1080/13880200701498952

[3] Davis JK. Oxidative stress: The paradox of aerobic life. Biochemical Society Symposia. 1995;**61**:1-31. DOI: 10.1042/bss0610001

[4] Valko M, Leibfritz D, Moncol J, Cronin MT, Mazur M, Telser J. Free radicals and antioxidants in normal physiological functions and human disease. The International Journal of Biochemistry & Cell Biology. 2007;**39**(1):44-84. DOI: 10.1016/j.biocel.2006.07.001

[5] Fridovich I. Free Radicals in Biology. Vol. 1. New York: Academic Press; 1976

[6] Limón-Pacheco J, Gonsebatt Bonaparte ME. The role of antioxidants and antioxidant-related enzymes in protective responses to environmentally induced oxidative stress. Mutation Research, Genetic Toxicology and Environmental Mutagenesis. 2009;**674**(1-2):137-147. DOI: 10.1016/j.mrgentox.2008.09.015

[7] Nakamura H, Nakamura K, Yodai J. Redox regulation of cellular activation. Annual Review of Immunology. 1997;**15**:351-369. DOI: 10.1146/annurev.immunol.15.1.351

[8] Nimse SB, Pal D. Free radicals, natural antioxidants, and their reaction mechanisms. RSC Advances. 2015;**5**:27986. DOI: 10.1039/c4ra13315c

[9] Dean RT, Fu S, Stocker R, Davies MJ. Biochemistry and pathology of radical-mediated protein oxidation. Biochemistry Journal. 1997;**324**:1-18

[10] Rice-Evans C. Free radicals and antioxidants in normal and pathological processes. In: Oxidative Stress, Lipoproteins and Cardiovascular Dysfunction. London: Portland Press; 1995. pp. 1-32

[11] Halliwell B. Antioxidants in human health and disease. Annual Review of Nutrition. 1996;**16**:33-50. DOI: 10.1146/annurev.nu.16.070196.000341

[12] Fridovich I. Superoxide radical and superoxide dismutases. Annual Review of Biochemistry. 1995;**64**:97-112. DOI: 10.1146/annurev.bi.64.070195.000525

[13] Dringen R, Pawlowski PG, Hirrlinger J. Peroxide detoxification by brain cells. Journal of Neuroscience Research. 2005;**79**:157-165. DOI: 10.1002/jnr.20280

[14] Marklund SL. Extracellular superoxide dismutase and other superoxide dismutase isoenzymes in tissues from nine mammalian species. The Biochemical Journal. 1984;**222**:649-655. DOI: 10.1042/bj2220649

[15] Chelikani P, Fita I, Loewen PC. Diversity of structures and properties among catalases. Cellular and Molecular Life Sciences. 2004;**61**:192-208. DOI: 10.1007/s00018-003-3206-5

[16] Góth L, Rass P, Páy A. Catalase enzyme mutations and their association with diseases. Molecular Diagnosis. 2004;**8**:141-149. DOI: 10.2165/00066982-200408030-00001

[17] Morón ÚM, Castilla-Cortázar I. Protection against oxidative stress and "IGF-I deficiency conditions". In: Antioxidant Enzyme. In Tech; 2012

[18] Gill SS, Tuteja N. Reactive oxygen species and antioxidant machinery in abiotic stress tolerance in crop plants. Plant Physiology and Biochemistry. 2010;**48**:909-930. DOI: 10.1016/j.plaphy.2010.08.016

[19] Rayman MP. Selenium in cancer prevention: A review of the evidence and mechanism of action. The Proceedings of the Nutrition Society. 2005;**64**:527-542. DOI: 10.1079/PNS2005467

[20] Chen S, Wu K, Knox RJ. Structure-function studies of DT-daphorase (NQ01) and NRH: Quinone oxidoreductase (NQO2). Free Radical Biology & Medicine. 2000;**29**(3-4):276-284. DOI: 10.1016/S0891-5849(00)00308-7

[21] Namiki M. Antioxidants/antimutagens in food. Critical Reviews in Food Science and Nutrition. 1990;**29**:273-300. DOI: 10.1080/10408399009527528

[22] Gordon MH. The mechanism of antioxidant action *in vivo*. In: Food Antioxidants. London: Elsevier; Hudson BJF (eds). 1990. pp. 1-18

[23] Chipault JR. Antioxidants for food use. In: Lunderberg WO, editor. Autoxidation and Antioxidants. New York: Wiley; 1962. pp. 477-542

[24] Martínez-Valverde I, Periago MJ, Ros G. Significado nutricional de los compuestos fenólicos de la dieta. Archivos Latinoamericanos de Nutrición. 2000;**50**(1):5-18

[25] Paran E, Novack V, Engelhard YN, Hazan-Halevy I. The effects of natural antioxidants from tomato extract in treated but uncontrolled hypertensive patients. Cardiovascular Drugs and Therapy. 2009;**23**(2):145-151. DOI: 10.1007/s10557-008-6155-2

[26] Yoshida M, Sakai T, Hosokawa N, Marui N, Matsumoto K, Fujioka A, et al. The effect of quercitin on cell cycle progression and growth of human gastric cancer cells. FEBS Letters. 1990;**260**(1):10-13. DOI: 10.1016/0014-5793(90)80053-L

[27] Ranelletti FO, Ricci R, Larocca LM, Maggiano N, Capelli A, Scambia G, et al. Growth-inhibitory effect of quercetin and presence of type-II estrogen-binding sites in human colon-cancer cell lines and primary colorectal tumors. International Journal of Cancer. 1992;**50**(3):486-492. DOI: 10.1002/ijc.2910500326

[28] Scambia G, Ranelletti FO, Panici PB. Inhibitory effect of quercetin on OVCA 433 cells and presence of type II oestrogen binding sites in primary ovarian tumours and cultured cells. British Journal of Cancer. 1990;**62**:942-947

[29] Yoshida M, Yamamoto M, Nikaido T. Quercitin arrests human leukemic T-cells in late G_1 phase of the cell cycle. Cancer Research. 1992;**52**:6676-6681. DOI: 10.1038/srep24049

[30] Teofili L, Pierlli L, Lovino MS. The combination of quercetin and cytosine arabinoside synergistically inhibits leukemic cell growth. Leukemia Research. 1992;**16**(5):497-503. DOI: 10.1016/0145-2126(92)90176-8

[31] Ren W, Qiao Z, Wang H. Tartary buckwheat flavonoid activates caspase 3 and induces HL-60 cell apoptosis. Methods and Findings in Experimental and Clinical Pharmacology. 2001;**23**:427-432

[32] Sakakibara H, Honda Y, Nakagawa S, Ashida H, Kanazawa K. Simultaneous determination of all polyphenols in

vegetables, fruits, and teas. Journal of Agricultural and Food Chemistry. 2003;**51**:571-581

[33] Riemersma RA, Rice-Evans C, Tyrrell RM, Clifford MN, Lean ME. Tea flavonoids and cardiovascular health. Q JM. 2001;**94**:277-282. DOI: 10.1093/qjmed/94.5.277

[34] Foti MC. Antioxidant properties of phenols. The Journal of Pharmacy and Pharmacology. 2007;**59**(12):1673-1685. DOI: 10.1211/jpp.59.12.0010

[35] Leopoldini M, Marino T, Russo N, Toscano M. Antioxidant properties of phenolic compounds: H-atom versus electron transfer mechanism. The Journal of Physical Chemistry A. 2004;**108**: 4916-4922. DOI: 10.1021/jp037247d

[36] Peterson GL. Review of the folin phenol protein quantitation method of lowry, rosebrough, farr, randall. Analytical Biochemistry. 1979;**100**(2):201-220. DOI: 10.1016/0003-2697(79)90222-7

[37] Julkunen-Tiitto R. Chemotaxonomical screening of phenolic glycosides in northern willow twigs by capillary gas chromatography. Journal of Chromatography A. 1985;**324**:129-139. DOI: 10.1016/S0021-9673(01)81312-1

[38] Britton S, Liaaen-Jensen S, Pfander H, editors. Carotenoids: Handbook. Boston, MA, USA: Birkhäuser; 2004

[39] Landrum JT. Carotenoids: Physical, Chemical, and Biological Functions and Properties. Boca Raton, FL, USA: CRC Press; 2010

[40] Edge R, Truscott T. Singlet oxygen and free radical reactions of retinoids and carotenoids—A review. Antioxidants. 2018;**7**:5. DOI: 10.3390/antiox7010005

[41] Everett SA, Kundu SC, Maddix S, Willson RL. Mechanism of free-radical scavenging by the nutritional antioxidant β-carotene. Biochemical Society Transactions. 1995;**23**:230S. DOI: 10.1042/bst023230s

[42] Mortensen A. Scavenging of benzylperoxyl radicals by carotenoids. Free Radical Research. 2002;**36**:211-216. DOI: 10.1080/10715760290006501

[43] Mortensen A, Skibsted LH. Importance of carotenoid structure in radical-scavenging reactions. Journal of Agricultural and Food Chemistry. 1997;**45**:2970. DOI: 10.1021/jf970010s

[44] El-Agamey A, McGarvey D. Evidence for a lack of reactivity of carotenoid addition radicals towards oxygen: A laser flash photolysis study of the reactions of carotenoids with acylperoxyl radicals in polar and non-polar solvents. Journal of the American Chemical Society. 2003;**125**:3330-3340. DOI: 10.1021/ja027986s

[45] Frei B, England L, Ames BN. Ascorbate is an outstanding antioxidant in human blood plasma. Proceedings of the National Academy of Sciences. 1989;**86**:6377-6381. DOI: 10.1073/pnas.86.16.6377

[46] Linster CL, Van Schaftingen E. Vitamin C. Biosynthesis, recycling and degradation in mammals. The FEBS Journal. 2007;**274**:1-22. DOI: 10.1111/j.1742-4658.2006.05607.x

[47] Corti A, Casini AF, Pompella A. Cellular pathways for transport and efflux of ascorbate and dehydroascorbate. Archives of Biochemistry and Biophysics. 2010;**500**:107-115. DOI: 10.1016/j.abb.2010.05.014

[48] Abraham SE. Biochemistry of free radicals and antioxidants. Scholars Academic Journal of Biosciences. 2014;**2**(2):110-118

[49] Lee J, Koo N, Min DB. Reactive oxygen species, aging, and antioxidative

nutraceuticals. Comprehensive Reviews in Food Science and Food Safety. 2004;**3**(1):21-33. DOI: 10.1111/j.1541-4337.2004.tb00058.x

[50] Buettner GR, Jurkiewicz BA. Chemistry and Biochemistry of Ascorbic Acid. New York: Marcel Dekker; 1996

[51] Williams NH, Yandell JK. Reduction of oxidized cytochrome c by ascorbate ion. Biochimica et Biophysica Acta (BBA)-Bioenergetics. 1985;**810**:274-277. DOI: 10.1016/0005-2728(85)90142-2

[52] Marcus RA, Sutin N. Electron transfers in chemistry and biology. Biochimica et Biophysica Acta. 1985;**811**:265-232. DOI: 10.1016/0304-4173(85)90014-X

[53] Aruoma OI. Assessment of potential prooxidant and antioxidant actions. Journal of the American Oil Chemists' Society. 1996;**73**(12):172-204. DOI: 10.1007/BF02517962

[54] Huang D, Ou B, Prior RL. The chemistry behind antioxidant capacity assays. Journal of Agricultural and Food Chemistry. 2005;**53**:1841-1856. DOI: 10.1021/jf030723c

[55] Prior RL, Wu X, Schaich K. Standardized methods for the determination of antioxidant capacity and phenolics in foods and dietary supplements. Journal of Agricultural and Food Chemistry. 2005;**53**: 4290-4302. DOI: 10.1021/jf0502698

[56] Marco GJ. A rapid method for evaluation of antioxidants. Journal of the American Oil Chemists' Society. 1968;**45**:594-598. DOI: 10.1007/BF02668958

[57] Fukumoto LR, Mazza G. Assessing antioxidant and prooxidant activities of phenolic compounds. Journal of Agricultural and Food Chemistry. 2000;**48**:3597-3604. DOI: 10.1021/jf000220w

[58] Wayner DDM, Burton GW, Ingold KU, Locke S. Quantitative measurement of the total peroxyl radical trapping antioxidant capability of human blood plasma by controlled peroxidation. The important contribution made by plasma proteins. FEBS Letters. 1985;**187**(1):33-37. DOI: 10.1016/0014-5793(85)81208-4

[59] Winston GW, Regoli F, Dugas AJJ, Fong JH, Blanchard KA. A rapid gas chromatographic assay for determining oxyradical scavenging capacity of antioxidants and biological fluids. Free Radical Biology & Medicine. 1998;**24**(3):480-493. DOI: 10.1016/S0891-5849(97)00277-3

[60] Bors W, Michel C, Saran M. Inhibition of the bleaching of the carotenoid crocin: A rapid test for quantifying antioxidant activity. Biochimica et Biophysica Acta. 1984;**796**:312-319. DOI: 10.1016/0005-2760(84)90132-2

[61] Cao G, Sofic E, Prior RL. Antioxidant and prooxidant behavior of flavonoids: Structure-activity relationships. Free Radical Biology & Medicine. 1997;**22**:749-760. DOI: 10.1016/S0891-5849(96)00351-6

[62] Brand-Williams W, Cuvelier ME, Berset C. Use of a free radical method to evaluate antioxidant activity. LWT- Food Science and Technology. 1995;**28**:25-30. DOI: 10.1016/S0023-6438(95)80008-5

[63] Re R, Pellegrini N, Proteggente A, Pannala A, Yang M, Rice-Evans C. Antioxidant activity applying and improved ABTS radical cation decolorization assay. Free Radical Biology & Medicine. 1999;**26**:1231-1237. DOI: 10.1016/S0891-5849(98)00315-3

[64] Singleton VL, Orthofer R, Lamuela-Raventós RM. Analysis of total phenols and other oxidation substrates and antioxidants by means of folin-ciocalteu reagent. Methods in Enzymology.

1999;**299**(1):152-178. DOI: 10.1016/S0076-6879(99)99017-1

[65] Benzie IFF, Strain JJ. The ferric reducing ability of plasma (FRAP) as a measure of antioxidant power: The FRAP assay. Analytical Biochemistry. 1996;**239**:70-76. DOI: 10.1006/abio.1996.0292

[66] Roginsky V, Lissi EA. Review of methods to determine chain-breaking antioxidant activity in food. Food Chemistry. 2005;**92**(2):235-254. DOI: 10.1016/j.foodchem.2004.08.004

[67] Bartosz G, Janaszewska A, Ertel D, Bartosz M. Simple determination of peroxyl radical-trapping capacity. International Union of Biochemistry and Molecular Biology. 1998;**46**(3):519-528. DOI: 10.1080/15216549800204042

[68] Valkonen M, Kuusi T. Spectrophotometric assay for total peroxyl radical-trapping antioxidant potential in human serum. Journal of Lipid Research. 1997;**38**(4):823-833

[69] Ghiselli A, Serafini M, Maiani G, Azzini E, Ferro-Luzzi A. A fluorescence-based method for measuring total plasma antioxidant capability. Free Radical Biology & Medicine. 1995;**18**:29-36. DOI: 10.1016/0891-5849(94)00102-P

[70] Whitehead TP, Thorpe GHG, Maxwell SRJ. Enhanced chemiluminescent assay for antioxidant capacity in biological fluids. Analytica Chimica Acta. 1992;**266**(2):265-277. DOI: 10.1016/0003-2670(92)85052-8

[71] Bastos EL, Romoff P, Eckert CR, Baader WJ. Evaluation of antiradical capacity by H_2O_2–hemin-induced luminol chemiluminescence. Journal of Agricultural and Food Chemistry. 2003;**51**(25):7481-7488. DOI: 10.1021/jf0345189

[72] Lichtenthaler R, Marx F. Total oxidant scavenging capacities of common European fruit and vegetable juices. Journal of Agricultural and Food Chemistry. 2005;**53**:103-110. DOI: 10.1021/jf0307550

[73] Ordoudi SA, Tsimidou MZ. Crocin bleaching assay step by step: Observations and suggestions for an alternative validated protocol. Journal of Agricultural and Food Chemistry. 2006;**54**:1663-1671. DOI: 10.1021/jf052731u

[74] Ordoudi SA, Tsimidou MZ. Crocin bleaching assay (CBA) in structure-radical scavenging activity studies of selected phenolic compounds. Journal of Agricultural and Food Chemistry. 2006;**54**:9347-9356. DOI: 10.1021/jf062115d

[75] Seeram NP, Aviram M, Zhang Y, Henning SM, Feng L, Dreher M, et al. Comparison of antioxidant potency of commonly consumed polyphenol-rich beverages in the United States. Journal of Agricultural and Food Chemistry. 2008;**56**(4):1415-1422. DOI: 10.1021/jf073035s

[76] Jacobo-Velázquez DA, Cisneros-Zeballos L. Correlations of antioxidant activity against phenolic content revisited: A new approach in data analysis for food and medicinal plants. Journal of Food Science. 2009;**74**(9):R107-R113. DOI: 10.1111/j.1750-3841.2009.01352.x

[77] Huang D, Ou B, Hampsch-Woodill M, Flanagan J, Prior R. High-throughput assay of oxygen radical absorbance capacity (ORAC) using a multichannel liquid handling system coupled with a microplate fluorescence reader in 96-well format. Journal of Agricultural and Food Chemistry. 2002;**50**: 4437-4444. DOI: 10.1021/jf0201529

[78] Huang D, Ou B, Hampsch-Woodill M, Flanagan JA, Deemer EK. Development and validation of oxygen radical absorbance capacity

assay for lipophilic antioxidants using randomly methylated β-cyclodextrin as the solubility enhancer. Journal of Agricultural and Food Chemistry. 2002;**50**:1815-1821. DOI: 10.1021/jf0113732

[79] Blois MS. Antioxidant determinations by the use of a stable free radical. Nature. 1958;**181**: 1199-1200. DOI: 10.1038/1811199a0

[80] Sánchez-Moreno C, Larrauri JA, Saura-Calixto F. A procedure to measure the antiradical efficiency of polyphenols. Journal of the Science of Food and Agriculture. 1998;**76**(2): 270-276. DOI: 10.1002/(SICI)1097-0010(199802)76:2<270::AID-JSFA945>3.0.CO;2-9

[81] Gramza A, Pawlak-Lemańska K, Korczak J, Wasowicz E, Rudzinka M. Tea extracts as free radical scavengers. Polish Journal of Environmental Studies. 2004;**14**(6):861-867

[82] Prakash A. Antioxidant activity. Medallion Laboratories Analytical Progress. 2001;**19**(2):1-6

[83] Sendra JM, Sentandreu E, Navarro JL. Reduction kinetics of the free stable radical 2,2-diphenyl-1-picrylhydrazyl (DPPH$^{\bullet}$) for determination of the antiradical activity of citrus juices. European Food Research and Technology. 2006;**223**:615-624. DOI: 10.1007/s00217-005-0243-3

[84] Beserra Almeida MM, Machado de Sousa PH, Campos Arriaga AM, Matias do Prado G, Carvalho Magalhaes CE, Arraes Maia G, et al. Bioactive compounds and antioxidante activity of fresh exotic fruits from norheastern Brazil. Food Research International. 2011;**44**:2155-2159. DOI: 10.1016/j.foodres.2011.03.051

[85] Lutz M, Hernández J, Henríquez C. Phenolic content and antioxidant capacity in fresh and dry fruits and vegetables grown in Chile. Cyta-Journal of Food. 2015;**13**(4):541-547. DOI: 10.1080/19476337.2015.1012743

[86] Prevc T, Segatin N, Ulrih NP, Cigic B. DPPH assay of vegetable oils and model antioxidants in protic and aprotic solvents. Talanta. 2013;**109**:13-19. DOI: 10.1016/j.talanta.2013.03.046

[87] Guo W, Trust B. Phenolic acid composition and antioxidante potencial of insoluble and soluble dietary fibre extracts derived from select whole-grain cereals. Foodservice Research International. 2013;**51**(2):518-525. DOI: 10.1016/j.foodres.2013.01.008

[88] Ancerewicz J, Miglavaca E, Carrupt PA, Testa B, Bree F, Zinin R, et al. Structure property relationship of trimetadizine derivatives and model compounds as potential antioxidants. Free Radical Biology & Medicine. 1998;**25**(1):113-120. DOI: 10.1016/S0891-5849(98)00072-0

[89] Min DB. Lipid oxidation of edible oil. In: Akoh K, Min DB, editors. Food Lipids: Chemistry, Nutrition and Biotechnology. New York: Marcel Dekkar; 1998

[90] Magalhães LM, Segundo MA, Reis S, JLFC L. Automatic method for determination of total antioxidant capacity using 2, 2-diphenyl-1-picrylhydrazyl assay. Analytica Chimica Acta. 2006;**558**:310-318. DOI: 10.1016/j.aca.2005.11.013

[91] Polášek M, Skala P, Opletal L, Jahodář L. Rapid automated assay of anti-oxidation/radical-scavenging activity of natural substances by sequential injection technique (SIA) using spectrophotometric detection. Analytical and Bioanalytical Chemistry. 2004;**379**(5-6):754-758. DOI: 10.1007/s00216-004-2559-4

[92] Milardovic S, Ivekovic D, Rumenjak V, Bozidar SG. Use of DPPH$^{\bullet}$/DPPH

redox couple for biamperometric determination of antioxidant activity. Electroanalysis. 2005;**17**(20):1847-1853

[93] Cheng Z, Moore J, Yu L. High-throughput relative DPPH radical scavenging capacity assay. Journal of Agricultural and Food Chemistry. 2006;**54**(20):7429-7436. DOI: 10.1021/jf0611668

[94] Sethiya NK, Raja MK, Mishra SH. Antioxidant markers based TLC-DPPH differentiation on four commercialized botanical sources of Shankhpushpi (a Medhya Rasayana): A preliminary assessment. Journal of Advanced Pharmaceutical Technology & Research. 2013;**4**(1):25-30. DOI: 10.4103/2231-4040.107497

[95] Shi S, Zhou H, Zhang Y, Huang K. Hyphenated HSCCC-DPPH· for rapid preparative isolation and screening of antioxidants from *Selaginella moellendorffii*. Chromatographia. 2008;**68**:173-178. DOI: 10.1365/s10337-008-0716-1

[96] Pulido R, Bravo L, Saura-Calixto F. Antioxidant activity of dietary polyphenols as determined by modified ferric reducing/antioxidant power assay. Journal of Agricultural and Food Chemistry. 2000;**48**:3396-3402. DOI: 10.1021/jf9913458

[97] Arnous A, Makris DP, Kefalas P. Effect of principle polyphenolic components in relation to antioxidant characteristics of aged red wines. Journal of Agricultural and Food Chemistry. 2001;**49**:5736-5742. DOI: 10.1021/jf010827s

[98] Schleisier K, Harwat M, Böhm V, Bitsch R. Assessment of antioxidant activity by using different *in vitro* methods. Free Radical Research. 2002;**36**(2):177-187. DOI: 10.1080/10715760290006411

[99] Silva MM, Santos MR, Caroco C, Rocha R, Justino C, Mira L. Structure-antioxidant activity relationships of flavonoids: Re-examination. Free Radical Research. 2002;**36**(11):1219-1227. DOI: 10.1080/198-1071576021000016472

[100] Miller NJ, Rice-Evans CA, Davies MJ, Gopinathan V, Milner AA. Novel method for measuring antioxidant capacity and its application to monitoring the antioxidant status in premature neonates. Clinical Science. 1993;**84**:407-412. DOI: 10.1042/cs0840407

[101] Miller NJ, Rice-Evans CA. Total antioxidant status in plasma and body fluids. Methods in Enzymology. 1994;**234**:279-293. DOI: 10.1016/0076-6879(94)34095-1

[102] Miller NJ, Rice-Evans CA. Spectrophotometric determination of antioxidant activity. Redox Report. 1996;**2**:161-171. DOI: 10.1080/13510002.1996.11747044

[103] Shalaby EA, Shanab SMM. Comparison of DPPH and ABTS assay for determining antioxidant potential of water and methanol extracts of *Spirulina platensis*. Indian Journal of Geo-Marine Sciences. 2013;**42**(5):556-564

[104] Rubalya VS, Neelamegam P. Antioxidant potential in vegetable oil. Research Journal of Chemistry and Environment. 2012;**16**(2):87-94

[105] Braca A, Fico G, Morelli I, De Simone F, Tome F, De Tommasi N. Antioxidant and free radical scavenging activity of avonol glycosides from different aconitum species. Journal of Ethnopharmacology. 2003;**86**(1):63-67. DOI: 10.1016/S0378-8741(03)00043-6

[106] Ismail A, Marjan ZM, Foong CW. Total antioxidant activity and phenolic content in selected vegetables. Food Chemistry. 2004;**87**(4):581-586. DOI: 10.1016/j.foodchem.2004.01.01

[107] Chaiyasit W, Elias RJ, McClements DJ, Decker EA. Role of physical structures in bulk oils on lipid oxidation. Critical Reviews in Food Science and Nutrition. 2007;**47**:299-317. DOI: 10.1080/10408390600754248

[108] Gülcin I. Antioxidant activity of food constituents: And overview. Archives of Toxicology. 2012;**86**: 345-391. DOI: 10.1007/ s00204-011-0774-2

[109] Mihaljevic B, Katušin-Ražem B, Ražem D. The re-evaluation of the ferric thiocyanate assay for lipid hydroperoxides with special considerations of the mechanical aspects. Free Radical Biology & Medicine. 1996;**21**(1):53-63. DOI: 10.1016/0891-5849(95)02224-4

Chapter 3

Effect of the Ozonization Degree of Emu Oil over Healing: An Emerging Oxidation Treatment

Daniel Martin Márquez López, Tomás A. Fregoso-Aguilar, Jorge A. Mendoza-Pérez and Sergio O. Flores-Valle

Abstract

This chapter deals with the ozonization process of the emu oil, the objective of this study was to quantitatively determine the peroxide value (PV) to measure the degree of ozonation, the peroxide value measures the number of peroxide groups in the ozonized oil. The ozone oxidizes the unsaturated chemical functions present in the oil giving a high cure rate for epidermal wounds. The healing process is not completely understood and there are different approaches, therefore, it was determined qualitatively if it has healing and inflammation properties, but the results of our studies have shown that the length and width of the wounds were healing quickly thanks to the peroxidation rate of the oils. In addition, both tests were correlated to obtain a greater appreciation of their functions, the mechanism involves a decrease in the inflammation of the wounds and stimulates the process of scar formation.

Keywords: ozonization, emu oil, peroxide value, healing, inflammation

1. Introduction

The skin is a fibroelastic membrane, considered the "outer covering of the body"; It is an organ that performs a wide range of functions including thermoregulation, protection against external aggressions, the absorption of ultraviolet radiation and the production of vitamin D. Additionally, it has an important function of immune recognition, it is an effective protection barrier against pathogenic microorganisms, being the largest organ of the integumentary system and a powerful receptor of sensory stimuli [1]. The frequent exposure to environmental aggressions makes this organ susceptible to suffer injuries that compromise its integrity altering the normal development of its functions [2]. One of the factors that compromise the continuity of this tissue are chronic wounds such as pressure ulcers (PPU), which have been a public health problem that mainly affects those persons who must remain in bed for long periods of time as consequence of chronic diseases [3] or acute dermatitis [4], which affects all human races and more frequently women. Pressure ulcers (PPU) can be presented at any age; however, it predominates in childhood, being more frequent before 5 years of age and persists in adulthood in up to 60–70% of patients [5]. Emu oil is known for the use that the natives of Australia gave it as a remedy to alleviate different ailments for 200 years [6]. In the First World War, ozonated oils were used for therapeutic purposes, as well as the healing of wounds and fissures [7].

Ozonated oils showed their role as modulators of wound healing [8]. The reaction of ozone with the unsaturations present in the fatty acids and other free acids of natural oils generate products such as ozonides and peroxides with germicidal activity and tissue regeneration [9]. The application of ozonated vegetable oil for wound healing quantification in mice, has shown that this oil must be ozonated until a "mean degree" of peroxidation is reached (PV = 1631 ± 64 mEq/kg) [10]. On the other hand, the periodic application of completely ozonated olive oil (iodine value = 0) caused in the skin hypersensitivity to contact and loss of hair in the application zone [11]. Furthermore, it is commonly observed that these ozonated oils present a delayed action [12]. A few crude oils from vegetable origin have the property of healing, once ozonized they acquire this property [13]. The search in the main platforms of scientific information on the ozonization of oils of animal origin throws information that lacks depth to know the effects of the products or by-products in the human body, which does not allow to find a relationship between different ozonized oils, in order to develop a synthetic ozonized oil. Therefore, a need is created to develop research that help to clarify the mechanisms of action of ozonized animal oil, for its greater compression and create the possibility of application. The objective of this work is to quantitatively determine the peroxide value (PV) to measure the degree of ozonation, determine qualitatively if it has healing and inflammation properties, in addition, correlate both tests to obtain a greater appreciation of its functions.

2. Methodology and materials

2.1 Ozonization of emu oil

The experiments were carried out at pressure and room temperature in a semi-continuous type reactor. A constant temperature of ±2°C below the melting temperature of 16°C was maintained.

The ozone is fed continuously and is bubbled to the oil contained in a jacketed reactor, water exert as cooling fluid through a recirculation bath. The reactor is designed in the lower part with a porous ceramic plate (diffuser), an output at the top for monitoring the remain ozone leaving the reactor and has a step valve used to obtain samples at 2, 5, 7 and 10% of ozone.

Ozone is generated from oxygen (acquired from INFRA) with a purity of 99.5%, by means of an ozone generator "AZCO". The refined grade A Willow Springs emu oil was used as raw material, which was applied the extraction technology as described by Marquez [14]. The ozone/oxygen mixture from the generator is introduced to the reactor from the bottom and is evenly distributed in the aqueous solution by means of the diffuser. In the upper part of the reactor there is an output that is connected to a gas phase ozone analyzer BMT-930 connected to a computer that receives the data to be processed in "MATLAB", and generates a graph of the concentration of ozone at the exit of the reactor against time (ozonogram) [7, 15]. The working conditions were: oil weight: 9 g, initial ozone concentration: 30 ± 0.5 mg/L, ozone flow: 0.5 L/min.

2.2 Peroxide value (PV)

This method is based on the determination in the test solution of the amount of peroxides contained by means of a titration based on the ISO 3960: 2017 standard.

The peroxide index indicates the milliequivalents of oxygen in the form of peroxide per kilogram of fat or oil.

A mass of 5.0 ± 0.05 g of sample is determined inside the flask, 30 cm^3 of acetic acid-chloroform solution is added and stirred until the sample is completely dissolved.

With a Mohr pipette, 0.5 ml of saturated potassium iodide solution is added; it is stirred and allowed to stand for 1 min, after which 30 ml of water are added. It is slowly and carefully titrated with 0.1 N sodium thiosulfate solution; shake vigorously after each addition, until it has a slightly yellow coloration; then add 0.5 ml of starch indicator solution and titration is continued without stirring until the blue color disappears. If the 0.1 N solution of sodium thiosulfate is less than 0.5 ml, repeat the determination using 0.01 N sodium thiosulfate solution.

Perform a blank test in the same conditions in which the sample test was carried out. In addition, the milliliters of 0.1 N thiosulfate solution used in the titration should be noted in each case and should not exceed 0.1 ml of thiosulfate. The determinations are made in duplicate at least [16].

The peroxide value is calculated by expressing the milliequivalents of peroxide contained in a kilogram of fat or oil by means of the following equation:

$$PV = (A - A_1) \times N \times \left(\frac{1000}{M}\right) \tag{1}$$

where PV = peroxide value; A = milliliters of sodium thiosulfate solution spent in the titration of the sample; A_1 = ml of sodium thiosulfate solution spent in the titration of the blank; N = normality of the sodium thiosulfate solution; M = mass of the sample in grams.

2.3 ^{31}P NMR

^{31}P NMR analysis was performed in triplicate and was based on the method of Lehnhardt. A detergent solution was prepared containing: sodium cholate (10% w/w), EDTA (1% w/w) and phosphonomethylglycine (PMG) as an internal standard for quantification (0.3 g/l); pH was adjusted to 7.1 using sodium hydroxide. The detergent solution was an aqueous solution containing 20% D_2O for deuterium field-frequency lock capability. Sample was mixed with detergent solution (750 μl) by vortexing, then dispersed by ultrasonication with occasional shaking at 60°C for up to 10 min. The amount of sample used depended on its phospholipid content (lecithin standard 15 mg, cream polar lipid 15 mg, BPC60 powder 50 mg, BPC60 lipid 15 mg, lipid-depleted BPC60 residue powder 70 mg, PC700 20 mg, beta serum powder 60 mg, liquid beta serum 200 μl in 500 μl detergent). When required, pH adjustment was made with aqueous NaOH after the sample was fully dispersed in the detergent. The solution was then transferred to a 5 mm NMR tube for analysis. The mixture was then transferred to a 5 mm NMR tube and the ^{31}P-NMR spectra were recorded. The NMR spectral data were acquired in a Bruker 400 MHz system using a delay of 25 s between 90° pulses and a line widening of 4.0 Hz. A minimum of 200 transients were acquired for each sample at room temperature [17]. The ^{31}P-NMR had a standard deviation of ±1.20%. A minimum of 200 transients were acquired for each sample at room temperature [17].

The chemical species at approximately 132.2 ppm had two TMDP groups and, therefore, two phosphorus atoms bound to it, doubling the NMR signal. For this reason, to obtain the moles of water, the peak area at approximately 132.2 ppm was halved and then it was added to the peak area at approximately 15.9 ppm.

2.4 Intensive wound healing activity in vivo

2.4.1 Experimental species

Male NIH mice of 60 days of age, weighing between 25 and 30 g, were maintained in separate cages in a room under controlled conditions with temperature at 23 ± 2°C, in a light cycle for 12 hours: dark cycle for 12 hours with free access to water and full commercial food.

The mice were used after a 3-day acclimation period to the laboratory environment.

Throughout the experiments, the animals were processed in accordance with ethical guidelines for the care of laboratory animals. The study was approved by the Brazilian College of Animal Experimentation (BCAE) protocol n° 050/2012.

2.4.2 Experimental groups

The animals were divided into five groups consisting of 6 animals: Group A: untreated mice (control).

Group B–E: cutaneous wounds treated topically with a single application of approx. 0.074 g of OEO at 2%, OEO at 5%, OEO at 7% and OEO at 10% respectively.

Histomorphometric and histopathological analyzes were performed on the 3rd postoperative day. The animals of each subgroup were euthanized on the pre-established day for the end of the experiment with an intraperitoneal injection of pentobarbital in deep anesthesia.

2.4.3 Model for split skin wounds

This test was carried out according to the methodology described by Pradeep et al. [18] with some modifications. To perform the surgical procedure, the animals were weighed and then anesthetized with a specific dose of pentobarbital (60 mg/kg BW). After being placed in the prone position, the animals were shaved with a comb of the 1.2 mm hair removal machine. The antisepsis was performed with 70% alcohol along the dorsal midline of the cervical region. A cylindrical fragment of the skin was removed from the midline of the dorsal region with a 10 mm diameter biopsy punch. The depth of the wound of the skin included the epidermis, the derma, the hypoderm and the muscular layer, so that the superficial fascia was exposed.

2.4.4 Treatment

After the surgery, the skin wounds were treated topically with approx. 0.074 g of OEO at 2%, OEO at 5%, OEO at 7% and OEO at 10% respectively, the control group does not make any application. The animals were treated every third day, during pre-established periods.

The clinical course of skin wounds was monitored daily for the presence of secretions, scabs, necrosis and secondary infections. At the end of the experiment, the mice were euthanized as previously described.

2.4.5 Statistics analysis

The results obtained from each group were analyzed statistically using a one-way ANOVA test. The GraphPad Prism 4.0 software (GraphPad, San Diego, CA, USA) and SPSS 18.0 (SPSS Inc., Chicago, IL, USA) were used. The differences were considered statistically significant with $P < 0.05$.

2.5 Injury inflammation activity in vivo

NIH male mice between 25 and 30 g were used. For all the 30 mice the feed is removed 12 hours before the test (water ad libitum). On the day of the test the animals are randomly distributed in batches with six mice each, marked and weighed (BW = body weight).

The saline solution was administered subcutaneously in the bearing of the left leg (LL) while the carrageenan was administered in the right leg (RL), with an indelible nib was marked the site in which the injections were applied, and the measurement was carried out. The injection was applied directing the liquid and the tip of the needle towards the toes of the leg. Great care was taken not to confuse the syringes of saline solution with that of carrageenan or the right and left paw, this could produce deficiencies in the analysis of results [19].

With the help of a Vernier the thickness of each leg was measured in the previously made mark. The first measurement will be made 15 min after carrageenan is administered. This procedure was repeated at times of 30, 50 and 120 min. The difference between the measurements of the right leg minus left leg for each rat will be obtained using:

$$Inflammation = RL - LL \quad (2)$$

At the end of the test, the animals were returned to their original cage to be delivered to the storekeeper for slaughter in accordance with the norms: NOM-033-ZOO-1995 (humane slaughter of domestic and wild animals), NOM-062- ZOO1-999 (technical specifications for the production care and use of laboratory animals) and NOM-087-Ecol-1995 (final disposal of biological products, excreta and corpuses).

3. Results and discussions

3.1 Emu oil composition

Triglycerides are the main components of vegetable oils; their distributions of fatty acid esters differ according to the characteristics of the seeds. The compositions of the avocado and emu oils are shown in **Table 1**. As observed in this table the avocado and emu oils have similar compositions of oleic acid (C18: 1) and linoleic acid (C18: 2), becoming its main components. In the following, "fatty acids" refers to free fatty acids and their dispersed esters in triglycerides.

3.2 Emu oil ozonization

The Emu oil was ozonated until the ozone reaction was completed, that is, when the exit ozone concentration was equal to the inlet concentration (62 min for the

Fatty acids (%)	Avocado oil	Emu oil	Human skin
Palmitoleic C16:1	3–9	3.2	3.8
Stearic C18:0	0.4–1.0	10.1	11.2
Oleic C18:1	56.0–74.0	51.6	30.8
Linoleic C18:2	10.0–17.0	13.2	15.1
Linolenic C18:3	ND-2.0	0.5	0.3
Arachidonic C20:0	ND	0.1	—
Gadoleic C20:1	ND	0.5	—
Phospholipids	1.0	—	—

Table 1.
Lipid composition of oils.

experimental conditions). The latter was controlled by the ozonogram, with the graph representing the ozone that was not consumed during the ozonation process. In **Figure 1**, the ozone of the emu oil can be observed, which indicates that the oil contains oxidizable substrate.

3.3 Peroxide value

Figure 2 shows a gradual increase in the PV with respect to a gradual increase of the ozonation time due to the composition of the fatty chain of triglycerides of the oil and the generation of peroxide bonds.

Ozone reacts with the carbon–carbon double bonds of unsaturated fatty acids and triglyceride present in emu oil to form important products such as trioxolanes and peroxides, which are responsible for decrease of inflammatory activity and help stimulate tissue repair. At low levels, reactive oxygen species (such as H_2O_2) generated by ozonation, which have a short shelf life, are non-radical oxidants capable of acting as ozone messengers responsible for promoting wound healing.

The PVs are obtained after 24 h of reaction. Emu oil only had a PV of 250 mEq O_2/kg of oil, while the PV of ozonated emu oil was much higher with a range of 2700–2900 mEq O_2/kg of oil. These results show that during the synthesis of the OEO, almost all the carbon double bonds in the olive oil reacted with the ozone molecules, generating peroxidic species to increase the PV. After 24 h of reaction, the hydroperoxides, the hydrogen peroxides, the polymeric peroxides and other organic peroxides in OEO had reacted with the iodide to form iodine. According to Günaydın, the reaction time is a very important factor in oils with high peroxide content, and must be greater than 2 min [20].

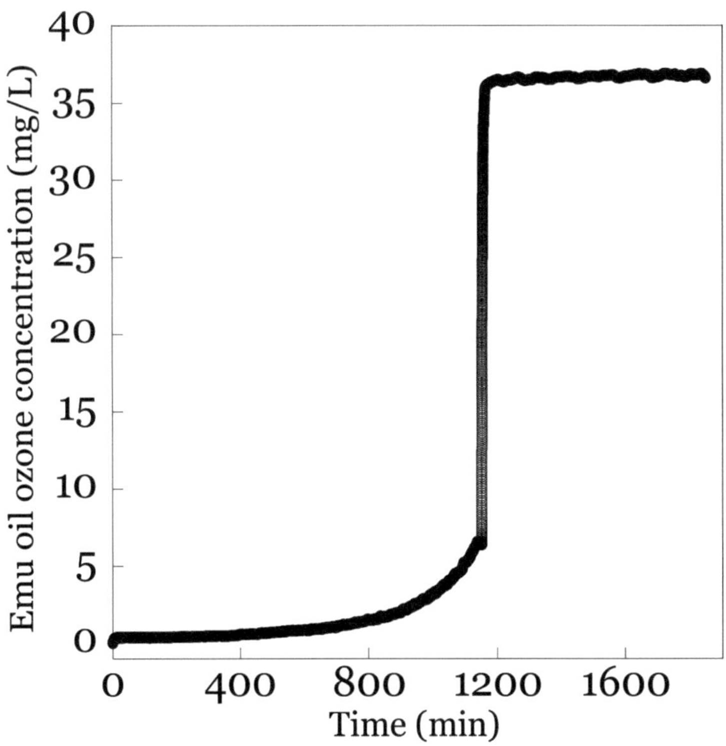

Figure 1.
Ozonogram of emu oil.

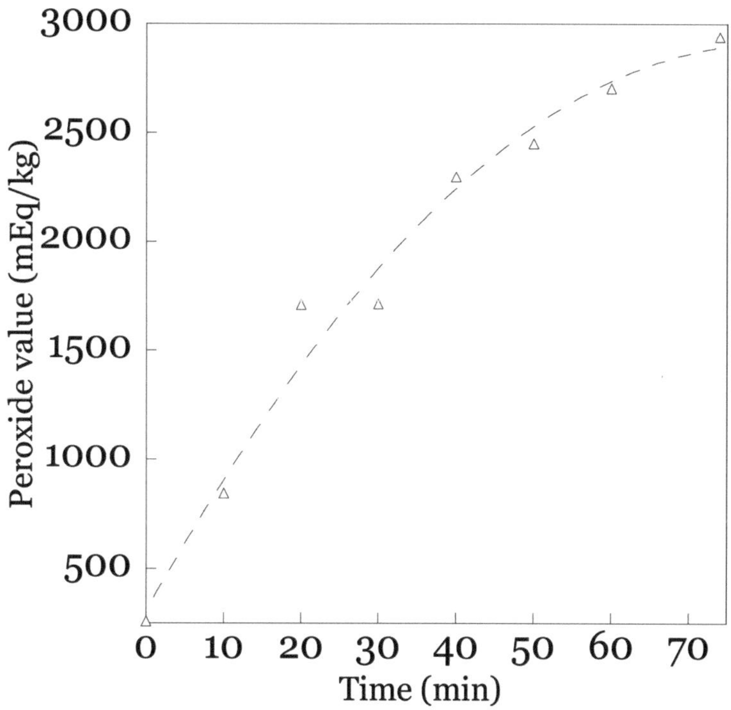

Figure 2.
Peroxide value graph with R^2 = 0.9798.

The spectrum of ^{31}P NMR is also shown in **Figure 3**, Where we can observe a peak that is in the range of the chemical change from 0 to −15 which represents the peak of phosphonomethylglycine used as an internal standard for quantification, which indicates that the emu oil does not have any type of phospholipid, the adipose part of the skin has phospholipids, ozonized vegetable-based oils also have phospholipids, once applied these, the phospholipids of the skin come in contact with the phospholipids of the oil of ozonized vegetable origin and send the order to close the pore to avoid invasion.

3.4 Healing

The effect on cleavage and incisional wound of the ozonized emu oil at 2% produced a minimal significant decrease in the period of epithelialization compared to the control. The treatment also showed a significant decrease in wound contraction (50%) compared to the control as shown in **Table 2**. In the incision wound model, it produced an increase in resistance to wound breakage in comparison with the control group as shown in **Figure 4**.

The effect on the excision and the incision wound across the width of the wound produced a decrease in the period of epithelialization compared to the control. The treatment showed a significant decrease in wound contraction (50%) compared to the control. In the incision wound model, both along and across the width of the wound produced an increase in the resistance to rupture of the wound compared to the control group as shown in **Figure 5**.

The weight and body temperature of each mouse were measured, and it was found that in the mice with weight and body temperature over time they ended in mortality.

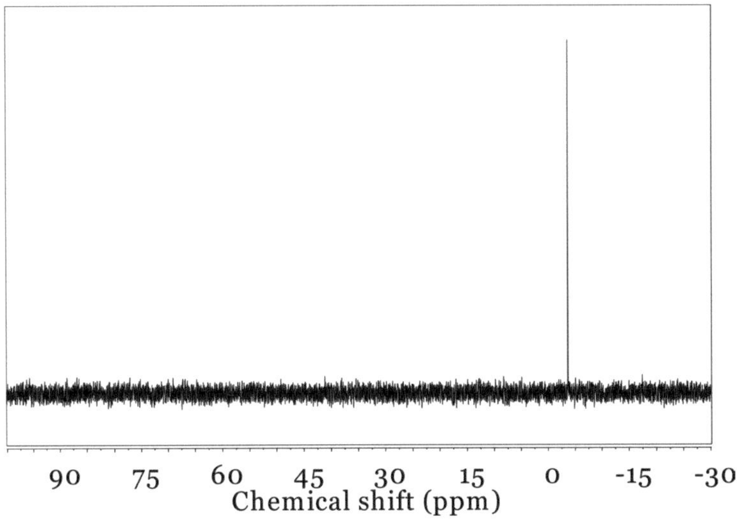

Figure 3.
The ^{31}P-NMR spectra for the refined emu oil.

Emu oil at 2%					
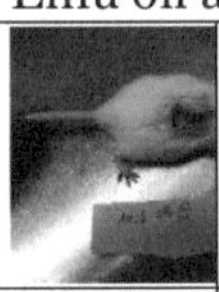	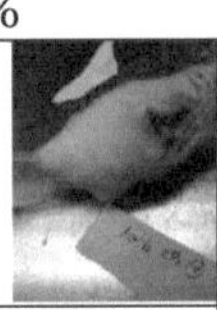	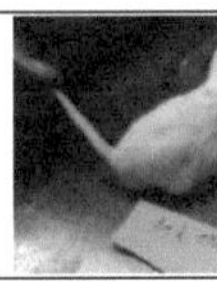	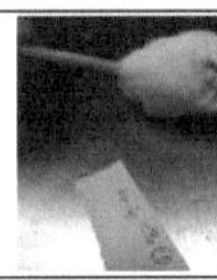	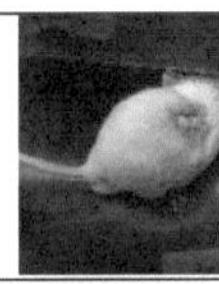	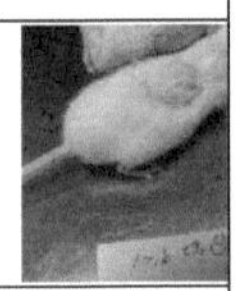
Day 1	Day 2	Day 3	Day 4	Day 5	Day 6
Grupo Control					
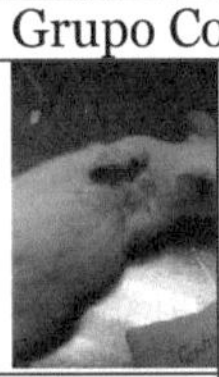	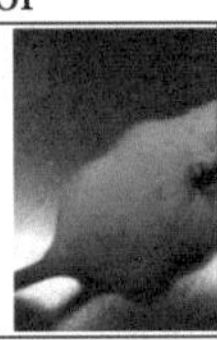	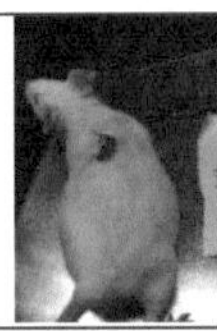	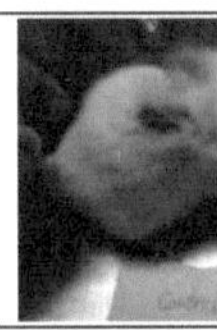	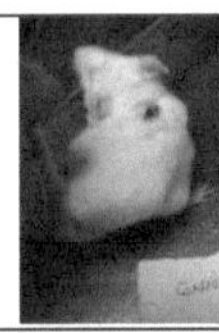	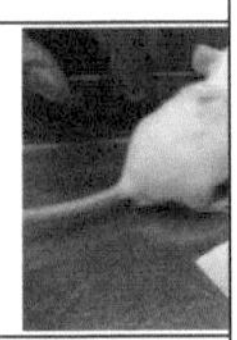
Day 1	Day 2	Day 3	Day 4	Day 5	Day 6

Table 2.
Healing processes.

3.5 Inflammation

Inflammation studies were carried out in each model, with one leg as control and the other as comparative of inflammation, ozonized emu oils of 2% and 7% concentration were taken, the averages of each mouse were obtained with their respective standard error. A gradual decrease in emu ozonized oil at 2% was observed with respect to 7% emu ozonized oil, as seen in **Figure 6**, in addition to comparing with the control group, which is found in **Figure 7**, a decrease in significant inflammation of the right leg.

In **Figure 7**, the normal decrease in inflammation in the left leg (control) of the animals is noted; aspect that served to evaluate the inflammation of the right leg that were administered with carrageenan and that is observed in Eq. (2) and the **Figure 6**.

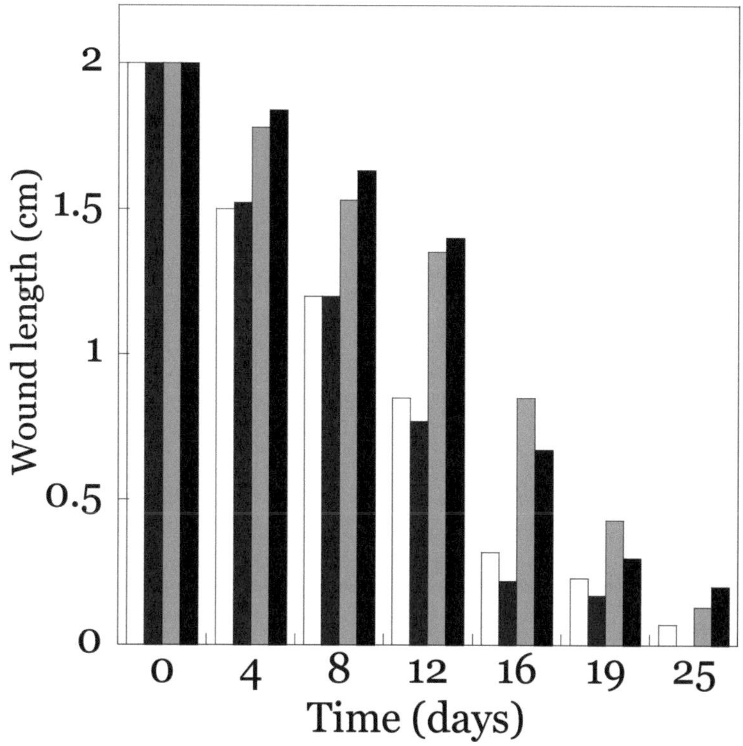

Figure 4.
Wound length for the control group (□) and the ozonized emu oil groups at 2% (▮), 7% (▮) and 10% (■).

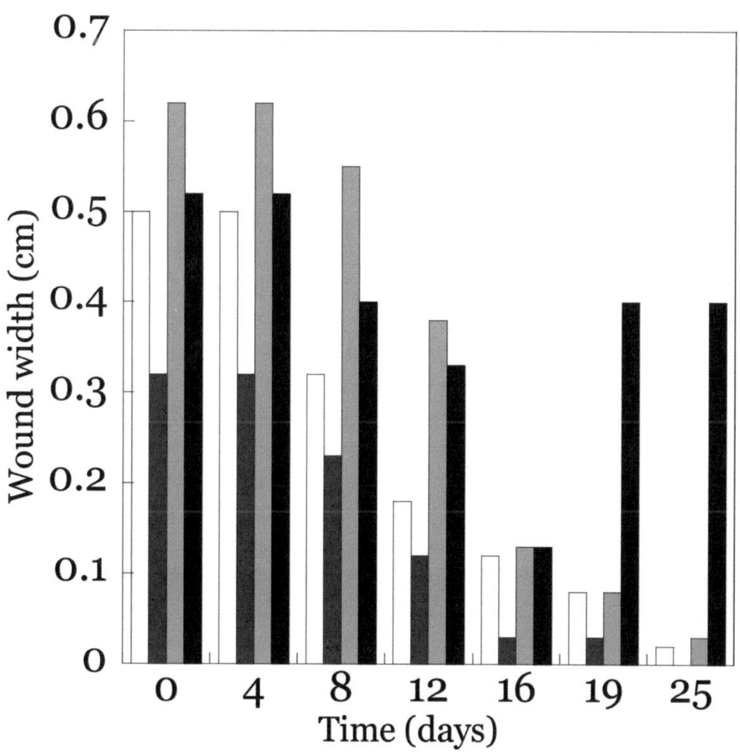

Figure 5.
Wound width healing for the control group (□) and the ozonized emu oil groups at 2% (▮), 7% (▮) and 10% (■).

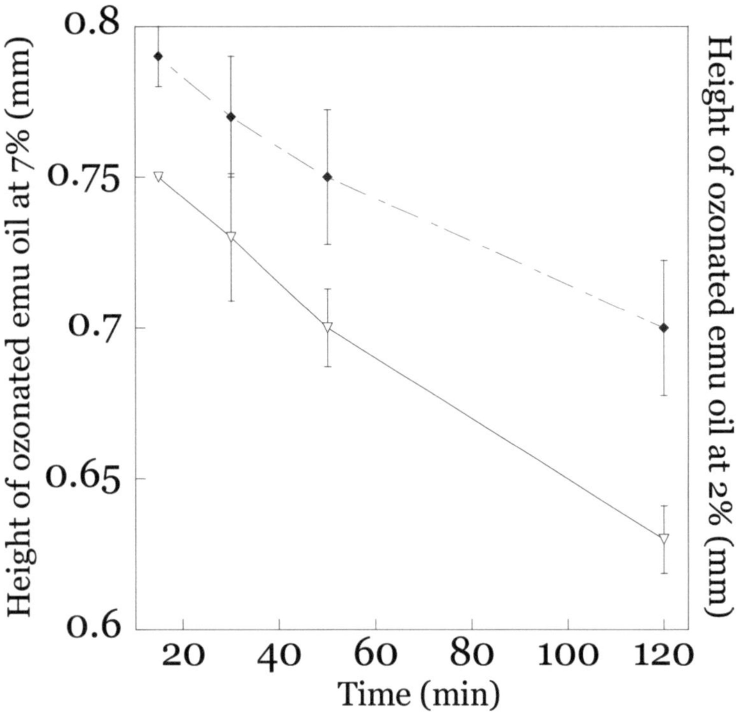

Figure 6.
Comparison of the inflammation height of emu oil at 7% (∇) height of inflammation of emu oil at 2% (◆) on the right leg.

3.6 Discussion of wound healing and inflammation

The reaction of ozone with the unsaturations present in the fatty acids and other free acids of the Emu oil generate products such as ozonides and peroxides. These products may enhance the topical absorption in the mouse skin, because the ozonized emu oil does not have phospholipids.

As it is known, in the processes of tissue damage and inflammation there is a rupture of the phospholipids that constitute the membranes of the cells or their organelles, leading to the activation of the phospholipase A2 which, in turn, is responsible for transforming the membrane phospholipids in arachidonic acid, main precursor through the action of enzymes such as cyclooxygenases, of prostaglandins with proinflammatory activity [21, 22]. This results in the activation of various nociceptor and anti-inflammatory pathways [23]. There are also many drugs aimed for inhibiting the inflammation and pain associated with these damages, but only some are also directed towards the aspect of tissue healing. Consequently, and considering the above, in this work we focus in the study of a biological (natural) product that could present these two characteristics: such as the emu oil subjected to the ozonation method described in the methodology. According to the results shown here, in the healing aspect, only the emu oil concentration at 2% had a significant effect on tissue repair; something that was not observed with the concentrations of 7 and 10%; so, it can be said that the optimal healing concentration was 2%. The fact that an adequate healing does not occur at higher concentrations may depend on the content of other factors not determined in this study, such as factors of plaquetary aggregation, anticoagulants, growth factors, etc. [24], which would be represented in a lesser proportion in the oil, in relation to its content of fatty acids. Obviously, to verify this, more profound studies would have to be done to detect the

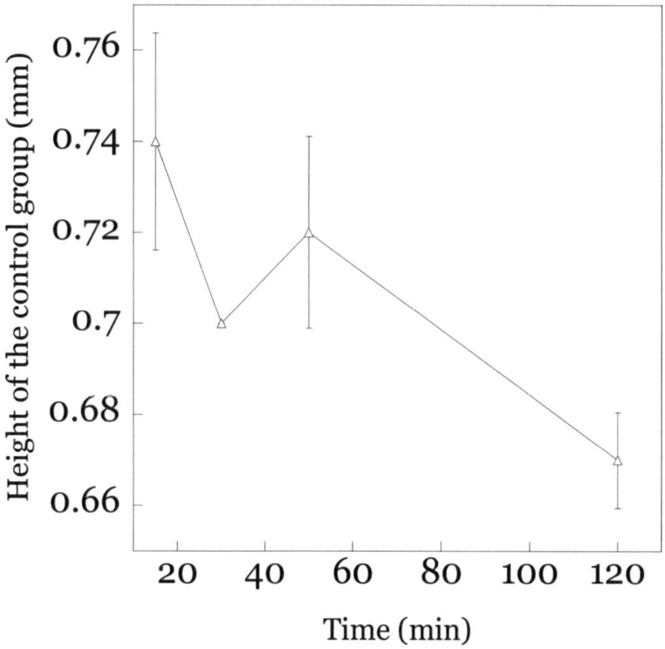

Figure 7.
Inflammation height of the control group (Δ) in the left leg.

presence of such factors that promote an accelerated closing of the wound, increases the neoepithelial thickness and the migration of macrophage-histiocyte cells. However, it is logical to consider that, as with many drugs in allopathic therapy, the dose-response effects do not follow a directly proportional trend, but there is a dose (in our case a concentration) to which the maximum healing response is promoted and none therapeutic effect is observed, although it is increased to dosage, this gives rise to future replications of the experiment with concentrations closer to 2%.

On the other hand, it was remarkable to find that with the two emu oil concentrations tested (2 and 7%), the anti-inflammatory effect was directly related to the concentration used in the mice. This may be related to the content of other fatty acids of emu oil, in addition to the linoleic which is known to participate in the anti-inflammatory actions of some commercial preparations (search for bibliography of this); because having higher content of fatty acids (e.g. stearic, palmitic and even oleic), and be submitted to the ozonation process described in previous paragraphs, it would confer to the tested concentrations a greater capacity to prevent the formation of proinflammatory prostaglandins as some interleukins, prostaglandin E2 and different leukotrienes. There is also the possibility that the ozonizing process conferred inhibitory activity on the inductive cyclooxygenases present in the membrane (COX-2) and that the inhibition of prostaglandin formation was carried out at that level, but for this, they would also have to be make more specific studies; however, the possibility is posed.

4. Conclusions

The present study was conducted to evaluate whether ozonized emu oil could promote wound healing in experimentally induced lesions in mice. The results of the present study also corroborate the use of emu oil for Vedic healing in folk medicine for the treatment of wounds.

Topically applied Vedic healing promoted resistance to wound breakage, wound contraction and period of epithelialization in different models of experimental wounds.

The phase of inflammation, macrophagia, fibroplasias and collagenation are intimately intertwined. Therefore, an intervention in any of these phases by medications could lead to the promotion or depression of the healing phase of the collage.

Acknowledgements

The corresponding author thanks to CONACYT for the grant awarded. All the authors thank the Instituto Politécnico Nacional (IPN) for the financial support given through the projects: SIP 20181685; SIP 20180081.

Appendices and nomenclature

LL	inflammation in the left leg (mm)
OEO	ozonized emu oil
PMG	phosphonomethylglycine, g/l
PPU	pressure ulcers
PV	peroxide value, mEq peroxide/kg of oil
RL	inflammation in the right leg (mm)

Author details

Daniel Martin Márquez López[1*], Tomás A. Fregoso-Aguilar[2], Jorge A. Mendoza-Pérez[2] and Sergio O. Flores-Valle[1]

1 Green Chemistry Laboratory, ESIQIE, National Polytechnic Institute, México, Mexico

2 National School of Biological Sciences, ENCB, National Polytechnic Institute, México, Mexico

*Address all correspondence to: dmarquezl0400@hotmail.com

References

[1] Martin P, Nunan R. Cellular and molecular mechanisms of repair in acute and chronic wound healing. The British Journal of Dermatology. 2015;**173**(2):370-378

[2] Ligresti C, Sasso F, Jahaj E, Ruka E. Wound bed preparation: Standards of care and predictability of the healing time of chronic wounds. Orthoplastic Surgery & Orthopedic Care International Journal. 2018;(7):1

[3] Tamayo-Rendon CM, Palacio-Grisales C, Osorio-Pabon CM, Roman-Giraldo JE, Rodriguez-Castrillon LC. Behaviour of pressure ulcers in services and intensive care unit special care unit in a high complexity clinical Medellin during the first half of 2014. Revista Ces Salud Publica. 2015;**6**(1):27-34

[4] Fernández-Viadero C, Jiménez-Sanz M, Fernández-Pérez A, Verduga-Vélez R, Crespo-Santiago D. Inflammation and oxidation: Predictive and/or causative factors. Revista Española de Geriatría y Gerontología. 2016;**51**(1):27-33

[5] Jegal J, Park NJ, Jo BG, Bong SK, Jegal H, Yang MH, et al. Anti-atopic properties of gracillin isolated from dioscorea quinqueloba on 2,4-dinitrochlorobenzene-induced skin lesions in mice. Nutrients. 2018;**10**(9):1-12

[6] Mashtoub S. Potential therapeutic applications for emu oil. Lipid Technology. 2017;**29**(3-4):28-31

[7] Guerra-Blanco P, Poznyak T, Chairez I, Brito-Arias M. Correlation of structural characterization and viscosity measurements with total unsaturation: An effective method for controlling ozonation in the preparation of ozonated grape seed and sunflower oils. European Journal of Lipid Science and Technology. 2015;**117**(7):988-998

[8] Kent J, Bommaraju T, Barnicki S. Handbook of Industrial Chemistry and Biotechnology. Cham, London: Springer; 2017

[9] Sagai M, Bocci V. Mechanisms of action involved in ozone therapy: Is healing induced via a mild oxidative stress? Medical Gas Research. 2011;**1**(29):1-19

[10] Valacchi G, Lim Y, Belmonte G, Miracco C, Zanardi I, Bocci V, et al. Ozonated sesame oil enhances cutaneous wound healing in SKH1 mice. Wound Repair and Regeneration. 2011;**19**(1):107-115

[11] Pai SA, Gagangras SA, Kulkarni SS, Majumdar AS. Potential of ozonated sesame oil to augment wound healing in rats. Indian Journal of Pharmaceutical Sciences. 2014;**76**(1):87-92

[12] Kendall AC, Kiezel-Tsugunova M, Brownbridge LC, Harwood JL, Nicolaou A. Lipid functions in skin: Differential effects of n-3 polyunsaturated fatty acids on cutaneous ceramides, in a human skin organ culture model. Biochimica et Biophysica Acta - Biomembranes. 2017;**1859**(9 Pt B): 1679-1689

[13] Afshar M, Ghaderi R, Zardast M, Delshad P. Effects of topical emu oil on burn wounds in the skin of balb/c mice. Dermatology Research and Practice. 2016;**2016**:6

[14] Márquez R, Repiso L, Sala A, Sallé L, Silvera C. Estudio de una tecnología de extracción y fraccionamiento de aceite de ñandú de alta calidad para su utilización en la industria cosmética y farmacéutica. Innotec. 2007;**1**(2):4-6

[15] Guerra-Blanco P, Poznyak T, Perez A, Gomez YMGY, Bautista-Ramirez ME, Chairez I. Ozonation degree of vegetable oils as the factor of their

anti-inflammatory and wound-healing effectiveness. Ozone: Science & Engineering. 2017;**39**(5):374-384

[16] ISO-3960:2017. Determination of Peroxide Value—Iodometric (Visual) Endpoint Determination. 5th ed. 2017. p. 10

[17] David K, Kosa M, Williams A, Mayor R, Realff M, Muzzy J, et al. ^{31}P-NMR analysis of bio-oils obtained from the pyrolysis of biomass. Biofuels. 2014;**1**(6):839-845

[18] Pradeep Y, Raju B, Reema R. Evaluation of wound healing effect of a polyherbal formulation by different cutaneous wound models. Pharmacology. 2012;**1**:973-980

[19] González M, Ospina L, Rincón J. Actividad antiinflamatoria de extractos y fracciones de *Myrcianthes leucoxila*, *Calea prunifolia*, *Curatella americana* y *Physalis peruviana peruviana* en los modelos edema auricular por tpa, edema plantar por carragenina y artritis inducida por colágeno. Bios. 2011;**10**(1):9-18

[20] Günaydın Y, Sevim H, Tanyolaç D, Gürpınar ÖA. Ozonated olive oil with a high peroxide value for topical applications: In-vitro cytotoxicity analysis with L929 cells. Ozone: Science & Engineering. 2018;**40**(1):37-43

[21] Powell WS, Rokach J. Biosynthesis, biological effects, and receptors of hydroxyeicosatetraenoic acids (HETEs) and oxoeicosatetraenoic acids (oxo-ETEs) derived from arachidonic acid. Biochimica et Biophysica Acta. 2015;**1851**(4):340-355

[22] Ricciotti E, FitzGerald GA. Prostaglandins and inflammation. Arteriosclerosis, Thrombosis, and Vascular Biology. 2011;**31**(5):986-1000

[23] West SJ, Bannister K, Dickenson AH, Bennett DL. Circuitry and plasticity of the dorsal horn—toward a better understanding of neuropathic pain. Neuroscience. 2015;**300**(6):254-275

[24] Singer AJ, Clark RA. Cutaneous wound healing. The New England Journal of Medicine. 1999;**341**(10):738-746

Chapter 4

Antioxidant Compounds from Agro-Industrial Residue

Beatriz Hernández-Carlos, Norma Francenia Santos-Sánchez, Raúl Salas-Coronado, Claudia Villanueva-Cañongo and Paula Cecilia Guadarrama-Mendoza

Abstract

Agro-industrial residues are a potential source of antioxidant compounds, which in general are phenolic compounds with a large chemical variability. The structure and the complexity of the phenolic compounds (polyphenols) determine their antioxidant capacity, pretreatments, and extraction methods. This chapter gives an overview of the chemical complexity of the phenolic compounds found in extractable and non-extractable fractions of agro-industrial residues, and representative compounds that are present in such residues are shown. Moreover, extraction methods described in this review showed the use of nonconventional technologies and chemical, enzymatic, or thermic treatments, useful to transform non-extractable polyphenols (NEP) to extractable polyphenol (EP) and then apply the EP extraction methods and recover antioxidants.

Keywords: agro-industrial residues, total phenol content, extractable and non-extractable polyphenols

1. Introduction

The agro-industry produces a huge amount of waste, such as peels and seeds from fruits (juice industry), coffee husks, coffee pulp, spent coffee grounds, cocoa husks, cocoa bean shells, acerola bagasse, soybean expeller, rice straw, wheat straw, and sugar bagasse. Most of these wastes contain value-added substances such as phenol-type compounds, which are important for their antioxidant activity. Phenolic compounds possess an aromatic ring, bearing one or more hydroxyl substituents, and whether they have low or high molecular weights (from one to several aromatic rings), all of them are generally referred to as polyphenols. The chemical complexity of polyphenols and the ease of extraction from vegetal tissues divide them into two main groups. The first group is comprised of low-molecular-weight phenols (LMWP) such as flavonoids, hydroxycinnamic acids, stilbenes, and benzoic acids, which are found in free form or as glycosides (**Figure 1**) [1–3]. They are easily extracted by aqueous-organic solvents which is why they are named extractable polyphenols (EP). The second group of compounds are low- or high-molecular-weight polyphenols that include (i) lignans which are phenolic acids or flavonoids associated with the cell wall, such as highly condensed phenylpropanoids [4] and (ii) tannins of high-molecular-weight polyphenols, which can be polymers

 IntechOpen

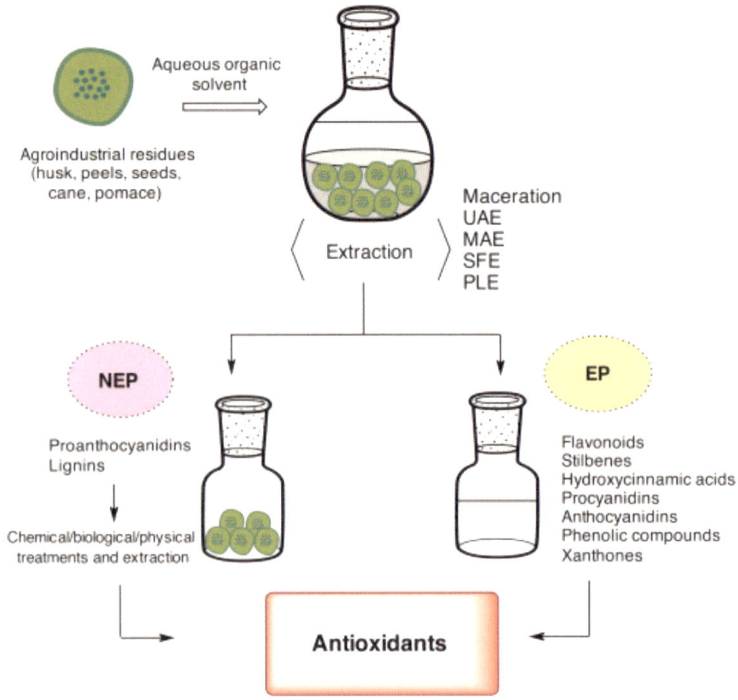

Figure 1.
Extractable (EP) and non-extractable polyphenols (NEP) from ARs.

of phenolic acids and sugars (hydrolysable tannins) or polymers of polyhydroxyflavan-3-ol (condensed tannins or proanthocyanidins) [5]. Due to structural complexity, low solubility, and matrix or vegetal tissue availability, these polyphenols are not easy to extract and therefore are considered non-extractable polyphenols (NEP).

EP and NEP from agro-industrial residues (ARs) represent sources of value-added compounds with potential uses as ingredients in functional foods [6] or dietary supplements due to their health benefits, including antioxidant activity [7–10].

Some problems associated with the recovery of antioxidant phenols or polyphenols are the low availability from matrix (NEP), chemical complexity (NEP), low extraction yields (NEP and EP), and the reduction of antioxidant activity during the extraction process (NEP and EP). All of them present challenges to be overcome for the best use of ARs and economic feasibility. In this review, chemical complexity, extraction methods, and antioxidant activity described in the most recent bibliography are presented. Research in the use of agro-industrial waste involves applying nonconventional extraction methods and establishing conditions that prevent the degradation of polyphenols and, consequently, the loss of antioxidant activity.

Phenolic compounds with antioxidant potential in ARs described to date can be grouped into five classes according to the number of carbon atoms in the basic skeleton: C_6C_1, C_6C_3, $C_6C_1C_6$, $C_6C_2C_6$, and $C_6C_3C_6$ [11]. There are benzoic acids **1–6** (C_6C_1), hydroxycinnamic acids **7–14** (C_6C_3), benzophenones **15–16** and xanthones **17–18** ($C_6C_1C_6$), stilbenes **19–26** ($C_6C_2C_6$), flavan-3-ols **27–30**, anthocyanidins **31–35**, flavonols **36–40**, flavanones **41–45**, flavones **46–49**, isoflavones **50–55** and dihydrochalcone **56** ($C_6C_3C_6$) **Figure 2**. **Table 1** shows low-molecular-weight phenolic compounds and their occurrence in ARs,

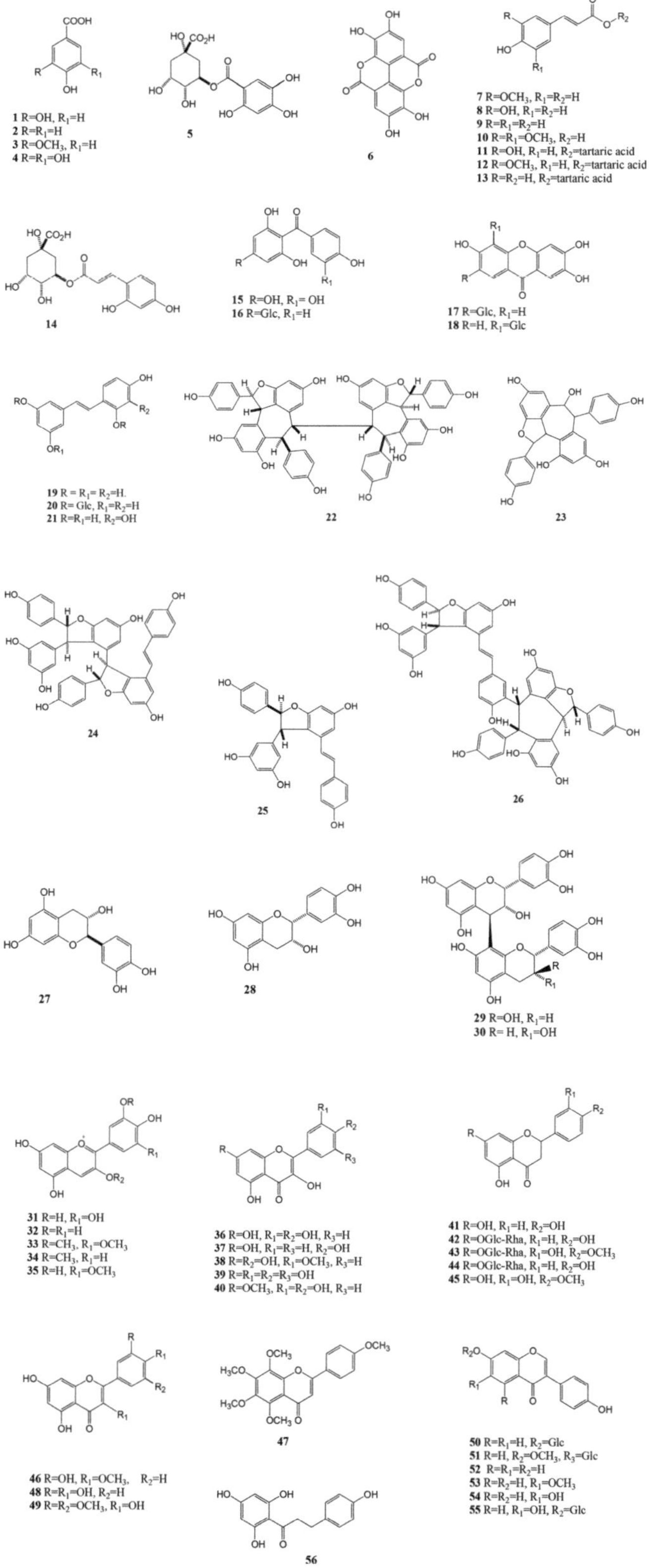

Figure 2.
Structures of low-molecular-weight polyphenols obtained from Ars [14, 31, 50–53].

Polyphenol	Example of ARs
Benzoic acids	
Protocatechuic acid **1**	Mandarin peels [14], grape bagasse [22], spent ground coffee grounds [23], grape pomace [24], sugarcane bagasse [25, 26]
p-Hydroxybenzoic acid **2**	Mandarin peels [14]
Vanillic acid **3**	Mandarin peels [14]
Gallic acid **4**	Mango peels and seeds [17]
Gallic acid derivates theogallin **5** and ellagic acid **6**	Orange peel [18], acerola bagasse [12], Vidal grape pomace [27], jocote [19], grape pomace [24]
Hydroxycinnamic acids and derivates	
Ferulic acid **7**	Coffee pulp [13], grape seed oil press residues [28], Vidal grape pomace [27], pomegranate seeds [29]
Caffeic acid **8**	Grape seed oil press residues [28], grape pomace [24]
p-Coumaric acid **9**	Grape seed oil press residues [28], mandarin peels [14], acerola bagasse [12], Vidal grape pomace [27]
Sinapic acid **10**	Mandarin peels [14], grape pomace [24]
Caftaric acid **11**	Grape seed oil press residues [28], grape pomace [24]
Fertaric acid **12**	Vidal grape pomace [27], seed oil press residues [28], grape pomace [24]
Coutaric acid **13**	Seed oil press residues [28], grape pomace [24]
Caffeoylquinic **14**, coumaroylquinic, and feruloylquinic acids	Coffee pulp [13], apple fiber [3], Saskatoon berry pomace [15], mandarin peels [14], acerola bagasse [12], green coffee seed residue [30], pear fiber [3], jocote [19]
Benzophenones	
Maclurin **15**, riflophenone **16**	Mango peels [17]
Xanthone	
Mangiferin **17**, isomangiferin **18**	Mango peels [17, 31]
Stilbenes	
Trans-resveratrol **19**	Grape pomace [24], grape skin [21], grape cane [32]
Trans-piceid **20**, *cis*-piceid and piceatannol **21**	Grape skin [21], grape cane [32]
Hopeaphenol **22** and isohopeaphenol, ampelopsin **23**, miyabenol C **24**, *trans*-ε-viniferin **25**, r-2-viniferin **26**, and ω-viniferin	Grape cane [32]
Flavan-3-ols	
(+)-Catechin **27**	Vidal grape pomace [27], cocoa husk [20], pomegranate seeds [29]
(−)-Epicatechin **28**	Vidal grape pomace [27], cocoa husk [20], acerola bagasse [12]
Procyanidins B1 **29**, procyanidins B2 **30**	Grape skins [21], grape pomace [24], Vidal grape pomace [27], pomegranate seeds [29]
Anthocyanidin	
Delphinidin **31**	Saskatoon berry pomace [15], blueberry waste [34], grape pomace [24]

Polyphenol	Example of ARs
Cyanidin **32**	Saskatoon berry pomace [15], grape skin [21], blueberry waste [33]
Malvidin **33**	Grape skin [21], blueberry waste [33]
Peonidin **34**	Grape skin [21], grape pomace [24], blueberry waste [33]
Petunidin **35**	Grape pomace [24], blueberry waste [33]
Flavonol	
Quercetin **36** and glycosides	Saskatoon berry pomace [15], Vidal grape pomace [27], pear fiber [3], grape skin [21], mango peels [31], jocote peels [19], grape pomace [24], lemon pomace [34]
Kaempferol **37** and glycosides	Vidal grape pomace [27], grape skin [21], mango peels [31], jocote [19], lemon pomace [35], pomegranate seeds [29]
Isorhamnetin **38**, glycosides	Apple fiber [3], grape skin [21]
Myricetin **39** glycosides	Grape skin [21]
Rhamnetin **40** glycosides	Mango peels [27], jocote peels [19]
Flavanone	
Naringenin **41**	Orange peels [18], lemon pomace [34]
Naringin **42**	Orange peels [18], lemon pomace [34], yuzu peels (*Citrus junos*) [16]
Hesperidin **43**	Orange peels [18], lemon pomace [34], yuzu peels (*Citrus junos*) [16]
Narirutin **44**	Orange peels [18]
Hesperetin **45**	Orange peels [18], lemon pomace [34]
Flavone	
Diosmetin **46**	Orange peels [18], sugarcane bagasse [25, 26]
Tangeritin **47**	Orange peels [18]
Luteolin **48**	Cocoa bean shells [35]
Tricin **49**	Milled rice straw extract [36], sugarcane bagasse [25, 26]
Isoflavones	
Daidzin **50**, glycitin **51**, daidzein **52**, glycitein **53**, genistein **54**	Soybean okara [37]
Genistin **55**	Soybean okara [37], cherry pomace [38], sugarcane bagasse [26]
Dihydrochalcone	
Phloretin **56** and glycosides	Apple fiber [3], yuzu peels (*Citrus junos*) [16]

Table 1.
Polyphenols described in agro-industrial residues.

mainly pomace, peels, seeds, and fibers from fruits such as acerola (*Malpighia*) [12], coffee [13], mandarin oranges (*Citrus*) [14], berries [15], yuzu (*Citrus*) [16], mangoes [17], apples [3], pears [3], oranges [18], jocote (*Spondias purpurea* L.) [19], cocoa husks [20], and grapes [21].

2. Extractable polyphenols (EP)

The applied methodologies in the use of ARs to obtain EP depend on residue type and polyphenol stability. For example, acerola bagasse contains water [39], and if the extraction procedure is not done quickly, the residue will need to be dried to avoid microbiological contamination without affecting polyphenol stability. On the other hand, the probable water content of cocoa husk is low, and therefore, the polyphenols' extraction procedures are direct because it is a solid residue. Therefore, drying and extraction technologies or methodologies are necessary to obtain suitable yields of EP with proven antioxidant activity. The description of the drying and extraction methodologies of the EP will focus on the work with anthocyanidins because they are unstable compounds and the conditions of drying or extraction for anthocyanins are important to avoid their decomposition.

2.1 Waste drying

Valorization studies showed acerola bagasse (*Malpighia emarginata* DC) is a good source of antioxidants due to total phenol content (TPC), which ranges from 0.44 to 10.82 g gallic eq/100 g dm (dry matter) [39–41], while the contents of anthocyanins ascorbic acid and proanthocyanidins are 1.002 ± 0.014, 1.002 ± 0.014, and 0.7985 ± 0.0213 g/100 g dw, respectively, and the antioxidant activity evaluation by DPPH• method showed 113.7 ± 0.4 μmol trolox/g dw. However, this residue contains water and therefore must be dried for efficient handling. The drying of the residue has been carried out by hot air (60–80 °C, 4–6 m/s). This procedure showed moderate retention of phenolic (26–31%), anthocyanins (23–36%), and proanthocyanidins (21%) compounds [41]. Better results were obtained using a roto-aerated dryer (115 °C, 2.25 m/s) with a pretreatment of the sample (sprayed with ethanol), and total phenol compounds (TPC) increased 104.6% with respect to fresh residue [42]. A more recent drying method for acerola bagasse is dehydration in a thick-layer dryer, where drying was done at low temperatures (31.7 °C, 230 min, 0.4 m/s or 60 °C, 159.3 min, 0.4 m/s), which were enough to obtain a dry residue with TPC values similar to those obtained in fresh residue (2352.4 ± 57.23 mg gallic acid/100 g dm) [42]. Drying studies of other ARs are described for grape and olive waste using thin-layer drying (air temperature 20–110 °C) [43, 44], and sustainable drying strategies such as the use of solar dryers have been described [45].

2.2 ARs extraction

Generally, EP extraction procedures are done using mixtures of water-organic solvents and assisted by microwave (MAE), heating, and ultrasound (UAE). In recent years, pressurized liquid extraction (PLE) and supercritical fluid extraction (SFE) have been applied, which could be better options because polyphenols are not exposed to severe conditions that promote degradation reactions. In addition, temperature control is a common method to assist the extraction procedures. For example, anthocyanidins, procyanidins, and flavonols were obtained from grape skins using MAE and UAE at 50 ± 5 °C. This work also demonstrated that the yields obtained by MAE with UAE were improved up to 40% (86.39–121.18 mg/100 g dm) [21]. Acid conditions have also been tested to improve the extraction of anthocyanins (anthocyanidin glycosides) from grape peels separated from red grape pomace from vintages 2001 to 2002. The extraction was made in two steps. First, the residue was macerated (2 h) with methanol/HCl 0.1 (v/v) with oxygen reduced in the mixture to dissolve polar polyphenols. Then extraction with an organic solvent was done to recover less polar polyphenols. Anthocyanin yields found were better (5967–131, 868 mg/kg dm) [24] than those obtained from grape skins from fresh fruits (1211.8 mg/kg dm) [21] due to previous thermic and enzymatic treatments during wine production, which helped release anthocyanins.

Effects of temperature, time, and solvent concentration on polyphenol extraction from grape marc showed better extraction yields with the increase of water (30–50%) in the ethanol-water mixtures, maintaining the temperature at 60 °C for shorter periods (<8 h) to avoid polyphenol degradation [46]. Similar ethanol-water mixtures (40.4 and 55.4%) were used to extract the major components of grape cane: *trans*-resveratrol **19**, *trans*-ε-viniferin **25,** and ferulic acid **7** (**Figure 2**). However, a higher temperature (84 °C) was necessary to obtain the highest antioxidant activities (260.8 and 1378.7 μmol TE/g TEAC and ORAC methods) [47]. Anthocyanins extraction from grape skins, stems, and seeds was effective at 70 °C with ethanol-water mixtures, (1:1) and assisted with pulsed electric fields (PEF) (9 kV, 15 s), ultrasound (35 kHz, 70 °C, 1 h), and high hydrostatic pressurization (600 MPa, 70°C, 1 h). The extraction yields for PEF were 81 and 25% higher than those obtained by ultrasound and hydrostatic pressurization [48]. A combination of methods has also been used, such as the consecutive application of UAE (4 min, 80 °C, 20 kHz, 80 W) and SFE (8 MPa, 40 °C, CO_2/ethanol) for polyphenols extraction from grape marc. The ultrasound treatment increased mass transfer and accelerated access of solvent (CO_2/ethanol) to vegetal tissues, and TPC was increased 27% (2736 ± 11 mg to 3493 ± 61 GAE/100 g dw) [49]. SFE with different conditions (90% CO_2, 5% ethanol, 5% water, 20 MPa, 40 °C) was more efficient than pressurized liquid extraction (PLE) in experiments with blueberry waste. Anthocyanidin yields were 808 ± 0.1 mg/100 g and 248 ± 0.2 mg/100 g for SFE and PLE (20 MPa, 50% water, pH 2, 40 °C) extractions, respectively [33]. PLE with increase of pressure and temperature and change of solvent (65 °C, 10 MPa, 75% ethanol) was shown to be more useful in the extraction of gallic acid **4** together with flavanones **41–45** from orange peels. The TPC obtained was 14.9 ± 0.7 mg GAE/g dm [18].

Polyphenols different from anthocyanins, such as phenolic acids (147.4–492.7 g/kg), gallic acid **4** (93.1–353.7 mg/kg), and flavonoids (2.52–13.5 mg/kg), were obtained with acidified methanol from residues of grape (*Vitis vinifera* L.) seed oil production [28], while protocatechuic acid **1** and chlorogenic acid **14** were extracted with hot water (92 ± 3 °C, 2 min) [13]. Other solvents used for EP extraction are acetone/water mixtures (80%, 3 h stirring) to obtain flavonol **37**, **40** glycosides and xanthones **17–18** from lyophilized mango peels (**Table 1** and **Figure 2**) [31]. In general, EP extraction is made with water-organic solvents and assisted by conventional and nonconventional methods. However, when extraction conditions are severe as when heating above 70 °C, acid extraction or ultrasound exposure for long periods of time, then these conditions are also useful for obtaining NEP, where the objective is promoting the breakdown of chemical bonds.

3. Non-extractable polyphenols (NEP)

Non-extractable polyphenols (tannins and lignins) are low- or high-molecular-weight compounds associated with vegetal tissue macromolecules; therefore, they are retained in the residue matrix during the extraction process. Depending on the monomeric structures and chemical reactivity of tannins, these are grouped in condensed and hydrolysable tannins. Condensed tannins are polyhydroxyflavan-3-ols oligomers and polymers linked by carbon-carbon bonds between flavanol units. These are also known as proanthocyanidins because the butanol/HCl/heat treatment produces a red anthocyanidin [54]. Hydrolysable tannins are multiple esters of gallic acid with glucose and products of oxidative reactions, and they can be soluble (EP) or non-soluble (NEP) (**Figure 3**) [55]. Lignin is a phenylpropanoid (C_6C_3) polyphenol where the monomeric units are *p*-coumaryl **71**, coniferyl, and sinapyl. Occurrence of monomeric units in lignin varies according to the taxonomic origin of the ARs, e.g., gymnosperms or angiosperms [56].

Non-extractable polyphenols are common in almost all ARs and represent significant polyphenol percentages of total phenol content (TPC) in vegetal tissues. For example, NEP quantification in peels from apple, banana, kiwi, mandarin, mango, nectarine, orange, pear, and watermelon showed that, of the total phenols found, 7–82% correspond to NEP [58]. Currently research in appropriate methodologies for the extraction of NEP is a priority topic because of the economic advantages of the use of ARs. Some examples of research on the best conditions for the extraction of NEP from ARs are those for the use of cocoa by-products, which involve extractions assisted by ultrasound [20, 35], thermic treatment [59, 60], hydrodynamic cavitation [35], pressurized liquids [50], pulsed electric field [61], subcritical water hydrolysis [62], and solid fermentation [63]. There are also reports on detailed chemical studies of the NEP structure thanks to modern analytical instrumentation, such as liquid chromatography (LC) coupled to matrix-assisted

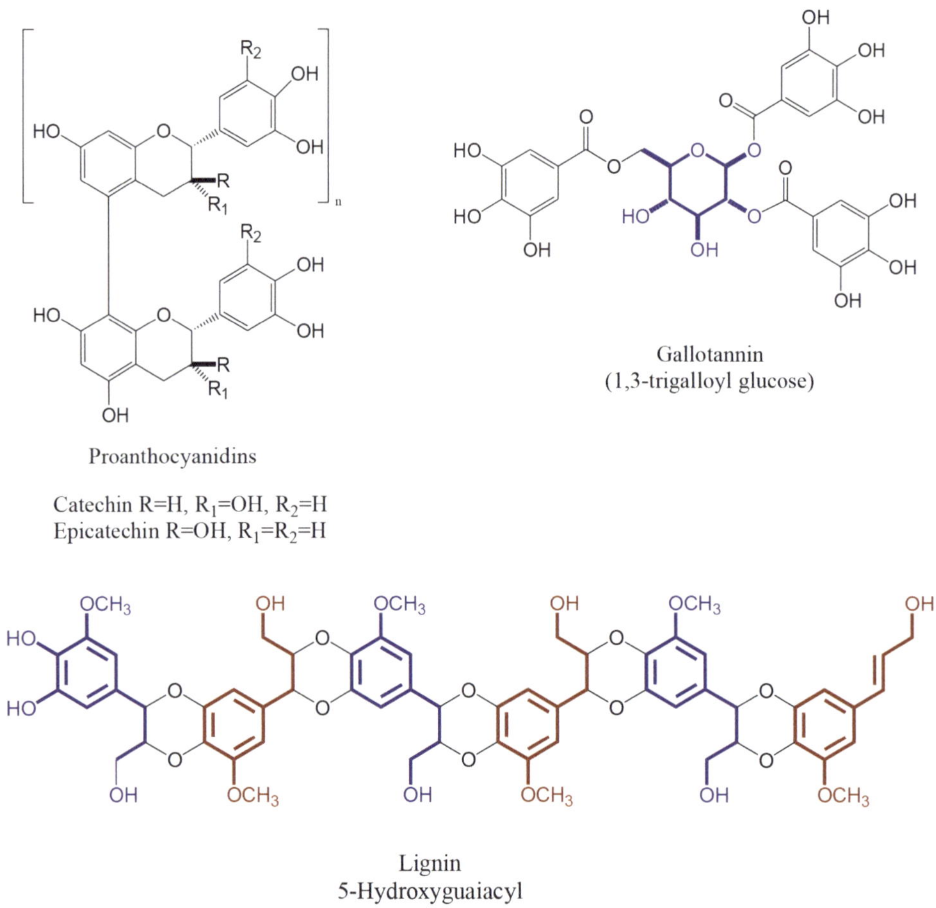

Figure 3.
Structures of condensed tannins (proanthocyanidins), hydrolysable tannins (gallotannins), and lignin (5-hydroxyguaiacyl residue) [55, 57].

laser desorption/ionization time-of-flight mass spectrometry (MALDI-TOF-MS), electrospray/ionization time-of-flight mass spectrometry (ESI-TOF-MS), LC × LC coupled to tandem mass spectrometry, pyrolysis/gas chromatography/mass spectrometry (Py/GC/MS), and nuclear magnetic resonance (NMR), which has been key to making detailed chemical studies of high-molecular-weight polyphenols [36, 64–66]. In the following paragraphs, some examples of chemical studies of NEP are presented to give an overview of the structural complexity that exists in them.

3.1 Tannins

Studies in pomegranate by-products led to the identification of several polyphenols. EP was extracted with acetone 70% (ultrasound-assisted 20 min, 30 °C), and NEP was previously subjected to basic hydrolysis of insoluble residues before extraction under the same conditions. Ellagic acid **6** and monogalloyl-hexoside **57** were the main compounds, in addition to ellagic acid derivates, valoneic acid bilactone I and II **58**, punicalagin **59** and isomers, trigalloylglucopiranose I and II, and granatin, among 34 hydrolysable tannins described in **Figure 4**. Moreover, condensed tannins such as procyanidin dimers **30** and gallocatechin (or catechin) hexoside were described. Antioxidant activity for polyphenol (EP and NEP) fractions was 0.12–3.58 mmol TE/g dm (DPPH) and 5.34–208.73 μmol TE/g dm (ABTS radical-scavenging activity) [66]. Oligomeric proanthocyanidins such as dimer, trimer, tetramer, pentamer, and hexamer units (MW 600, 889, 1177, 1465, and 1753 amu) were identified in coffee pulp by MALDI-TOF-MS analysis. Extraction of these tannins was made with acid aqueous acetone [67]. Acetone/water also was used to extract anthocyanidins from litchi pericarp (*Litchi chinensis*), after its incubation with *Aspergillus awamori*. Total extractable tannin recovery was increased up to 59%, and ESI-TOF-MS analysis revealed *A. awamori* degraded B-type condensed tannin and showed low capacity to degrade the condensed tannin A-type.

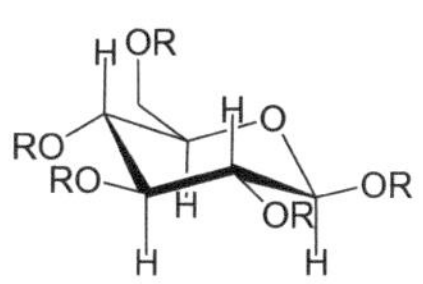

57

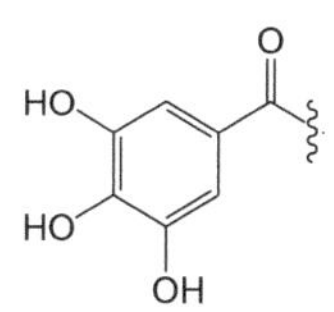

Galloyl group

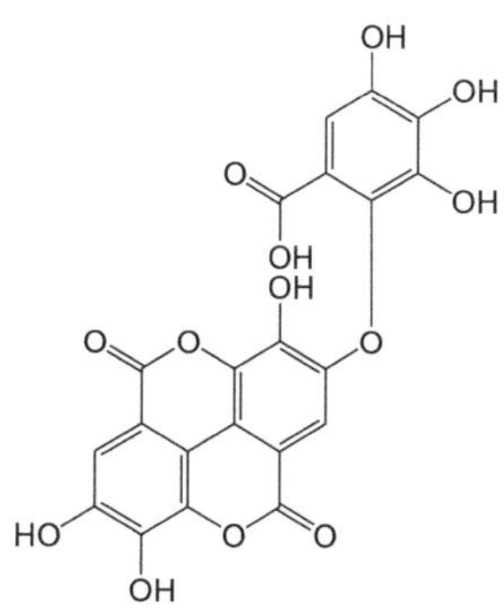

58

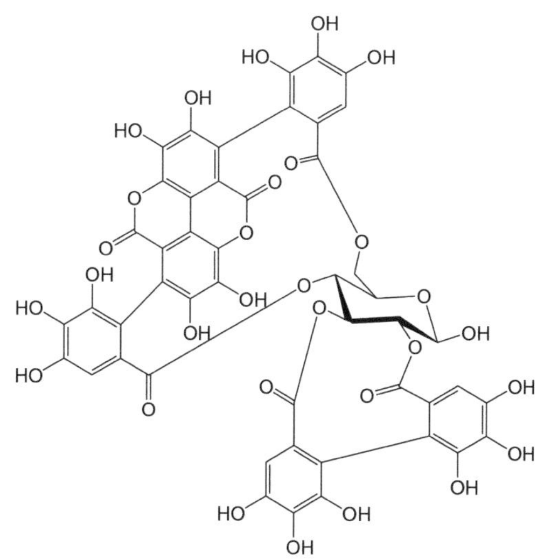

59

Figure 4.
Hydrolysable tannins identified in pomegranate by-products [55, 69].

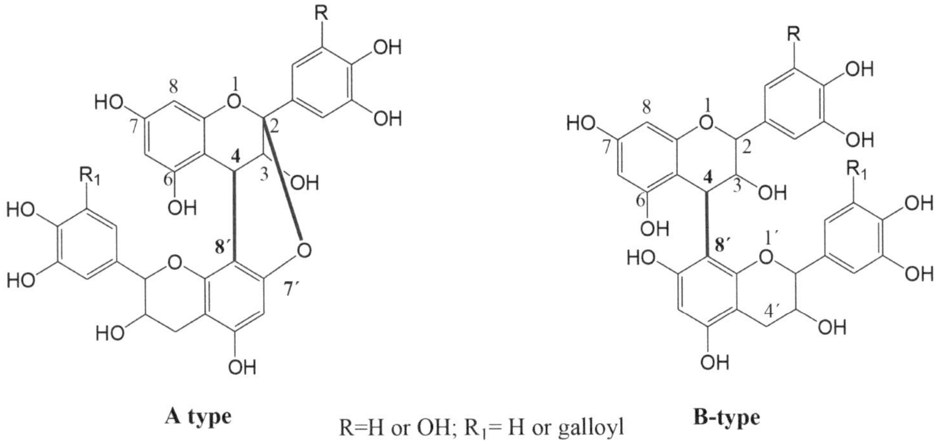

Figure 5.
Condensed A- and B-type condensed tannins. A-type C4-C8 couple C2-O-C7 linkage and B-type C4-C8 linkage [68].

Differences between both compound types are C4-C8 couple C2-O-C7′ linkages for A-type tannin, while C4-C8 linkages are found in B-type tannin (**Figure 5**) [68].

3.2 Lignin

Studies of chemical composition of NEP corresponding to lignin were made for that recovered from black liquor (BL) and milled rice straw extract (RSE). BL is produced from basic hydrolysis/heat of rice straw (straw alkali oxygen cooking). Lignin and phenolics from rice straw were obtained by Soxhlet extraction (ethanol/benzene 1:2, v/v, 8 h). Detailed studies by infrared and nuclear magnetic resonance spectroscopy showed a number of residues from rice straw lignin, including β-O-4'ethers **60**, β-O-4'ethers with acylated γ-OH **61**, phenylcoumarans **62**, resinols **63**, dibenzodioxocyns **64**, α,β-diaryl ethers **65**, tricin units **66**, Cα-oxidized guaiacyl unit **67**, syringyl units **68**, Cα-oxidized syringyl **69**, *p*-hydroxyphenyl units **70**, *p*-coumaroyl **71**, guaiacyl units **72**, feruloyl **73**, cinnamyl alcohol end-groups **74,** and cinnamyl aldehyde end-groups **75** (**Figure 6**). Antioxidant evaluation (DPPH• and ABTS• methods) showed lignin from BL had a better radical-scavenging ability than RSE, which was due to the release of *p*-hydroxyphenyl units by rice straw alkali oxygen cooking. This process caused the destruction of tricin [70]. Lignin and phenolics could also be extracted from milled rice straw by hydrothermal treatment (210 °C) to release cellulosic components, delignification (ethanol/water 60.5%, 130 °C) to fractionate the lignocellulosic biomass and separation (nanofiltration cutoff 280 Da) to isolate the polyphenols [71].

Extraction of NEP from residues that come from industrial processes has been done using methodologies applied to EP because they were released by the industrial process involved. For example, polyphenolics from sugarcane bagasse were extracted with 95% ethanol (maceration 7d) and *p*-coumaric acid; tricin **66**, luteolin, tricin 7-*O*-β-glucopiranoside, diosmetin **46**, 6-*C*-glucoside, and protocatehuic acid **1** (**Figure 2**) were isolated from ethanol extracts (ethanol 95%, 7d, maceration). TPC from extract was 3.0 mg GAE/100 mg dm [25]. Antioxidant activities (ORAC assay) of tricin **49**, *p*-coumaric **9**, and protocatechuic **1** acids were 9.76 ± 1.01, 7.22 ± 0.73, and 6.40 ± 0.62 μmol TE/μmol, respectively. Phenols yields were from <0.2 to 2.12 mg/kg dm. Other compounds reported in this residue were genistein **52** (15.22 ± 1.28 mg/g), genistein **53** (trace), and

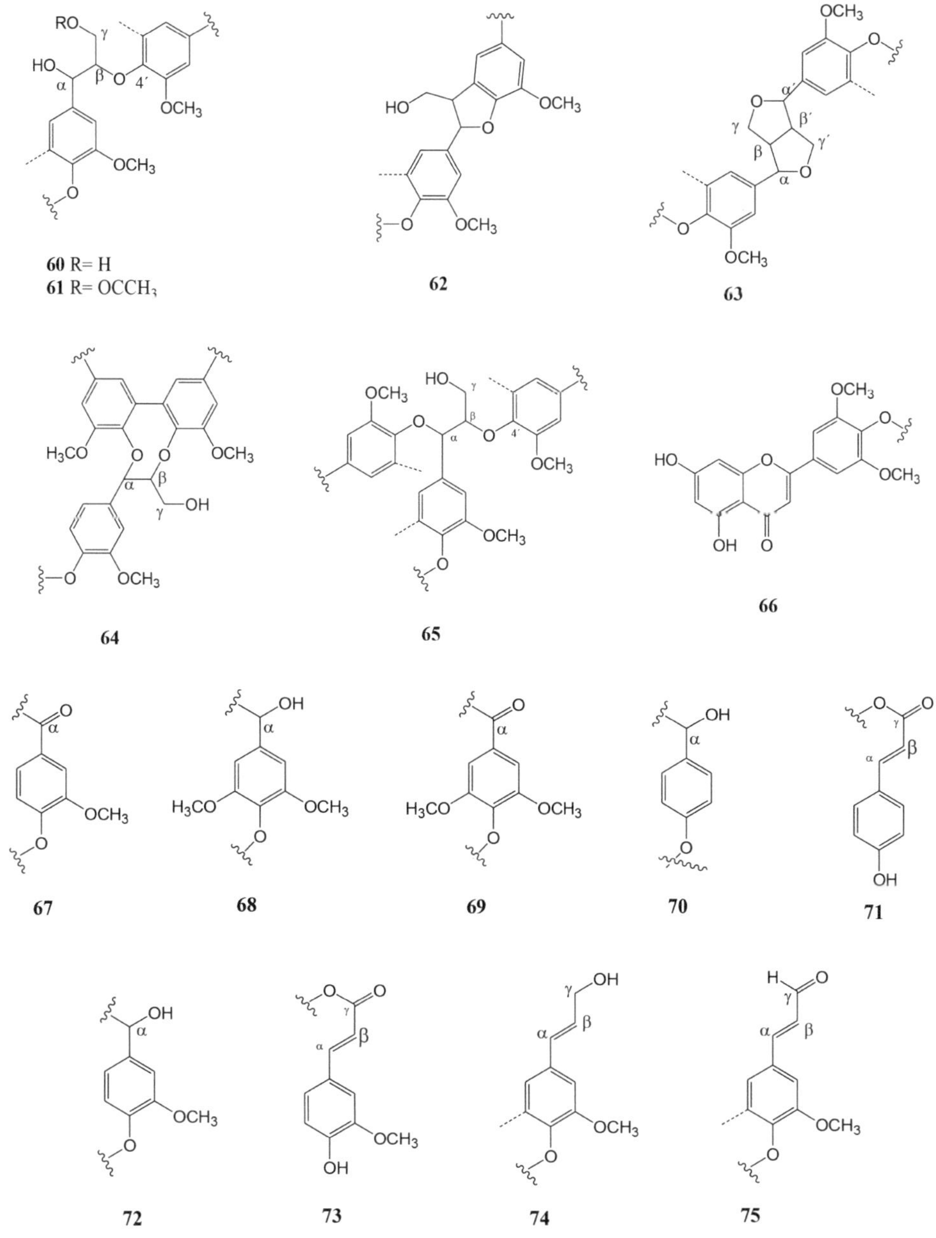

Figure 6.
Residues identified in lignin from rice straw [70].

quercetin **36** (9.98 0.40 mg/g DW) [26]. Polyphenol recovery was improved (117.1%) when residue was treated with glacial acetic acid and hydrogen peroxide at 60 °C for 7 h and later subjected to hydrolysis with xylanase (*Clostridium thermocellum* ATCC 27405). The antioxidant activity was increased 73% (695.8 ± 105.3 μmol trolox eq./L) [72].

Other residue that has undergone industrial processes enough to release polyphenols is the lignin from the ozone, soaking aqueous ammonia pretreatment of wheat. Py/GC/MS analysis showed the presence of 17 phenolic compounds derived from guaiacyl **72**, syringyl **68**, and *p*-hydroxyphenyl **70** units in ratios of 65.09, 23.36, and 11.5%, respectively, the main compounds being Phenol 2-methoxy (guaiacol) **76**, phenol 2-methoxy-4-vinyl (4-vinylguaiacol) **77**, and 2,6-dimethoxy phenol (syringol) **78**. The residue was identified as a potential source of antioxidants because it showed 86.9 ± 0.34% of inhibition of DPPH radicals similar to that of commercial BHT 103.3 ± 1% [36].

4. Antioxidant activity (AA) and extraction methods

Antioxidant activity (AA) obtained from AR's extracts varies according to the residue type and the extraction method. In case of cocoa residues, UAE (methanol/water 1:1 and acetone water 7:3) showed better method than maceration because AA was improved 8.8% (EC_{50} 0.0486 ± 0.0018 mg/mL) in comparison with that obtained from maceration with the same solvents (EC_{50} 0.0533 ± 0.0022 mg/mL), while total phenol content (TPC) was 41.96% higher (**Table 2**) [20]. Extracts with high TPC (55 mg GAE/g) but low AA values (EC_{50} 8.18 mg/mL) were obtained by hydrothermal treatment (170 °C, 30 min) [60], in comparison with those values for extracts obtained by UAE and maceration. Thermic treatment

Residue/ref.	Extraction method	Antioxidant activity	TPC/(dry matter)
Cocoa husk [20]	UAE 25 kHz, 30 min, MeOH/H_2O 1:1, and acetone/water 7:3	EC_{50} 0.0486 ± 0.0018 mg/mL (DPPH)	25.34 ± 1.82 mg GAE/g
	Maceration MeOH/H_2O 1:1, 2 h stir, acetone/water 7:3	EC_{50} 0.0533 ± 0.0022 mg/mL (DPPH) Ascorbic acid 0.0243 ± 0.0009 mg/mL	17.85 ± 1.33 mg GAE/g
Cocoa husk [60]	Hydrothermal, 170 °C, 30 min	EC_{50} 8.18 mg/mL (DPPH)	55 mg GAE/g
Cocoa bean shells [61]	Extraction EtOH/water rotatory agitation 25 °C with a pretreatment time of 11.99 μs, number of pulses of 991.28, PEF strength of 1.74 kV cm^{-1}, ethanol 39.15%, 118.54 min	101.1–321.97 μM TE/g (DPPH)	17.88–55.16 mg GAE/g
Cocoa bean shells [35]	UAE EtOH/water (70:30), 15 min, 150 W, 19.9 kHz, 40 °C	EC_{50} 66.9 ± 2.4 μg/mL and 235.3 ± 8.4 μM TE/g (DPPH)	125 mg GAE/g
Cocoa bean shells [50]	PLE EtOH, 10.35 MPa, 90 °C, 30 min	65 ± 2 μM TE/g (DPPH) 84 ± 4 μM TE/g (FRAP)	10 ± 0.3 mg ECE/g
Cocoa bean shells [35]	Hydrodynamic cavitation and Hex/EtOH/H_2O mixtures (30:49:21) scale-up reactor	EC_{50} 62.0 ± 3.1 μg/mL (DPPH) and 256.7 ± 9.9 μM TE/g (DPPH)	197.4 mg GAE/g
Cocoa bean shells [63]	Solid state fermentation with *Penicillium roqueforti* and EtOH/water extraction	81.3% inhibition (DPPH) 23.2 μM ferrous sulfate/g (FRAP)	926.6 ± 61 mg GAE/100 g
Acerola bagasse [12]	MeOH 50%, 80 °C, 15 min	405.11 ± 1.83 μM TE/Lg (Rutin 1473.07 ± 21.39 μM TE/Lg) (ABTS)	nd
Acerola bagasse [41]	Water and stirring 30 min	21.7–24.0 μM TE/g (DPPH)	2710.2–3171.9 mg GAE/100 g

Residue/ref.	Extraction method	Antioxidant activity	TPC/(dry matter)
Coffee pulp [13]	Water, 92 ± 3 °C, 2 min	EC_{50} 18–27 μg/mL (ABTS) 82–153 μg/mL (DPPH)	7.61–17.40 mg GAE/L
Coffee husk [23]	SFE 200 bar/323.15 K, CO_2 + 8% EtOH	EC_{50} 630 μg/mL (DPPH) 141 ± 1 μM TE/g (ABTS)	36 ± 1 mg CAE/g
	UAE, EtOH	EC_{50} 235.1 μg/mL (DPPH) 161 ± 3 μM TE/g (ABTS)	133.3 ± 0.6 mg CAE/g
Spent coffee grounds [23]	SFE 200 bar/323.15 K, CO_2 + 4% EtOH	EC_{50} 516.2 μg/mL (DPPH) 169 ± 3 μM TE/g (ABTS)	57 ± 3 mg CAE/g
	Soxhlet extraction, EtOAc	EC_{50} 202.23 μg/mL (DPPH) 160.13 ± 13 μM TE/g (ABTS)	182.6 ± 28.2 mg CAE/g
Coffee silver skin [1]	Hydroalcoholic solvent (50%) at 40°C, 60 min	326.0 ± 5.7 mg TE/L (DPPH) 1791.9 ± 126.3 mg FSE/L (FRAP)	302.5 ± 7.1 mg GAE/L
Spent coffee grounds [73]	Solid state fermentation with *Bacillus clausii* (37 °C, 39 h), defatted (hexane) and EtOH/water (80:20) extraction (orbital shaker, 30 °C, 50 rpm, 3 h)	17.894 μM TE/100 g (ABTS)	1051 mg GAE/ 100 g Increased 36%
Blueberry waste [33]	SFE 90% CO_2, 5% H_2O, 5% EtOH, 20 MPa	1658 ± 160 μM TE/g (DPPH) 199 ± 20 μM TE/g (ABTS)	134 ± 11 mg GAE/g Wet matter
	PLE 40 °C, 20 MPa, 15 min, 5 mL cell, EtOH/water 1:1	1746 ± 71 μM TE/g (DPPH) 66 ± 1 μM TEAC/g (ABTS)	90 ± 2 mg GAE/g Wet matter
Grape cane [47]	Water/EtOH 40.4 and 55.4%, 84 °C	238.6 μM TE/g (ABTS) 1259.6 μM TE/g (ORAC)	8.93 mg resveratrol eq./g
Grape cane [32]	Acetone/water 6:4, room temperature	1700–5300 μM TE/g (ORAC)	Stilbene total content 2.62–3.30 mg/g
Grape skins [21]	MAE, 600 W, 2450 MHz, 50 ± 5 °C, water/EtOH/phosphoric acid 50:50:1	nd	Stilbenes 1.5 mg/ 100 g
	UAE, 130 W, 40 kHz, 50 ± 5°C, water/ EtOH/phosphoric acid 50:50:1	nd	Stilbenes 0.71 mg/ 100 g
Soybean okara [37]	Solid state fermentation with *Saccharomyces cerevisiae* r. f. *bayanus* 72 h. Water/MeOH (80%) extraction	24.04 mM TE/g (DPPH) 20.65 mM TE/g (ABTS) Increase 15%	116 mg GAE/10 g

*UAE, ultrasound-assisted extraction; EC_{50}, effective concentration at 50%; PLE, pressurized liquid extraction; PEF, pulsed electric field; SFE, supercritical fluid extraction; TPC, total phenol content; MeOH, methanol; EtOH, ethanol; AcOEt, ethyl acetate; CAE, chlorogenic acid equivalent; GAE, gallic acid equivalent; ABTS, 2,2′-azino-*bis*(3-ethylbenzothiazoline-6-sulfonic acid) diammonium salt; DPPH, 2,2-diphenyl-1-picrylhydrazyl; ORAC, oxygen radical absorbance capacity; MAE, microwave-assisted extraction; TE, trolox equivalent; FRAP, ferric-reducing antioxidant power; FSE, ferrous sulfate equivalent; nd, not described*

Table 2.
Antioxidant activity and extraction methods in agro-industrial residues.

improves yields of polyphenols because it promotes release of NEP, but polyphenols can loss their antioxidant capacity. A method that significantly improved the TPC without reducing the AA of the extracts is the hydrodynamic cavitation (HC), which was used to assist polyphenols extraction from cocoa bean shells with hexane/ethanol/water mixtures [35]. The authors compared the efficiency of this method with UAE (ethanol/water); AA were similar (EC_{50} 62 ± 3.2 and 66.9 ± 2.4 μg/mL), while TPC was 125 and 197.4 mg GAE/g for extracts obtained by UAE and HC, respectively.

In general, SFE (with the optimal conditions) is an extraction method more convenient in order to avoid degradation reactions and therefore reduces the AA of extracts. Blueberry waste extracts were obtained by SFE (90% CO_2, 5% H_2O, 5% ethanol, 20 MPa) and PLE (40 °C, 20 MPa, 15 min). Both methods showed extracts with similar AA (1658 ± 160 and 1746 ± 71 μM TE/g), but SFE yields extracts with TPC 48% more higher (134 ± 11 mg GAE/g) than those from PLE (90.2 ± 2 mg GAE/g) (**Table 2**) [33]. However, extracts obtained by UAE (ethanol) and Soxhlet (ethyl acetate) from coffee residues showed better AA values (EC_{50} 235.1 and 202.23 μg/mL) than those observed in the extracts obtained by SFE (200 bar/ 323.15 K, CO_2 + 8 or 4% ethanol) (EC_{50} 630 and 516.2 μg/mL) [23].

Pretreatments as solid-state fermentation before polyphenolic extraction have shown effects on TPC and AA, for example, in spent coffee grounds, an increase in TPC and AA of 36%, and 15% were observed in fermented extracts by *Bacillus clausii* followed by ethanol/water extraction [73]. The same increase in AA was observed when soybean residues were subjected to solid-state fermentation using *Saccharomyces cerevisiae* (20.39–24.04 mM TE/g) [37]. However, the use of *Penicillium roqueforti* in this fermentation type with cocoa shells showed a weak increase of AA from 79.2 to 81.3% (2.6%) and the reduction of TPC from 2120 ± 20 mg GA/100 g to 926.6 ± 61 mg/100 g (56%) [63].

Grape cane residues are rich in stilbene compounds, which can be extracted with mixtures of water/ethanol or acetone/water, and their antioxidant activities depend on stilbene type present in extracts, e.g., quantitative structure-antioxidant activity relationship studies showed structural facts as planar geometry of *trans*-isomers has direct relation with the AA because polyphenols increase their free radical-stabilizing properties [74]. This may explain why AA is lower in extracts with higher stilbene contents; water/ethanol extracts with 8.93 mg resveratrol eq./g showed an AA of 1259.6 μM TE/g (ORAC), while acetone/water extracts with stilbene total content of 2.62–3.30 mg/g showed from 1700 to 5300 μM TE/g. Therefore, stilbene extraction accelerated by temperature can have consequences on stereoisomer content and therefore on the AA. Extraction of grape skins at 50 °C assisted by MAE and UAE showed better stilbenes contents for MAE (1.5 mg/ 100 g), but authors did not describe the AA [21]. Heat resistance phenol compounds and with significant AA are those found in residues previously treated to release NEP such as **56**, **76**-**79** [36, 75] (**Figures 2** and 7). For example, apple pulp was subjected to reflux with water for 2 h, and the EtOAc extract showed an AA of IC_{50}

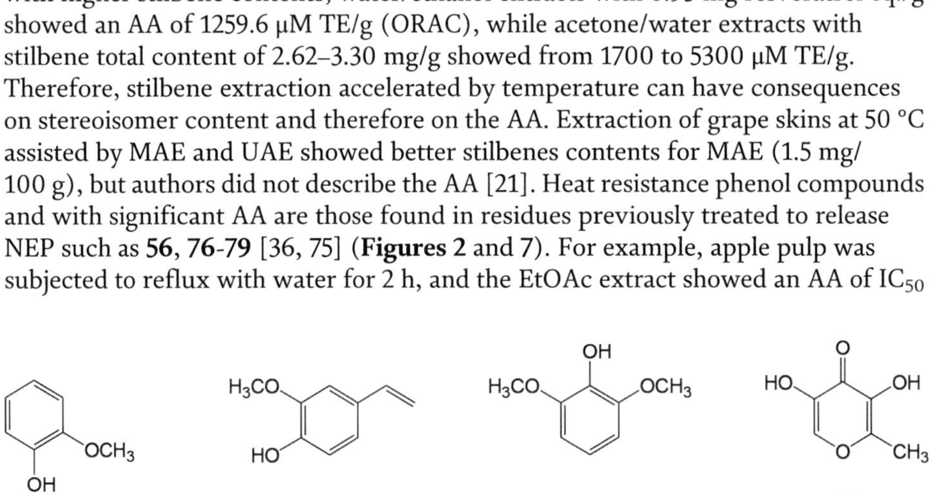

76 **77** **78** **79**

Figure 7.
Heat resistance phenol compounds identified in ARs [36, 75].

10.59 ± 2.77 μg/mL (DPPH), while 5-hydroxymaltol **79**, isolated from AcOEt extract, showed an IC_{50} value of 8.22 ± 1.83 μg/mL, which was 48 times higher than α-tocopherol (IC_{50} 0.17 ± 0.04 μg/mL) [75].

5. Conclusions

Most of the bibliography related to the study of waste is focused on the search for conditions for the greater extraction of polyphenols from ARs and evaluating the feasibility of using these residues as a source of antioxidants. To evaluate the extraction efficiency of the proposed methods, the content of total phenols (TCP), the quantification and/or identification of specific polyphenols and determination of AA have been described. Antioxidant activity of polyphenols varies mainly by the temperature, which could promote the compound degradation or only small structural changes, mainly with anthocyanidins and stilbenes. Extraction methods applied to ARs described in this review showed the use of nonconventional technologies such as SFE and LPE for EP extraction while chemical, enzymatic, or thermic hydrolysis has been used to transform NEP to EP to apply the EP extraction methods and recover antioxidants. Moreover, significant contributions to the knowledge of the chemistry of ARs are summarized and representative compounds are shown that cover most types of phenols that exist in the plant kingdom and that are present in such residues. The chemical structures of 79 low-molecular-weight compounds, mainly EP and some examples of tannin and lignin residues, are described. Therefore, the use of ARs to recover polyphenols is growing due to the knowledge of ARs chemistry and to the development of nonconventional extraction methods and more efficient dry methods.

Acknowledgements

The authors thank Carol Ann Hayenga for her assistance with English language in the preparation of this manuscript. The Technological University of the Mixteca provided support.

Conflict of interest

The authors declare that there are no conflicts of interests regarding the publication of this chapter.

Author details

Beatriz Hernández-Carlos*, Norma Francenia Santos-Sánchez, Raúl Salas-Coronado, Claudia Villanueva-Cañongo and Paula Cecilia Guadarrama-Mendoza
Technological University of Mixteca, Huajuapan de León, Oaxaca, México

*Address all correspondence to: bhcarlos@mixteco.utm.mx

References

[1] Costa AS, Alves RC, Vinha AF, Barreira SV, Nunes MA, Cunha LM, et al. Optimization of antioxidants extraction from coffee silver skin, a roasting by-product, having in view a sustainable process. Industrial Crops and Products. 2014;**53**: 350-357. DOI: 10.1016/j.indcrop.2014.01.006

[2] Peralbo-Molina A, Priego-Capote F, Luque de Castro MD. Tentative identification of phenolic compounds in olive pomace extracts using liquid chromatography-tandem mass spectrometry with a quadrupole-quadrupole-time-of-flight mass detector. Journal of Agricultural and Food Chemistry. 2012;**60**:11542-11550. DOI: 10.1021/jf302896m

[3] Delpino-Rius A, Eras J, Vilaró F, Cubero MÁ, Balcells M, Canela-Garayoa R. Characterization of phenolic compounds in processed fibers from the juice industry. Food Chemistry. 2015; **172**:575-584. DOI: 10.1016/j.foodchem.2014.09.071

[4] Lapierre C. Application of new methods for the investigation of lignin structure. In: Forage Cell Wall Structure and Digestibility, (Forage Cell Walls). Madison, WI: ASA, CSSA, SSSA; 1993. pp. 133-166. DOI: 10.2134/1993.foragecellwall.c6

[5] Pérez-Jiménez J, Saura-Calixto F. Fruit peels as sources of non-extractable polyphenols or macromolecular antioxidants: Analysis and nutritional implications. Food Research International. 2018;**111**:148-152. DOI: 10.1016/j.foodres.2018.05.023

[6] Martirosyan DM, Singh J. A new definition of functional food by FFC: What makes a new definition unique? Functional Foods in Health and Disease. 2015;**5**:209-223. DOI: 10.31989/ffhd.v5i6.183

[7] Frémont L. Biological effects of resveratrol. Life Sciences. 2000;**66**: 663-673. DOI: 10.1016/S0024-3205(99)00410-5

[8] Kong JM, Chia LS, Goh NK, Chia TF, Brouillard R. Analysis and biological activities of anthocyanins. Phytochemistry. 2003;**64**:923-933. DOI: 10.1016/S0031-9422(03)00438-2

[9] Macrae WD, Towers GN. Biological activities of lignans. Phytochemistry. 1984;**23**:1207-1220. DOI: 10.1016/S0031-9422(00)80428-8

[10] Lee S, Monnappa AK, Mitchell RJ. Biological activities of lignin hydrolysate-related compounds. BMB Reports. 2012;**45**:265-274. DOI: 10.5483/BMBRep.2012.45.5.265

[11] Mann J, Davison RS, Hobbs JB, Benthorpe DV, Harbone JB. Natural Products. 1st ed. Longman: Addison Wesley; 1995. p. 455

[12] Rezende Marques T, Aparecida Caetano A, Avelar Rodrigues LM, Assaid Simão A, Andrade Machado GH, Duarte Corrêa A. Characterization of phenolic compounds, antioxidant and antibacterial potential the extract of acerola bagasse flour. Acta Scientiarum. Technology. 2017;**39**:143-148. DOI: 10.4025/actascitechnol.v39i2.28410

[13] Duangjai A, Suphrom N, Wungrath J, Ontawong A, Nuengchamnong N, Yosboonruang A. Comparison of antioxidant, antimicrobial activities and chemical profiles of three coffee (*Coffea arabica* L.) pulp aqueous extracts. Integrative Medicine Research. 2016;**5**: 324-331. DOI: 10.1016/j.imr.2016.09.001

[14] Ma YQ, Chen JC, Liu DH, Ye XQ. Simultaneous extraction of phenolic compounds of citrus peel extracts: Effect of ultrasound. Ultrasonics

Sonochemistry. 2009;**16**:57-62. DOI: 10.1016/j.ultsonch.2008.04.012

[15] Li R, Hettiarachchy N, Rayaprolu S, Eswaranandam S, Howe B, Davis M, et al. Phenolics and antioxidant activity of Saskatoon berry (*Amelanchier alnifolia*) pomace extract. Journal of Medicinal Food. 2014;**17**:384-392. DOI: 10.1089/jmf.2012.0278

[16] Assefa AD, Saini RK, Keum YS. Extraction of antioxidants and flavonoids from yuzu (*Citrus junos* Sieb ex Tanaka) peels: A response surface methodology study. Journal of Food Measurement and Characterization. 2017;**11**:364-379. DOI: 10.1007/s11694-016-9405-1

[17] Dorta E, González LMG, Sánchez-Moreno C, de Ancos B. Screening of phenolic compounds in by-product extracts from mangoes (*Mangifera indica* L.) by HPLC-ESI-QTOF-MS and multivariate analysis for use as a food ingredient. Food Research International. 2014;**57**:51-60. DOI: 10.1016/j.foodres.2014.01.012

[18] Barrales FM, Silveira BPDPM, Ruviaro AR, Paulino BN, Pastore GM, Martinez J. Recovery of phenolic compounds from citrus by-products using pressurized liquids—An application to orange peel. Food and Bioproducts Processing. 2018;**112**:9-21. DOI: 10.1016/j.fbp.2018.08.006

[19] Engels C, Gräter D, Esquivel P, Jiménez VM, Gänzle MG, Schieber A. Characterization of phenolic compounds in jocote (*Spondias purpurea* L.) peels by ultra-high-performance liquid chromatography/electrospray ionization mass spectrometry. Food Research International. 2012;**46**:557-562. DOI: 10.1016/j.foodres.2011.04.003

[20] Quiroz-Reyes CN, Aguilar-Méndez MA, Ramírez-Ortíz ME, Ronquillo-De Jesús E. Comparative study of ultrasound and maceration techniques for the extraction of polyphenols from cocoa beans (*Theobroma cacao* L.). Revista Mexicana de Ingeniería Químic. 2013;**12**:11-18

[21] Crupi P, Dipalmo T, Clodoveo ML, Toci AT, Coletta A. Seedless table grape residues as a source of polyphenols: Comparison and optimization of non-conventional extraction techniques. European Food Research and Technology. 2018;**244**:1091-1100. DOI: 10.1007/s00217-017-3030-z

[22] Farías-Campomanes AM, Rostagno MA, Meirele MAA. Production of polyphenol extracts from grape bagasse using supercritical fluids: Yield, extract composition and economic evaluation. The Journal of Supercritical Fluids. 2013;**77**:70-78. DOI: 10.1016/j.supflu.2013.02.006

[23] Andrade KS, Gonçalvez RT, Maraschin M, Ribeiro-do-Valle RM, Martínez J, Ferreira SR. Supercritical fluid extraction from spent coffee grounds and coffee husks: Antioxidant activity and effect of operational variables on extract composition. Talanta. 2012;**88**:544-552. DOI: 10.1016/j.talanta.2011.11.031

[24] Kammerer D, Claus A, Carle R, Schieber A. Polyphenol screening of pomace from red and white grape varieties (*Vitis vinifera* L.) by HPLC-DAD-MS/MS. Journal of Agricultural and Food Chemistry. 2004;**52**:4360-4367. DOI: 10.1021/jf049613b

[25] Zheng R, Su S, Li J, Zhao Z, Wei J, Fu X, et al. Recovery of phenolics from the ethanolic extract of sugarcane (*Saccharum officinarum* L.) bagasse and evaluation of the antioxidant and antiproliferative activities. Industrial Crops and Products. 2017;**107**:360-369. DOI: 10.1016/j.indcrop.2017.05.050

[26] Zheng R, Su S, Zhou H, Yan H, Ye J, Zhao Z, et al. Antioxidant/antihyperglycemic activity of phenolics

from sugarcane (*Saccharum officinarum* L.) bagasse and identification by UHPLC-HR-TOFMS. Industrial Crops and Products. 2017;**101**:104-114. DOI: 10.1016/j.indcrop.2017.03.012

[27] Luo L, Cui Y, Zhang S, Li L, Suo H, Sun B. Detailed phenolic composition of Vidal grape pomace by ultrahigh-performance liquid chromatography-tandem mass spectrometry. Journal of Chromatography B. 2017;**1068**: 201-209. DOI: 10.1016/j.jchromb.2017.10.031

[28] Maier T, Schieber A, Kammerer DR, Carle R. Residues of grape (*Vitis vinifera* L.) seed oil production as a valuable source of phenolic antioxidants. Food Chemistry. 2009;**112**:551-559. DOI: 10.1016/j.foodchem.2008.06.005

[29] He L, Xu H, Liu X, He W, Yuan F, Hou Z, et al. Identification of phenolic compounds from pomegranate (*Punica granatum* L.) seed residues and investigation into their antioxidant capacities by HPLC-ABTS+ assay. Food Research International. 2011;**44**: 1161-1167. DOI: 10.1016/j.foodres.2010.05.023

[30] Castro ACCM, Oda FB, Almeida-Cincotto MGJ, Davanço MG, Chiari-Andréo BG, Cicarelli RMB, et al. Green coffee seed residue: A sustainable source of antioxidant compounds. Food Chemistry. 2018;**246**:48-57. DOI: 10.1016/j.foodchem.2017.10.153

[31] Berardini N, Fezer R, Conrad J, Beifuss U, Carle R, Schieber A. Screening of mango (*Mangifera indica* L.) cultivars for their contents of flavonol O- and xanthone C-glycosides, anthocyanins, and pectin. Journal of Agricultural and Food Chemistry. 2005; **53**:1563-1570. DOI: 10.1021/jf0484069

[32] Guerrero RF, Biais B, Richard T, Puertas B, Waffo-Teguo P, Merillon JM, et al. Grapevine cane's waste is a source of bioactive stilbenes. Industrial Crops and Products. 2016;**94**:884-892. DOI: 10.1016/j.indcrop.2016.09.055

[33] Paes J, Dotta R, Barbero GF, Martínez J. Extraction of phenolic compounds and anthocyanins from blueberry (*Vaccinium myrtillus* L.) residues using supercritical CO_2 and pressurized liquids. The Journal of Supercritical Fluids. 2014;**95**:8-16. DOI: 10.1016/j.supflu.2014.07.025

[34] Di Donato P, Taurisano V, Tommonaro G, Pasquale V, Jiménez JMS, de Pascual-Teresa S, et al. Biological properties of polyphenols extracts from agro industry's wastes. Waste and Biomass Valorization. 2018;**9**:1567-1578 DOI: 10.1007/s12649-017-9939-4

[35] Grillo G, Boffa L, Binello A, Mantegna S, Cravotto G, Chemat F, et al. Cocoa bean shell waste valorization; extraction from lab to pilot-scale cavitational reactors. Food Research International. 2019;**115**: 200-208. DOI: 10.1016/j.foodres.2018.08.057

[36] Azadfar M, Gao AH, Bule MV, Chen S. Structural characterization of lignin: A potential source of antioxidants guaiacol and 4-vinylguaiacol. International Journal of Biological Macromolecules. 2015;**75**:58-66. DOI: 10.1016/j.ijbiomac.2014.12.049

[37] Santos VAQ, Nascimento CG, Schimidt CA, Mantovani D, Dekker RF, da Cunha MAA. Solid-state fermentation of soybean okara: Isoflavones biotransformation, antioxidant activity and enhancement of nutritional quality. LWT-Food Science and Technology. 2018;**92**:509-515. DOI: 10.1016/j.lwt.2018.02.067

[38] Kołodziejczyk K, Sójka M, Abadias M, Viñas I, Guyot S, Baron A. Polyphenol composition, antioxidant capacity, and antimicrobial activity of the extracts obtained from industrial sour cherry pomace. Industrial Crops

and Products. 2013;**51**:279-288. DOI: 10.1016/j.indcrop.2013.09.030

[39] Silva PB, Duarte CR, Barrozo MA. Dehydration of acerola (*Malpighia emarginata* DC) residue in a new designed rotary dryer: Effect of process variables on main bioactive compounds. Food and Bioproducts Processing. 2016; **98**:62-70. DOI: 10.1016/j.fbp.2015.12.008

[40] Resende-Marques TR, Corrêa AD, Lino JBDR, Abreu CMPD, Simão AA. Chemical constituents and technological functional properties of acerola (*Malpighia emarginata* DC.) waste flour. Food Science and Technology. 2013;**33**: 526-531. DOI: 10.1590/S0101-20612013005000085

[41] Nóbrega EM, Oliveira EL, Genovese MI, Correia RT. The impact of hot air drying on the physical-chemical characteristics, bioactive compounds and antioxidant activity of acerola (*Malphigia emarginata*) residue. Journal of Food Processing and Preservation. 2015;**39**:131-141. DOI: 10.1111/jfpp.12213

[42] Silva DI, Silva NC, Mendes LG, Barrozo MA. Effects of thick-layer drying on the bioactive compounds of acerola residues. Journal of Food Process Engineering. 2018;**41**:e12854. DOI: 10.1111/jfpe.12854

[43] Doymaz I, Akgün NA. Study of thin-layer drying of grape wastes. Chemical Engineering Communications. 2009;**196**:890-900. DOI: 10.1080/00986440802668422

[44] Celma AR, Rojas S, Lopez F, Montero I, Miranda T. Thin-layer drying behavior of sludge of olive oil extraction. Journal of Food Engineering. 2007;**80**:1261-1271. DOI: 10.1016/j.jfoodeng.2006.09.020

[45] Montero I, Blanco J, Miranda T, Rojas S, Celma AR. Design, construction and performance testing of a solar dryer for agroindustrial by-products. Energy Conversion and Management. 2010;**51**: 1510-1521. DOI: 10.1016/j.enconman.2010.02.009

[46] Spigno G, Tramelli L, De Faveri DM. Effects of extraction time, temperature and solvent on concentration and antioxidant activity of grape marc phenolics. Journal of Food Engineering. 2007;**81**:200-208. DOI: 10.1016/j.jfoodeng.2006.10.021

[47] Karacabey E, Mazza G. Optimization of antioxidant activity of grape cane extracts using response surface methodology. Food Chemistry. 2010;**119**:343-348. DOI: 10.1016/j.foodchem.2009.06.029

[48] Corrales M, Toepfl S, Butz P, Knorr D, Tauscher B. Extraction of anthocyanins from grape by-products assisted by ultrasonics, high hydrostatic pressure or pulsed electric fields: A comparison. Innovative Food Science & Emerging Technologies. 2008;**9**:85-91. DOI: 10.1016/j.ifset.2007.06.002

[49] Da Porto C, Natolino A, Decorti D. The combined extraction of polyphenols from grape marc: Ultrasound assisted extraction followed by supercritical CO_2 extraction of ultrasound-raffinate. LWT-Food Science and Technology. 2015;**61**:98-104. DOI: 10.1016/j.lwt.2014.11.027

[50] Okiyama DC, Soares ID, Cuevas MS, Crevelin EJ, Moraes LA, Melo MP, et al. Pressurized liquid extraction of flavanols and alkaloids from cocoa bean shell using ethanol as solvent. Food Research International. 2018;**114**: 20-29. DOI: 10.1016/j.foodres.2018.07.055

[51] Rivière C, Papastamoulis Y, Fortin PY, Delchier N, Andriamanarivo S, Waffo-Teguo P, et al. New stilbene dimers against amyloid fibril formation. Bioorganic & Medicinal Chemistry Letters. 2010;**20**:3441-3443. DOI: 10.1016/j.bmcl.2009.09.074

[52] Sharma K, Mahato N, Cho MH, Lee YR. Converting citrus wastes into value-added products: Economic and environmently friendly approaches. Nutrition. 2017;**34**:29-46. DOI: 10.1016/j.nut.2016.09.006

[53] Choi SY, Ha TY, Ahn JY, Kim SR, Kang KS, Hwang IK, et al. Estrogenic activities of isoflavones and flavones and their structure-activity relationships. Planta Medica. 2008;**74**:25-32. DOI: 10.1055/s-2007-993760

[54] Schofield P, Mbugua DM, Pell AN. Analysis of condensed tannins: A review. Animal Feed Science and Technology. 2001;**91**:21-40. DOI: 10.1016/S0377-8401(01)00228-0

[55] Domínguez-Rodríguez G, Marina ML, Plaza M. Strategies for the extraction and analysis of non-extractable polyphenols from plants. Journal of Chromatography A. 2017;**1514**:1-15. DOI: 10.1016/j.chroma.2017.07.066

[56] Sette M, Wechselberger R, Crestini C. Elucidation of lignin structure by quantitative 2D NMR. Chemistry-A European Journal. 2011;**17**:9529-9535. DOI: 10.1002/chem.201003045

[57] Ragauskas AJ, Beckham GT, Biddy MJ, Chandra R, Chen F, Davis MK, et al. Lignin valorization: Improving lignin processing in the biorefinery. Science. 2014;**344**:1246843. DOI: 10.1126/science.1246843

[58] Pérez-Jiménez J, Díaz-Rubio ME, Saura-Calixto F. Non-extractable polyphenols in plant foods: Nature, isolation, and analysis. In: Watson RR, editor. Polyphenols in Plants. Academic Press: Elsevier; 2014. pp. 203-218. DOI: 10.1016/C2011-0-08711-2

[59] Adjin-Tetteh M, Asiedu N, Dodoo-Arhin D, Karam A, Amaniampong PN. Thermochemical conversion and characterization of cocoa pod husks a potential agricultural waste from Ghana. Industrial Crops and Products. 2018;**119**:304-312. DOI: 10.1016/j.indcrop.2018.02.060

[60] Hernández C, Morales Sillero A, Fernández-Bolaños J, Bermúdez Oria A, Azpeitia Morales A, Rodríguez-Gutiérrez G. Cocoa bean husk: Industrial source of antioxidant phenolic extract. Journal of Science and Food Agriculture. 2019;**99**:325-333. DOI: 10.1002/jsfa.9191

[61] Barbosa-Pereira L, Guglielmetti A, Zeppa G. Pulsed electric field assisted extraction of bioactive compounds from cocoa bean shell and coffee silverskin. Food and Bioprocess Technology. 2018;**11**:818-835. DOI: 10.1007/s11947-017-2045-6

[62] Mayanga-Torres PC, Lachos-Perez D, Rezende CA, Prado JM, Ma Z, Tompsett GT, et al. Valorization of coffee industry residues by subcritical water hydrolysis: Recovery of sugars and phenolic compounds. The Journal of Supercritical Fluids. 2017;**120**:75-85. DOI: 10.1016/j.supflu.2016.10.015

[63] Lessa OA, dos Santos Reis N, Leite SGF, Gutarra MLE, Souza AO, Gualbert SA, et al. Effect of the solid-state fermentation of cocoa shell on the secondary metabolites, antioxidant activity, and fatty acids. Food Science and Biotechnology. 2018;**27**:107-113. DOI: 10.1007/s10068-017-0196-x

[64] Arapitsas P. Hydrolysable tannin analysis in food. Food Chemistry. 2012;**135**:1708-1717. DOI: 10.1016/j.foodchem.2012.05.096

[65] Toro-Uribe S, Montero L, López-Giraldo L, Ibáñez E, Herrero M. Characterization of secondary metabolites from green cocoa beans using focusing-modulated comprehensive two-dimensional liquid chromatography coupled to tandem mass spectrometry. Analytica Chimica Acta. 2018;**1036**:204-213. DOI: 10.1016/j.aca.2018.06.068

[66] Ambigaipalan P, de Camargo AC, Shahidi F. Phenolic compounds of pomegranate byproducts (outer skin, mesocarp, divider membrane) and their antioxidant activities. Journal of Agricultural and Food Chemistry. 2016; **64**:6584-6604. DOI: 10.1021/acs.jafc.6b02950

[67] Ramirez-Coronel MA, Marnet N, Kolli VK, Roussos S, Guyot S, Augur C. Characterization and estimation of proanthocyanidins and other phenolics in coffee pulp (*Coffea arabica*) by thiolysis-high-performance liquid chromatography. Journal of Agricultural and Food Chemistry. 2004;**52**: 1344-1349. DOI: 10.1021/jf035208t

[68] Lin S, Li Q, Yang B, Duan X, Zhang M, Shi J, et al. Transformation of litchi pericarp-derived condensed tannin with *Aspergillus awamori*. International Journal of Molecular Sciences. 2016;**17**: 1067. DOI: 10.3390/ijms17071067

[69] Mämmelä P, Savolainen H, Lindroos L, Kangas J, Vartiainen T. Analysis of oak tannins by liquid chromatography-electrospray ionisation mass spectrometry. Journal of Chromatography A. 2000;**891**:75-83. DOI: 10.1016/S0021-9673(00)00624-5

[70] Jiang B, Zhang Y, Gu L, Wu W, Zhao H, Jin Y. Structural elucidation and antioxidant activity of lignin isolated from rice straw and alkali-oxygen black liquor. International Journal of Biological Macromolecules. 2018;**116**: 513-519. DOI: 10.1016/j.ijbiomac.2018.05.063

[71] Moniz P, Serralheiro C, Matos CT, Boeriu CG, Frissen AE, Duarte LC, et al. Membrane separation and characterisation of lignin and its derived products obtained by a mild ethanol organosolv treatment of rice straw. Process Biochemistry. 2018;**65**:136-145. DOI: 10.1016/j.procbio.2017.11.012

[72] Mandelli F, Brenelli LB, Almeida RF, Goldbeck R, Wolf LD, Hoffmam ZB, et al. Simultaneous production of xylooligosaccharides and antioxidant compounds from sugarcane bagasse via enzymatic hydrolysis. Industrial Crops and Products. 2014;**52**:770-775. DOI: 10.1016/j.indcrop.2013.12.005

[73] Rochín-Medina JJ, Ramírez K, Rangel-Peraza JG, Bustos-Terrones YA. Increase of content and bioactivity of total phenolic compounds from spent coffee grounds through solid state fermentation by *Bacillus clausii*. Journal of Food Science and Technology. 2018; **55**:915-923. DOI: 10.1007/s13197-017-2998-5

[74] Mikulski D, Molski M. Quantitative structure-antioxidant activity relationship of trans-resveratrol oligomers, trans-4, 4′-dihydroxystilbene dimer, trans-resveratrol-3-O-glucuronide, glucosides: Trans-piceid, cis-piceid, trans-astringin and trans-resveratrol-4′-O-β-D-glucopyranoside. European Journal of Medicinal Chemistry. 2010;**45**:2366-2380. DOI: 10.1016/j.ejmech.2010.02.016

[75] Demirci MA, Ipek Y, Gul F, Ozen T, Demirtas I. Extraction, isolation of heat-resistance phenolic compounds, antioxidant properties, characterization and purification of 5-hydroxymaltol from Turkish apple pulps. Food Chemistry. 2018;**269**:111-117. DOI: 10.1016/j.foodchem.2018.06.147

Chapter 5

The Bioaccessible Reducing Capacity of Buckwheat-Enhanced Wheat Breads Estimated by Electrochemical Method

Danuta Zielińska

Abstract

The application of cyclic voltammetry (CV) technique for the determination of bioaccessible reducing capacity of buckwheat-enhanced white wheat breads (BEWWBs) and buckwheat-enhanced dark wheat breads (BEDWBs) was addressed. Buckwheat flour (BF) or flour from roasted buckwheat groats (BFR) were used to substitute white (WWF) or dark wheat flour (DWF) at 10, 20, 30, and 50% w/w on total flour basis in bread formula. The study showed that substitution of 10, 20, 30, and 50% of WWF or DWF by BF or BFR in bread formula resulted in almost linear increase of the reducing capacity of BEWWBs and BEDWBs. After digestion of BEWWBs, the bioaccessible reducing capacity was up to fivefold higher than the reducing capacity of the corresponding undigested breads, and in all cases was also higher than that noted for a soluble fraction of the digestible portion of white wheat bread (WWB). In contrast, the bioaccessible reducing capacity of BEDWBs was only up to twofold higher but in all cases did not exceed the value noted for digested dark wheat bread (DWB). Our results indicate that CV methodology is suitable for obtaining rapid electrochemical profile of a bread sample after digestion useful for evaluation of their selected functional properties.

Keywords: wheat bread, buckwheat, digestion, cyclic voltammetry, bioaccessible reducing capacity

1. Introduction

In recent years, common buckwheat is gaining interest in the development of new food products due to health-promoting, biofunctional properties, gluten freeness, and its high nutritional value [1]. The high nutritional value of buckwheat attributed to a balanced amino acid composition and high contents of vitamin B_1 and B_2, lysine, flavonoids, phytosterols, soluble carbohydrates, D-*chiro*-inositol, fagopyritols, and thiamin-binding proteins has been described [2]. Buckwheat is also rich in antioxidant compounds such as flavonoids, phenolic acids, tocopherols, reduced glutathione, inositol phosphates, and melatonin [3, 4]. Therefore, based on the above evidences, ingredients derived from buckwheat could be attractive for the bakery industry [5].

Wheat flour is usually used in bread making, but more often it is demonstrated that the usage of buckwheat flour as an ingredient in bakery goods can provide beneficial health effects [6–11]. The buckwheat-enhanced wheat bread is an attractive model of polyphenol-rich bread for an in vitro investigation of the impact of digestion on the bioaccessible reducing/antioxidative capacity as well as on the potential bioaccessibility of wide spectrum of bioactive compounds. The selection on buckwheat flour for formula of model polyphenol-enriched breads was due to the several publications indicating the potential use of buckwheat flour as a functional ingredient in bakery product formulations [12].

Several methods to measure antioxidant properties have been proposed and were recently reviewed [13–17]. Among others, scavenging of stable radicals such as DPPH and ABTS, oxygen radical absorbance capacity (ORAC), total radical-trapping antioxidant parameter (TRAP), ferric-reducing antioxidant power (FRAP), and cupric ion (Cu^{2+})-reducing power (CUPRAC) were employed in foods [13]. Electrochemical methods, used for the determination of reducing activity, have been still developing. Among different electrochemical techniques, the most widely used for this purpose is cyclic voltammetry (CV). The main advantage of CV is its capability to rapidly observe the total redox behavior over a wide potential range without the necessity of measuring the specific reducing capacity of each component alone. In contrast to the abovementioned methods, electrochemical assays are low-cost and usually do not require time-consuming sample preparation. CV is based on the analysis of the anodic current (AC) waveform, which is a function of the reactive potential of a given compound in the sample or a mixture of compounds. The CV tracing indicates the ability of a compound to donate electrons at the potential of the anodic wave [18]. A CV also provides information describing the integrated reducing capacity without the specific determination of the contribution of each individual component. Therefore, in the past couple of years, CV has been suggested as an instrumental methodology for the evaluation of the reducing capacity of various food products [16, 19–21]. From the current point of view, the electrochemical methods should be used to assess the reducing capacity of food in vitro to cover all aspects of antioxidant efficacy in vivo [22, 23]. Recently it was demonstrated that that in vitro digestion of buckwheat-enhanced wheat breads was the crucial step in the formation of the antioxidant capacity due to the release of the high amount of phenolic compounds [24].

Since the use of electrochemical methods ensures the measurement of the bioaccessible reducing capacity of food as it could occur in vivo, the objective of this work was to show an application of a cyclic voltammetry (CV) technique for determination of the bioaccessible reducing capacity of a soluble fraction from a digestible portion of buckwheat-enhanced wheat breads.

2. Materials and methods

2.1 Chemicals and reagents

α-Amylase (A1031-5KU), pepsin (P7000), pancreatin (P7545), bile salts extract (B8631), and 6-hydroxy-2,5,7,8-tetramethylchroman-2-carboxylic acid (Trolox) were purchased from Sigma-Aldrich (St. Louis, MO, USA). All other reagents were from POCH, (Gliwice, Poland). Water was purified with a Milli-Q-system (Millipore, Bedford, USA).

2.2 Buckwheat-enhanced wheat bread preparation

White wheat flour (WWF), dark wheat flour (DWF), and buckwheat flour (BF) from common buckwheat var. Kora were purchased from a healthy food store in Olsztyn, Poland. The flour from roasted buckwheat groats (BFR) originated from a local company in Poland. BF or BFR were used to replace WWF or DWF or at level of 10, 20, 30, and 50% (w/w). Buckwheat-enhanced white wheat breads (BEWWBs), buckwheat-enhanced dark wheat breads (BEDWBs), and reference white (WWB) and dark wheat bread (DWB) were baked in a laboratory bakery. **Table 1** shows the buckwheat-enhanced wheat bread formulation and baking conditions. Three pieces of each type of bread were baked. Samples were freeze-dried, milled and sieved through a mesh of 0.6 mm, and then were stored at −20°C before using for analysis.

2.3 Preparation of buckwheat-enhanced wheat bread crude extracts for measurement of reducing capacity by cyclic voltammetry (CV)

The lyophilized and milled bread samples (0.25 g) were extracted in triplicate at 25°C with 5 mL of 67% aqueous methanol using Thermomixer comfort (Eppendorf, Germany) by shaking at 1400 rpm for 60 minutes [24]. Next, samples were centrifuged for 5 minutes (16,100 × *g*, 4°C) (5415 R centrifuge, Eppendorf, Germany). After that, the 67% methanol extracts were directly used to determine the reducing capacity.

Ingredient and conditions	**Substitution level (%)**				
	0	**10**	**20**	**30**	**50**
BEWWBs					
WWF (g)	350	315	280	245	175
BF (g)	–	35	70	105	175
BFR (g)	–	35	70	105	175
BEDWBs					
DWF (g)	350	315	280	245	175
BF (g)	–	35	70	105	175
BFR (g)	–	35	70	105	175
Water (mL)	228	228	228	228	228
	250	250	250	250	250
Salt (g)	3.5	3.5	3.5	3.5	3.5
Yeast (g)	10.5	10.5	10.5	10.5	10.5
Fermentation					
Temperature (°C)	37	37	37	37	37
Time (min)	90	90	90	90	90
Pieces of dough (g)	250	250	250	250	250
Proofing (75% rh)					
Temperature (°C)	37	37	37	37	37
Time (min)	25	25	25	25	25
Baking					
Temperature (°C)	250	250	250	250	250
Time (min)	30	30	30	30	30

BEWWBs, buckwheat-enhanced white wheat breads; BEDWBs, buckwheat-enhanced dark wheat breads; WWF, white wheat flour; DWF, dark wheat flour; BF, buckwheat flour; BFR, buckwheat flour from roasted groats.

Table 1.
Buckwheat-enhanced wheat bread formulation and baking conditions.

2.4 In vitro digestion of buckwheat-enhanced wheat breads

The buckwheat-enhanced wheat breads were in vitro digested as described in details [25] with some modifications. The protocol included three steps: saliva (pH 7.0), gastric (pH 2.0), and intestinal digestion (pH 7.5). Briefly, 10 g of lyophilized and milled buckwheat-enhanced wheat breads and reference wheat breads were suspended in 80 mL of deionized water. An α-amylase solution (77 U/mg solid) was added to the samples at a proportion of 3.25 mg/10 g of sample dry matter (d.m.) in 1 mM $CaCl_2$, pH 7.0. Then, samples were shaken in a water bath at 37°C for 30 minutes. For the gastric digestion, the pH was reduced to 2.0 with 6 N HCl, and pepsin solution (738 U/mg) was added in the amount of 0.5 g/10 g of sample d.m. in 0.1 N HCl. The incubation was continued under the same conditions for 120 minutes. In the next step, the pH was adjusted to 6.0 with 6 M NaOH, and a mixture of pancreatin (activity 8×USP) and bile salts extract was added. Subsequently, the pH was increased to 7.5 with 6 M NaOH, and water buffered to a pH of 7.5 was introduced to obtain a final volume of 150 mL. Then, the samples were incubated at 37°C for 120 minutes. After incubation, the digestive enzymes were inactivated by heating at 100°C for 4 minutes and cooled for centrifugation at 5000 rpm for 60 minutes at 4°C in an MPV-350R centrifuge (MPW Med. Instruments, Warsaw, Poland). The supernatants obtained were freshly used for the evaluation of the bioaccessible reducing capacity of buckwheat-enhanced wheat breads.

2.5 Measurement of reducing capacity of buckwheat-enhanced wheat breads by cyclic voltammetry (CV)

The cyclic voltammogram (CV tracing) provides information describing the integrated reducing capacity without the specific determination of the contribution of each electroactive component. It is based on the analysis of the anodic current (AC) waveform, which is a function of the reductive potential of a given compounds in the extract. The total reducing capacity of the sample is a function combining two sets of parameters. The first is the biological oxidation potential, whereas the second is the intensity of the anodic AC current (Ia), reflecting the concentration of the components. However, more often the area under the AC wave (S; related to the total charge) is calculated since it is a better parameter reflecting the reducing capacity of the sample [18].

In this study, the cyclic voltammetry experiments were performed in 67% methanol bread crude extracts and soluble fraction obtained after digestion mixed with 0.1 M sodium acetate-acetic buffer (pH 4.5) at ratio 1:1 (v/v) according to Zielińska et al. [26]. The sodium acetate-acetic buffer acted also as a supporting electrolyte for cyclic voltammetry measurements. A micro-electrochemical cell (with total volume of 200 μL), made all of Teflon, was used during the course of this experiment. Three electrodes, a glassy carbon (GC) working electrode (BAS MF-2012, 3 mm diameter), an Ag/AgCl (3.5 M KCl) reference, and a Pt (0.5 mm diameter coiled Pt wire) counter electrode, constituted the cell. Working electrode was hand-polished with 0.05 μm alumina-water paste (BAS CF-1050), using BAS (MF-1040) polishing cloth, and then rinsed with ultrapure water and methanol. The cyclic voltammetry experiment was performed in the range of 100–1100 mV at a potential sweep rate of 100 mV s^{-1} at room temperature using a potentiostat/galvanostat G 750 (Gamry Ins., USA). The area under the anodic current (AC) waveform of the voltammogram (S) related to the total charge was calculated as it was shown for dark wheat bread extract (**Figure 1**). The cyclic voltammograms of Trolox solutions over the concentration range of 0.05–2.5 mM were determined. The reducing capacity of buckwheat-rich wheat breads was expressed in terms of μmol Trolox equivalent (TE)/g of dry matter (DM).

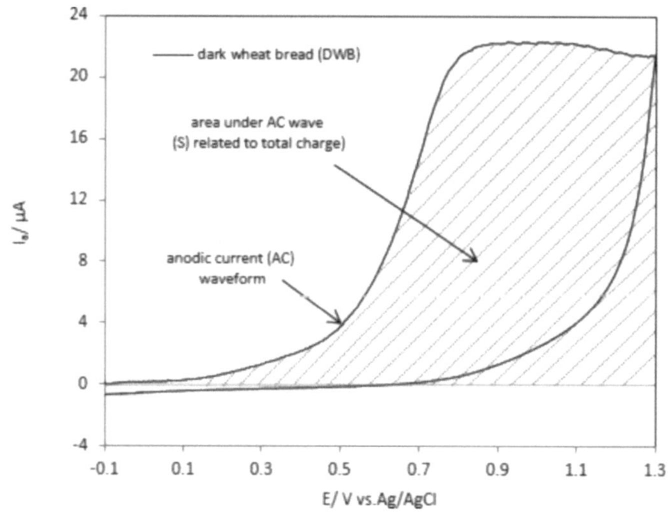

Figure 1.
Cyclic voltammogram of undigested dark wheat bread extract (DWB). The area under the anodic current (AC) waveform related to the total charge is indicated, and the mode of its calculation is presented. Measurements were performed with 67% methanol extract of DWB (100 mg/mL) mixed with 0.1 M sodium acetate-acetic buffer (pH 4.5) at ratio 1:1 (v/v) and scan rate 100 mV s^{-1}.

2.6 Statistical analysis

Results of the chemical analyses are illustrated as mean values and the standard deviation of three independent measurements. Fisher least significant difference (LSD) test at a significance level of $p < 0.05$ was performed for post hoc comparison. The Statistica ver. 5.0 software was used (General Convention and Statistica, StatSoft, USA, 1995).

3. Results and discussion

3.1 Reducing capacity of buckwheat-enhanced wheat breads

This reducing capacity of BEDWBs and BEWWBs was based on the electrochemical behavior and chemical properties of the electroactive compounds present in bread [27].

The cyclic voltammograms of 67% MeOH extracts from BEWWBs and BEDWBs breads before digestion were recorded as shown in **Figure 2**. The shape of the anodic waves was typically due to the response of several antioxidants with different oxidation potentials [11, 28]. The study showed that the substitution of WWF or DWF at levels of 10, 20, 30, and 50% w/w on total flour basis caused almost linear increase of the reducing capacity of undigested BEWWBs and BEDWBs breads (**Figure 3**). For example, the highest level of WWF substitution (50%) by BF resulted in almost fivefold increase in the reducing capacity, while the effect of substitution with BFR at 50% level was even higher, being above eightfold as compared to the reference WWB. Similarly, the reducing capacity of BEDWBs was higher than noted for DWB. It was found that substitution of DWF by BF or BFR at levels of 10, 20, 30, and 50% w/w on total flour basis caused a lower increase of the reducing capacity of BEDWBs as compared to BEWWBs. The highest level of DWF substitution (50%) by BF of BFR resulted in 2.2 and 2.6-fold increase of the reducing capacity of BEDWBs as compared to the reference DWB. These findings are in agreement with those provided by Lin et al. [6] which showed a fivefold

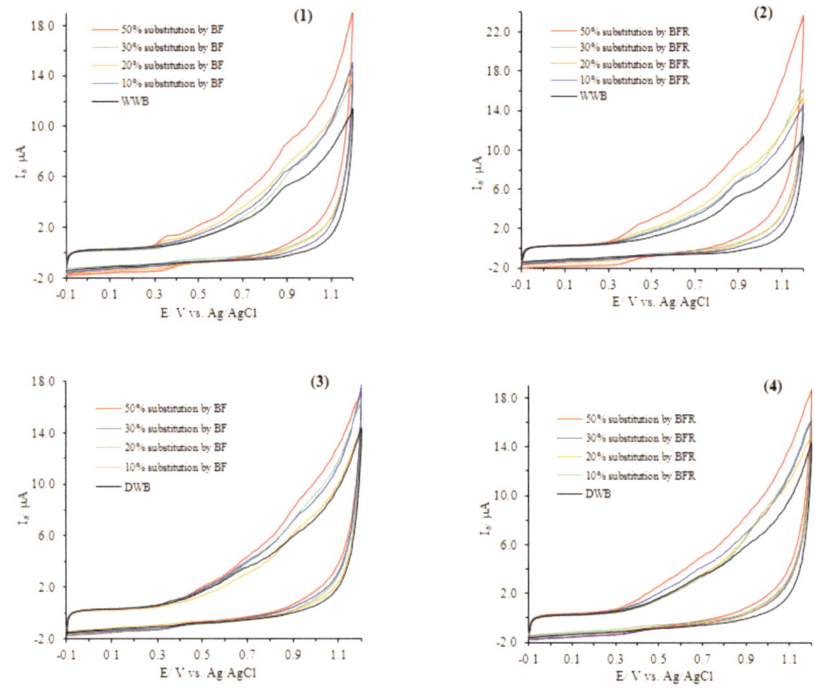

Figure 2.

Cyclic voltammograms of undigested buckwheat-enhanced white wheat breads (BEWWBs) and undigested buckwheat-enhanced dark wheat breads (BEDWBs). Upper figure, BEWWBs with (1) BF and (2) BFR substitution; lower figure, BEDWBs with (3) BF and (4) BFR substitution. Measurements were performed with 67% methanol extracts (100 mg/mL) mixed with 0.1 M sodium acetate-acetic buffer (pH 4.5) at ratio 1:1 (v/v) and scan rate 100 mV s^{-1}. The higher total charge under anodic current wave indicates a higher reducing capacity of the investigated bread extracts.

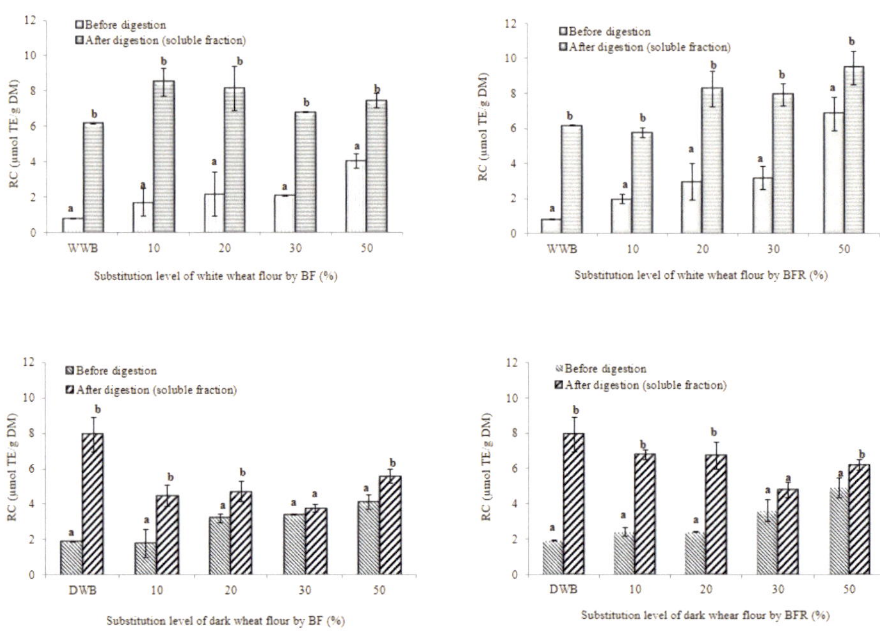

Figure 3.

Reducing capacity of buckwheat-enhanced white wheat breads (BEWWBs) and buckwheat-enhanced dark wheat breads (BEDWBs) before and after digestion in vitro. Upper figures, BEWWBs with BF and BFR substitution; lower figures, BEDWBs with BF and BFR substitution.

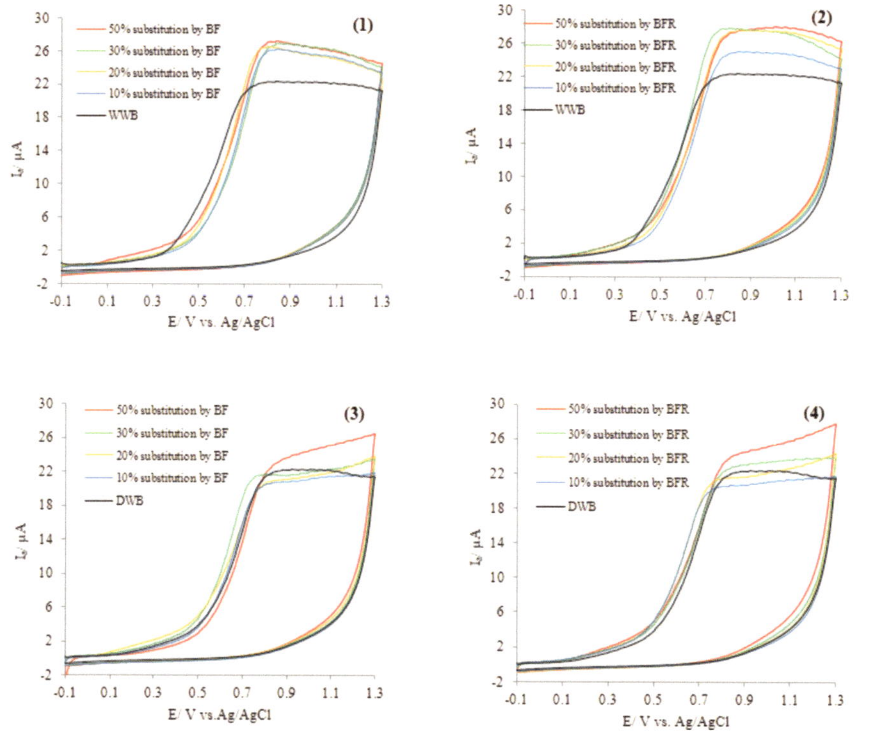

Figure 4.
Cyclic voltammograms of soluble fraction obtained after digestion of buckwheat-enhanced white wheat breads (BEWWBs) and buckwheat-enhanced dark wheat breads (BEDWBs). Upper figure, BEWWBs with (1) BF and (2) BFR substitution; lower figure, BEDWBs with (3) BF and (4) BFR substitution. Measurements were performed with soluble fraction obtained after digestion mixed with 0.1 M sodium acetate-acetic buffer (pH 4.5) at ratio 1:1 (v/v) and scan rate 100 mV s^{-1}.

increase in reducing power of buckwheat-enriched wheat bread at 15% substitution level using flour from unhusked buckwheat.

The cyclic voltammograms of soluble fraction obtained after digestion of BEWWBs and BEDWBs breads were recorded as shown in **Figure 4**. Comparison of the cyclic voltammograms recorded for undigested bread (**Figure 2**) with those recorded for soluble fraction obtained after digestion (**Figure 4**) showed broadened anodic waves due to the response of several reducing compounds with different oxidation potentials, including mainly released from the bread matrix phenolics compounds as described by Szawara-Nowak et al. [24]. After digestion of BEWWBs, the reducing capacity was higher by 21% (at substitution level of 50% by BF) and by 53% (at substitution level of 50% by BFR) than the reducing capacity of the corresponding digested reference WWB (**Figure 3**). In contrast, after digestion of BEDWBs, the reducing capacity was lower by 20% (substitution level of 50% by BF) and by 22% (substitution level of 50% by BFR) than the reducing capacity of the corresponding digested reference DWB. In contrast to digested BEWWBs, the reducing capacity of digested BEDWBs in all cases of substitution did not exceed the value noted for digested DWB. Available evidences based on the recent studies clearly indicate that the observed increase of reducing capacity of digested buckwheat-enhanced white and dark wheat breads was due to the release of phenolics from their conjugation forms as well as cell wall matrices. Szawara-Nowak et al. [18] showed significantly higher content of total phenolic compounds after in vitro gastrointestinal digestion of buckwheat-enhanced wheat breads as compared to the undigested ones. Moreover, the other scientists also demonstrated that simulated gastrointestinal conditions significantly increased the total phenolic compounds of extracts obtained from wheat whole grains and their flour, germ, and bran fractions [7, 29, 30]. It should be also pointed out that as the higher reducing capacity was observed in breads formulated with participation of BFR than BF, then a contribution of MRPs originating from this ingredient can be suggested [31].

It should be mentioned that practical limitation of applied CV methodology was that the working electrode. It had to be frequently cleaned to remove residues of sample from its surface and to maintain its sensitivity. However, the advantage of CV was related not to do requiring the use of reactive chemicals.

3.2 Bioaccessible reducing capacity of buckwheat-enhanced white and dark wheat breads

From a nutrition perspective, the definition of bioaccessibility is the fraction of a compound that is released from the food matrix in the gastrointestinal lumen and used for intestinal absorption [32]. This definition can be extended for the functional properties of food since it is closely related to the bioaccessibility of compounds responsible for the formation of this functional property. The in vitro digestion model has been widely used to study the complex multistage process of human digestion [33]. Bioaccessibility is a major factor that should be taken into account when assessing the potential health benefits of functional foods. Different contributors affect bioaccessibility. It can be affected by the composition of the digested food matrix, the synergisms and antagonisms of the different components, and the pH, temperature, and texture of the matrix [34]. Bioactive compounds are susceptible to multiple effects during digestion due to the effects of pH and enzymes, and in the present study, the bioaccessible reducing capacity of buckwheat-enhanced wheat breads was determined for the first time after an in vitro digestion by cyclic voltammetry method.

The reducing capacity of the digested BEWWBs and BEDWBs was significantly higher than those noted for the undigested corresponding breads (**Figure 3**). Therefore, for better evaluation of the bioaccessible reducing capacity in vitro, we introduced the reducing capacity bioaccessibility index (PRC):

$$PRC = RC_{GD}/C_{bread}.$$

where RC_{GD} is the reducing capacity after simulated gastrointestinal digestion (GD) and RC_{bread} is the reducing capacity of BEWWBs, BEDWBs, WWB, and DWB, respectively.

PRC value > 1 indicates high bioaccessibility; PAC value < 1 indicates low bioaccessibility. The similar factor was introduced by Gawlik-Dziki et al. [35] as a useful parameter to study the bioaccessibility of phenolics from coffee and coconut. The PRC values of BEWWBs and BEDWBs are shown in **Figure 5**. PRC ranged from 5.0 to 1.8 for digested BEWWBs with participation of BF and from 2.9 to 1.4 for digested BEWWBs with participation of BFR. The PRC index ranged from 2.5 to 1.4 for digested BEDWBs with participation of BF and from 2.8 to 1.3 for digested BEDWBs with participation of BFR. These values indicate high bioaccessible reducing capacity of buckwheat-enhanced wheat breads. It was also found that the reducing capacity bioaccessibility index (PRC) for BEWWBs and BEDWBs depends on the level of substitution WWF or DWF by BF or BFR. As the level of substitution was higher, then the PRC was lower despite of the high reducing capacity of bread samples. This finding indicates that not only real value of reducing capacity but also its bioaccessibility should be taken into account when functional properties of buckwheat-enhanced wheat breads are proposed for consumers. Therefore, the substitution level of wheat flours by BF or BFR at level up to 20–30% seems to be the best well-balanced.

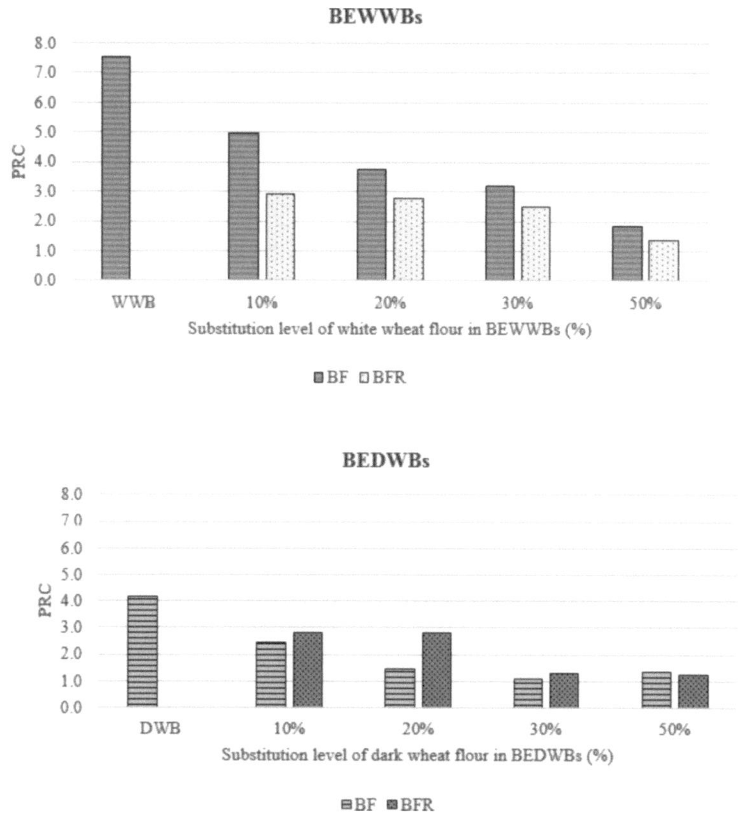

Figure 5.
The reducing capacity bioaccessibility index (PRC) of buckwheat-enhanced white wheat breads (BEWWBs) and buckwheat-enhanced dark wheat breads (BEDWBs).

4. Conclusions

The use of cyclic voltammetry allowed to show higher reducing capacity of digested in vitro buckwheat-enhanced wheat breads as compared to the undigested ones. Therefore, the bioaccessible reducing capacity of buckwheat-enhanced wheat breads seems to be an important factor characterizing the functional properties of bread among others. The reducing capacity bioaccessibility index (PRC) of buckwheat-enhanced wheat breads allowed to indicate the beneficial level of wheat flour substitution by buckwheat flours. The CV methodology is suitable for screening studies and allows obtaining a rapid electrochemical profile of a bread sample after digestion useful for evaluating their selected functional properties such as bioaccessible reducing capacity as proposed in this study.

Acknowledgements

This work was supported by grant no. 1346/B/P01/2010/38 from the National Science Centre.

Conflict of interests

The author declares that there are no conflict of interests regarding the publication of this paper.

Author details

Danuta Zielińska
Department of Chemistry, University of Warmia and Mazury in Olsztyn, Olsztyn, Poland

*Address all correspondence to: danuta.zielinska@uwm.edu.pl

References

[1] Kiprovski B, Mikulic-Petkovsek M, Slatnar A, Veberic R, Stampar F, Malencic D, et al. Comparison of phenolic profiles and antioxidant properties of European *Fagopyrum esculentum* cultivars. Food Chemistry. 2015;**185**:41-47

[2] Zielinska D, Zielinski H. Low molecular weight antioxidants and other biologically active components of buckwheat seeds. The European Journal of Plant Science and Biotechnology. 2009;**3SI**:29-38

[3] Zielinski H, Michalska A, Piskuła MK, Kozłowska H. Antioxidants in thermally treated buckwheat groats. Molecular Nutrition and Food Research. 2006;**50**:824-832

[4] Jiang P, Burczynski F, Campbell C, Pierce G, Austria JA, Briggs CJ. Rutin and flavonoid contents in three buckwheat species *Fagopyrum esculentum*, *F. tataricum*, and *F. homotropicum* and their protective effects against lipid peroxidation. Foodservice Research International. 2007;**40**:356-364

[5] Angioloni A, Collar C. Nutritional and functional added value of oat, Kamut®, spelt, rye and buckwheat versus common wheat in breadmaking. Journal of the Science of Food and Agriculture. 2011;**91**:1283-1292

[6] Lin LY, Liu HM, Lin SD, Mau JL. Quality and antioxidant property of buckwheat enhanced wheat bread. Food Chemistry. 2009;**112**:987-991

[7] Gawlik-Dziki U, Dziki D, Baraniak B, Lin R. The effect of simulated digestion in vitro on bioactivity of wheat bread with Tartary buckwheat flavones addition. LWT–Food Science and Technology. 2009;**42**:137-143

[8] Wronkowska M, Zielińska D, Szawara-Nowak D, Troszyńska A, Soral-Śmietana M. Antioxidative and reducing capacity, macroelements content and sensorial properties of buckwheat-enhanced gluten-free bread. International Journal of Food Science and Technology. 2010;**45**:1993-2000

[9] Zhang ZL, Zhou ML, Tang Y, Li FL, Tang YX, Shao JR, et al. Bioactive compounds in functional buckwheat food. Food Research International. 2012;**49**:389-395

[10] Giménez-Bastida JA, Zielinski H. Buckwheat as a functional food and its effects on health. Journal of Agricultural and Food Chemistry. 2015;**63**:7896-7913

[11] Szawara-Nowak D, Zielińska D, Wiczkowski W, Zieliński H. Antioxidant capacity of buckwheat enhanced wheat breads determined by updated methodology. Oxidation Communications. 2015;**38**:1591-1603

[12] Li SQ, Zhang QH. Advance in the development of functional foods from buckwheat. Critical Reviews in Food Science and Nutrition. 2001;**41**:451-464

[13] Gulcin I. Antioxidant activity of food constituents: An overview. Archives of Toxicology. 2012;**86**:345-391

[14] Sanchez-Moreno C. Review: Methods used to evaluate the free radical scavenging activity in foods and biological systems. Food Science and Technology International. 2002;**8**:121-137

[15] Magalhaes LM, Segundo MA, Reis S, Lima JLFC. Methodological aspects about in vitro evaluation of antioxidant properties. Analytica Chimica Acta. 2008;**613**:1-19

[16] Zielinski H, Zielinska D, Kostyra H. Antioxidant capacity of a new crispy type food products determined by updated analytical strategies. Food Chemistry. 2012;**130**:1098-1104

[17] Carocho M, Ferreira ICFR. A review on antioxidants, prooxidants and related controversy: Natural and synthetic compounds, screening and analysis methodologies and future perspectives. Food and Chemical Toxicology. 2013;**51**:15-25

[18] Chevion S, Roberts MA, Chevion M. The use of cyclic voltammetry for the evaluation of antioxidant capacity. Free Radical Biology and Medicine. 2000;**28**:860-870

[19] Giménez-Bastida JA, Zieliński H, Piskuła MK, Zielińska D, Szawara-Nowak D. Buckwheat bioactive compounds, their derived phenolic metabolites and their health benefits. Molecular Nutrition and Food Research. 2017;**61**:1-10

[20] Gulaboski R, Mirceski V, Mitrev S. Development of a rapid and simple voltammetric method to determine total antioxidative capacity of edible oils. Food Chemistry. 2013;**138**:116-121

[21] Arteaga JF, Ruiz-Montoya M, Palma A, Alonso-Garrido G, Pintado S, Rodriguez-Mellad JM. Comparison of the simple cyclic voltammetry (CV) and DPPH assay for the determination of antioxidant capacity of active principles. Molecules. 2012;**17**:5126-5138

[22] Zieliński H, Ciesarová Z, Kukurová K, Zielińska D, Szawara-Nowak D, Starowicz M, et al. Effect of fermented and unfermented buckwheat flour on functional properties of gluten-free muffins. Journal of Food Science and Technology. 2017;**54**:1425-1432

[23] Peñas E, Zielińska D, Gulewicz P, Zieliński H, Frias J. Vitamin C, phenolic compounds and antioxidant capacity of broccoli florets grown under different nitrogen treatments combined with selenium. Polish Journal of Food and Nutrition Sciences. 2018;**68**:179-186

[24] Szawara-Nowak D, Bączek N, Zieliński H. Antioxidant capacity and bioaccessibility of buckwheat-enhanced wheat bread phenolics. Journal of Food Science and Technology. 2016;**53**:621-630

[25] Delgado-Andrade C, Conde-Aguilera JA, Haro A, De La Cueva SP, Rufián-Henares JA. A combined procedure to evaluate the global antioxidant response of bread. Journal of Cereal Science. 2010;**56**:239-246

[26] Zielińska D, Szawara-Nowak D, Ornatowska A, Wiczkowski W. Use of cyclic voltammetry, photochemiluminescence and spectrophotometric methods for the measurement of the antioxidant capacity of buckwheat sprouts. Journal of Agricultural and Food Chemistry. 2007;**55**:9891-9898

[27] Zielińska D, Szawara-Nowak D, Zielinski H. Determination of the antioxidant activity of rutin and its contribution to the antioxidant capacity of diversified buckwheat origin material by updated analytical strategies. Polish Journal of Food and Nutrition Sciences. 2010;**60**:315-321

[28] Szawara-Nowak D, Zielińska D, Zieliński H, Wronkowska M. Antioxidant properties of dark wheat bread with added exogenous buckwheat flours addition. In: Waisundara V, Shiomi N, editors. Superfood and Functional Food–An Overview of Their Processing and Utilization. Chapter 13. Intech: Rijeka, Croatia. 2017. pp. 273-289. ISBN 978-953-51-2920-2. DOI: 10.5772/65411

[29] Liyana-Pathirana CM, Shahidi F. Antioxidant activity of commercial soft and hard wheat (*Triticum aestivum L.*) as affected by gastric pH conditions. Journal of Agricultural and Food Chemistry. 2005;**54**:1256-1264

[30] Chandrasekara A, Shahidi F. Bioaccessibility and antioxidant potential of millet grain phenolics as

affected by simulated in vitro digestion and microbial fermentation. Journal of Functional Foods. 2012;**4**:226-237

[31] Zielinski H, Michalska A, Amigo-Benavent M, del Castillo M, Piskula MK. Changes in protein quality and antioxidant properties of buckwheat seeds and groats induced by roasting. Journal of Agricultural and Food Chemistry. 2009;**57**:4771-4776

[32] Rein MJ, Renouf M, Cruz-Hernandez C, Actis-Goretta L, Thakkar SK, da Silva Pinto M. Bioavailability of bioactive food compounds: A challenging journey to bioefficacy. The British Journal of Clinical Pharmacology. 2013;**75**:588-602

[33] Li H, Deng Z, Liu R, Loewen S, Tsao R. Bioaccessibility, in vitro antioxidant activities and in vivo anti-inflammatory activities of a purple tomato (*Solanum lycopersicum* L.). Food Chemistry. 2014;**159**:353-360

[34] Fernàndez-Garcìa E, Carvajal-Lérida I, Pérez-Gàlvez A. *In vitro* bioaccessibility assessment as a prediction tool of nutritional efficiency. Nutrition Research. 2009;**29**:751-760

[35] Gawlik-Dziki U, Durak A, Jamioł M, Świeca MI. Interactions between antiradical and anti-inflammatory compounds from coffee and coconut affected by gastrointestinal digestion—In vitro study. LWT–Food Science and Technology. 2016;**69**:506-514

Chapter 6

Antioxidants in Date Fruits and the Extent of the Variability of the Total Phenolic Content: Review and Analysis

Abdulameer Allaith

Abstract

The date fruit is economically important agricultural commodity, as well as a staple food in many countries in the Arab world, North Africa, and the Middle East. Recent interest in its nutritional, health, and therapeutic attributes is manifested by the rise in scientific publications. Dates of various cultivars are widely publicized and highly ranked as rich sources of natural antioxidant constituents and antioxidant activity. Such publicity, justified or otherwise, is sometimes accompanied by misconceptions and claims of cultivar- and/or country-wise superiority. This chapter examines these claims using a dataset generated from scientific studies published over the last three decades focusing on the total phenolic (TP) content of three stages of date maturity, with emphasis on the last stage, Tamer. The dataset contains TP values (mg GAE/100 g DM) from 18 countries and 243 cultivars and included 583 entries. It only examines variability of TP values. Statistical analysis indicates a great variability of TP content, both within a particular cultivar and among different cultivars. Claims of cultivar- and country-wise superiority and very high ranking of date antioxidant activity are not substantiated. The chapter also discusses various causes of high variability and calls for a collaboration work to address the issue.

Keywords: antioxidant, antioxidant activity, date palm, dates, dried fruits, phenolic compounds, polyphenolics

1. Introduction

The date palm, the tree and the fruit alike, enjoys a high place in the hearts and minds of the people of the Arab region, in particular, and the Middle East in general and of the three major regional religions (Islam, Christianity, Judaism). A place where the mythological and the cognitive are highly intertwining and intersecting, culturally, religiously, and historically, in a clear indication of the depth of this tree's roots in the soul and civilization of this part of the world. The foundations on which this status is based may be lacking in validity and may be somehow exaggerated but cannot be ignored.

This tree, which enjoys a status of sanctity, due to many religious verses, conversations, and curses, was a staple food for the farmers in their ranches, the divers looking for pearls in the deep sea away from land for several months, and for the mobile

Bedouin in the deserts in the cold winter and in the high heat during their winter/summer traveling trips. With respect to common food consumption, the lives of people, in this area, were centered around few simple things, and their day may begin and end with eating dates supplemented with few additional foods such as milk, meat, and fish. The temporal and spatial presence of dates in the residences was overwhelming in the Arabian Peninsula and, archeologically, very well documented in many locales [1].

At present, global production statistics show increasing interest in dates as an economic commodity with a good financial return [2]. Scientifically, researchers have also increased their academic interest in studying different aspects of the date tree and its fruit using recent approaches and methodologies. The phytochemicals, antioxidant efficacies, and health of common dried fruits, including dates, have recently been reviewed [3]. The phenolic antioxidant properties and benefits in date fruits have recently been reviewed [4]. The biochemistry of the ripening process in dates as the main deriving source of metabolic variation has been recently reported [5].

Nutritionally, date fruits provide quick and high energy (~280–330 kcal/100 g) due to its high content of simple carbohydrates, mainly glucose, fructose, and sucrose [6]. They are also rich sources of fibers and potassium, among other nutrients. In recent years, there have been several reviews of the nutritional attributes of dates [6, 7]. The health and therapeutical attributes of dates have also been recently reviewed by [8–10]. These attributes include anticancer, anti-inflammatory, antimicrobial, antioxidant, antimutagenic, gastroprotective, hepatoprotective, immunostimulant, and nephroprotective activities. Of these, the antioxidant property appears to be of a high interest and, currently, is being explored at different levels using different methodological approaches including the metabolomics studies [11].

Because of this scientific activity, knowledge of the antioxidant properties of dates and the importance of dates as a good source of antioxidants has substantially increased. This knowledge, however, has been accompanied by claims and misconceptions, mostly are unsubstantiated and/or justified, rather, unfortunately confusing and questionable. Such claims include, but not limited to (1) claims of country-wise (or regional-wise) superiority of dates, (2) claims of antioxidant superiority of certain cultivars, and (3) claims of high ranking of dates among other dried fruits and natural products.

The main aim of this chapter is to review the current state of knowledge of the antioxidants in date fruits, with emphasis on dry stage (Tamer), and the issues pertinent to the huge quantitative discrepancy of total phenolic (TP) content in an attempt to find answers to questions that directly address the abovementioned issues/claims. This chapter singles out TP content as the only antioxidant parameter understudy due to space and time limitation; hence the analysis is a preliminary. Further analysis of TP content in relation to other related parameters and factors is highly needed and is to be seen.

2. The date palm

2.1 The tree and cultivars

The date palm (*Phoenix dactylifera* L.) is among the first domesticated perennial plants with some fossil records showing that the tree has existed for about 50 million years [12]. It has been growing in the Arabian Peninsula, the Middle East, North Africa, and South Asia for about 5000 years [12]. Generally, it is characterized by its ability to tolerate relatively high temperatures, salinity, and drought [13]. To produce dates, the date palm tree has a strict requirement to relatively a hot and lengthily summer. The date palm belongs to the family Arecaceae and is a dioecious flowering plant which can live for 100 years [13, 14]. Usually, artificial pollination of the date palm starts late February to early March [15]. Fruit development and ripening stages are cultivar-dependent (see next section). It is a common practice to classify cultivars into early, mid, and late cultivars where fruit maturation takes place in June, August, and late September, respectively. Worldwide, the number of date cultivars is large (2000–3000) [16], and at the country level, the number may range between 300 and 600 cultivars in the known major country producers [16]. Within each country, the number of cultivars with significant commercial importance is very limited (10–30). Generally, names of cultivars are, country (or regional)-dependent, with some names of cultivars being traded widely. The same cultivar may have different names in different countries.

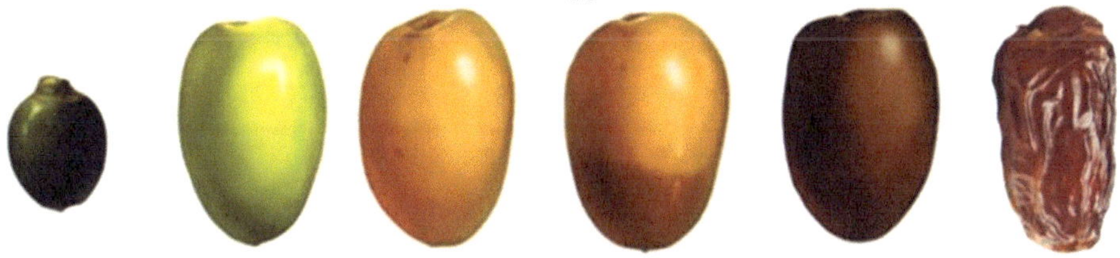

Figure 1.
Stages of maturation of date palm fruits. Re-drawn from Al-Mssallem et al. [17].

Parameter	Developmental (maturation) stages of date fruits				
	Hababouk	**Kimri**	**Khalal**	**Rutab**	**Tamar**
Moisture (%)		85	50–60	35–45	20–25
Duration (weeks)	5 weeks	9–14	3–5	Varies	Stable
Maturation and growth rate	Very early slow	Fast fruit enlargement	Full size, crunchy	Ripe, soft	Ripe, sun-dried
Color	Green	Green, unripe	Yellow or red	Varies	Golden grown to dark blue
Texture		Hard	Hard	Soft	Soft, semihard, hard
Edibility	Inedible	Inedible	Inedible with exceptions	Edible	Edible
TN (%)[a]			100	58–64	28–36
TP (%)[a]			100	45–57	40–51[b]
TF (%)[a]			100	40–88	22–70[b]
FRAP (%)[a]			100	30–72	25–55[b]
DPPH (%)[a]			100	55–76	39–60[b]

TN = tannins, TP = total phenolics, TF = total flavonoids, CT = condensed tannins[a]*All values are expressed as percent since data points of the included parameters vary greatly, with values of Khalal stage taken as 100%. These percentages were calculated from a limited number of published studies.*
[b]*Few published studies reported rather higher values in Tamer than Rutab.*

Table 1.
Chemical and physical characteristics of the developmental (maturation) stages of date fruits in relation to antioxidant properties.

2.2 The date palm fruit

The date palm fruit, the date, is a berry or drupe consisting of a single inedible seed (pit) surrounded by a fibrous, parchment-like endocarp, a fleshy mesocarp, and the fruit skin (pericarp) [13, 15]. Usually, the fruit is oblong, though great variation exists in shape, size, color, as well as in quality and texture. Weight of dates ranges between 4 and 36 g; length, 2–7.5 cm; diameter, 1.3–4 cm; and volume, 5–19 cm. The edible part of the date represents 85–92% of the total fruit weight. The development of the date passes through five distinct morphological stages, widely known by their Arabic names: Hababouk (Habanbo), Kimri, Khalal (Besser), Rutab, and Tamer (**Figure 1**, **Table 1**). At full size, Khalal, the color of dates is either yellow or red, with different shading and hues, with the yellow-colored dates representing the majority (> 80%). Date maturation starts 10–15 weeks after pollination and takes place over an extended period lasting for about 6–8 months. This process requires developmental competence and high heat. Dates of some cultivars can be eaten starting from the Khalal stage; others can only be eaten during or after attaining some degree of ripening. Antioxidant properties of dates are directly and indirectly influenced by the physiological aspects and developmental stages (**Table 1**).

3. Antioxidant in dates

3.1 The issue of large variability of total phenolic content

Over the past two decades, several studies on antioxidant properties of date fruits have been published. These studies have contributed to increase our knowledge and understanding of these properties and the importance of dates as a food and its medical, therapeutical, and health virtues. However, the foresight of these studies finds great variations of levels and values of studied parameters of antioxidant of these results, which confuses the researcher/reader, leading to some skepticism and casting doubt.

To illustrate the magnitude of the problem and the importance of attempting to overcome this wide disparity, I will review here what Hammouda et al. [17] recently noted while comparing their findings with results of a previous published. Hammouda et al. [18] estimated the TP of two date cultivars from three geographical origins using an HPLC methodology and reported an average of 154 mg/whole fruit (or 126.3 mg/edible part of the fruit, average weight of a fruit was 10.2 g). When they compared their findings with values reported on the widely cited study of Al-Farsi and Lee [6], which reported that TP ranged between 194 and 240 mg/100 g of fruit, corresponding to ~19–24 mg per fruit, they concluded that (a quote): "We consider that our estimation better reflects the real concentration of total polyphenols in dates as phloroglucinolysis–HPLC is the only quantification method that takes into account the nonextractable PCs which represent the major part of polyphenols in dates and which are not quantified when a colorimetric assay is performed on a methanol extract."

Many researchers have faced a similar situation and may have reached similar conclusions, as evidenced by many comparative studies. Recently, Mishra et al. [19] reviewed and analyzed the abnormalities associated with reporting the antioxidant activity using DPPH methods. Whether one agrees or disagrees with the above statement made by [18] is not the issue here. The issue is that whether the huge disparity of experimentally obtained and numerically reported values of antioxidants and antioxidant activity on date fruits really reflect the phenomena of natural variability or a manifestation of otherwise.

In the following section, the total phenolic (TP) content reported in the literatures by many groups will be statistically analyzed. Selection of the TP content to illustrate the extent of variability and diversity of the antioxidant in dates is largely based on its commonality and convenience. The majority of the published studies dealing with antioxidants and antioxidant activity of dates (other plant based produces as well) reports TP as the prime parameter. Furthermore, TP content is highly correlated with many assays used to estimate antioxidant activity (ABTS, DPPH, FRAP, etc.).

Estimation of TP is usually performed using the well-established Folin–Ciocalteu (FC) colorimetric method or one of its variants with gallic acid (GA) being widely used as a standard for calibration [19]. Results are usually expressed as mg GAE/g or 100 g. The FC method is based on electron transfer reactions between the phenolic antioxidant(s) and the FC reagent. It is not specific for TP determination and is prone to interfering compounds presented in the sample leading to biased estimation. Reducing sugars which are present in high concentration in dates and ascorbic acid, which is present in substantial level at some developmental stages, are examples of these interfering compounds [20]. Most of the published studies reporting TP in dates did not adequately address this issue.

3.2 Sources and preparation of dataset

Data used in this analytical review are of secondary type. They include the total phenolic (TP) content of 243 cultivars from 18 countries, covering the three potentially edible maturity stages, Khalal, Rutab, and Tamer (**Figure 1**). The selection of these datasets was based solely on relatedness and availability at the time of the preparation of this review. Values of TP were either copied and pasted from the published sources or extracted from graphs by using the online site WebPlotDigitizer [21]. A partial list of selected studies with some parameters of antioxidants and antioxidant activity is given in **Table 2**. **Table 3** lists countries of the recruited studies.

Most published values of TF were reported as sampled (i.e., the fresh or dry weight of the edible portion of the date fruits). To make them comparable and meaningful, these weight values were recalculated and presented on a dry matter (DM) basis. When given, moisture content was used to calculate the moisture fraction, hence the DM. In the absence of moisture content, the following general moisture contents were used: Khalal (66%), Rutab (43%), and Tamer (22%). When oven-dried or lyophilized samples were indicated, the moisture content used value was 15%. Samples of date syrup and wasted dates were also included since they usually possess similar TP content.

3.3 Data cleaning

The name of the same date cultivar in different countries may have different spellings. An example of this is the cultivar Barhi which has the following synonymous: Berhi = Burhi = Barhee = Barhy; Deglet Nour = Deglet Noor; Sokary = Sukkari = Sukari; and Sofry = Sufry = Suffry. It was very essential for the analysis to designate a single spelling for the same cultivar.

Outliers were statistically detected and removed from analysis. Removing of statistically detected outliers, at this stage of analysis, was based on convenience, simplifying the analysis, to examine their effects on estimates. Their analysis requires a more rigorous methodology, and perhaps these extreme values may represent a reality.

3.4 Statistical analysis

Excel (Microsoft) and SPSS (IBM, version 23) were used for statistical analysis which included estimates of central tendency and variability.

Country	Author (no. cultivar)	Parameter		Stg.	Mean (SD, range)	References
Algeria	Benmeddour et al., 2013 (10)	TP (mg GAE/100 g DW)		T	493.15 (294.90; 226–954)	[22]
		TF T(mg QE/100 g DW)		T	102.7 (94.45, 15.2–299)	
		CT (mg CE/100 g DW)		T	243.75 (139.62, 82.8–525.1)	
	Mansouri et al., 2005 (7)	TP (mg GAE/100 g FW)		T	4.70 (1.996, 2.5–8.4)	[23]
Egypt	Farag et al., 2014 (21)	TP (mg GAE/ 100 g DW)	(Low)	T	273.57 (40.53, 233–349)	[24]
			(Med)	T	449.57 (115.42, 437–622)	
			(High)	T	1332.83 (271.06, 1100–1898)	
			(Overall)	T	638.48 (473.12, 233–1898)	
Iran	Biglari et al., 2008 (8)	TP (mg GAE/100 g DW)		R	21.61 (45.27, 2.4–141.4)	[25]
		TF (mg CE/100 g DW)		R	12.57 (26.18, 1.6–81.2)	
		FRAP (umol/100 g DW)		R	65.46 (121.79, 11.6–387.3)	
		TEAC (umol TE/100 g DW)		R	97.99 (152.43, 22.8–500.3)	
	Mortazavi et al., 2015 (9)	TP (mg GAE/100 g FW)		K	126.04 (61.58, 57.8–262.8)	[26]
				R	57.41 (20.47, 23.5–94.1)	
				T	76.04 (18.87, 38.2–103.9)	
KSA	Farag et al., 2016 (18)	TP (mg GAE/100 g DW)		T	439.39 (559.37, 93–255)	[27]
	Hamad et al., 2015 (12)	TP (mg GAE/100 g DW)		T	17.52 (3.62, 10.5–22.1)	[11]
		TF (mg CE/100 g DW)		T	2.12 (0.51, 1.2–2.8)	
	Al-Turki et al., 2010 (5)	TP (mg GAE/100 g FW)		T	418.12 (55.18, 315.68–508.01)	[28]
	Hatem et al., 2018 (4)	TP (mg GAE/100 g FW)		K	4.92 (1.00, 3.26–5.94)	[29]
				R	6.95 (2.63, 2.49–9.23)	
				T	6.15 (1.23, 4.25–7.65)	
		DPPH (IC50: mg/ml)		K	4.62 (0.36, 4.1–5.1)	
				R	2.96 (1.53, 2.0–5.4)	
				T	4.0 (0.60, 3.4–5.0)	

Country	Author (no. cultivar)	Parameter	Stg.	Mean (SD, range)	References
Morocco	Taouda et al., 2014 (13)	TP (mg GAE/100 g DW)	T	2.68 (0.86, 1.5–4.5)	[30]
		TF (mg/100 g DW)	T	0.066 (0.094, 0.01–0.38)	
		DPPH (IC50: ug/ml)	T	17.43 (6.71, 7.5–33)	
	Bouhlali et al., 2017 (8)	TP (mg GAE/100 g DW)	T	466.26 (66.54, 331.9–537.1)	[31]
		TF (mg RE/100 g DW)	T	124.12 (53.06, 68.9–208.53)	
		CT (mg CE/100 g DW)	T	75.25 (11.86, 57.6–92.1)	
		FRAP (umol TE/100 g DW)	T	640.96 (157.8, 406.6–860.9)	
		DPPH (IC50: mg/ml)	T	3.94 (1.31, 2.1–6.2)	
		ABTS (umol TE/100 g DW)	T	621. 54 (124.8, 383.9–846.9)	
Oman	Al-Farsi et al., 2005 (3)	TP (mg GAE/100 g FW)	T	246.67 (80.45, 134–343)	[32]
	Singh et al., 2013 (6)	TP (mg GAE/100 g DM)	T	172.5 (56.84, 81–235)	[33]
Pakistan	Nazeem et al., 2011 (21)	TP (mg GAE/100 g DW)	T	216.22 (45.78, 141.9–297.0)	[34]
	Haider et al., 2013 (10)	TP (mg GAE/100 g DW)	K	459.92 (62.89, 349–571.3)	[35]
			R	211.076 (55.08, 102.8–265.3)	
			T	120.48 (47.46, 50.2–184.1)	
		DPPH (IC50: mg/ml)	K	0.59 (0.13, 0.47–0.86)	
			R	1.06 (0.32, 0.75–0.98)	
			T	1.86 (0.55, 1.4–2.9)	
Tunisia	El-Arem et al., 2012, (4) El-Arem et al., 2013 (5)	TP (mg GAE/100 g FW)	K	482.27 (93.14, 303.17–602.28)	[36] [37]
			R	362.93 (49.57, 278.8–435.4)	
			T	269.96 (60.17, 182.2–375.5)	
		TF (mg CE/100 g DW)	K	232.0 (53.91, 109.79–307.59)	
			R	144.49 (45.30, 79.6–231.0)	
			T	94.81 (24.77, 52.8–140.5)	
		CT (mg CE/100 g DW)	K	189.82 (68.66, 86.0–276.8)	
			R	121.1 (46.57, 65.3–198.2)	
			T	81.13 (22.24, 40.1–110.5)	

Country	Author (no. cultivar)	Parameter	Stg.	Mean (SD, range)	References
Tunisia	El-Arem et al., 2017 (3)	ABTS (mmol TE/100 g FW)	K	1.36 (0.03, 1.3–1.4)	[38]
			R	1.26 (0.07, 1.2–1.4)	
			T	1.13 (0.10, 1.0–1.3)	
		DPPH (AE = 1/EC50)	K	3.54 (0.63, 2.7–4.1)	
			R	2.54 (0.36, 2.1–2.7)	
			T	1.76 (0.42, 1.4–2.4)	
USA	Al-Turki et al., 2010 (10)	TP (mg GAE/100 g FW)	T	318.19 (61.75, 22.7–491.3)	[28]

Information are alphabetically arranged based on country.

Table 2.
Mean, SD, and range of selected parameters of antioxidant constituency (TP, TF, CT) and antioxidant activity (ABTS, DPPH, FRAP) extracted from selected published studies demonstrating the large reported variability.

Country	References	No.	Country	References	No.
Algeria	[22, 23, 39, 40]	4	Morocco	[30, 31, 65–68]	5
Bahrain	[41, 42]	2	Oman	[32, 33, 69, 70]	4
Egypt	[24, 43–45]	4	Palestine	[74]	1
Iran	[25, 26, 46–49]	6	Pakistan	[34, 35, 71–73]	5
Iraq	[50]	1	Spain	[75–77]	3
Israel	[51]	1	Sudan	[78]	1
KSA	[11, 27–29, 52–62]	14	Tunisia	[36–38, 78–86]	13
Malaysia	[63]	1	USA	[28, 87]	2
Mauritania	[64]	1	Yemen	[89]	1

Table 3.
Countries and number of recruited studies used to collect and analyze data points of TP content in date fruits.

4. Result

4.1 Descriptives

The total TP entries was 583, from 74 studies collected from 18 countries, consisting of 102 (17.9%), 118 (20.7), and 350 (61%) entries for Khalal, Rutab, and Tamer stages, respectively. More than 50% of the entries came from five countries (n, %): Pakistan (126, 21.61), KSA (125, 21.44), Tunisia (59, 10.12), Iran (47, 8.06), and Algeria (35, 6). The apparent number of included cultivars was 250, with Khalas (5.5%), Khadhrawi (4.3%), Barhi (3.1%), Hallawi (2.7%), Deglet Nour (2.4%), and Medjool (2%) being the most represented. Descriptive statistics, including estimates of centrality and dispersion, are presented in **Table 4** for data with and without outliers. The proportion of detected outliers was 1.96, 8.5, and 6.3% for the three maturation stages, respectively. As expected, the mean and median of TP content were higher in Khalal stage than the final maturation stage, Tamer. Removing outliers greatly improved the statistics of dispersion (SD, SEM, range, variance) as well as the kurtosis, skewness, and CL.

	Khalal		Rutab		Tamer	
	WO	NO	WO	NO	WO	NO
Count	104	102	119	108	360	339
Mean	994.92	935.98	368.67	228.62	446.97	240.93
SEM	111.83	105.85	38.74	18.05	59.00	10.18
Median	791.37	777.28	247.98	177.71	232.05	217.65
SD	1140.46	1068.99	422.65	182.33	1119.40	187.45
Variance	1300651.78	1142745.95	178630.03	33244.77	1253049.41	35137.96
Kurtosis	34.75	46.91	5.59	−0.71	47.66	−0.12
Skewness	4.95	5.85	2.21	0.55	6.55	0.71
Range	9785.41	9785.41	2228.61	663.80	10303.70	858.83
Minimum	9.59	9.59	4.33	4.33	0.14	0.14
Maximum	9795.00	9795.00	2232.94	668.13	10303.85	858.97
CL (95.0%)	221.79	209.97	76.72	35.81	116.02	20.03
CV	114.63	114.21	114.64	79.75	250.44	77.80
Q1	343.18	336.73	102.54	87.72	93.89	84.90
Q2	791.37	777.28	247.98	233.64	233.33	217.65
Q3	1298.02	1281.76	470.23	440.04	388.64	351.12

WO = with outliers included, NO = outliers not included.

Table 4.
Estimates of centrality and variability of the values of TP content (expressed as mg GAE/100 g DM) recruited in this work and obtained from studies listed on **Table 2**.

Khalal stage exhibited higher variation than Rutab and Tamer. The distribution of the TP values was not normal and rightly skewed for the three stages. **Figure 2** depicts the frequency and cumulative frequency density (CFD) of the TP values of the Tamer stage. Similar patterns are also seen for the Khalal and Rutab stages (not shown). More than 50% of the values of TP content were below 260 mg GAE/100 g DM.

Figure 3A and **B** depicts the spread of numerical values of the TP content in dates at Tamer stages against the country of origin of dates and cultivar, respectively. These figures, as well as data given in **Table 2**, provide clear evidence against claims and misconceptions of the antioxidant superiority of a particular date cultivar due to its country of origin or cultivar. Low and high values of TP content can be found for a specific date cultivar in a single country.

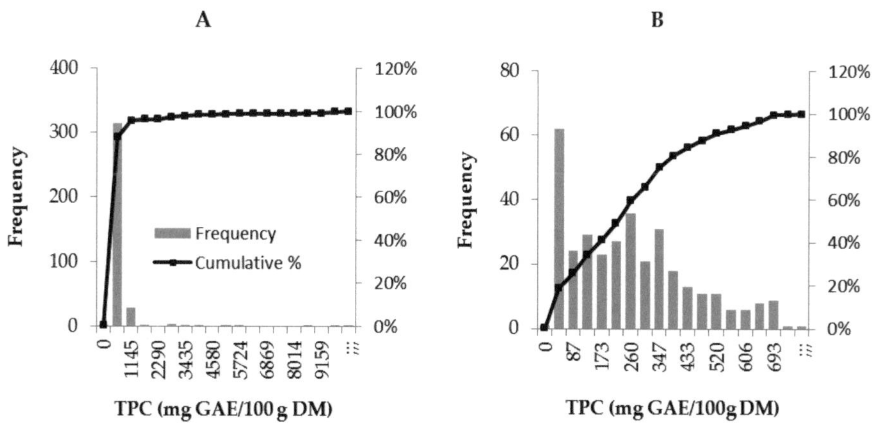

Figure 2.
Histogram and cumulative frequency density (CFD) of the TP content of the Tamer stage. (A) With outliers included, n = 360 and (B) outliers removed, n = 339.

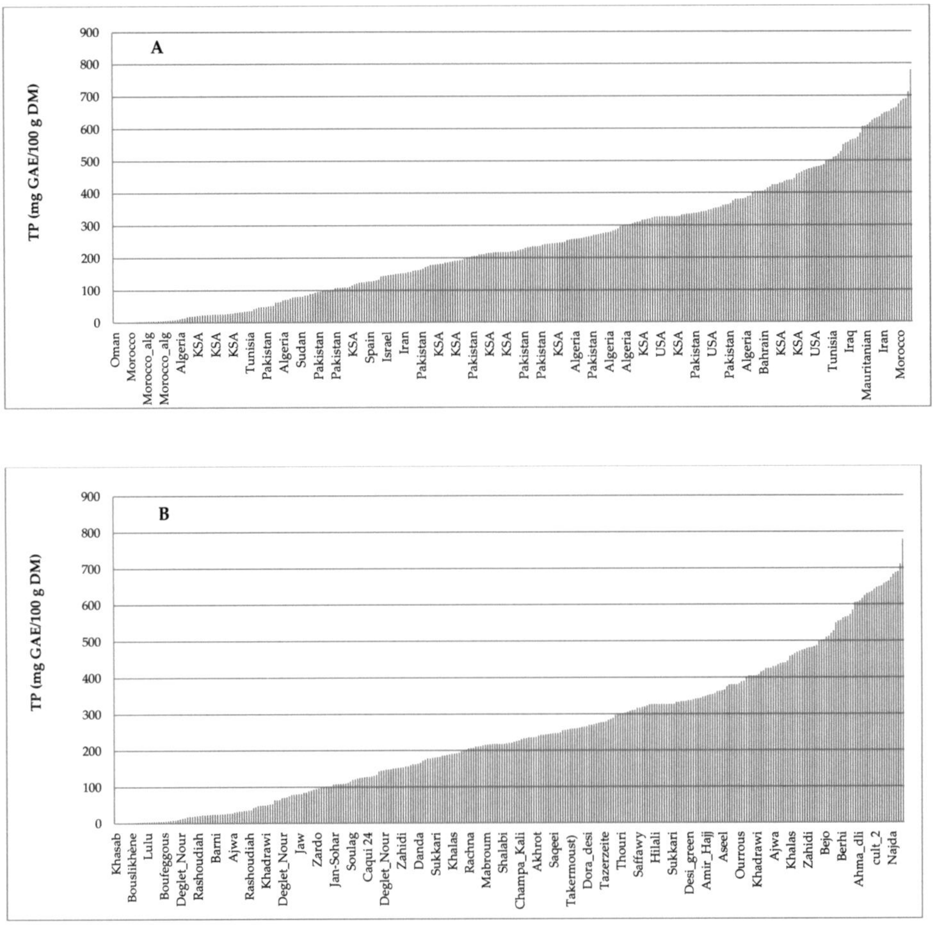

Figure 3.
Distribution of the values of TP content in Tamer stage arranged ascendingly according to the country of origin (A) and cultivar (B). Outliers were removed.

	Ajwa	Barhi	Khadhrawi	Khalas	Mejdool	Zahidi	Deglet Nour	Average
Count	9	4	10	20	7	7	13	10
Mean	178.48	254.50	274.79	158.10	265.45	251.96	159.52	220
SEM	70.05	89.86	61.51	34.75	61.84	64.58	34.47	60
Median	49.94	253.26	266.58	112.48	289.46	153.12	108.55	176
SD	210.15	179.71	194.50	155.39	163.62	170.87	124.28	171
Variance	44162.2	32295.9	37829.8	24145.3	26772.8	29195.4	15445.5	29,978
Range	577.66	319.39	477.41	458.12	468.4	407.66	363.74	439
Minimum	6.80	96.05	50.28	0.20	3.33	72.11	3.33	33
Maximum	584.46	415.44	527.69	458.32	471.72	479.77	367.07	472
CL (95.0%)	161.53	285.96	139.14	72.72	151.32	158.02	75.10	149
CV (%)	117.74	70.61	70.78	98.28	61.64	67.82	77.91	81
Country	2	5	7	4	5	5	5	5

Table 5.
Estimates of centrality and variability of reported TP values (expressed as mg GAE/100 g DM) of selected date cultivars from different countries.

	Ajwa (KSA)	Rashoudiah (KSA)	Sukkari (KSA)	Khalas (KSA)	Khalas (Oman)	Faradh (Oman)	Khasab (Oman)	Khalas (Oman)	Khalas (KSA)	Ajwa (KSA)
Count	7	3	11	13	5	5	4	5	13	7
Mean	195.48	141.60	280.46	148.11	109.03	155.57	71.68	109.03	148.11	195.48
SEM	89.26	60.87	54.46	43.82	61.34	90.67	59.66	61.34	43.82	89.26
Median	28.35	185.90	327.06	26.12	33.94	35.63	18.92	33.94	26.12	28.35
SD	236.17	105.42	180.63	157.99	137.17	202.74	119.31	137.17	157.99	236.17
Variance	55776.74	11114.00	32625.96	24961.62	18814.52	41102.45	14235.21	18814.52	24961.62	55776.74
Range	577.66	196.39	557.09	450.47	295.96	439.52	248.57	295.96	450.47	577.66
Minimum	6.8	21.26	8.44	7.85	0.20	0.23	0.14	0.20	7.85	6.8
Maximum	584.46	217.65	565.53	458.32	296.15	439.74	248.72	296.15	458.32	584.46
CL (95.0%)	218.423	261.89	121.35	95.47	170.31	251.73	189.85	170.31	95.47	218.423
CV (%)	120.81	74.45	64.40	106.67	125.80	130.32	166.46	125.80	106.67	120.81

Table 6.
Statistics of centrality and variability of reported TP values (expressed as mg GAE/100 g DM) of selected date cultivars taken from different studies from two countries (KSA and Oman).

4.2 Variability of TP values of selected date cultivars from different countries

Table 5 presents estimates of variability and central tendency of TP content of selected date cultivars reported from different countries. Normally, in nutritional epidemiology, the variance represents the true variability of nutrient content. The variability of continuous type of results produced experimentally by some assays is evaluated by the CV rather than SD, since the CV is a standardization of the SD (CV = SD/mean * 100). Using CV allows for direct comparison of estimates of variability regardless of the magnitude of the level of analyte under investigation. In many biological fields, a twofold difference in measurements of the same sample can be acceptable as the upper limit of variability. Furthermore, a CV of 40% can be tolerated in nutrient estimation for food labeling and nutrient intake calculation [90]. Since there is no reference value or a benchmark for the variability of TP content in dates to compare with, the above recommendation may be used to facilitate comparison. The variance and CV, as well as other estimates of dispersion, are very large. The largest variance was found for Ajwa, whereas Deglet Nour exhibited the lowest variance. The CV was even more pronounced as an evidence of the vast variability, with some cultivar possessing CV values of more than 100%. Estimates presented on **Table 5** demonstrate the extent of variability of the TP content values regardless of the country.

Table 6 presents similar statistics based on data obtained from studies originated from a single country for a particular date cultivar. This table illustrates the extent of variability of the TP content within a country. For example, TP values of Khalas cultivar from two countries (Saudi Arabia and Oman) showed large variation within cultivar and between the two countries, while the TP values of selected date cultivars taken from different studies carried out within that country are similar. Again, all estimates of variability are indicative of the large disparity of the published TP values. Notably, Ajwa cultivar of Saudi Arabia, which is grown almost exclusively in the holy city, Al-Madina Al-Munawara, possessed the largest CV (%) among the listed four cultivars.

5. Discussion

5.1 Variability of TP value and its implication

In the fields of public health, nutrition, and nutritional epidemiology, reliable and accurate estimates of concentration of a nutrient in a food commodity is important for estimating the daily consumption (intake) for an individual within a population, as well as for setting the average, upper, and lower limits of that nutrient for official recommendations and guidelines. The TP content is neither (yet) considered as a nutrient nor as a single chemical compound that can be reduced to the level of an officially declared nutrient such as ascorbic acid and treated similarly. TP is rather an experimentally measured value representing a chemical measure for an inherently great numbers of diverse groups of secondary metabolites or phytochemicals, simple and polyphenols, with many biological functions vital for the survival of their producers (plants) and for their consumer. Although TP is not a single entity, but, theoretically (and hypothetically) speaking, it is similar, in a way, to the groups of foods (proteins, carbohydrates, and lipids) which are characterized by high diversity of its nature, structure, and consistency. For this, one may be allowed to deal with TP content in a similar way, taking into consideration that TP content, at present, is not among the macro- and micronutrients.

Admittedly, large variation widely exists in biological measurements. In nutritional sciences, nutrient variability is a common place. A nutrient may vary in its numerical values for many reasons, and the magnitude of variation can be very large [92]. In the analysis of the already published values of the TP content date fruits for a large number of cultivars from different countries, regions, and continents, it can be concluded that the magnetite of variation in all edible stages, and in the Tamer stage in particular, is very high, in the order of hundreds, when extreme values and outliers are removed, and perhaps in thousands when these values are included.

This situation represents an unfavorable challenge for researchers, nutritionists, end users, and policy makers alike. To illustrate, a researcher may ask of the typical value of TP content of the date fruit in general or a typical value for a specific cultivar. In fact, in the literature, it is common to declare nutritional values of dates based on one or two cultivars with the assumption that these are true representative of the vast majority of cultivars, i.e., [91].

Does such variability is due to natural variation, or should we take into consideration the uncertainty, or a combination of both? This remains unclear and needs to be answered. While variability is defined as the occurrence of multiple values for a quantity at different locations and refers to the inherent heterogeneity or diversity of data in an assessment, uncertainty refers either to the lack of knowledge of the value of some quantity (qualitative uncertainty) or the usage of non-precise measurement methods of (quantitative uncertainty) may come from the use [93]. The source of uncertainty can be of many types including random errors, sampling, and measurement errors. Variability can be characterized but cannot be reduced, whereas uncertainty can be reduced, which, if appropriately applied, can lead to increased confidence in the estimates [93].

The variability of the values of the TP content for date fruits is evident by the various estimates of dispersion (see **Tables 4–6**). Causes of such dispersion are not known nor can be investigated unless the experimental conditions of the actual analysis can be traced back. In such situation, with little or no knowledge about of the data quality and the associated errors, one may speculate that data of the values of TP of dates do not merely reflect a natural variation, but element(s) of uncertainty cannot be excluded.

5.2 Sources of variability of antioxidant activity in dates

Variation in antioxidants and antioxidant activity is not limited to variation due to cultivars, maturity stage, and geographical or agronomical conditions. Rather, antioxidant activity varies between dates within the same bunch and even within the same fruit. In the following section, some of causes of the antioxidant will be presented.

5.2.1 Variation of antioxidant properties due to maturity stage

Many studies examined the effect of maturity stage in the antioxidant consistency and activity [25, 35–38, 41, 54, 73, 74]. There is a general agreement that the highest antioxidant activity is found in Khalal stage and the lowest in Tamer stage. Sourial et al. [94] reported data of five cultivars exhibiting a sigmoidal decline of tannins. The remaining tannin content at Tamer stage represented 33–43% of that at Rutab and Khalal stages. The kinetics of degradation of total phenolic content during these three stages was also reported [42]. TP content declines to follow first-order reaction in the Tamer stage which represents between 25 and 40% of the Khalal stage. Generally, red cultivars at Khalal stage possess greater antioxidant activity than yellow cultivars.

5.2.2 Variation of antioxidant properties within a single date fruit

Date fruits harvested from the same bunch at the same time may possess different levels of antioxidants, though may be statistically insignificant (need further studies). Within the same bunch, dates are differentially exposed to sunlight. Sunlight affects biosynthesis of simple and polyphenolic compounds including flavonoids. In many fruits, biosynthesis of polyphenolic compounds is an adoptive process [95]. High light induces the expression of many early and late genes involved in biosynthesis of flavonoids. Dates located inside the bunch are the least to receive sunlight, compared to those at the peripheral. This is also valid with regard to different bunches within the same tree.

Within a single date fruit, the distribution of antioxidants in the tissues is not homogenous. Guo et al. [96] reported that the peel of unspecified date cultivar possessed 2.4 times higher antioxidant activity than the pulp, 16.69 compared to 6.98 mmol/100 g WW (FRAP assay), respectively. A recent study by Djouab et al. [97], using Tamer of the yellow Algerian cultivar Mesh Degla, showed that the level of TP in the whole flesh, peel, brown tissue, and white tissue was 206, 247.3, 185.2, and 66.63 mg GAE/100 g DM, respectively. In this study, the antioxidant activity followed the same trend. Generally, fruit peels possess higher antioxidant than the flesh [96]. Depending on date cultivar, peel may contribute between 50 and 70% of the antioxidant, despite constituting only 3–5% of the total edible weight. Due to their vital biological role as protectants, many potent polyphenolic antioxidants are essentially localized in the peel, particularly during Khalal stage, leading to higher antioxidant activity. Furthermore, the white tissue of the flesh, the most inner part, possesses the least antioxidant/activity as compared to other tissues. Within the brownish tissue, condensed tannins are, usually, stored in the stone cells.

5.2.3 Variation of antioxidant activity due to diverse polyphenolic composition

Antioxidant property in plant-based food is largely due to the natural polyphenolic antioxidants. Redox properties of these natural antioxidants make them function as reducing agents, free radical scavengers, hydrogen donors, chelators, and metal. The phenolic consistency of date fruits, including flavonoids, has been recently studied by many research groups [18, 22–24, 38, 62, 68–70, 74, 98–100].

Phenolic acids found in dates belong mainly to benzoic or cinnamic acid derivatives. However, the distribution of phenolic acids varies considerably among different date cultivars. El-Arem et al. [38] reported a significant difference in the phenolic compounds amounts between maturation stages for the majority of cultivars. These groups identified two newly described phenolics in dates (hydroxyphenylacetic and phenylacetic acids). A contrasting example of the dynamic nature (or fluctuation) of phenolic acids in date fruits is cinnamic acid (CNA) which was also reported by this group [38]. CNA was not detected in the three maturity stages (K, R, T) of cultivars Gondi and Rotb Ahmar; however, it significantly increased during maturation of cultivar Gosbi and detected in comparable amount in R and T stages but not in K in the cultivar Khalt Dhahbi.

Farag et al. [24] recently identified 44 metabolites in 18 Saudi cultivars, of which 20 were flavonoids and 4 were hydroxycinnamates but also noted that several of previously reported predominant phenolic acids were not found in their study. While free phenolic acids are present in Rutab stage in most cultivars, albeit at lower concentration, the semidry cultivar Sukkari had no detectable free and glycosylated phenolic acids at Rutab stage and contained only esterified phenolics. Moreover, the fate of a particular phenolic acid or flavonoid differs between date cultivars (**Figure 4**). Among six different cultivars, Kursinszki et al. [98] reported that rhamnosyl

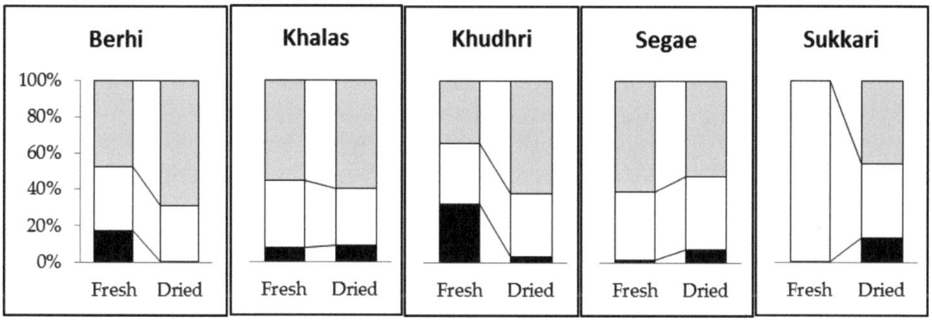

Figure 4.
Distribution of free (■), esterified (▩), and glycosylated (□) phenolic acids in five date fruits at two maturation stages Rutab (fresh) and sun-dried Tamer. Data extracted from Khojah [53].

hexosyl methyl luteolin was a major constituent in all of them, albeit at different levels, whereas hexosyl methyl luteolin sulfate was a major constituents in only three cultivars Khenaizi, Khalas, and Lulu. Among these cultivars, Lulu was characterized by being relatively low in flavonoid content. The Al-Medina dates were distinct by the presence of rhamnosyl hexosyl luteolin. A very recent detailed study by Abu-Reidah et al. [101] has identified 52 phenolic compounds in five various parts of the date palm tree including the edible portion (skin and pulp). The distribution (and the quantification) of phenolic compounds in the edible proton of the date fruit is of particular interest on this review. The combined number of peaks identified in pulp and skin was 22, of which 17 were found in pulp and 16 in skin, with 12 peaks being shared (~55%). Interestingly, the edible proton of dates was lacking of ferulic acid derivatives despite its known abundant in both, the skin and pulp. To the contrary, luteolin was only found in the skin, while its derivatives may be found, unequally, in both tissues. The methyl glycoside derivatives, which is consistent with specialization and functionality of the plant part, were also lacking from the edible portion.

5.2.4 Variation of antioxidants due to pollination, bagging, and thinning

Date palm tree is a dioecious monocotyledonous, and fertilization occurs either naturally or is carried out artificially. Pollens obtained from one cultivar can fertilize another cultivar. However, pollination has significant impacts in the physical and chemical properties of the resultant dates. It affects, among other things, the fruit set, size, time of ripening, seeds, eating quality, as well as the chemical constituency of the date including antioxidants, an effect known in plant science as metaxenia. Maryam [72] reported that pollen patents had the potential to significantly influence total phenolics in dates. Using eight male pollen patents to fertilize two different cultivars, the TP of Hallawi cultivar increased from 190 mg GAE/100 g in the control to 491 mg GAE/100 g and from 212 to 480 mg GAE/100 g in Khadhrawi cultivar. Similar effect was also found with ascorbic acid. Farag et al. [102] found that one of two pollinator types significantly increased the content of anthocyanin and ascorbic acid, but not tannins, over the other.

The practice of fruit thinning, either by reducing the number of fruits per bunch or the number of bunches per tree, leads to significant quality enhancement in dates. Several methods of thinning are available for date palm trees. This practice was found to reduce the tannins content in some date cultivars [103]. Bunch bagging of the same cultivar with perforated blue polyethylene increased ascorbic acid level, decreased the total soluble tannins concentrations and peroxidase activity, and had no significant effect on total phenolic content [104].

5.2.5 Variation of antioxidant priorities due to abiotic stress

In a study of the effect of sewage water irrigation of date palm tree in the antioxidant constituency of three Saudi date cultivars, Abdulaal et al. [105] reported higher levels of TP; TF; increased antioxidant activity using ABTS, DPPH, and the formation of phosphor-molybdenum complex test; as well as higher activities of peroxidase, polyphenol oxidase, and glutathione-S-transferase in dates irrigated with sewage water as compared to irrigation with municipal water. The increased level of these parameters was accompanied with higher accumulation of heavy metals (Cr, Cu, Fe, Mn, Pb, and Zn) in the sewage water-irrigated dates. The three studied cultivars showed differential responses regarding TP and TF. TP level in Agwa and Safawi increased by 28–30% over the control, while in Anbr cultivar it increased by only 8%. Furthermore, the extent of increase in TF in the three cultivars was somewhat similar (Agwa, 41%; Anbr, 50%; and Safawi, 50%). These results are suggestive of different response mechanisms and need further investigation.

Al-Busaidi et al. [106] recently reported that while the levels of Fe, Zn, and Ni were relatively higher in the treated sewage water irrigated than the groundwater irrigated, whereas the levels of Cu, Cd, Pb, and B were significantly higher in date fruits irrigated with groundwater than sewage water irrigated. These contradicting findings may be partially attributed to the level of treatment of sewage water used, i.e., secondary or tertiary treatment. In our own findings (unpublished) with locally grown several date cultivars, no significant difference was found in the accumulation of several heavy metals between groundwater and secondary-treated sewage water-irrigated dates.

5.2.6 Association of antioxidant consistency and antioxidant activity in date fruits

In vitro methods commonly used to estimate antioxidant activity include ABTS, DPPH, FRAP, and ORAC. Like many other plant-based foods, a clear relationship between the antioxidant content and antioxidant activity exists in date fruits, though its extent varies widely. For example, the DPPH method, widely used to estimate the radical scavenging activity of antioxidants was found [54] to be highly correlated to TP content in four Saudi cultivars, namely, Barhee (R^2 = 0.96), Khenazy (0.89), Helali (0.85), Lonet-Mesaed (0.64), but was not significantly correlated in Mejdool (0.46). In contrast, Medjool exhibited high correlation (R^2 = 0.91) between DPPH and total soluble tannin concentration. The correlation of DPPH and phenols, tannins, and flavonoid content of 12 products made from two Spanish date cultivars was also high, 0.765, 0.747, and 0.822, respectively [76]. On the other hand, plotting the IC50 (amount in µg/ml which gives 50% inhibition of DPPH quenching) of 18 cultivars from Saudi Arabia against their total phenolics showed a weak correlation (R^2 = 0.0341) [27]. These findings not only indicate that phenolic content plays as the major antioxidant in date fruits but also as a cause of the apparent variability of the date antioxidant activity.

6. Limitations of this work

Due to many constrains, this chapter addresses only one aspect of the variability of antioxidants in dates, namely, the TP content. The purpose of this chapter is to shed light and to expose the problem in the hope that other opportunities will be available to address the issue more comprehensively. The issue can be treated in depth with the inclusion of published values of other antioxidants as well as antioxidant activities. Potential and appropriate statistical tools to investigate the issue are within and between subject analysis of variability and multivariate analysis. Uncertainty as a potential source of variability of date antioxidants can also be examined.

7. Conclusion

Variability of levels of phytochemicals (plant-based) is a common phenomenon. However, the magnitude of such variability is influence by natural and artificial causes. Examination of values of the TP content in dates published over the last two decades reveals wide disparity that needs to be seriously addressed. This large variability creates a challenge that makes it difficult to deal with the validity and reliability of published values and may hinder or reduce its practical usefulness. Overcoming this problem and related issues requires collaboration between many groups from different countries. With many research teams interested in the date palm and its fruit (dates), this is possible and achievable and requires someone who takes the initiative.

Acknowledgements

The author wishes to thank Mrs. Batool Abdul Wahab, Department of Biology, College of Science, University of Bahrain, for her tremendous efforts during the preparation of this chapter, doing literature searching and collecting and making them available.

Author details

Abdulameer Allaith
Formerly at College of Science, University of Bahrain, Kingdom of Bahrain

*Address all correspondence to: biolaith@gmail.com

References

[1] Beech M. Archaeobotanical evidence for early date consumption in the Arabian gulf. Antiquity. 2000;**75**:83-89

[2] Msafiri M. Chapter 11. An overview of dates marketing. In: Manickavasagan A, Essa MM, Sukumar E, editors. Dates: Production, Processing, Food, and Medicinal Values. 1st ed. FL, USA; Taylor & Francis Group, CRC Press; 2012

[3] Chang SK , Alasalvar C, Shahidi F. Review of dried fruits: Phytochemicals, antioxidant efficacies, and health benefits. Journal of Functional Foods. 2016;**21**:113-132. DOI: 10.1016/j.jff.2015.11.034

[4] Arcot J, Khojah E. Phenolic acids in dates: Chemistry, properties and antioxidant benefits. In: Sun J, Prasad KN, Ismail A, Yang B, You X; Li L, editors. Polyphenols: Chemistry, Dietary Sources and Health Benefits. 1st ed. USA: Nova Science Publishers Inc.; 2013. pp. 369-376. Available from: http://www.novapublishers.com/

[5] Diboun I, Mathew S, Al-Rayyashi M, Elrayess M, Torres M, Halama A, et al. Metabolomics of dates (*Phoenix dactylifera*) reveals a highly dynamic ripening process accounting for major variation in fruit composition. BMC Plant Biology. 2015;**15**:291

[6] Al-Farsi MA, Lee CY. Nutritional and functional properties of dates: A review. Critical Reviews in Food Science and Nutrition. 2008 Nov;**48**(10):877-887. DOI: 10.1080/10408390701724264

[7] Al-Orf SM, Ahmed MHM, Al-Atwai N, Al-Zaidi H, Dehwah A, Dehwah S. Review: Nutritional properties and benefits of the date fruits (*Phoenix dactylifera* L.). Bulletin of the National Nutrition Institute of the Arab Republic of Egypt. 2012;**39**:97-129

[8] Ahmed A, Bano N, Tayyab M. Phytochemical and therapeutic evaluation of date (*Phoenix dactylifera*). A review. Journal of Pharmacy and Alternative Medicine. 2016;**9**:11-17

[9] Al-Alawi RA, Al-Mashiqri JH, Al-Nadabi JSM, Al-Shihi BI, Baqi Y. Date palm tree (*Phoenix dactylifera* L.): Natural products and therapeutic options. Frontiers in Plant Science. 2017;**8**:845. DOI: 10.3389/fpls.2017.00845

[10] Vayalil PK. Date fruits (*Phoenix dactylifera* Linn): An emerging medicinal food. Critical Reviews in Food Science and Nutrition. 2012;**52**:249-271. DOI: 10.1080/10408398.2010.499824

[11] Hamad I, Abd Elgawad H, Al Jaouni S, Zinta G, Asard H, Hassan S, et al. Metabolic analysis of various date palm fruit (*Phoenix dactylifera* L.) cultivars from Saudi Arabia to assess their nutritional quality. Molecules. 2015;**20**:13620-13641. DOI: 10.3390/molecules200813620

[12] The Worldwide Fruits. Available from: bhttps://www.worldwidefruits.com/phoenix-dactylifera-date-palm.html [Accessed: Nov 30, 2018]

[13] Al-Yahyai R, Manickavasagan A. An overview of date palm production. In: Manickavasagan A, Essa MM, Sukumar E, editors. Dates: Production, Processing, Food, and Medicinal Values. 1st ed. UK: CRC Press; 2012. pp. 3-12

[14] Zaid A, and de Wet PF. Botanical and systematic description of the date palm. In: Zaid A, Arias-Jiménez EJ, editors. Date Palm Cultivation. FAO Plant Production and Protection Paper. 156 Rev. 1. Rome, Italy. 2002. ISSN: 0259-2517, ISBN: 92-5-104863-0

[15] Barreveld, WH. Date palm products. FAO Agricultural Services Bulletin, No. 101, 1993, Food and Agriculture Organization of the United Nations, Rome

[16] Jaradat AA. Biodiversity of date palm, land use, land cover and soil sciences. In: Encyclopedia of Life Support Systems (EOLSS), Developed under the Auspices of the UNESCO. Oxford ,UK: Eolss Publishers; 2011. Available from: http://www.eolss.net [Accessed: Nov 30, 2018]

[17] Al-Mssallem IS, Hu S, Zhang X, Lin Q, Liu W, Tan J, et al. Genome sequence of the date palm *Phoenix dactylifera* L. Nature Communications. 2013;**4**:2274

[18] Hammouda H, Cherif JK, Malika Trabelsi-Ayadi M, Baron A, Sylvain GS. Detailed polyphenol and tannin composition and its variability in Tunisian dates (*Phoenix dactylifera* L.) at different maturity stages. Journal of Agricultural and Food Chemistry. 2013;**61**:3252-3263. DOI: 10.1021/jf304614j

[19] Mishra K, Ojha H, Chaudhury NK. Estimation of antiradical properties of antioxidants using DPPH assay: A critical review and results. Food Chemistry. 2012;**130**:1036-1043

[20] Bastola KP, Guragain YN, Bhadriraju V, Vadlani PV. Evaluation of standards and interfering compounds in the determination of phenolics by Folin-Ciocalteu assay method for effective bioprocessing of biomass. Am. J. Analytical Chemistry. 2017;**8**:416-431. DOI: 10.4236/ajac.2017.86032

[21] Rohatgi A. WebPlotDigitizer. Available from: https://automeris.io/WebPlotDigitizer/citation.html (Version: 4.1)

[22] Benmeddour Z, Mehinagic E, Le Meurlay D, Louaileche H. Phenolic composition and antioxidant capacities of ten Algerian date (*Phoenix dactylifera* L.) cultivars: A comparative study. Journal of Functional Foods. 2013;**5**:346-354. DOI: 10.1016/j.jff.2012.11.005

[23] Mansouri A, Embarek G, Kokkalou E, Kefalas P. Phenolic profile and antioxidant activity of the Algerian ripe date palm fruit (*Phoenix dactylifera*). Food Chemistry. 2005;**89**:411-420. DOI: 10.1016/j.foodchem.2004.02.051

[24] Farag MA, Mohsen M, Heinke R, Ludger A, Wessjohann LA. Metabolomic fingerprints of 21 date palm fruit varieties from Egypt using UPLC/PDA/ESI–qTOF-MS and GC–MS analyzed by chemometrics. Food Research International. 2014;**64**:218-226. DOI: 10.1016/j.foodres.2014.06.021

[25] Biglari F, Al Karkhi AF, Easa M. Antioxidant activity and phenolic content of various date palm (*Phoenix dactylifera*) fruits from Iran. Food Chemistry. 2005;**107**:1636-1641. DOI: 10.1016/j.foodchem.2007.10.033

[26] Mortazavi SMH, Azizollahi F, Moallemi N. Some quality attributes and biochemical properties of nine Iranian date (*Phoenix dactylifera* L.) cultivars at different stages of fruit development. International Journal of Horticultural Science and Technology. 2015;**2**(2): 161-171. Available from: https://ijhst.ut.ac.ir/article_56433.html

[27] Farag MA, Handoussa H, Fekry MI, Wessjohann LA. Metabolite profiling in 18 Saudi date palm fruit cultivars and their antioxidant potential via UPLCqTOF-MS and multivariate data analyses. Food & Function. 2016, 2016;**7**(2):1077-1086. DOI: 10.1039/c5fo01570g

[28] Al-Turki S, Shahb MA, Stushnoff CJ. Diversity of antioxidant properties and phenolic content of date palm (*Phoenix dactylifera* L.) fruits as affected by cultivar and location. Journal of Food, Agriculture and Environment. 2010;**8**:253-260

[29] Hatem A, Al-khalifa AR, Farouk A, Shaheen M. Effect of maturation stages on flavor profile

and antioxidant activity of date palm fruits (*Phoenix dactylifera*) grown in Saudi Arabia. International Journal of Pharmacology. 2018;**14**:407-414

[30] Taouda H, Chabir R, Errachidi F, Aarab L. Comparison of antioxidant activities and phenolic content of Moroccan date fruits. International Journal of Innovative Research in Science, Engineering and Technology. 2014;**3**(9):16121-16126. DOI: 10.15680/IJIRSET.2014.0309047

[31] Bouhlali EDT, Ramchoun M, Ghafoor K, Ennassir J, Zegzouti YF. Functional composition and antioxidant activities of eight Moroccan date fruit varieties (*Phoenix dactylifera* L.). Journal of the Saudi Society of Agricultural Sciences. 2017;**16**(3):257-264

[32] Al-Farsi M, Alasalvar C, Morris A, Baron M, Shahidi F. Comparison of antioxidant activity, anthocyanins, carotenoids, and phenolics of three native fresh and sun-dried date (*Phoenix dactylifera* L.) varieties grown in Oman. Journal of Agricultural and Food Chemistry. 2005;**53**:7592-7599. DOI: 10.1021/jf050579q

[33] Singh V, Guizani N, Essa M, Hakkim F, Rahman M. Comparative analysis of total phenolics, flavonoid content and antioxidant profile of different date varieties (*Phoenix dactylifera* L.) from Sultanate of Oman. International Food Research Journal. 2012;**19**:1063-1070

[34] Nadeem M, Rehman SU, Anjum FM, Bhatti IA. Textural profile analysis and phenolic content of some date palm varieties. Journal of Agricultural Research. 2011;**49**:525-539

[35] Haider MS, Khan IA, Jaskani MJ, Naqvi SA, Khan MM. Biochemical attributes of dates at three maturation stages. Emirates Journal of Food and Agriculture. 2014;**26**(11):953-962. DOI: 10.9755/ejfa.v26i11.18980

[36] El-Arem A, Behija SE, Beligh M, Lamia L, Manel I, Mohamed H, et al. Effects of the ripening stage on phenolic profile, phytochemical composition and antioxidant activity of date palm fruit. Journal of Agricultural and Food Chemistry. 2012;**60**:10896-10902 dx.doi.org. DOI: 10.1021/jf302602v

[37] El-Arem A, Saafi EB, Slama RB, Zayen N, Hammami M, Achour L. Phytochemical composition, antibacterial and antioxidant activities of common date palm (*Phoenix dactylifera* L.) fruit during three maturation stages. Tunisian Journal of Medicinal Plants and Natural Products. 2013;**10**(2):33-48

[38] El-Arem A, Saafi EB, Lahouar L, Bakhrouf A, Hammami M, Achour L. Antibacterial activity and principal analysis of chemical composition and antioxidant activity of Tunisian date palm (*Phoenix dactylifera* L.) fruit during ripening. Journal of Bioresources Valorization. 2017;**2**(1):21-33

[39] Louaileche H, Hammiche D, Hamoudi F. Total phenolic, flavonoid contents and in vitro antioxidant activity of Algerian date palm varieties: A comparative study. Am J. Food Science and Health. 2015;**1**(3):63-68

[40] Zineb G, Boukouada M, Djeridane A, Saidi M, Yousfi M. Screening of antioxidant activity and phenolic compounds of various date palm (*Phoenix dactylifera*) fruits from Algeria Mediterranean. Journal of Nutrition and Metabolism. 2012;**5**:119-126

[41] Allaith A. A. (2008). Antioxidant activity of Bahraini date palm (*Phoenix dactylifera* L.) fruit of various cultivars. International Journal of Food Science and Technology. 2008;**43**:1033-1040. DOI: 10.1111/j.1365-2621.2007.01558.x

[42] Al-Laith AA. Degradation kinetics of the antioxidant activity in date palm

(*Phoenix dactylifera* L.) fruit as affected by maturity stages. Arab Gulf Journal of Scientific Research. 2009;**27**:16-25

[43] Sakr MM, Abu Zeid IM, Hassan AE, Baz AGIO, Hassan WM. Identification of some date palm (*Phoenix dactylifera*) cultivars by fruit characters. Indian Journal of Science and Technology. 2010;**3**(3):338-343. ISSN: 0974-6846

[44] Ramadan BR, EL-Rify MNA, Abd El-Hamid AA, Abd El-Majeed MH. Effect of some treatments on chemical composition and quality properties of saidy date fruit (*Phoenix dactylifera* L.) during storage. Assiut Journal of Agricultural Sciences. 2016;**47**(5): 107-124. ISSN: 1110-0486

[45] Ibrahim FY, Khalil MM, Nezam EL-Din AAMM, Atieya KM. Studies on biological effect of some selected foods (un-pollinated siwi date, date palm pollen and doum fruit). Journal of Food and Dairy Sciences, Mansoura University. 2017:**8**(12):461-468

[46] Khanavi M, Saghari Z, Mohammadirad A, Khademi R, Hadjiakhoondi A, Abdollahi M. Comparison of antioxidant activity and total phenols of some date varieties. DARU. 2009;**1**(2):104-108

[47] Sadeghi Z, Valizadeh J, Shermeh OA. Antioxidant activity and total phenolic contents of some date varieties from Saravan region, Baluchistan, Iran. Journal of Medicinal Plant Research. 2015;**9**(4):78-83. DOI: 10.5897/JMPR2014.5676

[48] Shahdadi F, Mirzaei HO, Garmakhany AD. Study of phenolic compound and antioxidant activity of date fruit as a function of ripening stages and drying process. Journal of Food Science and Technology. 2015;**52**(3):1814-1819. DOI: 10.1007/s13197-013-1177-6

[49] Sharifi M, Bashtani M, Abasali Naserian A, Farhangfar H. Determination of chemical composition, mineral content, antioxidant capacity and rumen degradability in various varieties of wasted date palm. Italian Journal of Animal Science. 2017;**16**(3):507-514. DOI: 10.1080/1828051X.2017.1291285

[50] Matloob MH, Balakit AA. Phenolic content of various date palms fruits and vinegars from Iraq. International Journal of Chemical Sciences. 2016;**14**(4):1893

[51] Borochov-Neori H, Judeinstein S, Greenberg A, Volkova N, Rosenblat M, Aviram M. Antioxidant and antiatherogenic properties of phenolic acid and flavonol fractions of fruits of "Amari" and "Hallawi" date (*Phoenix dactylifera* L.) varieties. Journal of Agricultural and Food Chemistry. 2015;**63**:3189-3195. DOI: 10.1021/jf506094r

[52] El-Rayes DA. Characterization of three date palm cultivars based on RAPD fingerprints and fruit chemical composition. Environmental and Arid Land Agriculture Science. 2009;**20**:3-20

[53] Khojah EY. Development of a GC-MS method and analysis of phenolic acids in fruit and spice matrices and evaluation of their antioxidant capacity [thesis]. School of Chemical Engineering, The University of New South Wales Sydney, Australia: 2010

[54] Awad MA, Al-Qurashi AD, Mohamed SA. Antioxidant capacity, antioxidant compounds and antioxidant enzyme activities in five date cultivars during development and ripening. Scientia Horticulturae. 2011;**129**:688-693. DOI: 10.1016/j.scienta.2011.05.019

[55] Saleh EA, Tawfik MS, Abu-Tarboush HM. Phenolic contents and antioxidant activity of various date palm (*Phoenix dactylifera* L.) fruits from Saudi Arabia. Food and Nutrition

Sciences. 2011;**2**:1134-1141. DOI: 10.4236/fns.2011.210152

[56] Awad MA, Al-Qurashi AD. Gibberellic acid spray and bunch bagging increase bunch weight and improve fruit quality of 'Barhee' date palm cultivar under hot arid conditions. Scientia Horticulturae. 2012;**138**:96-100

[57] AL-Juhaimi F, Ghafoor K and Özcan MM. Physicochemical properties and mineral contents of seven different date fruit (*Phoenix dactylifera* L.) varieties growing from Saudi Arabia. Environmental Monitoring and Assessment. 2014;**186**:2165-2170. DOI: 10.1007/s10661-013-3526-3

[58] Al-Tamim EA. Study of anti-nutrients and antioxidant in date palm fruits (*Phoenix Dactylifera* L.) from Saudi Arabia and Egypt. Journal of American Science. 2014;**10**(3): 154-195. Available form: http://www.jofamericanscience.org

[59] Eid N, Enani S, Walton G, Corona G, Costabile A, Gibson G, et al. The impact of date palm fruits and their component polyphenols, on gut microbial ecology, bacterial metabolites and colon cancer cell proliferation. Journal of Nutritional Science. 2014;**3**:e46. DOI: 10.1017/jns.2014.16

[60] Nassar OM, Amin MA, Hassan ME, Nasr HA. Identifying the natural antioxidants and total phenols of some date varieties in Saudi Arabia. Biosciences Biotechnology Research Asia. 2016;**13**(2):865-872. Available from: http://www.biotech-asia.org/?p=12676

[61] Saleh AM, Awad M, El-Dengawy E-R FA, Abdel-Mageed HM, El-Badry MO, Salah HA, et al. Total phenolic and flavonoid contents and antioxidant activities of sixteen commercial date cultivars grown in Saudi Arabia. RSC Advances. 2016;**6**:44814-44819. DOI: 10.1039/c6ra02831d

[62] El-Rahman SNA. Al-Mulhem SI characteristic analysis, antioxidant components and antioxidant activity of date fruits, date seeds and palm shell. Clinical Medicine Case Reports. 2017;**1**:1-1

[63] Samad MA, Hashim SH, Simarani K, Yaacob JS. Antibacterial properties and effects of fruit chilling and extract storage on antioxidant activity, total phenolic and anthocyanin content of four date palm (*Phoenix dactylifera*) cultivars. Molecules. 2016;**21**:419. DOI: 10.3390/molecules21040419

[64] Lemine M, Mint F, Mohamed-Ahmed MVO, Ben Mohamed Maoulainine L, Bouna ZEAO, et al. Antioxidant activity of various Mauritanian date palm (*Phoenix dactylifera* L.) fruits at two edible ripening stages. Food Science & Nutrition. 2014;**2**:700-705. DOI: 10.1002/fsn3.167

[65] Bouhlali EDT, Alem C, Zegzouti YF. Antioxidant and anti-hemolytic activities of phenolic constituents of six Moroccan date fruit (*Phoenix dactylifera* L.) syrups. BTAIJ Journal. 2016;**12**(1):45-52

[66] Bouhlali EDT, Bammou M, Sellama K, Benlyas M, Alemb C, Filali-Zegzouti Y. Evaluation of antioxidant, antihemolytic and antibacterial potential of six Moroccan date fruit (*Phoenix dactylifera* L.) varieties. Journal of King Saud University Science. 2016;**28**(2):136-142

[67] Hasnaoui A, Elhoumaizi MA, Borchani C, Attia H, Besbes S. Physico-chemical characterization and associated antioxidant capacity of fiber concentrates from Moroccan date flesh. Indian Journal of Science and Technology. 2012;**5**(7):2954-2960

[68] Khalloukia F, Ricartea I, Breuera A, Owen RW. Characterization of phenolic compounds in mature Moroccan Medjool date palm fruits

(*Phoenix dactylifera*) by HPLC-DAD-ESI-MS. Journal of Food Composition and Analysis. 2018;**70**:63-71. DOI: 10.1016/j.jfca.2018.03.005

[69] Al-Harrasi A, Rehman NU, Hussain J, Khan AL, Al-Rawahi A, Gilani SA, et al. Nutritional assessment and antioxidant analysis of 22 date palm (*Phoenix dactylifera*) varieties growing in Sultanate of Oman. Asian Pacific Journal of Tropical Medicine. 2014, 2014;7:S591-S598. DOI: 10.1016/s1995-7645(14)60294-7

[70] Al-Harthi SS, Mavazhe A, Al Mahroqi H, Khan SA. Quantification of phenolic compounds, evaluation of physicochemical properties and antioxidant activity of four date (*Phoenix dactylifera* L.) varieties of Oman. Journal of Taibah University Medical Sciences. 2015;**10**(3):346-352

[71] Anjum FM, Bukhat SI, El-Ghorab AH, Khan MI, Nadeem M, Hussain S, et al. Phytochemical characteristics of date palm (*Phoenix dactylifera*) fruit extracts. Pakistan Journal of Food Sciences. 2012;**22**(3):117-127

[72] Maryam. Studies on metaxenial effect and use of molecular approaches for detection of hybrids, genetic diversity and sex in date palm (*Phoenix dactylifera* L.) [thesis]. Institute of Horticultural Sciences, Faculty of Agriculture, University of Agriculture, Faisalabad, Pakistan: 2014

[73] Haider MS, Khan IA, Jaskani MJ, Naqvi SA, Mateen S, Shahzad U, et al. Pomological and biochemical profiling of date fruits (*Phoenix dactylifera* L.) during different fruit maturation phases. Pakistan Journal of Botany. 2018;**50**(3):1069-1076

[74] Odeh I, Al-Rimawi F, Abbadi J, Obeyat L, Qabbajeh M, Hroub A. Effect of harvesting date and variety of date palm on antioxidant capacity, phenolic and flavonoid content of date palm (*Phoenix dactylifera*). Journal of Food and Nutrition Research. 2014;**2**(8):499-505

[75] Amorós A, Pretel M, Almansa M, Botella M, Zapata P, Serrano M. Antioxidant and nutritional properties of date fruit from Elche grove as affected by maturation and phenotypic variability of date palm. Food Science and Technology International. 2009;**15**:65-72. DOI: 10.1177/1082013208102758

[76] Martín-Sánchez AM, Cherif S, Ben-Abda J, Barber-Vallés X, PérezÁlvarez JÁ, Sayas-Barberá E. Phytochemicals in date co-products and their antioxidant activity. Food Chemistry. 2014;**158**:513-520. DOI: 10.1016/j.foodchem.2014.02.172

[77] Trigueros L, and Sendra E. Nutritional and antioxidant properties of date pastes and blanching water obtained from by-products of medjoul and confitera cultivars. Food Science and Technology. 2014;**2**(3):34-40. DOI: 10.13189/fst.2014.020302. Available from: http://www.hrpub.org

[78] Mohamed RM, Fageer AS, Eltayeb MM, Mohamed Ahmed IA. Chemical composition, antioxidant capacity, and mineral extractability of Sudanese date palm (*Phoenix dactylifera* L.) fruits. Food Science & Nutrition. 2014;**2**(5):478-489. DOI: 10.1002/fsn3.123

[79] Chaira N, Ferchichi A, Mrabet A, Sghairoun M. Chemical composition of the flesh and the pit of date palm fruit and radical scavenging activity of their extracts. Pakistan Journal of Biological Sciences. 2007;**10**:2202-2207

[80] Chaira N, Smaali MI, Martinez-Tomé M, Mrabet A, Murcia MA, Ferchichi A. Simple phenolic composition, flavonoid contents and antioxidant capacities in water-methanol extracts of Tunisian common date cultivars (*Phoenix dactylifera* L.).

International Journal of Food Sciences and Nutrition. 2009;**60**:316-329. DOI: 10.1080/09637480903124333

[81] Saafi EB, Louedi M, Elfeki A, Zakhama A, Najjar MF, Hammami M, et al. Protective effect of date palm fruit extract (*Phoenix dactylifera* L.) on dimethoate induced-oxidative stress in rat liver. Experimental and Toxicologic Pathology. 2011;**63**:433-441. DOI: 10.1016/j.etp.2010.03.002

[82] Mrabet A, Rodríguez-Arcos R, Guillen-Bejarano R, Chaira N, Ferchichi A, Jiménez-Araujo A. Dietary fiber from dimethoate Tunisian common date cultivars (*Phoenix dactylifera* L.): Chemical composition, functional properties, and antioxidant capacity. Journal of Agricultural and Food Chemistry. 2012;**60**:3658-3664. DOI: 10.1021/jf2035934|

[83] Kchaou W, Abbès F, Attia H, Besbes S. In vitro antioxidant activities of three selected dates from Tunisia (*Phoenix dactylifera* L.). Journal of Chemistry. 2014;**2014**:8 p. Article ID 367681. DOI: 10.1155/2014/367681

[84] Souli A, Sebai H, Rtibi K, Chehimi L, Sakly M, Amri M, et al. Effects of dates pulp extract and palm sap (*Phoenix dactylifera* L.) on gastrointestinal transit activity in healthy rats. Journal of Medicinal Food. 2014;**17**:782-786. DOI: 10.1089/jmf.2013.0112

[85] Mrabet A, Jiménez-Araujo A, Fernández-Bola-os J, Rubio-Senent F, Lama-Mu-oz A, Sindic M, et al. Antioxidant phenolic extracts obtained from secondary Tunisian date varieties (*Phoenix dactylifera* L.) by hydrothermal treatments. Food Chemistry. 2016;**196**:917-924. DOI: 10.1016/j.foodchem.2015.10.026

[86] Masmoudi-Allouche F, Touati S, Mnafgui K, Gharsallah N, El-Feki A, Allouche N. Phytochemical profile, antioxidant, antibacterial, antidiabetic and anti-obesity activities of fruits and pits from date palm (*Phoenix dactylifera* L.) grown in south of Tunisia. Journal of Pharmacognosy and Phytochemistry. 2016;**5**(3):15-22

[87] Al-Jasass FM, Siddiq M, Sogi DS. Antioxidants activity and color evaluation of date fruit of selected cultivars commercially available in the United States. Advances in Chemistry. 2015;**2015**:5

[88] Vinson JA, Zubik L, Bose P, Samman N, Proch J. Dried fruits: Excellent in-vitro and in-vivo antioxidants. Journal of the American College of Nutrition. 2005;**24**:44-50. DOI: 10.1080/07315724.2005.10719442

[89] Al-Shoaibi Z, Al-Mamary MA, AL-Habori MA, Al-Zubairi AD, and Abdelwahab SI. In vivo antioxidative and hepatoprotective effects of palm date fruits (*Phoenix dactylifera*). International Journal of Pharmacology. 2012;**8**:185-191. DOI: 10.3923/ijp.2012.185.191

[90] European Commission. Health and consumers directorate-general. Guidance document for competent authorities for the control of compliance with EU legislation. 2012

[91] United States Department of Agriculture Agricultural Research Service. National Nutrient Database for Standard Reference Legacy Release. Basic Report #: 09087, Dates, deglet noor. Available from: https://ndb.nal.usda.gov/ndb/foods/show/09087 [Accessed: Dec 2, 2018]

[92] Willett W. Nutritional Epidemiology. New York: Oxford University Press; 1998

[93] EPA U S. EPA ExpoBox, Chapter 2: Uncertainty and variability. In: Exposure Factors Handbook 2011 Edition (Final Report). U.S. Environmental Protection Agency, Washington, DC,

EPA/600/R-09/052F, 2011. Available from: https://archive.epa.gov/

[94] Sourial GF, Khalifa AS, Gaafar SI, Tewfik AA, Mousa AA. Evaluation of some selected date cultivars grown in Sharkiya Vine, Egypt, 2. Chemical Composition. Proceeding of the Second Symposium of the Date Palm in Saudi Arabia, Al-Ahsa, King Faisal University, Kingdom of Saudi Arabia. 1986, pp. 141-152

[95] Zoratti L, Karppinen K, Luengo Escobar A, Häggman H, Jaakola L. Light-controlled flavonoid biosynthesis in fruits. Frontiers in Plant Science. 2014;5:534. DOI: 10.3389/fpls.2014.00534

[96] Guo C, Yang J, Wei J, Li Y, Xu J, Jiang Y. Antioxidant activities of peel, pulp and seed fractions of common fruits as determined by FRAP assay. Nutrition Research. 2003;**23**:1719-1726. DOI: 10.1016/j.nutres.2003.08.005

[97] Djouab A, Benamara S, Gougam H, Amellal H, Hidous K. Physical and antioxidant properties of two Algerian date fruit species (*Phoenix dactylifera* L. and *Phoenix canariensis* L.). Emirates Journal of Food and Agriculture. 2016;**28**(9):601-608. DOI: 10.9755/ejfa.2015-12-1056

[98] Kursinszki L, Kalászh H, Szőke É, Adeghate E, Hassan MY, Adem A. Comparative analysis of six different brands of date fruits. Acta Chromatographica. 2011;**23**(4):603-610. DOI: 10.1556/AChrom.23.2011.4.6

[99] Hong YJ, Tomas-Barberan FA, Kader AA, Mitchell AE. The flavonoid glycosides and procyanidin composition of Deglet Noor dates (*Phoenix dactylifera*). Journal of Agricultural and Food Chemistry. 2006;**54**:2405-2411

[100] Nematallah KA, Ayoub NA, Abdelsattar E, Meselhy MR, Elmazar MM, El-Khatib AH, et al. Polyphenols LC-MS2 profile of Ajwa date fruit (*Phoenix dactylifera* L.) and their microemulsion: Potential impact on hepatic fibrosis. Journal of Functional Foods. 2018;**49**:401-411. DOI: 10.1016/j.jff.2018.08.032

[101] Abu-Reidah IM, Gil-Izquierdo A, Medina S, Ferreres F. Phenolic composition profiling of different edible parts and by-products of date palm (*Phoenix dactylifera* L.) by using HPLC-DAD-ESI/MS(n). Food Research International. 2017;**100**(Pt 3):494-500. DOI: 10.1016/j.foodres.2016.10.018

[102] Farag KM, Elsabagh AS, ElAshry HA. Fruit characteristics of "Zaghloul" date palm in relation to Metaxenic influences of used pollinator. American-Eurasian Journal of Agricultural & Environmental Sciences. 2012;**12**(7):842-855

[103] Lobo MG, Yahia EM and Kader AA. Biology and postharvest physiology of date fruit. In:Dates: Postharvest Science, Processing Technology and Health Benefits, 1st ed. Siddiq M, Aleid SM, Kader AA, editors, West Sussex, UK: John Wiley & Sons. 2014

[104] Khalil HA. Improving yield, fruit quality and storability of 'Zaghloul' date palm cultivar by pre-harvest sprays of some growth regulators and bunch bagging Egypt. Journal of Horticulture. 2015;**42**(2):8825-8832

[105] Abdulaal WH, Zeyadi M, Baothman OAS, Zamzami MA, Choudhry H, Almulaiky YQ, et al. Investigation of antioxidant and detoxifying capacities of some date cultivars (*Phoenix dactylifera* L.) irrigated with sewage water. RSC Advances. 2017;7:12953-12958. DOI: 10.1039/c6ra28760c

[106] Al-Busaidi A, Shaharoona B, Al-Yahyai R, and Ahmed M. Heavy metal concentrations in soils and date palms irrigated by groundwater and treated wastewater. Pakistan Journal of Agricultural Sciences. 2015;**52**(1):129-134

Chapter 7

Flavonoids and Phenolic Acids as Potential Natural Antioxidants

Biljana Kaurinovic and Djendji Vastag

Abstract

For centuries, aromatic herbs and spices have been added to different foods to improve the flavor and organoleptic properties. The use of aromatic plants and spices in phytotherapy is mostly related to different activities of their essential oils, such as antimicrobial, spasmolytic, carminative, hepatoprotective, antiviral, and anticarcinogenic activities. Furthermore, many studies point to strong antioxidant activities of aromatic plants and their essential oils. Knowing that phenolic compounds are the most responsible for the antioxidant activity, the amount of total phenolic contents and content of flavonoids have also been determined. In order to examine the antioxidant properties of five different extracts of *Laurus nobilis* L. leaves, various assays which measure free radical scavenging ability were carried out: 1,1-diphenyl-2-picrylhydrazyl, hydroxyl, superoxide anion, nitric oxide and hydroxyl radical scavenger capacity test, and lipid peroxidation assay. In all of the tests, only the EtOAc extract showed a potent antioxidant effect.

Keywords: aromatic plants, flavonoids, phenolic acids, ROS, oxidative stress

1. Introduction

The history of medicinal herb usage dates back to the distant past, many centuries and civilizations ago. Plants have played an important role in many cultures in the treatment of various diseases, and floral fragrances have been used to refine the spirit and body, to attract partners, and to establish a psychophysical balance. The first written testimonials on the use of herbs for treatment are found in China. Emperor Kin-Nong knew about 100 medicinal plants in 3000 years BC. One of the oldest classical medical texts of ancient China is "Pent-Sao," which was written 2500 years BC and is composed of 52 books; of which, two books are dedicated to herbal remedies. In the nineteenth century, medicinal and exotic plants have become lucrative, as more and more people began growing plants in their homes. China, Japan, and South America were overwhelmed by collectors from plant companies who looked for tropical plants to meet the needs of society. This instigated scientific pharmacy and the start of chemical and physiological research on medicinal herbs. It can be said that the nineteenth century was the century of alkaloids, because hundreds were isolated from plants from all over the world. The beginning of the twentieth century threatened medicinal herbs to be completely thrown out of use. Thus, "medicines" that have been successfully used for thousands of years have become subject to mockery and disdain. The expulsion of medicinal herbs from therapy can be compared to the darkness of the Middle Ages that had ruled Europe.

 IntechOpen

In the last four decades, especially in the developed countries of Europe and America, scientists have shown increasing interest in plant research. It is estimated that today about 60% of the total world population in treatment relies on herbs and natural products that are thus recognized as an important source of drugs [1]. Phytochemistry studies a huge variety of organic substances that have been discovered and which accumulate in plants. Furthermore, phytochemistry is also defining the structure of these compounds, their biosynthesis, metabolism, natural distribution, and biological activities [2]. An important place among them is occupied by aromatic plants, whose aroma is associated with the presence of essential oils and complex mixtures of volatile compounds, dominated by mono- and sesquiterpenes. In addition to essential oils, aromatic plants are characterized by the presence of plant phenolic compounds, primarily coumarins and phenylpropanoids, that have been shown to possess multiple pharmacological activities. Investigations of these secondary biomolecules intensified when some commercial synthetic antioxidants were found to exhibit toxic, mutagenic, and carcinogenic effects [3]. It was also found that excessive production of oxygen radicals in the body initiates the oxidation and degradation of polyunsaturated fatty acids. It is known that free radicals attack the highly unsaturated fatty acid membrane systems and induce lipid peroxidation, which is a key process in many pathological conditions and one of the reactions that cause oxidative stress. Particularly, the biological membrane lipids in the spinal cord and brain are vulnerable, because they contain high levels of polyunsaturated fatty acids. Moreover, the brain contains significant amounts of transitional prooxidant metals and consumes a lot of oxygen. These features facilitate the formation of oxygen radicals involved in the processes of aging, Alzheimer's and Parkinson's disease, ischemic heart damage, arthritis, myocardial infarction, arteriosclerosis, and cancer. Phenolic antioxidants "stop" free oxygen radicals and free radicals formed from the substrate by donating hydrogen atoms or electrons. Many plant species and aromatic plants have been tested because of their antioxidant and antiradical activities [4].

The aim of this chapter was to show the antioxidant role of phenolic acids and flavonoids presented in aromatic plants and to assess their potential capacity as scavengers of different free radicals.

2. Oxygen as a toxic molecule

Atmospheric oxygen (O_2) is present as a biradical with two unpaired electrons, which have the same spin quantum number and are located opposite the orbited orbits. This electronic structure of molecular oxygen determines its chemical reactivity and allows the absorption of individual electrons, with the formation of numerous intermediate, partially reduced oxygen species that are commonly referred to as reactive oxygen species (ROS) [5, 6]. These reactive oxygen species are able to react with basic cellular structures and biomolecules [7] and are responsible for the emergence of many diseases and degenerative damage [8].

The normal concentration of free radicals in the body is very low. However, the effects are very disruptive, as the chain reaction allows one free radical to cause changes in thousands of molecules and damage DNA, RNA, and enzymes in cell membranes and leads to the formation of lipoxygenation products before being inactivated. Which part of the cell (proteins, nucleic acids, membrane lipids, cytosolic molecules) or the extracellular component (hyaluronic acid, collagen) will react with free radicals depends on the nature of the radical and the site of its formation (e.g., cytosolic membranes, mitochondria, endoplasmic reticulum, peroxisome, cell membranes). Due to the presence of molecular oxygen in aerobic organisms and its ability to easily receive electrons, free radicals of oxygen origin start more reactions in the cell. The reactions responsible for their formation are respiration, processes of autoxidation of hydroquinone and catecholamine, reduced transition metals, some herbicides and drugs, as well as irradiation that causes water decomposition.

2.1 The role of ROS and RNOS in the onset of many diseases

Any disorder of oxygen species' regulation resulting from a disturbance in the balance between the formation of reactive oxygen metabolites and their elimination by the antioxidant protection system is the state of oxidative stress. In oxidative stress, the formation and accumulation of reactive metabolites are increased, resulting in oxidative processes of destruction of cellular components and genetic material.

2.1.1 Cardiovascular disease

ROS, RNOS, and LP are considered to be the major contributors to the etiology of atherosclerosis and various chronic disorders such as coronary disease, stroke, and ischemic dementia [9]. Antioxidants introduced through food can reduce the occurrence of cardiovascular diseases by inhibiting the production of free radicals and oxidative stress, protecting LDL from oxidation and aggregation, and inhibiting the synthesis of proinflammatory cytokines [10].

2.1.2 Neurodegenerative diseases

Oxidative stress often occurs in the brain, because although it represents only 2% of the body weight, the brain uses up to 20% of oxygen added. Also, the brain contains large amounts of polyunsaturated fatty acids subject to lipid peroxidation under conditions of high oxygen concentration [11, 12].

2.1.3 Carcinogenesis

Although there are insufficient facts to confirm that the presence of free radicals is necessary in the process of carcinogenesis, it is clear that they can lead to mutations, transformations, and cancers [13]. Regarding the development of cancer, the most important target for ROS is DNA. Carcinogenesis is the result of successive mutations in DNA molecules leading to uncontrolled growth and cell phenotypic modification. One of the first steps in this process is the direct interaction of electrophiles or free radicals with cellular DNA in which promutagen lesions develop. If no repair is performed, these lesions result in mutations in the next generation of cells [14]. An increased intake of antioxidants through diet or dietary supplements is associated with a reduction in the onset of cancer.

2.1.4 Aging

A reduced amount of free radicals or a reduction in the speed of their production postpones the aging process and a whole series of diseases related to the aging process [15]. A certain maximum life potential characterizes each animal species. There is a reciprocal correlation between the speed of oxygen consumption (and therefore the production of free radicals) and the maximum life potential. Some studies have shown that the aging process can be slowed by increased food intake that increases antioxidant capacity (e.g., fruit and vegetables) or by supplemental intake of vitamins E, C, and β-carotene [16].

3. Antioxidant protection systems

The process of oxidative modification of proteins, carbohydrates, DNA, and lipids is a universal mechanism of damage to the cell, especially at the membrane level. On the other hand, the numerous roles of free radicals in physiological processes make their creation a mandatory precondition of life, which is why a protective system has been established during evolutionary development. The basic role of this protection system is to reduce the amount and uncontrolled creation of free radicals and their precursors in the cell.

From a functional point of view, the antioxidant protection of the organism includes three levels of action:

1. Antioxidant protection systems that prevent the endogenous formation of free radicals. This level of protection is ensured by the spatial separation of processes in which free radicals are formed.

2. Engagement of the system in conditions of normal and enhanced formation of free radicals. According to the nature and method of action, antioxidants are divided into two types:

    a. Enzymatic (superoxide-dismutase, catalase, xanthine oxidase, peroxidase, glutathione peroxidase, glutathione reductase, glutathione-S-transferase). These enzymes make the so-called primary line of antioxidant protection.

    b. Nonenzymatic or the so-called secondary line of defense.

3. Enzymatic antioxidants involved in the reparation of oxidative damage of lipids, proteins, carbohydrates, and nucleic acids.

3.1 Phenolic compounds

During the evolution, the plants developed effective defense mechanisms against the harmful effects of visible, ultraviolet light and radiation and are a natural source of various antioxidants. Several thousands of biologically active secondary biomolecules of higher plants for phenolic compounds (vitamin E, flavonoids, biflavonols, benzophenones, xanthones, stilbene, quinones, betacities, phenolic acids, acetophenones, phenylpropanoids, coumarins, isocoumarins, chromones, phenols, and diterpenic alcohols) and different nitrogen compounds (alkaloids, amines, amino acids, and chlorophyll derivatives) have been shown to exhibit strong antioxidant activity, but antioxidant activity of essential oils of many spice plants is intense. Their significance is higher because it has been found that many synthetic antioxidants exhibit undesired effects after a prolonged use (e.g., some of them are withdrawn from the market as a possible carcinogen). These biomolecules exhibit their activity through various mechanisms: removing free radicals, binding metal ions, inhibiting enzymatic systems that produce free radical forms, increasing the concentration of biologically important endogenous antioxidants, and inducing the expression of a variety of genes responsible for the synthesis of enzymes that inhibit oxidative stress [14]. The term "herbal phenols" encompasses a wide range of plant substances that form one of the most numerous classes of secondary biomolecules that have a common characteristic of an aromatic ring carrying one or more hydroxyl groups as substituents, including functional derivatives (esters, glycosides, etc.). However, this broad definition also includes some non-phenolic substances. For this reason, it is recommended to combine a definition that includes a chemical description and a biogenetic origin. In nature, there are two general biosynthetic pathways for the synthesis of plant phenols: (1) a polyacetate route and (2) a phenylpropanoid route with scrub acid as an intermediate. Some phenols are formed by a combination of these two times [17].

The efficiency of phenolic compounds in protection against oxidative stress depends on their reactivity in relation to toxic oxygen species and the reactivity of phenoxy radicals relative to critical biomolecules. Chemical or enzymatic oxidation of phenolic components of plant tissue results in a dark color which is of particular importance in food technology. Their susceptibility to oxidation allows their use in the protection of fats and oils.

Phenolic compounds also increase the activity of antioxidant enzymes, thus indirectly affecting the concentration of harmful oxygen radicals in the living cell. In high concentrations, radical reactions such as DNA damage, superoxide anion production, etc. can also be act as a prooxidant [18].

3.1.1 Phenolic acids

The term "phenolic acid" includes hydroxy and other functional derivatives of benzoic acid (C_6—C_1) and cinnamic acid (C_6—C_3) [19, 20]. **Figures 1** and **2** give the structures of the basic representatives of these acids.

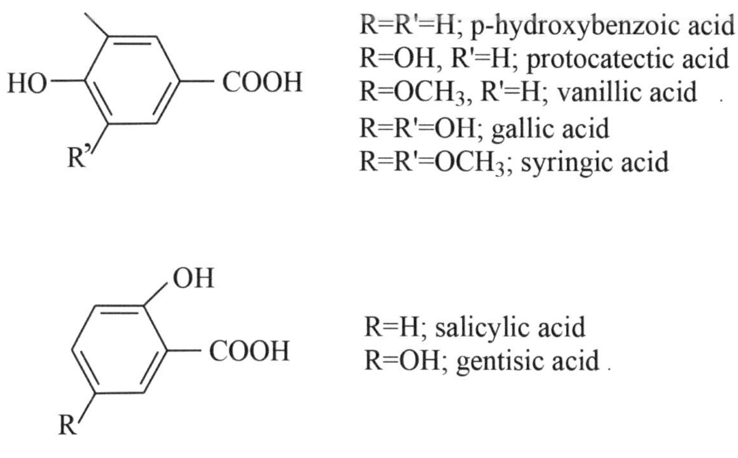

Figure 1.
Chemical compounds of basic benzoic acid derivatives.

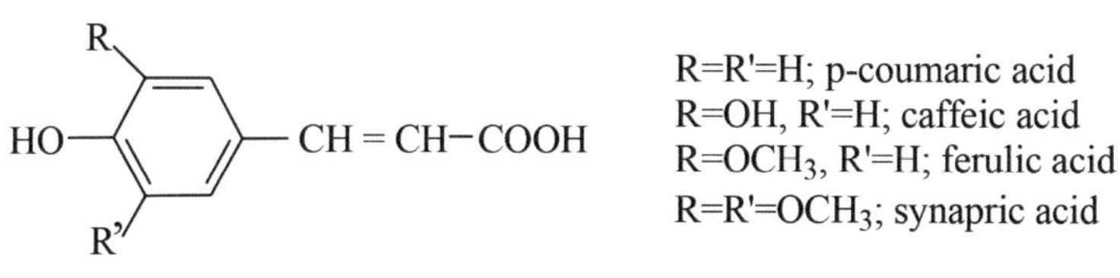

Figure 2.
Chemical formulas of basic derivatives of cinnamic acid.

Cinnamic acids, especially hydroxy-cinnamic acids, have the role of basic precursors in the biosynthesis of various plant phenols. The cinnamic acid and its derivatives are produced by condensation of the acidic acids with phosphoenolpyruvate to give the horizmic acid. Additional reactions of interconversion, decarboxylation, transamination, and disinfection lead to the formation of cinnamon (3-phenylpropenoic acid) and hydroxy-cinnamic acid. Subsequent reactions of hydroxylation, methoxylation, etc. produce cimetic acid derivatives such as p-coumaric acid (p-hydroxy cinnamic acid), β-acid (2,3-dihydroxy cinnamic acid), ferulic acid (2-methoxy-3-hydroxy cinnamic acid), and synapartoic acid (2,4-dimethoxy-3-hydroxy cinnamic acid).

The derivatives of cinnamic acid, in particular hydroxy-cinnamic acids, are the basis of the overall phenylpropanoid metabolism consisting of complex biochemical reactions which as a result supply the plant with important phenolic components [21].

3.1.2 Flavonoids

The term "flavonoids" was proposed by Geisman and Heinseiner [21] to describe all plant pigments having a C_6—C_3—C_6 skeleton, in which two benzene rings are linked via the C_3 unit. These natural products, varying in color from white to yellow, except anthocyanidins responsible for almost all pink and violet shades [20], are widely distributed in the plant kingdom with the exception of algae and fungi. So far, more than 4000 flavonoids have been found in plants, fruits, and vegetables [22]. The most common are seeds, citrus fruits, olive oil, tea, and red wine [23]. They are found in vacuoles, chloroplasts, and chromoplasts, in the form of glycosides, and in the extinct cells free of glycosides. The presence of OH groups directly linked to the carbon atoms of the benzene ring determines the antioxidant role of flavonoids, phenolic acids, and their esters. The expressed activity is shown by compounds with two hydroxyl groups, arranged as for catechol, and three hydroxyl groups arranged as in pyrogallol.

The structure of all flavonoids is based on the C_{15} skeleton of the chromatic structure for which the secondary ring (B) is attached (**Figure 3**) [24, 25].

Flavonoids are divided according to the substitution profile of the heterocyclic ring. In the classification of flavonoids, the oxidation state of the heterocyclic ring as well as the position of the secondary aromatic ring is taken into account. A total of about 12 subgroups of flavonoids are distinguished. The secondary (B) ring may be in position 2 (flavones, flavonols, dihydroflavonols, catechins, flavans, and

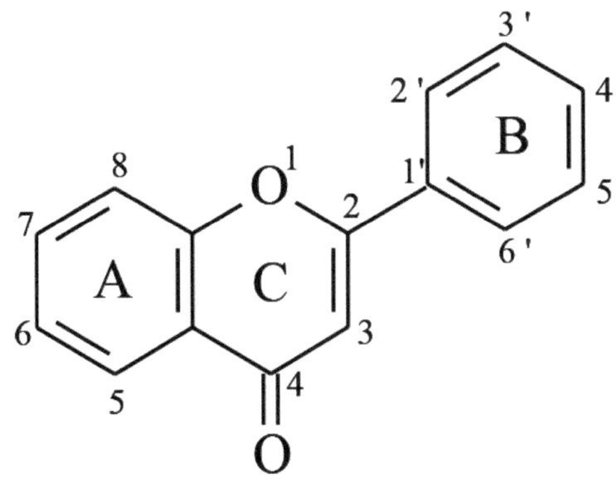

Figure 3.
Basic structure of flavonoids.

anthocyanidins), position 3 (isoflavonoids), or position 4 (4-phenyl-coumarins, neoflavonoids). In a few cases, the six-membered heterocyclic ring occurs in an open isomeric form (chalcones and dihydrochalcones) or is replaced by a five-membered ring.

The most widespread of all flavonoids are flavonols (3-hydroxyflavones) and flavones. The most commonly used flavonoids are quercetin, kaempferol, and myricetin. Quercetin is considered the most widespread component of all plant phenols. More than 100 glycosides of quercetin are known. Among flavonols there are about 200–300 known aglycons of these compounds [26].

3.1.3 The importance of phenolic compounds

Phenolic acids are important not only for ensuring the construction of lignin but also for regulating plant growth and disease resistance. Hydroxy-cinnamic acids are associated with the role of growth regulators and proteins in the development of certain diseases. In addition, it is possible that they are important for chloroplasts and the process of photosynthesis itself. Benzoic acid has been shown to inhibit photosynthesis in chloroplasts of spinach [17]. p-Coumaric acid is the most widespread compound among plant phenols. Furthermore, rosmarinic acid has antioxidant, anti-inflammatory, and antimicrobial effects. Its antioxidant effect is stronger than vitamin E. Rosemary acid prevents damage to cells caused by free radicals and reduces the risk of cancer and atherosclerosis. Unlike antihistamines, rosemary acid prevents the activation of immune system cells that cause swelling and fluid collection. It is used in the treatment of stomach ulcers, arthritis, cataracts, cancer, and bronchial asthma [27, 28]. Caffeic acid far exceeds other antioxidants because it reduces the production of α-toxin by more than 95%. It has been proven that high doses of coffee acids have a detrimental effect on the rats because they cause gastric papillomas. However, the combination of different antioxidants, including baconic acid, had a pronounced effect on the reduction of colon tumors in the same rats. The harmful effects of bicarbonate on human health are not known [29]. Calcium acid and its derivative caffeic acid phenethyl ester (CAPE) show a reduction in tumors and show anti-inflammatory and anticancer effects on ultraviolet-exposed skin, especially UVC and UVB rays [30]. Anticancer activity was observed in mice whose skin was treated with bee propolis and a papilloma-causing agent (TPA). CAPE significantly reduced the number of papillomas [31].

Flavonoids have a high ecological significance. They function as pigments that attract insect pollinators, not only as signal molecules for microorganisms that are useful for the plant but also as antimicrobial agents [32]. In this sense, yellow flavones and flavonols are particularly important. Because of the intense absorption of UV radiation, flavonoids protect the plant tissue from UV radiation, thereby influencing vital processes in chloroplasts.

In a pharmacological view, flavonoids show antiviral, antiallergic, antitumor, antibacterial, antifungal, and antithrombotic activity [33]. They act on blood vessels, namely, flavanones and catechins, that increase the resistance of the capillaries. They show an anti-inflammatory activity that depends on the structure of flavonoids [34]. The flavonoid anti-inflammatory activity was also confirmed by in vitro testing of the ability to inhibit lipoxygenase and cyclooxygenase [35]. Flavonoids eliminate pathological changes on capillaries and are used against diabetes, hypertension, and atherosclerosis. Flavonoids have been found to stimulate the secretion of bile and inhibit enzymes and enzymatic systems. Many flavonoids have antimicrobial and antiviral activity. A certain number of flavonoids show some cytotoxic activity. The common structural feature of cytotoxic flavonoids is trisubstituted ring A, methylation at position C4 [21].

For many flavonoids, high antioxidant activity has been demonstrated in various in vitro systems [36–38]. It has been shown that quercetin, rhamnetin, and isorhamnetin can reduce the amount of serum and liver cholesterol in addition to the in vivo antioxidant activity they show [39]. Flavonoids have been found to inhibit the activity of XOD and have the ability to capture superoxide radicals. Based on this, it is assumed that flavonoids can help in the treatment of gout and ischemia by reducing the amount of uric acid and superoxide anion of radicals in tissues [40]. Two flavonol glycoside-gallate esters showed inhibitory activity on human immunodeficiency virus-1 (HIV-1) integrase [41]. The HIV-1 integrase manages the process of incorporating viral DNA into the DNA of the host cell molecule, which is necessary for the virus to reproduce and produce virions. In this way, the inhibition of the given enzyme can be effective in anti-AIDS therapy. For example, quercetin has a beneficial effect on human health: it improves heart rate and reduces the risk of cancer. It has an anti-inflammatory and antiallergic effect. All of these effects are caused by a strong antioxidant effect of quercetin. Like many other flavonoids, quercetin inhibits the oxidation of LDL cholesterol, and its anti-inflammatory activity derives from inhibition of lipoxygenase enzyme and inhibition of inflammatory mediators. Quercetin also inhibits the release of histamine. Studies have shown that quercetin lowers the risk of prostate, uterine, breast, tissue, and colon cancer. It is presumed to reduce the production of uric acid by inhibiting XOD. It also shows NO inhibitory activity. Rutin has a strong antioxidant effect, as well as the ability to build chelates with metal ions (e.g., iron) and reduces Fenton's reaction in which harmful oxygen radicals are produced. It is supposed to stabilize vitamin C. If rutin is taken along with vitamin C, the activity of ascorbic acid increases. Rutin strengthens the capillaries, which helps people who easily bleed or get bruises. It prevents the formation of various edemas, which is an early symptom of a chronic vein disease. It has an anti-inflammatory effect. There are indications that rutin can inhibit some carcinogenic and precancerous conditions, prevent atherogenesis, and reduce the cytotoxicity of oxidized LDL cholesterol [22]. Furthermore, kaempferol prevents arteriosclerosis by inhibiting the oxidation of low-density lipoproteins and the formation of blood platelets. It has a role of a chemopreventive agent, which means it prevents the formation of cancer cells. Quercetin has a synergistic effect in reducing the proliferation of malignant cells, so treatment with quercetin and kaempferol combinations is more effective than their individual use [42]. In addition, tangeretin acts as an anticancer agent, and in in vitro studies, it has been shown to act against some forms of malignant cells. It strengthens the cell wall and protects it from attack. It also causes apoptosis of cells suffering from leukemia, while normal cells remain undamaged [43]. Tangeretin prevents tumor suppression of intercellular bonds when transmitting the signal [44]. In the G1 phase of the cell cycle, it "freezes" the cancer cells and prevents their replication. In short, in vitro studies have shown that tangerine exhibits antimutagenic, noniinvasive, and antiproliferative activity [45]. Animal studies have shown that tangeretin reduces cholesterol levels [46] and has a potentially protective effect from Parkinson's disease [47].

4. Lauraceae family

The Lauraceae family comprises over 2500 species, which occur within the subtropics and tropics of Eastern Asia and South and North America. Most species possess aromatic roots, stems, and fruits. One of the most well-known and most frequently used plants from this family is *Laurus nobilis* L., also called bay laurel.

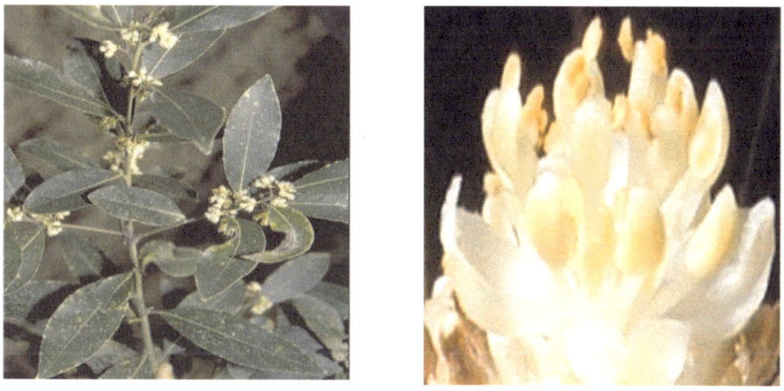

Figure 4.
Laurus nobilis L [21].

L. nobilis is a species held in high esteem since ancient times. It was dedicated to Apollo, the ancient Greek god of light, and a symbol of peace and victory used to make wreaths for emperors, generals, and poets (**Figure 4**) [48].

4.1 *Laurus nobilis* L.

Laurel is a tree or a large bush of pyramidal shape with aromatic, constantly green leaves and shiny gray corn. It reaches a height of up to 5.5 m, but the cultivated form is usually lower (1–3 m). The leaves are elliptical, fairly thick, leathery, and shiny green. Clusters of tiny, yellow, single-polar flowers appear in the spring. Berries (fruit) (*Lauri Fructus*), when dry, are black and wrinkled and contain two oval fat seeds. Laurel is cultivated in several cultivated forms: spp. *aurea* with yellowish young leaves, spp. *angustifolia* with narrow leaves (often called Vrbolik laurel), and spp. *undulata* with corrugated leaf edges. Laurel is commercially grown for aromatic leaves in Turkey, Algeria, Morocco, Portugal, Spain, Italy, France, and Mexico [49, 50].

The distillation of laurel leaves produces green-yellow volatile oil that contains a high percentage of oxidized components. Essential oil leaf (0.8–3%) contains mainly 1,8-cineol (50%) and then eugenol, acetyleugenol, methyl eugenol, α- and β-pinene, felsenren, linalool, geraniol, and terpineol. Dried berries can extract green mass (melting point about 30°C) containing several percent essential oils (0.6–10%), depending on the conditions of breeding and storage. Berries contain both volatile and fixed oils. The others are known under the common name "laurel oil" (Oleum Lauri expressum, Oleum laurinum, and Oleum Lauri unguinosum). As essential ingredients, the oil contains laurosterin, glycerol ester with lauric acid, and sesquiterpenoid (the costume and dehydrocostus lactone), while the rest is made up of fats: triglycerides with lauric, myristic, and elastic acids. As with leaves, the aroma is mainly due to terpenes (cineol, terpineol, α- and β-pinene, citral) but also cinnamic acid and its methyl ester [51].

The main flavonoids in bay leaf are quercetin, kaempferol, rutin, and their derivatives (**Figure 5**).

Kaempferol appears in the form of four nonpolar glycosides (**Figure 6**) [52, 53].

Laurus nobilis is characterized by the presence of the other important plant phenolic substances such as phenolic acids (rosmarinic and caffeic acids) (**Figure 7**).

As a medicinal plant, bay leaves and fruits have been employed against rheumatism, skin rashes, and earaches. In addition, it has been used as a stomachic, astringent, carminative, diaphoretic, stimulant, emetic, emmenagogue, abortifacient,

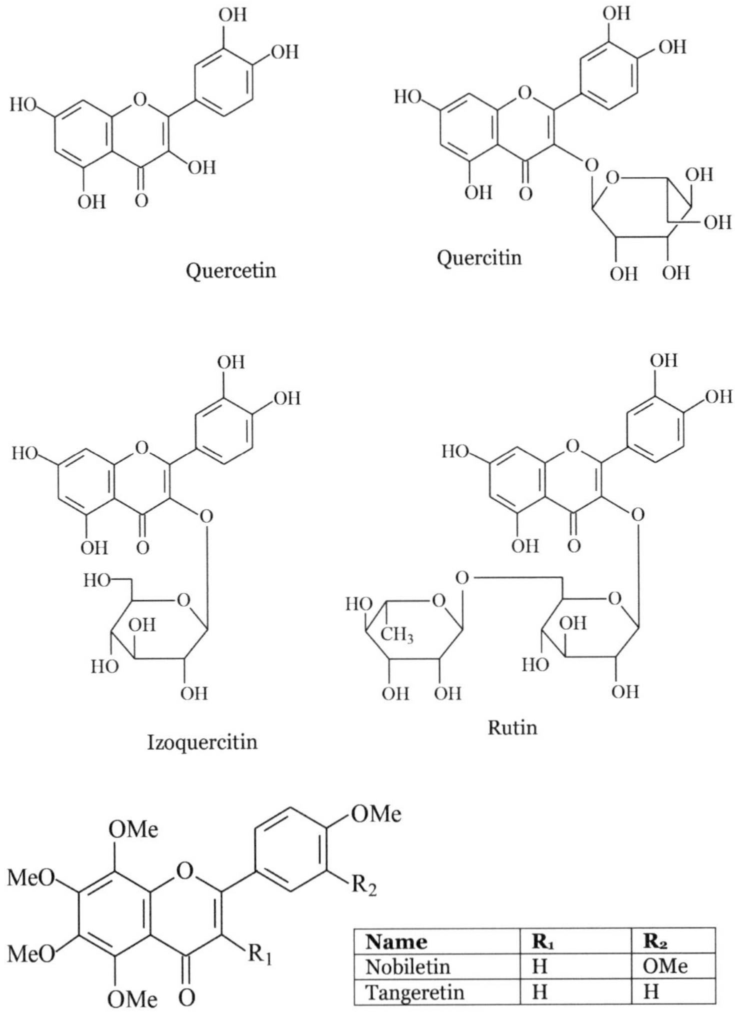

Name	R₁	R₂
Nobiletin	H	OMe
Tangeretin	H	H

Figure 5.
Structures of the main flavonoids present in L. nobilis [21].

and insect repellent. The essential oil is used by the cosmetic industry in creams, perfumes, and soaps.

Numerous investigations of qualitative composition of plant extracts have revealed the presence of high concentration of phenols in the extracts obtained using polar solvents [54]. The extracts that display the highest antioxidant activity have the highest concentration of phenols. Because of that, our research on laurel was recently extended to the comprehensive in vitro and in vivo studies of antioxidant activity of different extracts of leaves, to assess their potential capacity as scavengers of free radicals. Results of determination of total phenolic contents and total flavonoid contents in laurel leaf extracts are given in **Table 1**.

The amount of total phenolics in *L. nobilis* extracts ranged from 2.41 mg GAE/g d.w. (Et_2O extract) to 4.53 mg GAE/g d.w. (EtOAc extract). A significant amount of these compounds has also been observed in the n-BuOH extract (3.96 mg GAE/g d.e.). Furthermore, a considerable total flavonoid content was determined in the EtOAc and n-BuOH extracts. A little less amount of total flavonoids was determined in the $CHCl_3$ extract, while the smallest quantity of these compounds was found in the Et2O and H_2O extracts. HPLC-DAD analysis indicates a significant presence of flavonoids and phenolic in the EtOAc and n-BuOH extracts. Quercetin glycosides and flavonoids

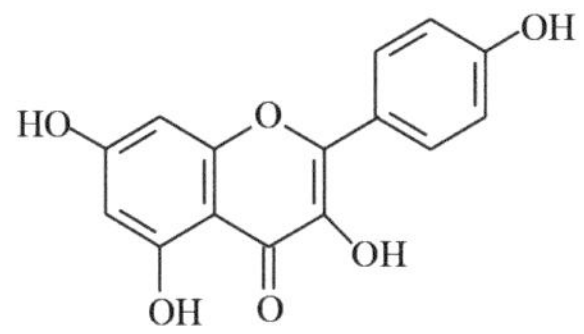

Kaempherol

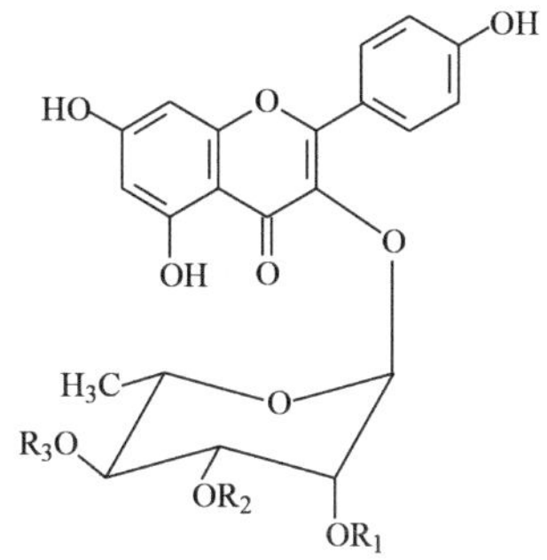

Name	R₁	R₂	R₃
Kaempherol-3-O-α-L-(3”,4”-di-E-p-kumaril)-ramnozid	H	E-p-kumaril	E-p-kumaril
Kaempherol-3-O-α-L-(2”,4”-di-E-p-kumaril)-ramnozid	E-p-kumaril	H	E-p-kumaril
Kaempherol-3-O-α-L-(2”,4”-di-Z-p-kumaril)-ramnozid	Z-p-kumaril	H	Z-p-kumaril
Kaempherol -3-O-α-L-(2”-E-p-kumaril)-ramnozid	E-p-kumaril	H	H

Figure 6.
Structures of kaempferol and its glucosides present in L. Nobilis [21].

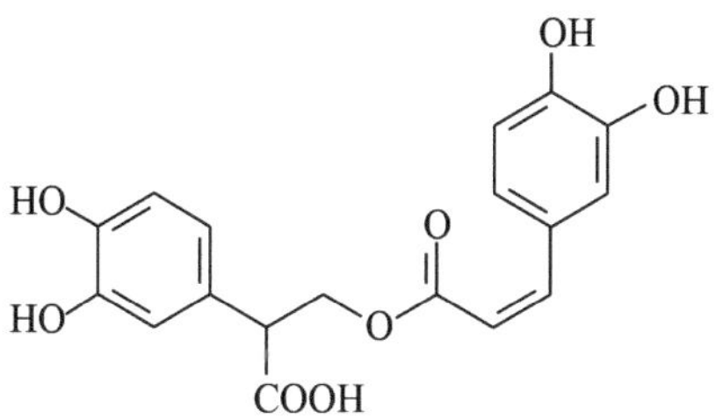

Rosmarinic acid

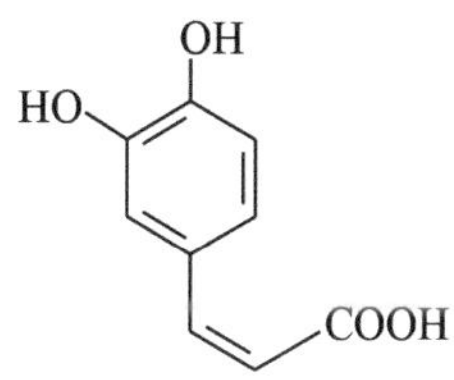

Caffeic acid

Figure 7.
Structures of two phenolic acids in L. nobilis.

Extracts	Et_2O	$CHCl_3$	EtOAc	n-BuOH	H_2O
Total phenolic content	2.41	2.85	4.53	3.96	3.20
Total flavonoid content	0.76	1.02	1.56	1.07	0.68

Table 1.
The amount of total phenolic contents (mg GAE/g d.w.) and content of total flavonoids (mg QE/g d.w.) in L. nobilis extracts.

(e.g., kaempferol-3-*O*-Glc) were detected in EtOAc extract. In addition, the presence of phenolic acids (such as caffeic acid) and flavonoids (rutin and kaempferol) was proven in the H_2O extract. The amount of flavonoids in extracts plays a significant role in their antioxidant capacity. Differences in flavonoid content between extracts and between plant organs can be explained by different numbers of secretory structures in various plant tissues [42, 55, 56].

It should be considered that the number of identified and quantified compounds in MeOH extract of *L. nobilis* L. has been expanded in the present work (**Table 2**).

The results indicate that the major bioactive compounds in *L. nobilis* extracts were kaempferol-3-O-glucoside, quercetin, and rutin. Phenolic acids were also

	Compounds	Extract
Phenolic acid	p-Hydroxybenzoic acid	38.46
	Protocatechuic acid	n.d.
	p-Coumaric acid	n.d.
	Vanillic acid	n.d.
	Gallic acid	n.d.
	Caffeic acid	16.18
	Quinic acid	n.d.
	Ferulic acid	n.d.
	Syringic acid	n.d.
	Chlorogenic acid	13.11
	Cinnamic acid	n.d.
Flavonoids	Apigenin	n.d.
	Naringenin	n.d.
	Luteolin	5.19
	Kaempferol	11.97
	Apigenin-7-O-β-glucoside	n.d.
	Luteolin-7-O-β-glucoside	n.d.
	Kaempferol-3-O-glucoside	56.15
	Quercetin-3-O-glucoside	31.18
	Rutin	17.44
	Quercetin	21.62
	Quercitrin	7.14

Table 2.
LC-MS-MS quantification of bioactive compounds presented in L. nobilis L. crude MeOH extract (μg/g d.w.).

observed in the high level, where the antioxidant, caffeic, and chlorogenic acids were found in the highest amount. Furthermore, p-hydroxybenzoic acid was also found in very high amount. The rest of the phenolic acids were not detected [57–59].

Furthermore, antioxidant activity was observed in the study of laurel leaf extracts in different solvents on the content of $DPPH^{\bullet}$, $O_2^{\bullet-}$, $NO^{\bullet}$, and $OH^{\bullet}$ radicals (**Table 3**).

The obtained results could point to strong quenching activities of flavonoids present in the leaves of laurel against DPPH radicals, and a high degree of correlation is observed between total phenol content and the ability of EtOAc extract to neutralize DPPH radicals. This is indicated by the fact that phenolic compounds

Extract	Et_2O	$CHCl_3$	EtOAc	n-BuOH	H_2O
DPPH radical	127.38	139.42	83.24	181.35	161.83
$O_2^{\bullet-}$ radical	327.60	429.43	163.57	288.64	486.32
NO radical	168.77	322.84	158.63	386.80	618.42
OH radical	442.84	241.18	121.84	213.36	187.65

Table 3.
IC50 values (μg/mL) of L. nobilis for different antioxidant assays.

play a key role in neutralizing free radical species which occurs by the mechanism of electron transfer. But, it can be supposed that such antiradical activity is also caused, besides flavonoids, by terpenoids, since nonpolar solvents also exhibited high antiradical potential. When investigating neutralization of $O_2^{\bullet -}$ and NO radicals, ethyl acetate extract has also exhibited the greatest ability of their scavenging. These results can be attributed to the presence of sesquiterpene lactones isolated from the plant that possess certain biological and pharmacological activity [60, 61]. Matsuda et al. [62] have also established that the methanolic extract from the leaves of *L. nobilis* was found to inhibit nitric oxide (NO) production in lipopolysaccharide (LPS)-activated mouse peritoneal macrophages. It was concluded that seven sesquiterpene lactones (costunolide, dehydrocostus lactone, eremanthine, zaluzanin C, magnolialide, santamarine, and spirafolide) potently inhibited LPS-induced NO production. Inhibition of NO radicals with laurel extracts is very significant, having in mind the ability to neutralize the superoxide anion radicals as well. The common reaction between superoxide anion radical and nitrogen oxide radical yields a very reactive peroxynitrite anion ($ONOO^-$) which is very active in reaction of nitrification of phenols—e.g., nitrification of thyroxine causes enzyme dysfunctions, and increased amounts of 3-nitrothyrozine were found in various pathological states [63]. If formation of nitroderivatives of thyroxine is prevented, the occurrence of these diseases due to oxidative stress is reduced. Ethyl acetate extract of laurel leaves is especially suited in this process since it neutralizes both superoxide anion radical and NO radical. Obtained results can be related to the experiments in which the total amount of phenols and flavonoids were determined (**Table 1**), which show that ethyl acetate extract of laurel leaf contains the largest amounts of total phenolic content and total flavonoid content. The cellular damage resulting from hydroxyl radical is strongest among free radicals. Hydroxyl radical can be generated by biochemical reaction. Superoxide radical is converted by superoxide dismutase (SOD) to H_2O_2, which can subsequently produce extremely reactive $OH^{\bullet}$ radicals in the presence of transition metal ions such as iron and cooper [64, 65]. A good antioxidant potential of neutralization OH radical was shown by the EtOAc (IC_{50} = 121.84 μg/mL) and H_2O (IC_{50} = 187.65 μg/mL) extracts. Such a good antioxidant activity of H_2O and EtOAc extracts is expected, because it is known that the antioxidant activity of phenols is primarily a result of the ability of these compounds to act as donors of hydrogen atoms removing free radicals with the formation of less reactive phenoxyl radicals [66]. The increased stability of the formed phenoxyl radicals primarily attributed to electron delocalization and the existence of multiple resonant forms. Researching dependence of activity on the structure was found to have three structural features as important factors of radical removal potential and/or antioxidant potential of flavonoids: (1) *o*-dihydroxy function of ring B, which serves as the target of radicals; (2) 2,3-double bond in conjugation with 4-oxo function, which is responsible for electron delocalization of the ring B; and (3) the additional presence of 3- and 5-hydroxyl groups for the maximum radical scavenging potential [67]. The positive relationship between increased hydroxylation and increased antioxidant activity of flavonoids was found in different lipid systems, such as oil and liposome systems. Also, for phenolic acids and coumarins, it has been shown that vicinal diol groups are important for radical scavenging capacity and that methoxylation or glycosylation of o-hydroxy group in the coumarins and esterification of phenolic acids reduce the antioxidant activity of these compounds [68]. For example, it was determined that rosmarinic acid has stronger antioxidant effect than vitamin E. Rosmarinic acid prevents cell damage caused by free radicals and reduces the risk of cancer and atherosclerosis. In contrast to the histamines, rosmarinic acid prevents activation of the immune system cells that cause swelling and fluid collection [27, 69]. Furthermore, the action of some flavonoids is based on their ability to chelate transition metal ions, thereby preventing the formation of radicals (initiators of LP), catching radical initiators of LP (ROS), scavenging lipid alkoxyl and lipid peroxyl radicals, and regenerating α-tocopherol by reduction of α-tocopherol radicals. Different metals have different binding affinities of the flavonoids. Thus, for example, iron has the highest binding affinity for 3-OH group of ring C, then catechol group ring B, and at the end of 5-OH group of ring A, while the copper ions bind to the first ring catechol group B [70]. Also, in the previous investigation, on *L. nobilis*, different groups of chemicals were isolated (luteolin, apigenin, alkaloids, monoterpene, and germacrane alcohols) [71].

5. Conclusions

One of the paradoxes of life on Earth is that, on the one hand, oxygen is necessary for the life of aerobic organisms. On the other hand, increased concentrations of oxygen and especially its reactive metabolites (reactive oxygen species) may lead to the development of numerous diseases. A major source of free radicals in biological systems is molecular oxygen (O_2). The results of our in vitro assays of examined five different extracts of *Laurus nobilis* leaves expressed significant protective effects on ROS (DPPH, $O_2^{\bullet-}$, NO, and OH radicals), which was found to be correlated to different compounds. HPLC-DAD analysis indicates a significant presence of flavonoids and phenolic in the EtOAc and n-BuOH extracts. Quercetin glycosides and flavonoids (e.g., kaempferol-3-*O*-Glc) were detected in EtOAc extract. In addition, the presence of phenolic acids (such as caffeic acid) and flavonoids (rutin and kaempferol) was proven in the H_2O extract. The amount of flavonoids in extracts plays a significant role in their antioxidant capacity, and it can be concluded that ethyl acetate proved to be the best solvent for extraction of plant material. Furthermore, it can be concluded that these extracts can be used in the preparation of various herbal medicines.

Acknowledgements

This work was supported by the Ministry of Science and Environmental Protection of the Republic of Serbia (Project No. 172058).

Conflict of interest

The authors declare that there is no conflict of interest.

DOI: http://dx.doi.org/10.5772/intechopen.83731

Author details

Biljana Kaurinovic* and Djendji Vastag
Department of Chemistry, Biochemistry and Environmental Protection,
University of Novi Sad, Republic of Serbia

*Address all correspondence to: biljana.kaurinovic@dh.uns.ac.rs

References

[1] Harvey A. Strategies for discovering drugs from previously unexplored natural products. Drug Discovery Today. 2000;**5**:294-300

[2] Harborne JB. Phytochemical Methods: A Guide to Modern Techniques of Plant Analysis. 3rd ed. London: Chapman & Hall; 1998. 110 p

[3] Namiki M. Antioxidants/ antimutagens in food. Food Science and Nutrition. 1990;**29**:273-300

[4] Gülçin I, Topal F, Çakmakçı R, Bilsel M, Gören AC, Erdogan U. Pomological features, nutritional quality, polyphenol content analysis, and antioxidant properties of domesticated and 3 wild ecotype forms of raspberries (*Rubus idaeus* L.). Journal of Food Science. 2011; **76**:585-593

[5] Halliwell B. Chloroplast Metabolism: The Structure and Function of Chloroplast in Green Leaf Cells. Oxford: Clarendon Press; 1984. pp. 180-206

[6] Halliwell B. Oxygen radicals as key mediators in neurological disease: Fact or fiction? Annals of Neurology. 1992; **32**(1):10-13

[7] Mimica-Dukić N. *In vivo* and *in vitro* study of antioxidant activity of plant extracts. Archive of Pharmacy. 1997;**5**: 475-493

[8] Marx JL. Oxygen free radicals linked to many diseases. Science. 1985;**204**: 235-238

[9] Knight JA. Diseases related to the oxygen derived free radicals. Annals of Clinical and Laboratory Science. 1995; **25**(2):111-121

[10] Kushi LH. Dietary antioxidant vitamins and death from coronary disease in postmenopausal women. The New England Journal of Medicine. 1996; **334**:1156-1162

[11] Behl C, Davis JB, Lesley R, Schubert D. Hydrogen peroxide mediates amyloid β-protein toxicity. Cell. 1994;**77**:817-827

[12] Romero FJ, Bosch-Morell F, Romero MJ, Jareno EJ, Romero B, Marin N. Lipid peroxidation products and antioxidants in human disease. Environmental Health Perspectives. 1998;**106**:1229-1234

[13] Simić MG. Mechanism of inhibition of free-radical processes in mutagenesis and carcinogenesis. Mutation Research. 1998;**202**:377-386

[14] Primiano T, Sutter RT, Kensler WT. Redox regulation of genes that protect against carcinogens. Comparative Biochemistry and Physiology. 1997; **118**(4):487-497

[15] Harman D. Free radical theory of aging. Mutation Research. 1992;**275**: 257-266

[16] Gutler RG. Antioxidant, aging and longevity. In: Pryor WA, editor. Free Radical in Biology. Orlando: Academic Press; 1984. pp. 102-107

[17] Đorđević VB, Pavlović DD, Kocić GM. Biohemija Slobodnih Radikala. Niš: Medicinski fakultet; 2000. 128 p

[18] Harborne JB. Plant phenolics. In: Dey PM, Harborne JB, editors. Methods in Plant Biochemistry. London, San Diego, New York, Boston, Sydney, Tokyo, Toronto: Academic Press; 1989. pp. 493-508

[19] Rice-Evans CA, Packer L. Flavonoids in Health and Disease. Boca Raton: CRC Press; 2003. pp. 1-43

[20] Kumar S, Pandey KA. Chemistry and biological activities of flavonoids:

An overview. The Scientific World Journal. 2013;(11-12):1-16

[21] Kaurinović B. Antioxidant activities of *Laurus nobilis* L. and *Melittis melissophyllum* L. extracts (in Serbian) [PhD thesis]. Novi Sad: PMF; 2008. 68 p

[22] Petri G, Krawczyk U, Kery A. Spectrophotometric and chromatographic investigation of bilberry anthocyanins for quantification purposes. Microchemical Journal. 1997; **55**:12-23

[23] Ohshima H, Yoshie Y, Auriol S, Gilbert I. Antioxidant and pro-oxidant actions of flavonoids: Effects of DNA damage induced by nitric oxide, peroxynitrite and nitroxyl anion. Free Radical Biology and Medicine. 1998;**25**: 1057-1065

[24] Amalesh S, Gouranga D, Sanjoy KD. Roles of flavonoids in plants. International Journal of Pharmacy and Pharmaceutical Sciences. 2011;**6**(1): 12-35

[25] Panche AN, Diwan AD, Chandra SR. Flavonoids: An overview. Journal of Nutritional Science. 2016;**5**:1-15

[26] Goufo P, Trindade H. Rice antioxidants: Phenolic acids, flavonoids, anthocyanins, proanthocyanidins, tocopherols, tocotrienols, c-oryzanol, and phytic acid. Food Science and Nutrition. 2014;**2**(2):75-104

[27] Shetty K. Biotechnology to harness the benefits of dietary phenolics; focus on Lamiaceae. Asia Pacific Journal of Clinical Nutrition. 1997;**6**:162-171

[28] Kaurinović B, Popović M, Vlaisavljević S, Rašeta M. Antioxidant activities of *Melittis melissophyllum L.* (Lamiaceae). Molecules. 2011;**16**: 3152-3167

[29] Peppercorn MA, Goldman P. Caffeic acid metabolism by gnotobiotic rats and their intestinal bacteria. PNAS. 1972;**69**(6):1413-1415

[30] Neradil J, Veselsk R, Slanina J. UVC-protective effect of caffeic acid on normal and transformed human skin cells in vitro. Folia Biologica. 2003;**49**: 197-202

[31] Huang MT, Ma W, Yen P, Xie JG, Han J, Frenkel K, et al. Inhibitory effects of caffeic acid phenethyl ester (CAPE) on 12-O-tetradecanoylphorbol-13-acetate-induced tumor promotion in mouse skin and the synthesis of DNA, RNA and protein in HeLa cells. Carcinogenesis. 1996;**17**(4):761-765

[32] Dixon AR, Steele LC. Flavonoids and isoflavonoids—A gold mine for metabolic engineering. Trends in Plant Science. 1999;**4**:394-400

[33] Middleton EJ. Biological properties of plant flavonoids: An overview. International Journal of Pharmacognosy. 1996;**34**(3):344-348

[34] Boonmuen N, Gong P, Ali Z, Chittiboyina AG, Khan I, Doerge DR, et al. Licorice root components in dietary supplements are selective estrogen receptor modulators with a spectrum of estrogenic and anti-estrogenic activities. Steroids. 2016;**105**:42-49

[35] Abad JM, Bermejo P, Villar A. The activity of flavonoids extracted from *Tanacetum microphyllum* DC. (Compositae) on soybean lipoxygenase and prostaglandin synthetase. General Pharmacology. 1995;**26**:815-819

[36] Morel I, Lescoat G, Cogrel P, Sergent O, Pasdeloup N, Brissot P, et al. Antioxidant and iron-chelating activities of the flavonoids catechin, quercetin and diosmetin on iron-loaded rat hepatocyte cultures. Biochemical Pharmacology. 1993;**45**:13-19

[37] Jimenez M, Garcia-Carmona F. Myricetin, an antioxidant flavonol is a

substrate of polyphenol oxidase. Journal of the Science of Food and Agriculture. 1999;**79**:1993-2000

[38] Pekkarinen SS, Heinonen IM, Hopia IA. Flavonoids quercetin, myricetin, kaempferol and (+)-catechin as antioxidants in methyl linoleate. Journal of the Science of Food and Agriculture. 1999;**79**:499-506

[39] Igarashi K, Ohmuma M. Effects of isorhamnetin, rhamnetin, and quercetin on the concentrations of cholesterol and lipoperoxide in the serum and liver and on the blood and liver antioxidative enzyme activities of rats. Bioscience Biotechnology and Biochemistry. 1995; **59**:595-601

[40] Cos P, Ying L, Callome M, Hu JP, Cimanga K, Van Poel B, et al. Structure-activity relationship and classification of flavonoids as inhibitors of xanthine oxidase and superoxide scavengers. Journal of Natural Products. 1998;**61**(1): 71-76

[41] Kim JH, Woo E, Shin C, Park H. A new flavonol glycoside gallate ester from acer okamotoanum and its inhibitory activity against human immunodeficiency Virus-1 (HIV1) integrase. Journal of Natural Products. 1998;**61**:145-148

[42] Acland ML, van de Waarsenburg S, Jones R. Synergistic antiproliferative action of the flavonols quercetin and kaempferol in cultured human cancer cell lines. In Vivo. 2005;**19**(1):69-76

[43] Hirano T, Abe K, Gotoh M, Oka K. Citrus flavone tangeretin inhibits leukaemic HL-60 cell growth partially through induction of apoptosis with less cytotoxicity on normal lymphocytes. The British Journal of Cancer. 1995; **72**(6):1380-1388

[44] Chaumont JP, Leger D. Campaign against allergic moulds in dwellings. inhibitor properties of essential oil geranium bourbon, citronellol, geraniol and citral. Annales Pharmaceutiques Françaises. 1992;**50**(3):156-166

[45] Kandaswami C, Perkins E, Soloniuk DS, Drzewiecki G, Middleton EJ. Antiproliferative effects of citrus flavonoids on a human squamous cell carcinoma in vitro. Cancer Letters. 1991; **56**(2):147-152

[46] Kurowska EM, Manthey JA. Hypolipidemic effects and absorption of citrus polymethoxylated flavones in hamsters with diet-induced hypercholesterolemia. Journal of Agricultural and Food Chemistry. 2004; **52**(10):2879-2886

[47] Datla KP, Christidou M, Widmer WW, Rooprai HK, Dexter DT. Tissue distribution and neuroprotective effects of citrus flavonoid tangeretin in a rat model of Parkinson's disease. Neuroreport. 2001;**12**(17):3871-3875

[48] Agati A, Azzarello E, Pollastri S, Tattini M. Flavonoids as antioxidants in plants: Location and functional significance. Plant Science. 2012;**96**: 67-76

[49] Basak SS, Candan F. Effect of *Laurus nobilis* L. essential oil and its main components on α-glucosidase and reactive oxygen species scavenging activity. Iranian Journal of Pharmaceutical Research. 2013;**12**(2): 367-379

[50] Cherrat L, Espina L, Bakkali M, Garcia-Gonzalo D, Pagan R, Laglaoui A. Chemical composition and antioxidant properties of *Laurus nobilis* L. and *Myrtus communis* L. essential oils from Morocco and evaluation of their antimicrobial activity acting alone or in combined processes for food preservation. Journal of the Science of Food and Agriculture. 2014;**96**(6):1197-1204

[51] Fiorini C, Fouraste I, David B, Bessiere J. Composition of the flower,

leaf and stem essential oils from *L. nobilis* L. Flavour and Fragrance Journal. 1997;**12**:91-93

[52] Caredda A, Marongiu B, Porcedda S, Soro C. Supercritical carbon dioxide extraction and characterization of *L. nobilis* essential oil. Journal of Agricultural and Food Chemistry. 2002; **50**:1492-1496

[53] Akgul A, Kivanc M, Bayrak A. Chemical composition and antimicrobial effect of Turkish laurel leaf oil. Journal of Essential Oil Research. 1989;**1**:277-280

[54] Fiorini C, David B, Fouraste I, Vercauteren J. Acylated kaempferol glycosides from *Laurus nobilis* leaves. Phytochemistry. 1998;**47**(5):821-824

[55] Škerget M, Kotnik P, Hadolin M, Rižner-Hraš A, Simonič M, Knez Ž. Phenols, proanthocyanidins, flavones and flavonols in some plant materials and their antioxidants activities. Food Chemistry. 2005;**89**:191-198

[56] Orčić D, Franciškovič M, Bekvalac K, Svirčev E, Beara I, Lesjak M, et al. Quantitative determination of plant phenolics in *Urtica dioica* extracts by high-performance liquid chromatography coupled with tandem mass spectrometric detection. Food Chemistry. 2014;**143**:48-53

[57] Čanadanović-Brunet J, Ćetković G, Djilas S, Tumbas V, Bogdanović G, Mandić A, et al. Radical scavenging, antibacterial, and antiproliferative activities of *Melissa officinalis* L. extracts. Journal of Medicinal Food. 2008;**11**:133-143

[58] Tucakov J. Healing with Herbs (Phytotherapy) (in Serbian). Beograd, Serbia: Rad; 1997. 34 p

[59] Kaurinović B, Popović M, Vlaisavljević S. In vitro and in vivo effects of *Laurus nobilis L.* leaf extracts. Molecules. 2010;**15**:3378-3390

[60] Fraga B. Natural sesquiterpenoids. Natural Product Reports. 2003;**20**: 392-413

[61] Kaurinović B, Popović M, Ćebović T, Mimica-Dukić N. Effects of *Calendula officinalis* L. and *Taraxacum officinale* Weber (Asteraceae) extracts on the production of OH• radicals. Fresenius Environmental Bulletin. 2003; **12**:250-253

[62] Matsuda H, Kagerura T, Toguchida I, Ueda H, Morikawa T, Yoshikawa M. Inhibitory effects of sesquiterpene from bay leaf on nitric oxide production in lipopolysaccharide-activated macrophages: Structure requirement and role of heat shock protein induction. Life Sciences. 2000;**66**: 2151-2157

[63] Groves JT. Peroxynitrite: Reactive, invasive, enigmatic. Current Opinion in Chemical Biology. 1999;**3**:226-235

[64] Hsu YC, Chan YP, Chang J. Antioxidant activity of extract from *Polygonum cuspidatum*. Biological Research. 2007;**40**:13-21

[65] Kaurinović B, Popović M, Vlaisavljević S, Schwartsowa H, Vojinović-Miloradov M. Antioxidant profile of *Trifolium pratense* L. Molecules. 2012;**17**:11156-11172

[66] Bors W, Heller W, Michel C, Saran M. Flavonoids as antioxidants: Determination of radical scavenging efficiences. Methods in Enzymology. 1990;**186**:343-355

[67] Pakkarinen SS, Heinonen IM, Hopia IA. Flavonoids quercetin, myricetin, kaemferol and (+)-catechin as antioxidants in methyl linoleate. Journal of the Science of Food and Agriculture. 1999;**79**:499-506

[68] Kaurinović B, Popović M, Vlaisavljević S, Trivić S. Antioxidant capacity of *Ocimum basilicum L.* and

Origanum vulgare L. extracts. Molecules. 2011;**16**:7401-7414

[69] Cotelle N. Role of flavonoids in oxidative stress. Current Topics in Medicinal Chemistry. 2001;**1**:569-590

[70] Popović M, Kaurinović B, Jakovljević V, Mimica-Dukić N, Bursać M. Effect of celery (*Apium graveolens*) extracts on some biochemical parameters of oxidative stress in mice treated with carbon tetrachloride. Phytotherapy Research. 2006;**20**: 531-537

[71] Vlaisavljevic S, Kaurinovic B, Popovic M, Vasiljevic S. Profile of phenolic compounds in *Trifolium pratense* L. extracts at different growth stages and their biological activities. International Journal of Food Properties. 2016;**20**(12):3090-3101

Section 2

Antioxidants Compounds and Diseases

Chapter 8

The Role of Endogenous Antioxidants in the Treatment of Experimental Arthritis

Katarina Bauerova, Jarmila Kucharska, Silvester Ponist, Lukas Slovak, Karol Svik, Vladimir Jakus and Jana Muchova

Abstract

The pathogenesis of rheumatoid arthritis is poorly understood; however, elevated oxidative stress has been described to be involved. In this chapter, we present experiments with endogenous molecules bearing antioxidative properties. In our studies, we used male Lewis rats, and the arthritis was induced with *Mycobacterium butyricum*. In the first experiment, we tested coenzyme Q_{10} (CoQ_{10}) in the oral daily dose of 100 mg/kg b.w. Markers of inflammation and total antioxidant status were corrected in the group supplemented. CoQ_{10} treatment significantly improved concentrations of the investigated endogenous antioxidants. Further as an important fact, we consider a good bioavailability of used CoQ_{10} formulation which was confirmed by increased CoQ concentrations in plasma, tissue, and mitochondria from skeletal muscles. In the second study, we describe the results with hyaluronic acid (HA) administered in oral daily doses of 0.5 mg and 5 mg/kg b.w. and of different molecular weights (0.43, 0.99, and 1.73 MDa). A notable antioxidative effect of HA was assessed: its administration increased the activities of antioxidant enzymes (superoxide dismutase and glutathione peroxidase) in erythrocytes and total antioxidant capacity of plasma and reduced the marker of oxidative damage to lipids—plasmatic lipid hydroperoxides. HA with the highest molecular weight showed the most significant effect.

Keywords: oxidative stress, antioxidants, coenzyme Q_{10}, hyaluronan, arthritis

1. Introduction

1.1 Involvement of oxidative stress in rheumatoid arthritis

Rheumatoid arthritis (RA) is the most common inflammatory rheumatic disease, affecting almost 1–2% of the world's population. Most of patients present rheumatoid factors, which are autoantibodies directed to the Fc fraction of immunoglobulin G and antibodies reacting with citrullinated peptides [1, 2]. The pathogenesis of RA is understood incompletely. Until now, there is a lack of optimal therapy against this disease. The disease is characterized by immunological dysfunction and chronic inflammation which results in synovial joint deformity and destruction. In the course of RA, the synovial membrane of diarthrodial joints is inflamed, and articular tissue is damaged which leads to severe functional disarrangement of the entire joint. The initial stages of RA synovitis are characterized by proliferation of the microvasculature and secondary edema. Eventually, this process matures into a progressive infiltration of immune cells, including B cells, T cells, and monocytes from the bloodstream. These immune cells are activated in the joint and differentiate and acquire mature phenotypes. The influx of immune cells is also associated with phenotypic changes in synoviocytes, the typical resident cells. Both fibroblast- and monocyte-derived synoviocytes proliferate extensively and participate in inflammatory process. Synovial proliferation, neovascularization, and leukocyte extravasation transform the normal synovium into an invasive tumor-like "pannus." The architecture of the microvasculature is highly dysregulated, and thus efficiency of oxygen supply to the synovium is poor [3]. This, alongside with increased metabolic turnover of the expanding synovial pannus, leads to oxidative stress (OS), altered cellular bioenergetics, and a hypoxic microenvironment, which further promotes synovial invasiveness and abnormal cell function within the joint [4]. Free radicals such as reactive oxygen species (ROS) and reactive nitrogen species (RNS) have distinct contribution to the destructive, proliferative synovitis of RA and play a prominent role in cell-signaling events (**Figure 1**).

However, few studies had clarified the role of free radicals in the etiopathogenesis of RA. Significant higher serum levels of ROS and RNS in RA patients in comparison with healthy subjects were described. Furthermore, strong positive correlation between ROS, RNS, and the clinical and biochemical markers of RA was observed [5]. In another study glycated, oxidized, and nitrated proteins and amino acids were detected in synovial fluid (SF) and plasma of arthritic patients with characteristic patterns found in early and advanced RA, with respect to healthy control [6]. Combination of estimates of oxidized, nitrated, and glycated amino acids with hydroxyproline and anti-cyclic citrullinated peptide antibody status in plasma provided a biochemical test of relatively high sensitivity and specificity for early-stage diagnosis and typing of arthritic disease. Advanced oxidation protein products (AOPPs) have been confirmed to accumulate in RA patients. A study of Ye et al. [7] demonstrated that AOPPs induce apoptosis of human chondrocyte via ROS-related mitochondrial dysfunction and endoplasmic reticulum stress pathways. These data implicate that AOPPs may represent a novel pathogenic factor that contributes to RA progression. Further it seems that an accurate redox balance is necessary to sustain an immune state that both prevents the development of overt autoimmunity and minimizes collateral tissue damage [8]. The inflamed joint

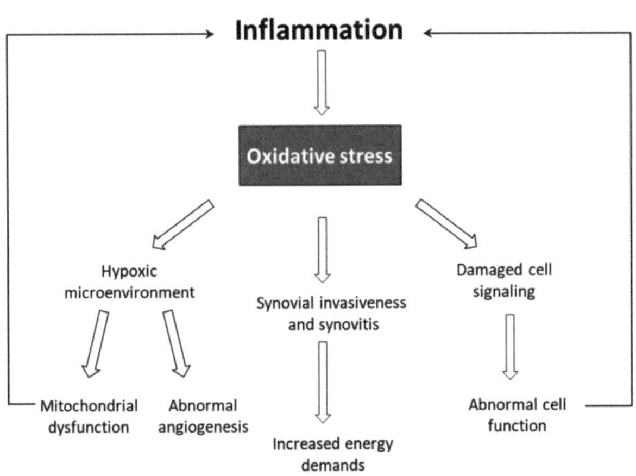

Figure 1.
Pathological changes in arthritic joint induced by oxidative stress.

is profoundly hypoxic, with evidence of oxidative damage and impaired mitochondrial dysfunction, as a result of abnormal angiogenesis and increased energy demands of the expanding synovial pannus [9]. In this hypoxic-inflammatory microenvironment, synovial cells adapt in order to survive through altering their cellular metabolism, which activates complex cross talk of key signaling pathways in the inflamed joint which further exacerbates inflammation. Thus, understanding the underlying mechanisms mediating hypoxia-induced pathways, OS, and subsequent cellular inflammation may provide a basis for novel therapies. It is well documented that ROS can activate different signaling pathways having a vital importance in the pathophysiology of RA [10].

Our chapter is focused on two main aims:

1. To verify the hypothesis that per oral supplementation of CoQ_{10} could affect inflammation in arthritic rats by regulating endogenous antioxidants and OS with detailed analysis performed in plasma and skeletal muscles.

2. To verify the hypothesis that hyaluronan per oral administration can restore the redox balance under the conditions of experimental arthritis. OS has been monitored in erythrocytes and in plasma. The effect of three different molecular weights of polysaccharides has been evaluated.

1.2 Role of antioxidant systems and endogenous antioxidants in remission of rheumatoid arthritis

Epidemiological studies have shown that RA occurs in previously healthy subjects who had low levels of circulating antioxidants [11], implying a pathogenic role of increased OS in the development of RA. Patients with RA have been reported to have lower serum levels of a variety of antioxidants, including vitamin E, vitamin C, β-carotene, selenium, and zinc, in comparison with healthy individuals [12]. In order to prevent the damaging effect of prooxidants, the body has an antioxidant defense system that protects cellular systems from oxidative damage [13]. Some common enzymes that are involved in the neutralization of free radicals are endogenous enzymatic antioxidants such as superoxide dismutase (SOD), glutathione peroxidase (GPx), catalase (CAT), glutathione reductase (GR), and peroxiredoxins. These enzymes neutralize hydrogen peroxide, yielding water (CAT, GPx) and oxygen (CAT) molecules. The nonenzymatic endogenous antioxidants taking part in the first line of defense belong to preventive antioxidants, and in blood plasma they are represented by metal-binding proteins as ceruloplasmin, ferritin, lactoferrin, transferrin, and albumin. These proteins inhibit the formation of ROS by binding with transition metal ions (e.g., iron and copper). Also, metallothionein plays an essential role in the prevention against ROS. The second line of defense against ROS involves nonenzymatic antioxidants that are represented by molecules characterized by the ability to rapidly inactivate radicals and oxidants. The third line of defense consists of repair mechanisms against damage caused by free radicals. This form of protection is provided by enzymatic antioxidants, which can repair damaged DNA and proteins, fight against oxidized lipids, stop chain propagation of peroxyl lipid radicals, and repair damaged cell membranes and molecules [14]. Dietary antioxidants (vitamins C and E, carotenoids, polyphenols, and biogenic elements) can affect the activity of endogenous antioxidants. Endo- and exogenous antioxidants may act synergistically to maintain or re-establish redox homeostasis. The major endogenous nonenzymatic low-molecular-mass antioxidants include glutathione, uric acid, melatonin, coenzyme Q, bilirubin, and polyamines. Considering the mechanism of antioxidant protection, the endogenous substances can be divided into true scavengers, metal-buffering proteins, and chelators of redox-stable metals [13]. This chapter is focused on evaluating coenzyme Q_{10} and hyaluronan of different molecular weight in experimental arthritis induced in rats.

2. Coenzyme Q_{10} supplementation and its contribution to therapy of arthritis

2.1 The protective properties of coenzyme Q

Chronic inflammation, systemic OS, and mitochondrial dysfunction are the main factors which participate in etiopathogenesis of arthritis. Mitochondria play a central role in ATP formation in the respiratory chain (**Figure 2**) and in maintaining redox homeostasis. OS processes are activated under pathological conditions. Oxidative damage of mitochondria may lead to the dysfunction of the respiratory chain which further increases ROS formation. Thus, mitochondrial dysfunction can contribute to the development of inflammatory human diseases [16].

The therapy of RA is an actual problem in clinical rheumatology due to the toxicity and side effects of antirheumatic drugs; therefore, new treatment options are being sought. Methotrexate (MTX), used in the treatment of RA, can induce hepatocellular injury. In combination with coenzyme Q_{10}, anti-arthritic effect of MTX was potentiated, and hepatotoxicity was suppressed [17]. Preservation of mitochondrial function could reduce OS and may represent a novel therapeutic approach in patients with inflammatory diseases. Progressive muscle atrophy and inflammatory myopathy in RA have been proposed to be mediated by disturbances of myofibrils and mitochondria [18]. Due to the unique properties, coenzyme Q_{10} (CoQ_{10}) can serve as a useful adjuvant in the management of arthritis. CoQ_{10}

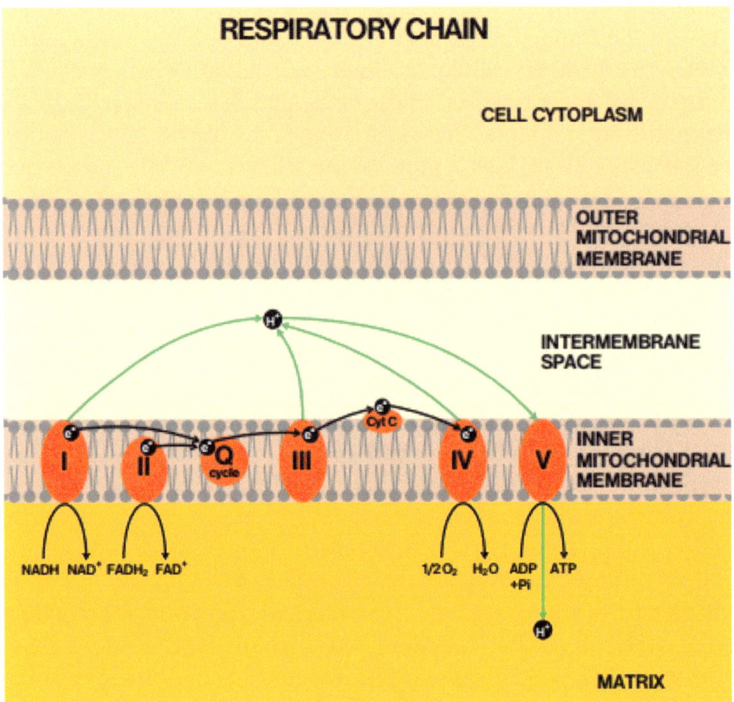

Figure 2.
Function of coenzyme Q in mitochondrial respiratory chain. With permission of [15].

is irreplaceable in mitochondrial bioenergetics; it participates as a cofactor of dehydrogenases in the transport of electrons and protons as well as in ATP production [19]. The respiratory chain located in the inner mitochondrial membrane is organized into five complexes (I, II, III, IV, and V). The transport of electrons from NADH and $FADH_2$ and production of electrochemical potential and proton gradients are necessary for the synthesis of ATP [20, 21]. Electrons are carried out from complexes I and II to complex III by coenzyme Q (CoQ). It has been demonstrated that lipoperoxidation is accompanied by reduced mitochondrial CoQ concentrations concomitantly with the decreased activities of respiratory chain enzymes, such as NADH- and succinate oxidases [22–24]. Increased levels of antioxidants have also been reported including CoQ in tissues as well as activities of antioxidant enzymes in experimental models of diseases associated with increased free radicals' generation such as diabetes mellitus [25–27]. The term "redox signaling" has been introduced to describe a regulatory process in which protective responses against oxidative damage are induced to reset the oxidant-antioxidant balance [28]. CoQ (ubiquinone) is the only lipophilic antioxidant to be biosynthesized; the main form in humans is CoQ_{10}, in rats' coenzyme Q_9 (CoQ_9) (**Figure 3**).

CoQ exerts its antioxidant function either directly on superoxide radicals or indirectly on lipid radicals, both singly and in cooperation with vitamin E [29]. Beneficial antioxidant and anti-inflammatory properties of CoQ_{10} were proved in RA patients [30]. Tocopherols are the subgroup of vitamin E, occurring in isomers α, β, γ, and δ. All tocopherols are potent antioxidants with lipoperoxyl radical-scavenging activities [31]. The main forms of tocopherols in humans are alpha-tocopherol (αT) and gamma-tocopherol (γT) (**Figure 4**).

The most significant difference in metabolism of αT and γT is preferential binding of αT by α-TTP (α-tocopherol transfer protein). The γT is metabolized mainly through cytochrome P450, and formed hydrophilic metabolites are excreted in urine [32]. Isoforms of vitamin E differentially regulate inflammation [33]. In contrast to αT, γT reacts with nitrogen radicals which are formed extensively in inflammatory diseases such as RA. Vitamin E has a potential role in skeletal muscle health, in regulation of OS and inflammation [34]. Low levels of vitamin E and

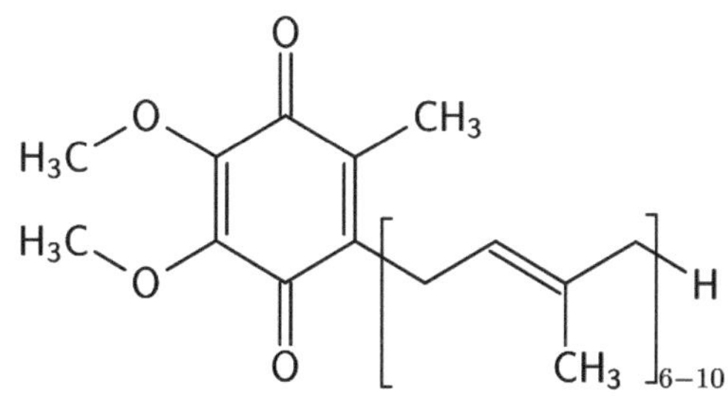

Figure 3.
Chemical structure of coenzyme Q.

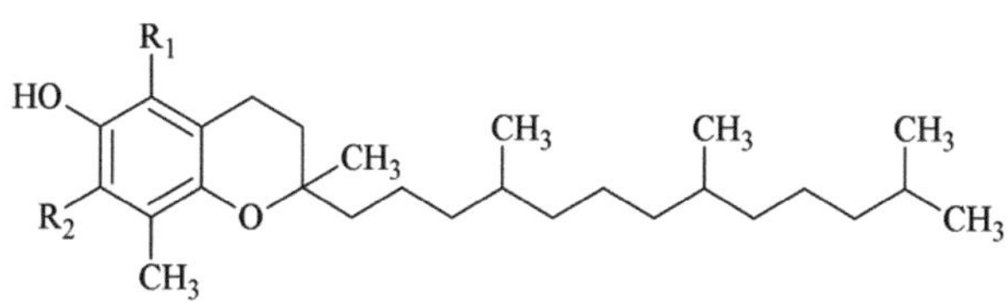

Figure 4.
Chemical structure of tocopherols. α-tocopherol: R1 = CH_3; R2 = CH_3; γ-tocopherol: R1 = H; R2 = CH_3.

other endogenous antioxidants have been considered as a risk factor for the development of RA [35]. We hypothesized that administration of CoQ_{10} could affect inflammation in arthritic rats by regulating the endogenous antioxidants and OS.

2.2 Experimental design of adjuvant arthritis with administration of coenzyme Q_{10}

Adjuvant arthritis (AA) was induced by intradermal injection of *Mycobacterium butyricum* in incomplete Freund's adjuvant to male Lewis rats [36, 37]. The experiment included healthy control animals (HC), arthritic animals (AA), and arthritic animals with administration of CoQ_{10} (liquid liposomal CoQ_{10}—LiQSorb®) in the oral daily dose of 100 mg/kg b.w. (AA-CoQ) by the use of gavage. The analyses were performed 28 days after the arthritis induction and in the beginning of CoQ_{10} supplementation. Concentrations of CoQ_9, CoQ_{10}, αT, and γT were determined by HPLC method with spectrophotometric detection at 275 nm (CoQ) and 295 nm (tocopherols), using external standards [38, 39]. Total CoQ_9 and CoQ_{10} (oxidized and reduced forms) in plasma was measured after oxidation with 1,4-benzoquinone [40]. Mitochondria from hind paw skeletal muscle tissue were isolated by means of differential centrifugation according to slightly modified methods [41, 42]. Mitochondrial proteins were estimated spectrophotometrically [43]. Data were collected and processed using CSW 32 chromatographic station (DataApex Ltd). Concentrations were calculated: in the plasma in μmol/l, in the tissue in nmol/g of wet weight, and in the mitochondria in nmol/mg of proteins. Total antioxidant status (TAS) in plasma was determined using the Randox Total Antioxidant Status kit with colorimetric detection at 600 nm. Markers of inflammation, C-reactive protein (CRP), and monocyte chemotactic protein-1 (MCP-1) were measured by ELISA. Data are expressed as mean ± SEM. Statistical significance between experimental groups was evaluated using Student's t-test, $p < 0.05$, which was considered as a significant result.

2.3 Evaluation of results of administration of coenzyme Q_{10} in experimental arthritis

AA for a period of 28 days significantly increased markers of inflammation—CRP and MCP-1—and decreased TAS (**Table 1**). Concentrations of total CoQ_9 (oxidized and reduced) and γT in plasma of AA rats increased significantly (**Table 2**).

In skeletal muscle tissue and mitochondria of AA rats, concentrations of oxidized form of coenzyme Q_9 ($CoQ_{9\text{-}OX}$) and αT decreased significantly and $CoQ_{10\text{-}OX}$ only slightly. Tissue γT increased compared to controls; in mitochondria the increase was marginally significant ($p = 0.077$), (**Tables 3** and **4**). Treatment of arthritic rats with CoQ_{10} (AA-CoQ) for 28 days partially suppressed inflammatory markers and increased TAS, but not statistically significant (**Table 1**). Elevated concentrations of total CoQ_9 and γT in plasma were corrected to control values. Concentration of CoQ_{10} in plasma increased extremely, demonstrating a good bioavailability of CoQ_{10} administered (**Table 2**). In tissue and mitochondria, concentrations of CoQ_9 and CoQ_{10} increased in comparison with AA rats and were comparable to controls. Concentrations of αT in tissue and mitochondria also increased, in the tissue at the limit of significance ($p = 0.071$) and in mitochondria without statistical significance (**Tables 3** and **4**).

Bioenergetic and antioxidant properties of CoQ_{10} are sufficiently described [44]. However, new research findings suggest that CoQ_{10} supplementation has also lowering effects on circulating inflammatory mediators, including CRP,

Plasma	CRP	MCP-1	TAS
	μg/ml	pg/ml	mmol/l
HC	457.4 ± 21.3	1462 ± 159.2	0.673 ± 0.037
AA	602.2 ± 10.7**	2925 ± 389.1**	0.529 ± 0028*
AA-CoQ	563.3 ± 14.5	2539 ± 144.1	0.562 ± 0.033

*p < 0.05.
**p < 0.01 vs. HC.

Table 1.
Markers of inflammation: C-reactive protein (CRP), monocyte chemotactic protein (MCP-1), and total antioxidant status (TAS) in plasma.

Plasma	$CoQ_{9\text{-}TOT}$	$CoQ_{10\text{-}TOT}$	αT	γT
	μmol/l	μmol/l	μmol/l	μmol/l
HC	0.328 ± 0.023	0.031 ± 0.004	19.9 ± 1.13	0.643 ± 0.051
AA	0.468 ± 0.044**	0.027 ± 0.003	21.6 ± 0.72	0.834 ± 0.060*
AA-CoQ	0.237 ± 0.016++	0.804 ± 0.069++	19.6 ± 1.07	0.678 ± 0.043+

*p < 0.05.
**p < 0.01 vs. HC.
+p < 0.05.
++p < 0.01 vs. AA.

Table 2.
Concentrations of total coenzyme Q_9 ($CoQ_{9\text{-}TOT}$), total coenzyme Q_{10} ($CoQ_{10\text{-}TOT}$), α-tocopherol (αT), and γ-tocopherol (γT) in plasma.

Tissue	$CoQ_{9\text{-}ox}$	$CoQ_{10\text{-}ox}$	αT	γT
	nmol/g ww	nmol/g ww	nmol/g ww	nmol/g ww
HC	43.1 ± 3.01	1.90 ± 0.160	23.0 ± 1.23	0.98 ± 0.042
AA	32.7 ± 2.49*	1.63 ± 0.187	18.7 ± 0.829*	1.39 ± 0.155*
AA-CoQ	40.9 ± 4.07	2.43 ± 2.52+	22.2 ± 1.42	1.07 ± 0.084

*p < 0.05 vs. HC.
+p < 0.05 vs. AA.

Table 3.
Concentrations of oxidized forms of coenzyme Q_9 ($CoQ_{9\text{-}OX}$), coenzyme Q_{10} ($CoQ_{10\text{-}OX}$), α-tocopherol (αT), and γ-tocopherol (γT) in the skeletal muscle tissue.

interleukin 6 (IL-6), and tumor necrosis factor α (TNF-α). Meta-analysis of clinical randomized controlled trials evaluated the effects of CoQ_{10} in some inflammatory diseases but with inconsistent results due to heterogeneity and limited number of studies [45].

In an experimental study, an antiarthritic effect of CoQ_{10} against induced gouty arthritis in rats was found [46]. CoQ_{10} treatment at the dosage 10 mg/kg/body weight for 3 days reduced paw edema, minimized lysosomal enzyme release, boosted antioxidant system, and suppressed lipid peroxidation. Protective mechanism of CoQ_{10} against cartilage degeneration induced by interleukin-1β was studied on isolated rat chondrocytes [47]. The study demonstrated the anticatabolic and cartilage protective potentials of CoQ_{10} by inhibition of overexpression of matrix

Mitochondria	$CoQ_{9\text{-}ox}$	$CoQ_{10\text{-}ox}$	αT	γT
	nmol/mg prt	nmol/mg prt	nmol/mg prt	nmol/mg prt
HC	3.28 ± 0.14	0.144 ± 0.01	0.305 ± 0.02	0.042 ± 0.01
AA	2.67 ± 0.13**	0.126 ± 0.01	0.216 ± 0.02*	0.058 ± 0.01
AA-CoQ	3.16 ± 0.08⁺⁺	0.149 ± 0.01⁺	0.289 ± 0.03	0.052 ± 0.01

$^{*}p < 0.05$.
$^{**}p < 0.01$ vs. HC.
$^{+}p < 0.05$.
$^{++}p < 0.01$ vs. AA.

Table 4.
Concentrations of oxidized forms of coenzyme Q_9 ($CoQ_{9\text{-}OX}$), coenzyme Q_{10} ($CoQ_{10\text{-}OX}$), α-tocopherol (αT), and γ-tocopherol (γT) in skeletal muscle mitochondria.

metalloproteinases which may represent a new approach in the treatment of patients with osteoarthritis. Administration of CoQ_{10} in the dose 100 mg/kg for 28 days suppressed cartilage degeneration by inhibiting inflammatory mediators and OS in an experimental model of rat osteoarthritis [48]. Beneficial effects of CoQ_{10} supplementation on inflammatory cytokines and OS in RA patients were proved. In the double-blind, randomized controlled clinical trial in patients with RA, CoQ_{10} supplementation with 100 mg/day for 2 months led to a significant decrease of malondialdehyde (MDA) formation and a nonsignificant increase of total antioxidant capacity, indicating beneficial effects on OS. CoQ_{10} also suppressed overexpression of inflammatory cytokines TNF-α significantly and IL-6 nonsignificantly [30].

Our results show that administration of CoQ_{10} to rats with induced adjuvant arthritis in the oral daily dose of 100 mg/kg b.w. for 28 days partially corrected inflammatory markers and TAS but without statistical significance (**Table 1**). CoQ_{10} treatment corrected concentration of CoQ_9 in plasma to control value (**Table 2**). In the skeletal muscle tissue and isolated mitochondria, concentrations of CoQ_9 and CoQ_{10} increased in comparison with AA rats and were comparable to controls. Concentrations of αT in tissue and mitochondria were also improved, in the tissue marginally significant and in mitochondria without statistical significance (**Tables 3** and **4**). Sufficient concentrations of CoQ together with αT, the main form of vitamin E, may be important in skeletal muscle function, in regulation of OS and inflammation. The role of vitamin E in regulation of diseases has been extensively studied in humans, animal models, and cell systems. It has been reported that isoforms of vitamin E may have opposing regulatory functions during inflammation, when supplementation with αT was anti-inflammatory and γT pro-inflammatory [33]. Different effects of vitamin E isoforms may result from differences in their metabolism, as αT is preferentially bound α-TTP (α-tocopherol transfer protein), while γT is metabolized mainly through cytochrome P450 and its concentrations in plasma and tissues are dependent on cytochrome P450 metabolism in the liver [49]. Our results show elevated concentrations of γT in plasma and skeletal muscle tissue of arthritic rats together with increased markers of inflammation and decreased TAS (**Tables 1–3**). This confirms the previous findings that inflammation and inhibition of the cytochrome P450 can increase γT concentration [50]. Treatment of arthritic animals with CoQ_{10} corrected elevated levels of γT to control values and showed beneficial effect on concentrations of αT, CoQ_9, and CoQ_{10} in the skeletal muscle tissue and mitochondria. This can help improve bioenergetic function of the skeletal muscle that is impaired by arthritic inflammatory

DOI: http://dx.doi.org/10.5772/intechopen.85568

process. Elevated concentrations of endogenous antioxidants can contribute to regulation of oxidative stress.

3. Hyaluronan in arthritis: regulation of inflammation through antioxidative effects

3.1 The protective properties of hyaluronan

OS is important in the pathogenesis of autoimmune diseases such as RA and in its experimental model-adjuvant arthritis. The control of inflammation and OS in arthritic patients by hyaluronic acid (HA) is one of the approaches to the treatment of RA, concentration of which is reduced in the synovial fluid of patients suffering from arthritis. The most important aspect from a treatment perspective is the fact that HA has been found to be safe and well tolerable. The widespread use of HA also leads to lower use of nonsteroidal anti-inflammatory drugs, which may be an advantage for patients. HA is a high-molecular-weight, ubiquitous glycosaminoglycan (GAG) that naturally occurs within the cartilage and synovial fluid [51]. It is an anionic linear polysaccharide composed of alternating N-acetyl D-glucosamine and D-glucuronic acid residues attached by β(1-4) and β(1-3) glycosidic bonds (**Figure 5**) with molecular mass ranging from 6.5 to 10.9 MDa [52]. It is structurally the simplest compound among GAGs. HA has hydrophilic groups which not only form hydrogen bonds with each other but also interact with water molecules.

In physiological solutions hyaluronan manifests very unusual rheological properties and has exceedingly lubricious and very hydrophilic properties. This is the reason why HA occurs in the salt form, hyaluronate, and is present in every connective tissue and organ such as the skin, synovial fluid, blood vessels, serum, brain, cartilage, heart valves, and the umbilical cord. Synovial fluid in particular has the highest concentration of HA (3–4 mg/ml) compared to anywhere else in the body [53]. HA plays important physiological roles in living organisms which makes it an attractive biomaterial for various medical applications [54, 55]. HA has several diverse physiological functions. Because of its hygroscopic properties, hyaluronan significantly influences hydration and the physical properties of the extracellular matrix. In addition to its function as a passive structural molecule, hyaluronan also acts as a signaling molecule by interacting with cell surface receptors resulting in the activation and modulation of signaling cascades that influence inflammatory processes, including the antioxidant scavenging of the ROS and/or RNS arising from polymorphonuclear nucleosides' respiratory bursts as well as cell migration,

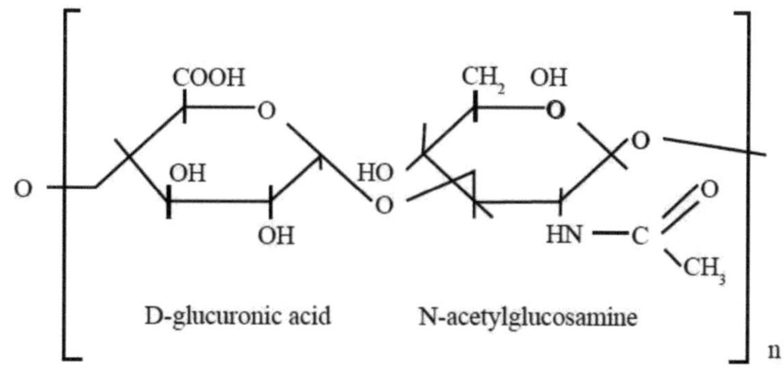

Figure 5.
Chemical structure of hyaluronan.

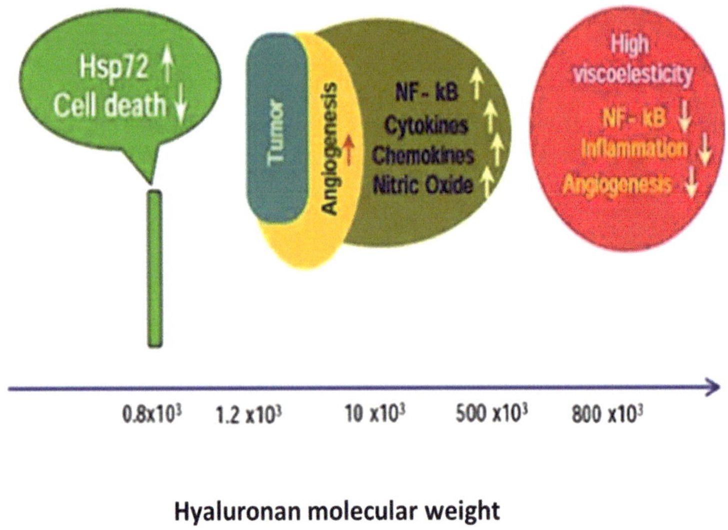

Figure 6.
Biological effects of hyaluronan oligosaccharides depend on their molecular weight.

proliferation, and gene expression [55]. Moreover, there is a brisk metabolism of HA in humans, with approximately one-third (around 5 g) of total HA were degraded and replaced daily predominantly by the reticuloendothelial system [56].

Many physiological effects of HA may be functions of its molecular weight. Already in the year 2000, Camenisch and McDonald [57] published an overview of the effects of HA, dependent on its molecular weight. HA of an average mass of 0.2 MDa prolonged survival of peripheral blood eosinophils in vitro but HA of the mass of 3–6 MDa had a much lower effect. This observation follows from several previous reports suggesting distinct angiogenic and pro-inflammatory biological activities of lower molecular weight HA or HA oligomers. Lower molecular weight HA, but not high-molecular-weight HA, stimulates the production of metalloelastase and expression of inducible nitric oxide synthase in rat liver endothelial and Kupffer cells. In addition, it has been reported that low-molecular-weight degradation products of HA elicit pro-inflammatory responses by modulating the toll-like receptor-4 or by activating the nuclear factor kappa B (NF-kB). In contrast, high-molecular-weight HA manifests an anti-inflammatory effect via CD receptors and by inhibiting NF-kB activation [58] (**Figure 6**). During progression of inflammation and OS in the joints, HA depolymerizes into lower molecular weight compounds (2.7–4.5 MDa) which consequently diminish the mechanical and viscoelastic properties of the synovial fluid [51] as well as activate different signaling pathways. Randomized, double-blinded, placebo-controlled trials have proven the effectiveness of HA (administered by the intra-articular injection or in the form of dietary supplements 48–240 mg/day) for the treatment of symptoms associated with synovitis [53].

Kogan et al. [59] suggest mechanisms, by which HA could exert its therapeutic effect: (i) restoration of elastic and viscous properties of the synovial fluid; (ii) induction of the endogenous synthesis of HA by synovial cells by the effect of exogenous HA, stimulation of chondrocyte proliferation, and inhibition of cartilage degradation; (iii) anti-inflammatory action of HA, since the therapy is associated with decreased inflammatory cell count in synovial fluid, modulation of cytokine expression, and reduction of ROS content; and (iv) analgesic effect. An important feature of HA is its antioxidant properties. The direct radical-scavenging properties of HA have been demonstrated in various experimental models. These results are in accord with the concept that hyaluronic acid mainly acts as a chemical ROS

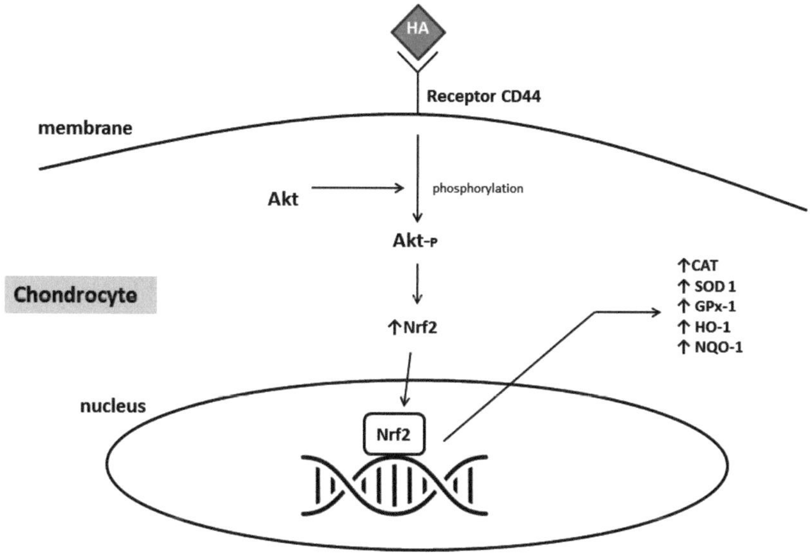

Figure 7.
Hyaluronan increases enzymatic antioxidant defense through Nrf2 upregulation. HA, hyaluronan; AKT, serine/threonine protein kinase; Nrf2, factor erythroid 2-related factor 2; CAT, catalase; SOD-1, superoxide dismutase-1; GPx-1, glutathione peroxidase; HO-1, hemeoxygenase-1; NQO-1, NAD(P)H (quinone)dehydrogenase 1.

and/or RNS scavenger in extracellular space [55]. In favor of a direct antiradical activity, there is also the ability of hyaluronic acid (biopolymer) to form a viscous, pericellular meshwork that restricts ROS movement in close proximity to cells and thus interferes with the oxidative cascade [55]. The presence of CD44 hyaluronate receptors on the plasma membrane of granulocytes, which mediate the internalization of the biopolymer via endocytosis, offers another key to interpretation of the HA antioxidant mechanism of action, that is, the reduction in ROS and/or RNS is caused by hyaluronic acid internalization and the intracellular neutralization of the radicals [60]. One important pharmacological function of HA is the reduction of cellular superoxide generation and accumulation through nuclear factor erythroid 2-related factor 2 (Nrf2) regulation, which is a master transcription factor in cellular redox reactions. Antioxidants and phase II detoxifying enzymes such as catalase (CAT), superoxide dismutase (SOD), heme oxygenase-1, glutathione S-transferase, glutathione peroxidase (GPx), and thioredoxin are coordinated at transcription level by Nrf2, so the hyaluronic acid could affect the activity and quantity of these antioxidant enzymes (**Figure 7**) [61].

The aim of this study was to compare the effect of different molecular weights of hyaluronic acid (0.43, 0.99, and 1.73 MDa) applied in two different doses (0.5 and 5 mg/kg b.w.), on the rat hind paw volume and parameters of OS: activity of antioxidant enzymes in erythrocytes (SOD, GPx, CAT), total antioxidant capacity, and concentration of lipid hydroperoxides (LPx, marker of oxidative damage to lipids) in plasma.

3.2 Experimental design of adjuvant arthritis with administration of hyaluronan

Male Lewis rats were randomly divided into groups according to the treatment they received:

(1) Not treated control groups (HC)

(2) Arthritic animals not treated with HA (AA)

(3) Arthritic animals treated with hyaluronic acid (HA) during 28 days:

(a) Group NHA (M_w(HA) = 0.43 MDa, in an oral daily dose of 0.5 mg/kg b.w.)

(b) Group 5NHA (M_w(HA) = 0.43 MDa, in an oral daily dose of 5 mg/kg b.w.)

(c) Group SHA (M_w(HA) = 0.99 MDa, in an oral daily dose of 0.5 mg/kg b.w.)

(d) Group 5SHA (M_w(HA) = 0.99 MDa, in an oral daily dose of 5 mg/kg b.w.)

(e) Group VHA (M_w(HA) = 1.79 MDa, in an oral daily dose of 0.5 mg/kg b.w.)

(f) Group 5VHA (M_w(HA) = 1.79 MDa, in an oral daily dose of 5 mg/kg b.w.).

Adjuvant arthritis was induced by a single intradermal injection of heat-inactivated *Mycobacterium butyricum* [36, 37]. Blood was collected to obtain plasma and erythrocytes. Total antioxidant capacity and concentration of LPx were determined in plasma. Isolated erythrocytes were washed three times with 0.15 mol/l NaCl solution. After centrifugation (900 × g, 5 min, 4°C), erythrocytes were hemolyzed by adding a triple volume of cold distilled water and stored at −20°C until further analyses. Activities of Cu/Zn-superoxide dismutase (SOD), glutathione peroxidase (GPx) and catalase (CAT), and the concentration of hemoglobin (Hb) were determined in the hemolysate of erythrocytes. From clinical parameters hind paw volume (HPV) was evaluated [62]. The activity of SOD was determined using a commercial kit. The results are expressed in U of SOD per mg Hb. The activity of GPx was also determined by a commercial kit. The results are expressed in μkat per g Hb. CAT activity was determined by a modified method according to [63], and the results are expressed in μkat per g Hb. The total antioxidant capacity of plasma was measured using the Trolox equivalent antioxidant capacity (TEAC) assay [64]. Quantification was performed using the dose-response curve for the reference of antioxidant Trolox, a water-soluble form of vitamin E. The results are presented as mmol of Trolox per ml of plasma. The level of LPx in plasma was measured using the method previously described by [64], and the results are presented in nmol per ml of plasma. The experimental data were expressed as the mean ± SEM. Statistical analysis was performed using Student's t-test. The limit for statistical significance was set at $p < 0.05$.

3.3 Evaluation of results of administration of hyaluronans in experimental arthritis

The onset of AA confirmed the increased hind paw volume in arthritic groups (data not shown). HA administration did not cause a significant reduction of HPV in any molecular weight and at any doses used. Parameters of OS are summarized in **Table 5**. Rats with AA had significantly higher activity of SOD and CAT in erythrocytes as well as higher concentration of LPx in comparison to HC group. Activity of GPx was marginally increased ($p = 0.054$) and TEAC was not changed.

The effect of hyaluronic acid on antioxidant enzyme activities, the total antioxidant capacity of plasma, and the effect on LPx concentration are summarized in **Table 6**. We have found significantly higher erythrocyte SOD activity after administration of HA in all molecular forms and doses, whereas GPx activity was significantly higher only after HA administration at the higher dose. At a lower

Parameter	HC	AA	P
SOD (U/mg Hb)	422.65 ± 15.93	546.48 ± 14.25	0.0001
GPx (μkat/g Hb)	51.10 ± 1.45	56.86 ± 2.26	0.054
CAT (μkat/g Hb)	2.61 ± 0.18	3.06 ± 0.09	0.044
TEAC (mmol/l)	4.01 ± 0.07	4.04 ± 0.09	n.s.
LPx (nmol/ml)	20.76 ± 3.55	53.34 ± 5.83	0.003

Control group (HC), arthritis group (AA), statistical significance (P).
Activities of superoxide dismutase (SOD), glutathione peroxidase (GPx) and catalase (CAT) in erythrocytes, total antioxidant capacity (TEAC), and concentration of lipoperoxides (LPx) in plasma were measured on the 28th day.

Table 5.
Oxidative stress markers in rats with adjuvant arthritis.

dose, we observed a significantly elevated GPx activity only in the SHA group (M_w(HA) = 0.99 MDa). For both enzymes, we have also noticed a significant difference between the effects of the same molecular forms of HA but administered at different doses. The higher HA dose (5 mg/kg b.w.) significantly increased the GPx activity compared to the lower dose (0.5 mg/kg b.w.).

Subanalysis based on the molecular weight of the administered HA revealed the higher SOD activity in the VHA group compared to NHA (p = 0.0013), in the 5SHA and 5VHA groups compared to 5NHA (p = 0.0025, respectively, p = 0.0308), and VHA compared to SHA (p = 0.0107). The higher GPx activity was found in SHA group in comparison to NHA (p = 0.0425), in 5SHA, respectively, 5VHA in comparison to 5NHA (p = 0.0217 respectively p = 0. 0058), and lower activity in VHA group in comparison to SHA (p = 0.0069). A similar trend was observed in the effect of HA on the total antioxidant capacity of plasma. The values of this parameter were increased in all groups but significantly only when HA was administered at a higher concentration.

Also, the higher HA dose significantly increased the total antioxidant capacity compared to the lower dose. Differences in the effect of HA with different molecular weights were seen only in the 5VHA group, whereas TEAC was significantly increased when compared to the 5NHA group (p = 0.0212). On the other hand, HA in all molecular weights and at both monitored doses significantly reduced CAT activity. The effect of different doses was found only in SHA and VHA groups, where the higher dose significantly reduced activity in SHA (p = 0.0004) and significantly increased activity in VHA (p = 0.0192). At higher doses, we found significant reductions of CAT activity in VHA compared to both NHA and SHA (p = 0.0018 and p = 0.0001) and in 5SHA compared to 5NHA (p = 0.0194). Concentration of LPx was significantly reduced in all monitored groups, with no differences in the effect of different molecular weights of HA or in the effect of doses.

Our study, for the first time, evaluated the ability of the HA to affect the activity of erythrocyte antioxidant enzymes, as well as total antioxidant capacity and LPx of rats with AA. We have found increased activities of antioxidant enzymes (SOD, GPx and CAT) in erythrocytes of AA rats with increased plasma LPx concentration. Administration of different molecular weights of HA (0.43, 0.99, and 1.73 MDa) applied in two different doses (0.5 and 5 mg/kg b.w.) resulted in a further increase in activities of these enzymes, but we observed a decreased concentration of plasma LPx.

Inflammatory diseases, including RA, are characterized by sustained overproduction of ROS, accompanied by disruption of the antioxidant defense system resulting in local and systemic OS development in the affected joint-synovial fluid [65], and in addition to the joints, plasma and some organs are affected [66]. The results of the present work showed that in spite of the increased antioxidant enzyme

Parameter	AA	NHA	5NHA	SHA	5SHA	VHA	5VHA
SOD (U/mg Hb)	546.48 ± 14.25	615.26 ± 23.00*	817.37 ± 28.45***	661.41 ± 24.34**	944.73 ± 41.35***	777.17 ± 30.91***	869.42 ± 34.96***
GPx (μkat/g Hb)	56.86 ± 2.26	55.53 ± 3.297	71.17 ± 3.76**	64.95 ± 2.65*	84.89 ± 4.20***	55.44 ± 1.40	93.52 ± 6.83***
CAT (μkat/g Hb)	3.06 ± 0.09	2.61 ± 0.15*	2.40 ± 0.08***	2.81 ± 0.12	2.06 ± 0.10***	2.02 ± 0.05***	2.28 ± 0.09***
TEAC (mmol/l)	4.04 ± 0.09	4.23 ± 0.09	4.57 ± 0.03**	4.07 ± 0.10	4.80 ± 0.24**	4.19 ± 0.10	4.73 ± 0.06**
LPx (nmol/ml)	53.34 ± 5.83	24.35 ± 1.19**	26.84 ± 1.70*	25.3 ± 4.67**	27.98 ± 3.45*	25.13 ± 5.53**	24.49 ± 2.67*

*$p < 0.05$.
**$p < 0.01$.
***$p < 0.001$ *vs. AA.*
NHA ($M_w(HA) = 0.43$ MDa, 0.5 mg/kg b.w.); 5NHA ($M_w(HA) = 0.43$ MDa, 5 mg/kg b.w.); SHA ($M_w(HA) = 0.99$ MDa, 0.5 mg/kg b.w.); 5SHA ($M_w(HA) = 0.99$ MDa, 5 mg/kg b.w.); VHA ($M_w(HA) = 1.79$ MDa, 0.5 mg/kg b.w.); 5VHA ($M_w(HA) = 1.79$ MDa, 5 mg/kg b.w.).
Activities of superoxide dismutase (SOD), glutathione peroxidase (GPx) and catalase (CAT) in erythrocytes, total antioxidant capacity (TEAC), and concentration of lipoperoxides (LPx) in plasma were measured on the 28th day.

Table 6.
Effect of hyaluronic acid on oxidative stress markers.

activities found in erythrocytes of rats with AA, lipid peroxidation in plasma is increased in comparison to control group. Lipid peroxides are generated at the site of tissue injury due to increased ROS production during chronic inflammation and diffuse into blood where they can be estimated [67]. Studies have reported raised levels of MDA, 4-hydroxynonenal, and other markers of oxidative lipid damage in the serum, plasma, and erythrocytes of RA patients [65, 68]. Kumar et al. [68] also found increased plasma SOD activity in patients with RA, similarly to Mazzetti et al. [69]. Similar results were found in early type 2 diabetes patients [70], where increased antioxidant defense in plasma and erythrocytes is explained as a potential mechanism that can overcome oxidative damage induced by ROS overproduction. There are some reports on erythrocyte SOD, CAT, and GPx activities in patients with RA or in rats with AA, but the results are controversial [71, 72]. It is possible that differences between different investigators' results, regarding antioxidant status, are due to differences in the stage of the disease. Chronic inflammation may deplete antioxidant defenses, whereas acute inflammation can upgrade them [73].

In our study, we did not notice a change in total plasma antioxidant capacity in the group of arthritic rats, similarly to Bracht et al. [66] in the mono-arthritic rats. Vijayakumar et al. [74] confirmed susceptibility of erythrocytes to peroxide stress. They have found not only elevated plasma lipid peroxidation but also the excessive lipid peroxidation in erythrocytes and erythrocyte membranes. In addition, they found decreased glutathione levels and GPx activity in plasma but increase in erythrocytes of RA patients as compared to healthy subjects. Superoxide radicals play an important role as a chemical mediator on the inflammatory response to RA. The increased activity of plasma SOD observed in the abovementioned studies as well as increased activity of SOD in erythrocytes observed in our study could therefore be found due to their function in dismutation of superoxide radicals excess. Thus, the activities of antioxidant enzymes in blood cells including erythrocytes could reflect the rate of OS in the affected cells. This could be a suitable approach for assessing the effect of therapy aimed to reduce inflammation and OS.

Our study demonstrated that HA (in all molecular weights and in both doses), orally administrated in a rat model of AA, affected all measured markers of OS. Furthermore, erythrocyte antioxidant markers including SOD and GPx, and total antioxidant capacity of plasma, increased significantly during 28 days of supplementation. On the other hand, we have found decreased erythrocyte CAT activity and plasma concentration of LPx. Based on our results, we cannot give a clear explanation how the HA can affect all observed parameters. Numerous studies have confirmed the effect of HA on the activity of these enzymes but in other cells and tissues and not in erythrocytes [75, 76]. It was confirmed that HA can reduce cellular superoxide generation and its accumulation through Nrf2 regulation which can induce transcription of antioxidant enzymes such as SOD, GPx, CAT, and others [61]. Supplementary to its primary role in cytoprotection, Nrf2 is also linked to differentiation, proliferation, growth, and apoptosis, and it is thought that Nrf2 has evolved from an original role in hematopoiesis and the regulation of cell differentiation from early lineages [77].

Based on this, we could assume that during proliferation and differentiation of hematopoietic stem cells, expression of antioxidant enzymes can be induced. In the induction of expression, the CD44 receptor, which binds HA and mediates its role as a signal molecule, could have importance. We could just speculate if the activities of antioxidant enzymes in erythrocytes reflect the effect of administered HA on the activities of these enzymes in other tissues as well. As we observed an increase in both SOD and GPx activities in erythrocytes of AA rats under HA supplementation, we anticipate a similar mechanism of HA action in other cells, e.g., in chondrocytes, where the increase in antioxidant potential could provide antioxidant protection of synovial fluid and reduction of lipoperoxidation not only in the synovium but also in the plasma as what we have found in our study. Also, the direct antioxidant ability of HA, which has been described, could contribute to the reduction of lipoperoxidation [55]. However, further studies need to be made to confirm these assumptions.

4. Conclusion

New treatment strategies based on blockade of cytokine pathways in late stages of RA are progressing. In spite of their benefits, long-time utilization of these blocking agents has indicated side effects. The antioxidant defense system includes endogenous (enzymatic and nonenzymatic) and exogenous (dietary) antioxidants that interact in establishing redox homeostasis in the body. Therapeutic benefits from antioxidant treatment are primarily bound to reduction of systemic OS.

CoQ_{10} treatment significantly improved concentrations of the investigated endogenous antioxidants (CoQ_9-total, CoQ_{10}-total, and gamma tocopherol in plasma). CoQ_{10} for its bioenergetic, antioxidant, and anti-inflammatory properties might be therapeutically useful for a long-term supplementary administration to patients with inflammatory diseases such as RA.

In our study, we have shown the ability of per orally administered HA to improve the antioxidant defense (SOD, GPx, and total antioxidant capacity of plasma). This therapeutic effect of HA could be a result of direct (intestinal absorption) and indirect (intestinal cell immunomodulatory) anti-inflammatory activities. Recent results have shown that dietary high-molecular-weight HA can be distributed to connective tissues. Dietary HA could be beneficial for joints, knee pain, relief of synovial effusion, or inflammation and improvement of muscular knee strength. HA also binds to toll-like receptor-4 (TLR4) in the luminal surface of the large intestine resulting in the downregulation of systemic proinflammatory cytokines.

However, further research is needed with endogenous antioxidants, mainly human studies, in order to establish an antioxidative treatment approach in inflammatory-based diseases such as RA.

Acknowledgements

The experiments were supported by APVV-15-0308, VEGA 2/0044/15, and VEGA 2/0115/19. In the experiment realization, Danica Mihalova, Jana Urgosova, Frantisek Drafi, Martina Horvathova, Kristina Farkasova, Anna Gvozdjakova, Olga Vancova, and Olga Ulicna were involved. Hyaluronan samples were purchased by cofounder and current CEO Vladimir Velebny (Contipro, Czech Republic). Thanks to Miloslav Zloh for the technical assistance in manuscript preparation.

Conflict of interest

The authors declare that they do not have any conflict of interest.

Author details

Katarina Bauerova[1,2,*], Jarmila Kucharska[3], Silvester Ponist[1], Lukas Slovak[1], Karol Svik[1], Vladimir Jakus[3] and Jana Muchova[3]

1 Institute of Experimental Pharmacology and Toxicology, Centre of Experimental Medicine, Slovak Academy of Sciences, Bratislava, Slovakia

2 Faculty of Pharmacy, Comenius University, Bratislava, Slovakia

3 Faculty of Medicine, Comenius University, Bratislava, Slovakia

*Address all correspondence to: katarina.bauerova@savba.sk

References

[1] Altindag O, Karakoc M, Kocyigit A, Celik H, Soran N. Increased DNA damage and oxidative stress in patients with rheumatoid arthritis. Clinical Biochemistry. 2007;**40**:167-171. DOI: 10.1016/j.clinbiochem.2006.10.006

[2] Kinne RW, Brauer R, Stuhlmuller B, Palombo-Kinne E, Burmester GR. Macrophages in rheumatoid arthritis. Arthritis Research. 2000;**2**:189-202. DOI: 10.1186/ar86

[3] Tas SW, Maracle CX, Balogh E, Szekanecz Z. Targeting of proangiogenic signalling pathways in chronic inflammation. Nature Reviews Rheumatology. 2016;**12**:111-140. DOI: 10.1038/nrrheum.2015.164

[4] Quinones-Flores CM, Gonzalez-Chavez SA, Del Rio ND, Pacheco-Tena C. Oxidative stress relevance in the pathogenesis of the rheumatoid arthritis: A systematic review. BioMed Research International. 2016;**2016**:6097417. DOI: 10.1155/2016/6097417

[5] Khojah HM, Ahmed S, Abdel-Rahman MS, Hamza AB. Reactive oxygen and nitrogen species in patients with rheumatoid arthritis as potential biomarkers for disease activity and the role of antioxidants. Free Radical Biology & Medicine. 2016;**97**:285-291. DOI: 10.1016/j.freeradbiomed.2016.06.020

[6] Ahmed U, Anwar A, Savage RS, Thornalley PJ, Rabbani N. Protein oxidation, nitration and glycation biomarkers for early-stage diagnosis of osteoarthritis of the knee and typing and progression of arthritic disease. Arthritis Research & Therapy. 2016;**18**:250. DOI: 10.1186/s13075-016-1154-3

[7] Ye W, Yhu S, Liao C, Xiao J, Wu Q, Lin Z, et al. Advanced oxidation protein products induce apoptosis of human chondrocyte through reactive oxygen species/mediated mitochondrial dysfunction and endoplasmic reticulum stress pathways. Fundamental & Clinical Pharmacology. 2017;**31**:64-74. DOI: 10.1111/fcp.12229

[8] Hoffmann MH, Griffiths HR. The dual role of reactive oxygen species in autoimmune and inflammatory diseases: Evidence from preclinical models. Free Radical Biology & Medicine. 2018;**125**:62-71. DOI: 10.1016/j.freeradbiomed.2018.03.016

[9] McGarry T, Biniecka M, Veale DJ, Fearon U. Hypoxia, oxidative stress and inflammation. Free Radical Biology & Medicine. 2018;**25**:15-24. DOI: 10.1016/j.freeradbiomed.2018.03.042

[10] Phull AR, Nasir B, Ul Haq I, Kim SJ. Oxidative stress, consequences and ROS mediated cellular signaling in rheumatoid arthritis. Chemico-Biological Interactions. 2018;**281**:21-136

[11] Filippin LI, Vercelino R, Marroni NP, Xavier RM. Redox signaling and the inflammatory response in rheumatoid arthritis. Journal of Clinical & Experimental Immunology. 2008;**152**:415-422. DOI: 10.1111/j.1365-2249.2008.03634.x

[12] Hagfors L, Leanderson P, Skoldstam L, Andersson J, Johansson G. Antioxidant intake, plasma antioxidants and oxidative stress in a randomized, controlled, parallel, Mediterranean diatery intervention study on patients with rheumatoid arthritis. Nutrition Journal. 2003;**2**:5. DOI: 10.1186/1475-2891-2-5

[13] Mironczuk-Chodakowska I, Witkowska AM, Zujko ME. Endogeneous non-enzymatic antioxidants in the human body. Advances in Medical Sciences. 2018;**63**:68-78. DOI: 10.1016/j.advms.2017.05.005

[14] Muftuoglu M, Mori M, de Souza-Pinto NC. Formation and repair of oxidative damage in the mitochondrial DNA. Mitochondrion. 2014;**17**:164-181. DOI: 10.1016/j.mito.2014.03.007

[15] Gvozdjakova A, editor. Mitochondrial Medicine: Mitochodrial Metabolism, Diseases, Diagnosis and Therapy. Netherlands: Springer Publisher; 2008. ISBN 978-1-4020-6713-6

[16] Lopez-Armada MJ, Riveiro-Naveira RR, Vaamonde-Garcia C, Valcarcel-Ares MN. Mitochondrial dysfunction and the inflammatory response. Mitochondrion. 2013;**13**:106-118. DOI: 10.1016/j.mito.2013.01.003

[17] Tawfik MK. Combination of coenzyme Q_{10} with methotrexate supresses Freund's complete adjuvant-induced synovial inflammation with reduced hepatotoxicity in rats: Effect on oxidative stress and inflammation. International Immunopharmacology. 2015;**24**:80-87. DOI: 10.1016/j.intimp.2014.018

[18] DePalma L, Chillemi C, Albanelli S, Rapali S, Bertoni-Freddari C. Muscle involvement in rheumatoid arthritis: An ultrastructural study. Ultrastructural Pathology. 2000;**24**:151-156. DOI: 10.1080/01913120050132886

[19] Crane FL, Navas P. The diversity of coenzyme Q function. Molecular Aspects of Medicine. 1997;**18**:1-6

[20] Mitchel P. The vital protonmotive role of coenzyme Q. In: Folkers K, Littarru GP, Yamagami T, editors. Biomedical and Clinical Aspects of Coenzyme Q. Vol. 6. Amsterdam: Elsevier Science Publishers BV; 1991. pp. 3-10. ISBN: 0-444-81152-4

[21] Ernster L, Dallner G. Biochemical, physiological and medical aspects of ubiquinone function. Biochimica et Biophysica Acta. 1995;**1271**:195-204

[22] Lenaz G, Fato R, Castellucio C, Cavazzoni M, Estronell E, Huertas JE, et al. An updating of the biochemical function of coenzyme Q in mitochondria. Molecular Aspects of Medicine. 1994;**15**:29-56

[23] Gvozdjakova A, Kucharska J. Implication of coenzyme Q depletion in heart transplantation. In: Kagan VE, Quinn DJ, editors. Coenzyme Q: Molecular Mechanisms in Health and Disease. CRC Press LLC, Boca Raton, London, New York, Washington, D.C.: CRC Press LLC; 2000. pp. 293-304. ISBN 0-8493-8732-9

[24] Kucharska J, Braunova Z, Ulicna O, Zlatos L, Gvozdjakova A. Deficit of coenzyme Q in heart and liver mitochondria of rats with streptozotocin-induced diabetes. Physiological Research. 2000;**49**:411-418. ISSN 0862-8408

[25] Jain SK, Levine SN. Elevated lipid peroxidation and vitamin E-quinone levels in heart ventricles of streptozotocin-treated diabetic rats. Free Radical Biology & Medicine. 1995;**18**:337-341

[26] Stefek M, Sotnikova R, Okruhlicova L, Volkovova K, Kucharska J, Gajdosik A, et al. Effect of dietary supplementation with the pyridoindole antioxidant stobadine on antioxidant state and ultrastructure of diabetic rat myocardium. Acta Diabetologica. 2000;**37**:111-117

[27] Kucharska J, Gvozdjakova A, Stefek M, Sotnikova R, Sumbalova Z. Adaptive changes of antioxidant status in development of experimental diabetes. Bratislava Medical Journal. 2001;**102**:515-519

[28] Droge W. Free radicals in the physiological control of cell function. Physiological Reviews. 2002;**82**:47-95. DOI: 10.1152/physrev.00018.2001

[29] Kagan VE, Fabisiak YP, Tyurina YY. Independent and concerted antioxidant functions of coenzyme Q. In: Kagan

VE, Quinn DJ, editors. Coenzyme Q: Molecular Mechanisms in Health and Disease. CRC Press LLC, Boca Raton, London, New York, Washington, D.C.: CRC Press LLC; 2000. pp. 119-129. ISBN 0-8493-8732-9

[30] Abdollahzad H, Aghdashi MA, Jafarabadi MA, Alipour B. Effects of coenzyme Q_{10} supplementation on inflammatory cytokines (TNF-α, IL-6) and oxidative stress in rheumatoid arthritis patients: A randomized controlled trial. Archives of Medical Research. 2015;**46**:527-533. DOI: 10.1016/j.aremed.2015.08.006

[31] Jiang Q, Christen S, Shigenaga MK, Ames BN. γ-Tocopherol, the major form of vitamin E in the US diet, deserves more attention. The American Journal of Clinical Nutrition. 2001;**74**:714-722. DOI: 10.1093/ajcn/74.6.714

[32] Jiang Q. Natural forms of vitamin E: Metabolism, antioxidant, and antiinflammatory activities and their role in disease prevention and therapy. Free Radical Biology & Medicine. 2014;**72**:76-90. DOI: 10.1016/j.freeradbiomed.2014.03.035

[33] Cook-Mills JM, McCary CA. Isoforms of vitamin E differentially regulate inflammation. Endocrine, Metabolic & Immune Disorders Drug Targets. 2010;**10**:348-366

[34] Chung E, Mo H, Wang S, Zu Y, Efakhani M, Rios SR, et al. Potential roles of vitamin E in age-related changed in skeletal muscle health. Nutrition Research. 2018;**49**:23-36. DOI: 10.1016/nutres.2017.09.005

[35] Knekt P, Heliovaara M, Aho K, Alfthan G, Marniemi J, Aromaa A. Serum selenium, serum alpha-tocopherol, and the risk of rheumatoid arthritis. Epidemiology. 2000;**11**:402-405

[36] Slovak L, Svik K, Mihalova D, Toth J, Czigle S, Paskova L, et al. Ferulaldehyde improves the effect of methotrexate in experimental arthritis. Molecules. 2017;**22**:191. DOI: 10.3390/molecules22111911

[37] Slovak L, Ponist S, Fedorova T, Logvinenko A, Levachova I, Samsonova O, et al. Evaluation of liposomal carnosine in adjuvant arthritis. General Physiology and Biophysics. 2017;**36**:471-479. DOI: 10.4149/gpb_2017014

[38] Lang JK, Gohil K, Packer L. Simultaneous determination of tocopherols, ubiquinols, and ubiquinones in blood, plasma, tissue homogenates, and subcellular fractions. Analytical Biochemistry. 1986;**157**:106-116

[39] Kucharska J, Gvozdjakova A, Simko F. Simvastatin decreased coenzyme Q in the left ventricle and skeletal muscle but not in the brain and liver in L-NAME-induced hypertension. Physiological Research. 2007;**56**:49-54

[40] Mosca F, Fattorini D, Bompadre S, Littarru GP. Assay of coenzyme Q_{10} in plasma by a single dilution step. Analytical Biochemistry. 2002;**305**: 49-54. DOI: 10.1006/abio.2002.5653

[41] Palmer JW, Tandler B, Hoppel CL. Biochemical properties of subsarcolemmal and interfibrillar mitochondria isolated from rat cardiac muscle. The Journal of Biological Chemistry. 1977;**252**(23):8731-8739

[42] Koves TR, Noland RC, Bates AL, Henes ST, Muoio DM, Cortright RN. Subsarcolemmal and intermyofibrilar mitochondria play distinct roles in regulating skeletal muscle fatty acid metabolism. American Journal of Physiology Cell Physiology. 2005;**288**:1074-1082. DOI: 0.1152/ajpcell.00391.2004

[43] Lowry DH, Rosenbrough NY, Farr AL, Randall RJ. Protein measurement with the Folin phenol

reagent. The Journal of Biological Chemistry. 1951;**193**:265-276

[44] Gvozdjakova A. In: Cornelissen G, Singh RB, editors. Recent Advances in Mitochondrial Medicine and Coenzyme Q_{10}. New York: Nova Science Publishers, Inc; 2018. p. 450. ISBN: 978-1-53613-149-9

[45] Fan L, Feng Y, Chen G-C, Qin L-Q, Fu C-L, Chen L-H. Effects of coenzyme Q_{10} supplementation on inflammatory markers: A systemic review and meta-analysis of randomized controlled trials. Pharmacological Research. 2017;**119**:128-136. DOI: 10.1016/j.phrs.2017.01.032

[46] Lavinya BU, Bardhan I, Prince SE. Efficacy of coenzyme Q_{10} in inhibiting monosodium urate crystal-induced inflammation in rats. European Journal of Pharmacology. 2016;**791**:589-594. DOI: 10/1016/j.ejphar.2016.09.036

[47] Li X, Guo Y, Huang S, He M, Liu Q, Chen W, et al. Coenzyme Q_{10} prevents the interleukin-1 beta induced inflammatory response via inhibition of MAPK signaling pathways in rat articular chondrocytes. Drug Development Research. 2017;**78**:403-410. DOI: 10.1002/ddr.21412

[48] Lee J, Hong YS, Jeong JH, Yang EJ, Jhun JY, Park MK, et al. Coenzyme Q_{10} ameliorates pain and cartilage degradation in a rat model of osteoarthritis by regulating nitric oxide and inflammatory cytokines. PLoS One. 2013;**8**:e69362. DOI: 10.1371/journal.pone.0069362

[49] Abe C, Uchida T, Ohta M, Ichikawa T, Yamashita K, Ikeda S. Cytochrome P450-dependent metabolism of vitamin E isoforms is a critical determinant of their tissue concentrations in rats. Lipids. 2007;**42**:637-645. DOI: 10.1007/s11745-007-3064-2

[50] Cooney RV, Franke AA, Wilkens LR, Gill J, Kolonel LN. Elevated plasma γ-tocopherol and decreased α-tocopherol in men are associated with inflammatory markers and decreased plasma 25-OH vitamin D. Nutrition and Cancer. 2008;**60**:21-29. DOI: 10.1080/01635580802404162

[51] Bowman S, Awad ME, Hamrick MW, Hunter M, Fulzele S. Recent advances in hyaluronic acid based therapy for osteoarthritis. Clinical and Translational Medicine. 2018;**7**:6. DOI: 10.1186/s40169-017-0180-3

[52] Altman RD, Manjoo A, Fierlinger A, Niazi F, Nicholls M. The mechanism of action for hyaluronic acid treatment in the osteoarthritic knee: A systematic review. BMC Musculoskeletal Disorders. 2015;**16**:321. DOI: 10.1186/s12891-015-0775-z

[53] Oe M, Tashiro T, Yoshida H, Nishiyama Y, Masuda Y, Maruyama K, et al. Oral hyaluronan relieves knee pain: A review. Nutrition Journal. 2016;**15**:11. DOI: 10.1186/s12937-016-0128-2

[54] Kim H, Jeong H, Han S, Beack S, Hwang BW, Shin M, et al. Hyaluronate and its derivatives for customized biomedical applications. Biomaterials. 2017;**123**:155-171. DOI: 10.1016/j.biomaterials.2017.01.029

[55] Braga PC, Dal Sasso M, Lattuada N, Greco V, Sibilia V, Zucca E, et al. Antioxidant activity of hyaluronic acid investigated by means of chemiluminescence of equine neutrophil bursts and electron paramagnetic resonance spectroscopy. Journal of Veterinary Pharmacology and Therapeutics. 2015;**38**:48-54. DOI: 10.1111/jvp.12141

[56] Fraser JR, Laurent TC, Laurent UB. Hyaluronan: Its nature, distribution, functions and turnover. Journal of Internal Medicine. 1997;**242**:27-33

[57] Camenisch TD, McDonald JA. Hyaluronan: Is bigger better. American Journal of Respiratory Cell and

Molecular Biology. 2000;**23**:431-433. DOI: 10.1165/ajrcmb.23.4.f201

[58] Campo GM, Avenoso A, Campo S, D'Ascola A, Nastasi G, Calatroni A. Molecular size hyaluronan differently modulates toll-like receptor-4 in LPS-induced inflammation in mouse chondrocytes. Biochimie. 2010;**92**:204-215. DOI: 10.1016/j.biochi.2009.10.006

[59] Kogan G, Soltes L, Stern R, Gemeiner P. Hyaluronic acid: A natural biopolymer with a broad range of biomedical and industrial applications. Biotechnology Letters. 2007;**29**:17-25. DOI: 10.1007/s10529-006-9219-z

[60] Halicka HD, Mitlitski V, Heeter J, Balazs EA, Darzynkiewicz Z. Attenuation of the oxidative burst-induced DNA damage in human leukocytes by hyaluronan. International Journal of Molecular Medicine. 2009;**23**:695-699

[61] Onodera Y, Teramura T, Takehara T, Fukuda K. Hyaluronic acid regulates a key redox control factor Nrf2 via phosphorylation of Akt in bovine articular chondrocytes. FEBS Open Bio. 2015;**5**: 476-484. DOI: 10.1016/j.fob.2015.05.007

[62] Gardi C, Bauerova K, Stringa B, Kuncirova V, Slovak L, Ponist S, et al. Quercetin reduced inflammation and increased antioxidant defense in rat adjuvant arthritis. Archives of Biochemistry and Biophysics. 2015;**583**:150-157. DOI: 10.1016/j.abb.2015.08.008

[63] Bergmeyer HU. Methods of Enzymatic Analysis. Volume III: Enzymes 1: Oxidoreductases, Transferases. Weiheim: VCH; 1987

[64] Re R, Pellegrini N, Proteggente A, Pannala A, Yang M, Rice-Evans C. Antioxidant activity applying an improved ABTS radical cation decolorization assay. Free Radical Biology & Medicine. 1999;**26**:1231-1237

[65] Łuczaj W, Gindzienska-Sieskiewicz E, Jarocka-Karpowicz I, Andrisic L, Sierakowski S, Zarkovic N, et al. The onset of lipid peroxidation in rheumatoid arthritis: Consequences and monitoring. Free Radical Research. 2016;**50**(3):304-313. DOI: 10.3109/10715762.2015.1112901

[66] Bracht A, Silveira SS, Castro-Ghizoni CV, Sa-Nakanishi AB, Oliveira MRN, Bersani-Amado CA, et al. Oxidative changes in the blood and serum albumin differentiate rats with monoarthritis and polyarthritis. SpringerPlus. 2016;**5**(1):36. DOI: 10.1186/s40064-016-1671-1

[67] Gutteridge JM. Lipid peroxidation and antioxidants as biomarkers of tissue damage. Clinical Chemistry. 1995;**41**:1819-1828

[68] Kumar V, Prakash J, Gupta V, Khan MK. Antioxidant enzymes in rheumatoid arthritis. Journal of Arthritis. 2016;**5**:206. DOI: 10.4172/2167-7921.1000206

[69] Mazzetti I, Grigolo B, Borzì RM, Meliconi R, Facchini A. Serum copper/zinc superoxide dismutase levels in patients with rheumatoid arthritis. International Journal of Clinical & Laboratory Research. 1996;**26**:245-249

[70] Savu O, Bradescu OM, Serafinceanu C, Iosif L, Tirgoviste CI, Stoian I. Erythrocyte caspase-3 and antioxidant defense is activated in red blood cells and plasma of type 2 diabetes patients at first clinical onset. Redox Report. 2013;**18**(2):56-62. DOI: 10.1179/1351000213Y.0000000040

[71] Staroń A, Mąkosa G, Koter-Michalak M. Oxidative stress in erythrocytes from patients with rheumatoid arthritis. Rheumatology International. 2012;**32**(2):331-334. DOI: 10.1007/s00296-010-1611-2

[72] Karatas F, Ozates I, Canatan H, Halifeoglu I, Karatepe M, Colakt R.

Antioxidant status and lipid peroxidation in patients with rheumatoid arthritis. The Indian Journal of Medical Research. 2003;**118**:178-181

[73] El-barbary AM, Khalek MAA, Elsalawy AM, Hazaa SM. Assessment of lipid peroxidation and antioxidant status in rheumatoid arthritis and osteoarthritis patients. The Egyptian Rheumatologist. 2011;**33**:179-185

[74] Vijayakumar D, Suresh K, Manoharan S. Lipid peroxidation and antioxidant status in blood of rheumatoid arthritis patients. Indian Journal of Clinical Biochemistry. 2006;**21**:104-108

[75] Mobasheri A, Biesalski HK, Shakibaei M, Henrotin Y. Antioxidants and osteoarthritis. In: Laher I, editor. Systems Biology of Free Radicals and Antioxidants. Vol. 133. Berlin, Heidelberg: Springer-Verlag; 2014. pp. 2997-3026. DOI: 10.1007/978-3-642-30018-9_130

[76] Ke C, Sun L, Qiao D, Wanga D, Zeng X. Antioxidant activity of low molecular weight hyaluronic acid. Food and Chemical Toxicology. 2011;**49**:2670-2675

[77] Bryan HK, Olayanju A, Goldring CE, Park BK. The Nrf2 cell defence pathway: Keap1-dependent and -independent mechanisms of regulation. Biochemical Pharmacology. 2013;**85**(6):705-717. DOI: 10.1016/j.bcp.2012.11.016

Chapter 9

Antioxidants as a Double-Edged Sword in the Treatment of Cancer

Majid Asadi-Samani, Najmeh Kaffash Farkhad, Mohammad Reza Mahmoudian-Sani and Hedayatollah Shirzad

Abstract

Antioxidant compounds are thought to prevent and treat diseases, especially cancer, under any circumstances. For this purpose, nature-based antioxidants nowadays are being commonly used to prevent and treat diseases. Indeed, phenolic compounds found in medicinal plants have opened a new horizon to prevent and treat diseases because of having antioxidant properties. However, some recent studies have reported that antioxidants are not absolute anticancer compounds and certain drugs have been reported to reduce levels of reactive oxygen species (ROS) in the cancer cells, i.e., their main action mechanism. It has been argued that increasing levels of ROS cause an increase in apoptosis rate and therefore can be considered an approach to treat fatal and hard-to-treat cancers. This chapter seeks to partly explain the role of ROS in progression or inhibition of cancer growth in addition to the role of antioxidants in preventing and treating this disease.

Keywords: reactive oxygen species, antioxidant, cancer, apoptosis

1. Introduction

Cancer kills many people worldwide every year. Even in developed countries such as the United States, the rate of mortalities of cancer is high yet [1]. Although nowadays cancer therapy has improved, since complete recovery of cancer patients following a single treatment is quite difficult, a multidisciplinary approach combined with surgery, chemotherapy, radiotherapy, and immunotherapy is usually utilized [2, 3]. However, some of these approaches cause several severe side effects in patients. Moreover, for many patients, current therapeutic approaches are successful only in delaying the time to disease progression rather than affecting long-term survival rates [4].

Many previous studies have shown that antioxidant supplementations are useful in cancer treatment [5]. An antioxidant substance in the cell is present at low concentrations and significantly reduces or prevents oxidation of the oxidizable substrates [6]. The researchers have evaluated highly complex antioxidant to protect the cells of the body against free radical damages [4]. However, some recent studies have reported that decreasing levels of cells' oxidants, as reactive oxygen species (ROS) increase, causes increase in apoptosis rate and therefore can be considered an approach to treat fatal and hard-to-treat cancers.

This chapter seeks to partly explain the role of ROS in progression or inhibition of cancer growth in addition to the role of antioxidants in preventing and treating this disease.

2. Oxidative stress in cancer

Among many factors that cause cancer, oxidative stress is one of the most principal and well-studied events that gives elevation to the conditions leading to tumor onset and progression [7, 8]. The oxidative stress and chronic inflammation processes are tightly coupled, and the failure to block these processes could result in genetic/epigenetic changes that drive the initiation of carcinogenesis [9]. Oxidative stress as an imbalance between the production and elimination of ROS causes excessive oxidative damage to macromolecules, cells, and tissues [10]. Oxidative/nitrosative stress-induced peroxidation of membrane lipids can be very damaging because it leads to alterations in the biological properties of the membrane, such as the degree of fluidity, and can lead to inactivation of membrane-bound receptors or enzymes, which in turn may disable normal cellular function and increment tissue permeability [11]. The main outcome of oxidative/nitrosative stress is damage to lipids, nucleic acids, and proteins that can induce a variety of cellular responses through generation of reactive species or can compromise cell health and viability, finally causing cell death via apoptosis or necrosis [5, 12].

3. Reactive oxygen species (ROS)

Free radicals are known as "any chemical species capable of independent existence that contains one or more unpaired electrons" [13]. Reactive oxygen species (ROS) are free radicals which are correlated with the oxygen atom (O) or their equivalents and have stronger reactivity with other molecules, rather than with O_2 [14]. When an imbalance between free radical and reactive metabolite production occurred, ROS are formed and can potentially exhibit a negative effect on the organism [15]. ROS is a collective term that includes the superoxide anion (O_2^-), hydrogen peroxide (H_2O_2), and hydroxyl radical ($HO^\cdot$) [14]. Radical formation in the body occurs via several mechanisms, involving both endogenous and environmental factors [11].

4. ROS in cancer

Cancer is a multistage process defined by initiation, promotion, and progression [16, 17], and oxidative stress interacts with all three stages. A little increase in the ROS level may cause a transient alteration in the cellular level, while a severe increase in ROS may result to irreversible oxidative damage and lead to cell death [18]. ROS can also promote carcinogenesis by inducing pro-oncogenic signaling pathways and DNA mutations. For instance, ROS may stimulate the phosphorylation of mitogen-activated protein kinase (MAPK), JUN N-terminal kinase (JNK) activation, cyclin D1 expression, and extracellular signal-regulated kinase (ERK), all of which are related to growth of tumor cells and survival [19].

Cancer cells generate ROS more abundantly than normal cells and cause elevated oxidative stress [20]. ROS can induce tumorigenicity and promote tumor progression via inducing DNA damage [21]. ROS induces gene mutations and structural changes in the DNA and results in DNA damage during the early stage

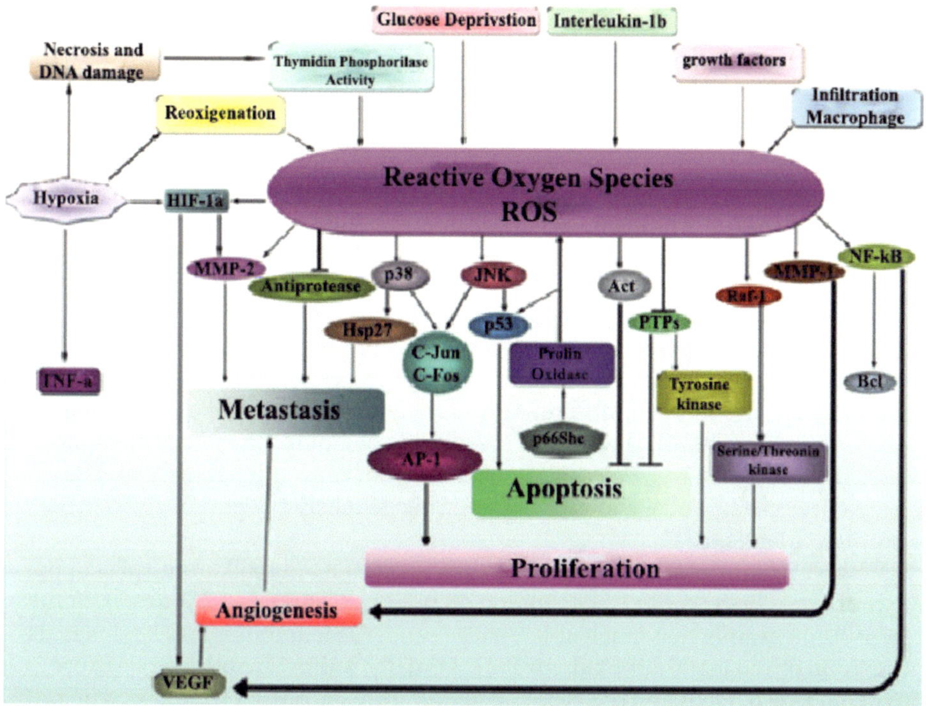

Figure 1.
Relation between ROS actions with promoting and fighting cancer [23].

of tumorigenicity. In addition to, ROS can increase cell proliferation and decrease apoptosis via modifying second-messenger systems, causing abnormal gene expression, and blocking cell communications. Finally, oxidative stress can add DNA alterations to initiate cell population and promote cancer progression [22].

ROS might function as a double-edged sword (**Figure 1**). A moderate increase of ROS may promote cell proliferation and survival. However, when the increase of ROS reaches a certain level (the toxic threshold), it can overwhelm the antioxidant capacity of the cells and result in cell death [23]. It is long thought that antioxidants can remove the ROS that is produced in normal cellular processes and can protect cells from oxidative damage.

Reactive oxygen species (ROS) can promote cellular processes to cancer. In addition, they can induce apoptosis. Actually, ROS might function as a double-edged sword.

5. Antioxidants as a double-edged sword in cancer

Antioxidants as chemicals that interact with neutralized free radicals can prevent them from causing damages. Antioxidants divide to two main subgroups including enzymatic and nonenzymatic antioxidants. Catalase, superoxide dismutase, and glutathione peroxidases are some of the most important enzymatic antioxidants [11]. Catalase (EC 1.11.1.6) as the first antioxidant enzyme was to be characterized and catalyzes conversion of hydrogen peroxide to water and oxygen. Superoxide dismutase (EC 1.15.1.1) is one of the most potent intracellular enzymatic antioxidants that catalyzes the conversion of superoxide anions to dioxygen and hydrogen peroxide. Glutathione peroxidases catalyze the oxidation of glutathione at the direction of a hydroperoxide, which may be hydrogen peroxide or another species such as a lipid hydroperoxide.

Also, flavonoids, alkaloids, coumarins, carotenoids, and vitamins such as E, A, C (ascorbic acid), and D3 are some of the most important nonenzymatic antioxidants that are usually available in many natural products [24].

Antioxidants are known as free radical scavengers. Examples of dietary antioxidants include beta-carotene, lycopene, and vitamins A, C, and E (alpha-tocopherol). Also, the mineral element selenium is often thought to be a dietary antioxidant. Moreover, natural compounds such as flavonoids, in particular ECGC and resveratrol, were shown to have a promising future as antioxidants and anticarcinogenic agents. These compounds can be consumed through fruits and vegetables [25]. In recent years, potential chemotherapeutic properties of antioxidants have been evaluated as a primary agent or in combination with an already established chemotherapeutic agent for different types of cancers. There is friction among researchers about the efficacy and safety of these complimentary treatments and their substantial role in protecting tumor cells from conventional therapy. The antioxidants can be endogenous or obtained exogenously as a part of a diet or as dietary supplements [11].

However, many natural compounds such as natural antioxidants display opposing properties in cancer cells, depending on their concentration (**Figure 2**). Some recent studies imply that much of late-stage cancer's incurability may be due to its possession of too many antioxidants [14]. Actually, antioxidants may also cause direct damage to DNA and the cell. Watson recently wrote that time has come to seriously ask whether antioxidant use predominately causes rather than prevents cancer [26].

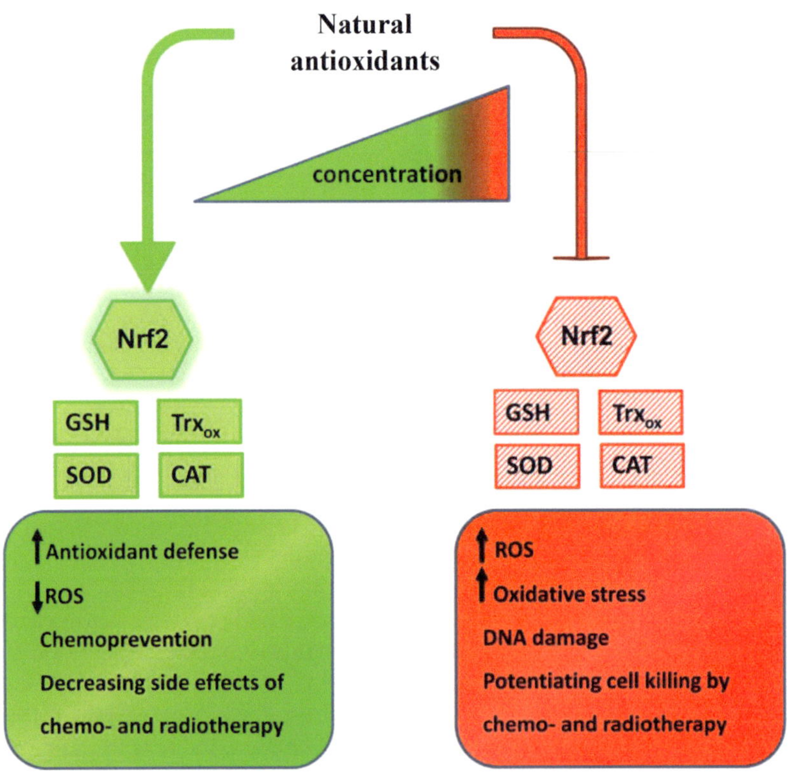

Figure 2.
Natural antioxidants act as a double-edged sword in cancer [28].

Some of these studies proposed that in some cases high-dose supplements of antioxidants may be related to health hazards. For example, high doses of beta-carotene may enhance the risk of lung cancer in smokers. Prostate cancer can occur in dealing with high doses of vitamin E [27]. Antioxidant supplements may also interact with some medications. Based on these new concepts, the continuous use of certain antioxidants such as glutathione, superoxide dismutase, catalase, and thioredoxin may serve as a barrier to apoptosis, the main anticancer mechanism, through excessively reducing ROS [11].

The excessive damages via ROS can be associated with changes in mitochondrial membrane permeability, which result in cytochrome C release and apoptotic death. Against, cancer cells boost their anti-apoptotic mechanisms like a nuclear factor kappa-light-chain-enhancer of activated B cell (NFκB) pathway to escape cell death [9]. Disruption of redox balance in cells causes activation of the transcription factors like nuclear factor erythroid 2-related factor 2 (Nrf2), NFκB, and activator protein 1 (AP-1) as redox-sensitive transcription factors [28]. Nrf2 transcription factor is the major driver of antioxidant expression that leads to protection against DNA damage, endogenous and exogenous hazards, and consequent cancer initiation [29, 30]. Nrf2 overexpresses in some types of human cancers including skin, head, and neck, squamous cell carcinoma, esophagus, pancreatic, gallbladder, prostate, colorectal, breast, lung, and ovary. The cytoprotective properties of the Nrf2 indicate that this pathway can be exploited by tumor cells to promote their survival [31, 32]. In the ROS-sensitive cancer cells, natural product-derived inhibitors of Nrf2 pathway can induce ROS that may result in cell death [28]. Many antioxidants such as polyphenols are significant groups of Nrf2 inhibitors.

Particularly in the case of cancer, the Nrf2 pathway has opposing properties: activating the pathway is vital for chemoprevention, but when the control is lost, it provides big consequences, so cancer cells result in fast proliferation, the escape of senescence and apoptosis, and resistance to chemotherapy and radiotherapy. Therefore, both activation and inhibition of Nrf2 activities can be beneficial [33]. As said above, natural products with antioxidant agents target Nrf2 pathway as an anticancer approach [28]. Several antioxidants may interact with other antioxidants that regenerate their primary properties; this mechanism is known as the "antioxidant network."

Opposing activities of natural products such as antioxidants in prevention and treatment of cancer depend on their concentration. At lower amounts, they often promote cells' antioxidant capacity via activating Nrf2-dependent signaling and enhancing expression of ROS scavengers. However, higher concentrations can inhibit antioxidant defense and induce oxidative stress.

6. Antioxidants and tumorigenesis

Genetic alterations that promote tumor cause to produce endogenous antioxidants [14]. In this process, Nrf2 is the main factor for the transactivation of involved genes in the maintenance of redox homeostasis [34]. As constitutive upregulation of Nrf2 factor has been reported for a variety of human cancer types, Nrf2 activity has been indicated to be necessary for proliferation of cancer cells [35–37], reprogramming of metabolism [38], chemoresistance [39], serine biosynthesis [36], as well as mRNA translation [37] in part through maintenance of redox homeostasis. Hi-activated pathway of Nrf2 increases the amount of cellular ROS scavengers. On the other hand, lowering stress burden via enhancing detoxifying force can affect the pathways that promote proliferation and growth [40, 41]. Blocking antioxidant activity in cancer cells decreases their ability to balance oxidative insult and might result in cell death [42]. In addition to Nrf2, the transcription factor p53 has also been shown to suppress ROS accumulation via directly regulating the expression of a variety of antioxidant genes including SOD2, GPX1, and CAT [14, 39] and through the induction of the metabolic TIGAR gene (TP53-inducible glycolysis and apoptosis regulator) [14].

Oxidative stress can happen due to reduction in enzymatic antioxidant activities. Moreover, it can occur due to ionizing, radiation, chemotherapy, aging, shear stress, cytokines, and growth factor receptor interactions [14]. Antioxidants and oxidative stress interact with the initiation, promotion, and progression of cancer [41]. Actually, the cell-damaging effects of free radicals can be balanced by antioxidants. Furthermore, as the fruits and vegetables are good sources of antioxidants, people who eat them more than others have a lower risk for various diseases such as heart and neurological diseases, and there is evidence that some types of vegetables and fruits in general protect against a number of cancers [43].

7. Advantages of using antioxidants as an anticancer approach

In addition to the standard anticancer treatment options such as chemotherapy, radiotherapy, and surgery, several natural products due to their antioxidant activities have been identified to have a potential for cancer prevention [44] and treatment [45].

In radiotherapy and chemotherapy, ROS and free radicals partly cause various adverse effects [46]. ROS generation causes various tissue or organ injuries; for example, doxorubicin and other anthracycline antibiotics are known to lead to cardiotoxicity [47]; cisplatin and other platinums lead to nephrotoxicity, ototoxicity, and peripheral neuropathy [48]; bleomycin leads to lung injury [49]; and alkylating agents cause DNA damage of drug-treated cells [50]. Tissue or organ injuries may also induce carcinogenesis [51]. Many previous studies reported that using antioxidants with these gold standard methods can significantly decrease these cellular damages. For instance, in one study that is reported by Askua et al., among the 49 studies, 46 examined the reduction of adverse effects by antioxidant supplementation; in 34 trials, possible reductions in chemotoxicities or radiotoxicities using antioxidant supplementation were reported; and only 1 RCT, using vitamin A, reported that supplementation possibly increased chemoinduced toxicities. The remaining 11 studies reported no significantly difference in toxicities between control and supplementation groups [51]. Further, the results of the Shanghai Breast Cancer Survival Study showed that consumption of multivitamins or vitamins such as C and E within 6 months of breast cancer diagnosis correlated with 18% decreased mortality and 22% decreased recurrence rate [52]. In addition, the Life After Cancer Epidemiology (LACE) cohort study results on effects of vitamins E and C and combination of carotenoid supplementation in breast cancer showed that vitamins E and C intake before and after breast cancer diagnosis was related to 22% reduced risk of all-cause mortality, 32% decreased breast cancer mortality, and 20% decreased recurrence risk [53].

8. Future therapeutic perspectives

We are approaching a new era wherein ROS biology and their effects in the physiopathology of cancer may be dissected with unprecedented detail, bringing potential therapeutic benefits derived from selective manipulations of cancer redox balance to be uncovered, paving the way to novel and exciting investigations in the fight against cancer [6]. Owing to the crucial roles of cancer stem cells in tumor initiation, disease recurrence, and drug resistance, the potential of using a redox-modulating strategy to eliminate this subpopulation of malignant cells could have major implications in cancer treatment. Redox adaptation is an important concept that, to a large degree, explains the mechanisms by which cancer cells survive under persistent endogenous ROS stress and become resistant to certain anticancer agents. Targeting these biochemical properties of cancer cells with redox-modulating strategies is a feasible therapeutic approach that may enable therapeutic selectivity and overcome drug resistance. Also, Nrf2 is arguably the most important regulator of the expression of molecules that have antioxidant functions within the cell [13]. Nrf2 controls the expression of these enzymes and is considered to be a master regulator of intracellular antioxidant responses. An increased Nrf2 activity in normal cells is protective and beneficial against oxidative stress, but cancer cells harness the ability of Nrf2 to survive under stress conditions [14]. Nrf2 activators, such as bardoxolone methyl CDDO-Me, have shown anticancer activity preclinically and are currently being tested in clinical trials [15]. Moreover, glutathione (GSH) metabolism seems to be the main target of currently used anticancer drugs. Combinations of GSH inhibitors (or other antioxidant inhibitors) with radiotherapy or chemotherapeutic drugs that cause cell death induced by oxidative stress may prove to be useful for more effectively killing cancer cells.

9. Conclusion

ROS/RNS protection in cancer is an important issue that attracts many scientists in recent years to discover the mechanism of action of various antioxidants. The idea that fruit and vegetable consumption alone is associated with a decreased risk of cancer is yet to be determined. This chapter shows that antioxidants, as previously reported, contribute to prevent and treat many types of cancer, but their anticancer effects are not absolute and depend on the time, amount, and conditions of their administration to treat different cancers. It is important that physicians make an integrated decision, based on the following consideration: (1) the background and state of the patient, (2) the antioxidant dosage and types, and (3) type of cancer and antitumor therapy. In addition, it is necessary to examine the safety and viability of antioxidants in pathological conditions and cancer therapy and that trials be performed with a single regimen, single type of cancer, and single antioxidant.

Author details

Majid Asadi-Samani[1*], Najmeh Kaffash Farkhad[2],
Mohammad Reza Mahmoudian-Sani[3] and Hedayatollah Shirzad[4*]

1 Medical Plants Research Center, Basic Health Sciences Institute, Shahrekord University of Medical Sciences, Shahrekord, Iran

2 Mashhad University of Medical Sciences, Mashhad, Iran

3 Research Center of Thalassemia and Hemoglobinopathy, Health Research Institute, Jundishapur University of Medical Sciences, Ahvaz, Iran

4 Cellular and Molecular Research Center, Basic Health Sciences Institute, Shahrekord University of Medical Sciences, Iran

*Address all correspondence to: biology_2011@yahoo.com and shirzad1951@yahoo.com

References

[1] Bray F, Ferlay J, Soerjomataram I, Siegel RL, Torre LA, Jemal A. Global cancer statistics 2018: GLOBOCAN estimates of incidence and mortality worldwide for 36 cancers in 185 countries. CA: A Cancer Journal for Clinicians. 2018;**68**(6):394-424

[2] Ito T, Urushima H, Sakaue M, Yukawa S, Honda H, Hirai K, et al. Reduction of adverse effects by a mushroom product, active hexose correlated compound (AHCC) in patients with advanced cancer during chemotherapy: The significance of the levels of HHV-6 DNA in saliva as a surrogate biomarker during chemotherapy. Nutrition and Cancer. 2014;**66**(3):377-382

[3] Stone JB, DeAngelis LM. Cancer-treatment-induced neurotoxicity—focus on newer treatments. Nature Reviews. Clinical Oncology. 2016;**13**(2):92-105

[4] Crawford S. Anti-inflammatory/antioxidant use in long-term maintenance cancer therapy: A new therapeutic approach to disease progression and recurrence. Therapeutic Advances in Medical Oncology. 2014;**6**(2):52-68

[5] Valko M, Leibfritz D, Moncol J, Cronin MT, Mazur M, Telser J. Free radicals and antioxidants in normal physiological functions and human disease. The International Journal of Biochemistry & Cell Biology. 2007;**39**(1):44-84

[6] Rahman K. Studies on free radicals, antioxidants, and co-factors. Clinical Interventions in Aging. 2007;**2**(2):219-236

[7] Sosa V, Moline T, Somoza R, Paciucci R, Kondoh H, LLeonart ME. Oxidative stress and cancer: An overview. Ageing Research Reviews. 2013;**12**(1):376-390

[8] Guina T, Biasi F, Calfapietra S, Nano M, Poli G. Inflammatory and redox reactions in colorectal carcinogenesis. Annals of the New York Academy of Sciences. 2015;**1340**(1):95-103

[9] Murata M, Thanan R, Ma N, Kawanishi S. Role of nitrative and oxidative DNA damage in inflammation-related carcinogenesis. Journal of Biomedicine & Biotechnology. 2012;**2012**:623019

[10] Halliwell B. Free radicals and antioxidants - quo vadis? Trends in Pharmacological Sciences. 2011;**32**(3):125-130

[11] Kurutas EB. The importance of antioxidants which play the role in cellular response against oxidative/nitrosative stress: Current state. Nutrition Journal. 2016;**15**(1):71

[12] Flora SJ. Structural, chemical and biological aspects of antioxidants for strategies against metal and metalloid exposure. Oxidative Medicine and Cellular Longevity. 2009;**2**(4):191-206

[13] Martin-Cordero C, Leon-Gonzalez AJ, Calderon-Montano JM, Burgos-Moron E, Lopez-Lazaro M. Pro-oxidant natural products as anticancer agents. Current Drug Targets. 2012;**13**(8):1006-1028

[14] Chio IIC, Tuveson DA. ROS in cancer: The burning question. Trends in Molecular Medicine. 2017;**23**(5):411-429

[15] Duracková Z. Some current insights into oxidative stress. Physiological Research. 2010;**59**(4):459-469

[16] Ames BN, Gold LS. Animal cancer tests and cancer prevention. Journal of the National Cancer Institute. Monographs. 1992;**12**:125-132

[17] Yang Y, Zhu Y, Xi X. Anti-inflammatory and antitumor action of hydrogen via reactive oxygen species. Oncology Letters. 2018;**16**(3):2771-2776

[18] Trachootham D, Alexandre J, Huang P. Targeting cancer cells by ROS-mediated mechanisms: A radical therapeutic approach? Nature Reviews. Drug Discovery. 2009;**8**(7):579-591

[19] Ranjan P, Anathy V, Burch PM, Weirather K, Lambeth JD, Heintz NH. Redox-dependent expression of cyclin D1 and cell proliferation by Nox1 in mouse lung epithelial cells. Antioxidants & Redox Signaling. 2006;**8**(9-10):1447-1459

[20] Szatrowski TP, Nathan CF. Production of large amounts of hydrogen peroxide by human tumor cells. Cancer Research. 1991;**51**(3):794-798

[21] Wang J, Yi J. Cancer cell killing via ROS: To increase or decrease, that is the question. Cancer Biology & Therapy. 2008;7(12):1875-1884

[22] Klaunig JE, Xu Y, Isenberg JS, Bachowski S, Kolaja KL, Jiang J, et al. The role of oxidative stress in chemical carcinogenesis. Environmental Health Perspectives. 1998;**106**(Suppl 1): S289-S295

[23] Salmaninejad A, Kangari P, Shakoori A. Oxidative stress: Development and progression of breast cancer. Tehran University Medical Journal. 2017;**75**(1):1-9

[24] Ghatreh-Samani M, Esmaeili N, Soleimani M, Asadi-Samani M, Ghatreh-Samani K, Shirzad H. Oxidative stress and age-related changes in T cells: Is thalassemia a model of accelerated immune system aging?. Central-European Journal of Immunology. 2016;**41**:116-124

[25] Asadi-Samani M, Kooti W, Aslani E, Shirzad H. A systematic review of Iran's medicinal plants with anticancer effects. Journal of Evidence-Based Complementary & Alternative Medicine. 2016;**21**:143-153

[26] Watson J. Oxidants, antioxidants and the current incurability of metastatic cancers. Open Biology. 2013;**3**(1):120144

[27] Antioxidants: MedlinePlus. Available at: https://medlineplus.gov/antioxidants.html.01/03/2018

[28] Sznarkowska A, Kostecka A, Meller K, Bielawski KP. Inhibition of cancer antioxidant defense by natural compounds. Oncotarget. 2017;**8**(9):15996-16016

[29] Rotblat B, Melino G, Knight RA. NRF2 and p53: Januses in cancer? Oncotarget. 2012;**3**:1272-1283

[30] Rotblat B, Southwell AL, Ehrnhoefer DE, Skotte NH, Metzler M, Franciosi S, et al. HACE1 reduces oxidative stress and mutant Huntingtin toxicity by promoting the NRF2 response. Proceedings of the National Academy of Sciences of the United States of America. 2014;**111**:3032-3037

[31] Kumar H, Kim I-S, More SV, Kim B-W, Choi D-K. Natural product-derived pharmacological modulators of Nrf2/ARE pathway for chronic diseases. Natural Product Reports. 2014;**31**:109-139

[32] Geismann C, Arlt A, Sebens S, Schäfer H. Cytoprotection "gone astray": Nrf2 and its role in cancer. OncoTargets and Therapy. 2014;**7**:1497-1518

[33] Marquardt JU, Gomez-Quiroz L, Arreguin Camacho LO, Pinna F, Lee Y-H, Kitade M, et al. Curcumin effectively inhibits oncogenic NF-κB signaling and restrains stemness

features in liver cancer. Journal of Hepatology. 2015;**63**:661-669

[34] Hayes JD, Dinkova-Kostova AT. The Nrf2 regulatory network provides an interface between redox and intermediary metabolism. Trends in Biochemical Sciences. 2014;**39**:199-218

[35] No JH, Kim YB, Song YS. Targeting nrf2 signaling to combat chemoresistance. Journal of Cancer Prevention. 2014;**19**:111-117

[36] DeNicola GM, Karreth FA, Humpton TJ, Gopinathan A, Wei C, Frese K, et al. Oncogene-induced Nrf2 transcription promotes ROS detoxification and tumorigenesis. Nature. 2011;**475**:106-109

[37] Chio II, Jafarnejad SM, Ponz-Sarvise M, Park Y, Rivera K, Palm W, et al. NRF2 promotes tumor maintenance by modulating mRNA translation in pancreatic cancer. Cell. 2016;**166**:963-976

[38] Mitsuishi Y, Taguchi K, Kawatani Y, Shibata T, Nukiwa T, Aburatani H, et al. Nrf2 redirects glucose and glutamine into anabolic pathways in metabolic reprogramming. Cancer Cell. 2012;**22**:66-79

[39] Zhang P, Singh A, Yegnasubramanian S, Esopi D, Kombairaju P, Bodas M, et al. Loss of Kelch-like ECH-associated protein 1 function in prostate cancer cells causes chemoresistance and radioresistance and promotes tumor growth. Molecular Cancer Therapeutics. 2010;**9**:336-346

[40] Cho J, Seo J, Lim CH, Yang L, Shiratsuchi T, Lee M-H, et al. Mitochondrial ATP transporter Ant2 depletion impairs erythropoiesis and B lymphopoiesis. Cell Death and Differentiation. 2015;**22**:1437-1450

[41] Singer E, Judkins J, Salomonis N, Matlaf L, Soteropoulos P, McAllister S, et al. Reactive oxygen speciesmediated therapeutic response and resistance in glioblastoma. Cell Death & Disease. 2015;**6**:e1601

[42] Mei H, Sun S, Bai Y, Chen Y, Chai R, Li H. Reduced mtDNA copy number increases the sensitivity of tumor cells to chemotherapeutic drugs. Cell Death & Disease. 2015;**6**:e1710

[43] Kooti W, Servatyari K, Behzadifar M, Asadi-Samani M, Sadeghi F, Nouri B, et al. Effective Medicinal Plant in Cancer Treatment, Part 2. Journal of Evidence-Based Complementary & Alternative Medicine. 2017;**22**:982-995

[44] Asadi-Samani M, Bagheri N, Rafieian-Kopaei M, Shirzad H. Inhibition of Th1 and Th17 Cells by Medicinal Plants and Their Derivatives: A Systematic Review. Phytotherapy Research. 2017;**31**:1128-1139

[45] Asadi-Samani M, Rafieian-Kopaei M, Lorigooini Z, Shirzad H. A screening of growth inhibitory activity of Iranian medicinal plants on prostate cancer cell lines. BioMedicine. 2018;**8**:8

[46] Mizutani H. Mechanism of DNA damage and apoptosis induced by anticancer drugs through generation of reactive oxygen species. Yakugaku Zasshi. 2007;**127**:1837-1842

[47] Hrelia S, Bordoni A, Angeloni C, Leoncini E, Biagi P. Nutritional interventions to counteract oxidative stress in cardiac cells. The Italian Journal of Biochemistry. 2004;**53**:157-163

[48] Jung M, Hotter G, Vinas JL, Sola A. Cisplatin upregulates mitochondrial nitric oxide synthase and peroxynitrite formation to promote renal injury. Toxicology and Applied Pharmacology. 2009;**234**:236-246

[49] Muecke R, Micke O, Schomburg L, Glatzel M, Reichl B, Kisters K, et al. Multicenter, phase III trial comparing selenium supplementation with observation in gynecologic radiation oncology: Follow-up analysis of the survival data 6 years after cessation of randomization. Integrative Cancer Therapies. 2014;**13**:463-467

[50] Block KI, Koch AC, Mead MN, Tothy PK, Newman RA, Gyllenhaal C. Impact of antioxidant supplementation on chemotherapeutic efficacy: A systematic review of the evidence from randomized controlled trials. Cancer Treatment Reviews. 2007;**33**:407-418

[51] Yasueda A, Urushima H, Ito T. Efficacy and interaction of antioxidant supplements as adjuvant therapy in cancer treatment: A systematic review. Integrative Cancer Therapies. 2016;**15**(1):17-39

[52] Nechuta S, Lu W, Chen Z, Zheng Y, Gu K, Cai H, et al. Vitamin supplement use during breast cancer treatment and survival: A prospective cohort study. Cancer Epidemiology, Biomarkers & Prevention. 2011;**20**(2):262-271

[53] Greenlee H, Kwan M, Kushi L, Song J, Castillo A, Weltzein E, et al. Antioxidant supplement use after breast cancer diagnosis and mortality in the Life After Cancer Epidemiology (LACE) cohort. Cancer. 2012;**118**(8):2048-2058

Chapter 10

Antioxidants at Newborns

Melinda Matyas and Gabriela Zaharie

Abstract

Humans possess defense mechanisms against free radicals: enzymatic and non-enzymatic antioxidants. Antioxidant defense is deficient in newborns and can be enhanced by the action of reactive oxygen species, generated by perinatal diseases such as respiratory distress or asphyxia. Prematurity itself will be associated with deficient antioxidant mechanisms, which are primarily enzymatic, but also non-enzymatic. Under oxidative stress conditions, antioxidant defense is overcome and thus, low-molecular weight free iron is released, which is not bound to transferrin and will play a role in Fenton's reaction, catalyzing lipid peroxidation. The generated ROS will in turn influence antioxidant defense mechanisms, stimulating their synthesis, as an adaptation mechanism of the body in response to the presence of increased ROS levels.

Keywords: antioxidants, newborn, oxidative stress

1. Aim

The aim of the current chapter is to review the antioxidant status particularities newborn, to present the antioxidant evaluation and current opinions on antioxidant treatment in newborns.

2. Introduction

The human body possesses defense mechanisms against free radicals, consisting of enzymatic and non-enzymatic antioxidants. Antioxidant defense is deficient in newborns and can be enhanced by the action of reactive oxygen species, generated by perinatal diseases such as neonatal respiratory distress or birth asphyxia. Prematurity itself will be associated with deficient antioxidant mechanisms, which are primarily enzymatic, but also non-enzymatic. Antioxidant defenses, especially enzymatic ones, develop during the last trimester of pregnancy. Consequently, premature newborns will not have sufficient antioxidant defense. Under oxidative stress conditions, antioxidant defense is overcome and thus, low-molecular weight free iron is released, which is not bound to transferrin and will play a role in Fenton's reaction, catalyzing lipid peroxidation [1, 9]. Reactive oxygen species (ROS) production occurs through various mechanisms, of which the most common are hyperoxia, reperfusion, and inflammation. The generated ROS will in turn influence antioxidant defense mechanisms, stimulating their synthesis, as an adaptation mechanism in response to the presence of increased ROS levels. In neonatology, a "free radical disease" is described, which includes a number of disorders:

bronchopulmonary dysplasia, retinopathy of prematurity, necrotizing enterocolitis, and periventricular leukomalacia [1, 8, 17].

In the case of perinatal asphyxia, ROS will exert a considerable harmful effect on the brain because antioxidant levels are low and there is an increased oxygen consumption during transition from fetal life to neonatal life [14, 15, 25]. Randomized studies on relatively large numbers of term newborns with asphyxia have demonstrated the importance of resuscitation with atmospheric air in limiting injury and improving the survival rate [13, 26].

3. Antioxidants classification

Antioxidants are most commonly classified into enzymatic and non-enzymatic systems. Depending on their solubility, non-enzymatic antioxidants are divided into water-soluble and lipid-soluble antioxidants.

The main enzymatic antioxidant systems are:

- *superoxide dismutase* (SOD)—an enzyme that detoxifies the superoxide anion;
- *catalase* (CAT)—detoxifies oxygenated water and has a protective antitumor role;
- *peroxidases*—myeloperoxidase (MPO), lipid peroxidase, glutathione peroxidase (GSH-Px)—mainly protect the liver;
- *glutathione peroxidase (GPx) intracellular selen-protein that reduces hydrogen peroxide to glutathione disulfide and water*;
- *the system of cytochrome oxidases*, which reduce oxygen; they play a role in reducing the amount of oxidant or potentially oxidant substances; they can be released into the blood and extracellular fluid.

The main non-enzymatic antioxidant systems are represented by:

- the reduced-oxidized glutathione redox cycle;
- vitamin E—which intercepts the peroxyl radical;
- vitamin C;
- carotenoids—alpha-carotene, a precursor of vitamin A, is 10 times more effective than beta-carotene;
- selenium;
- uric acid and urates;
- bilirubin;
- cysteine-rich metallothioneins;
- metal-binding proteins: albumin, transferrin, ferritin, lactoferrin, and ceruloplasmin;

- amino acids such as histidine, taurine, cysteine which ensures protection against toxic aldehydes present in cigarette smoke, methionine which protects the colon;

- Heme proteins and heme-binding proteins—hemopexin, haptoglobin, porphyrin, carnosine, estrogens, coenzyme Q10, polyamines, saturated fatty acids, flavonoids which stabilize the cell membrane and are used in eye diseases, phenols, and polyphenols. Ceruloplasmin is an extracellular copper-transport protein.

3.1 Antioxidant enzymes

The most important antioxidant enzymes in newborns are: superoxide dismutase, catalase, and glutathione peroxidase.

Superoxide dismutase has three forms: MnSOD located in mitochondria, copper-zinc superoxide dismutase (Cu/ZnSOD) in the cytoplasm, and extracellular superoxide dismutase (EC-SOD). In newborns, the last one is located intracellularly in the cytoplasm, unlike in adults, where it is located extracellularly, as indicated by its name [23, 27].

Superoxide dismutase has the role of converting the highly toxic superoxide radical to hydrogen peroxide and water. Catalase and glutathione peroxidase convert hydrogen peroxide to water.

In the absence of catalase, a cascade reaction is triggered with the formation of hydroxyl radicals, which requires the presence of iron metal ions (Fe^{2+}) and copper Cu^{2+}, known as the Haber-Weiss reaction:

$$H_2O_2 + Fe^{2+} \rightarrow OH^{\bullet} + OH^{-} + Fe^{3+} \quad (1)$$

The hydroxyl radical resulting from this reaction will attack the structures of the cell, causing its destruction.

In the intrauterine period, there is an interaction between the fetus, placenta, and uterus, which requires a redox signal with a role in maintaining the balance of this interaction and allowing the development of antioxidant systems in the fetal period.

The decrease in lipid peroxidation in the placenta with the evolution of pregnancy is an indirect marker of the development of antioxidant mechanisms with the increase of gestational age [18].

Normal vascular development is conditioned by the activity of nitric oxide controlled by nitric oxide synthase. Nitric oxide plays a role in regulating the activity of antioxidant enzymes.

The protective role of SOD was demonstrated in experimental groups of animals—rats—at the Physiology Department of the University of Medicine, Cluj-Napoca, Romania [16]. The authors studied lipid peroxides as oxidative stress parameters by measuring malondialdehyde (MDA) and ceruloplasmin using the Ravin test [16].

The animals exposed to hypobaric hypoxia had, immediately after SOD administration, significantly increased malondialdehyde (MDA) values, which were close to the values found in unprotected animals exposed to hypobaric hypoxia. At 24 hours after SOD administration, in animals exposed to hypoxia, the values of MDA as a marker of lipid peroxidation were significantly decreased, being lower than those of the control group. In the case of ceruloplasmin, values were significantly lower in protected compared to unprotected animals [16].

The preterm neonate is born before the antioxidant systems capable of neutralizing ROS are formed. Birth itself is an oxidative stress-inducing factor, which will cause, in conjunction with other factors mentioned before such as hypoxia, hyperoxia, reperfusion, or inflammation, the rapid exhaustion of impaired defense mechanisms in the premature newborn. Transplacental nutrient supply has an important role in the formation of antioxidant defense mechanisms. However, this supply is limited in the case of preterm neonates. Chorioamnionitis present in a relatively great number of premature births is an induction factor for MnSOD mRNA in fetal membranes. Antenatal corticosteroids, in addition to their role in early lung, brain, and intestinal maturation, influence stimulation of the activity of antioxidant enzymes: SOD, catalase, and glutathione transferase [25, 29].

The endogenous surfactant has SOD and catalase in its composition. Their antioxidant role in the surfactant is to prevent surfactant lipid peroxidation and inactivation following the oxidative attack of ROS. These enzymes with antioxidant effects are not found in similar amounts in the exogenous surfactant used for the treatment of respiratory distress [30].

It is important to identify newborns at risk for oxidative stress in order to initiate early antioxidant therapy with a view to limiting oxidative stress progression. Since oxidative stress can frequently start during the intrauterine period, finding antioxidant therapies for the mother with an impact on the newborn is essential.

3.2 Non-enzymatic antioxidants

Vitamins have an antioxidant role. Among water-soluble vitamins, vitamin C is the most studied. The most extensively studied lipid-soluble vitamins in neonates are vitamins A and E.

Vitamin A acts on retinol-binding proteins and on retinoic acid receptors. The main actions of retinol consist of maintaining epithelial integrity, regulating growth and proliferation, and modulating the levels of ceruloplasmin, a protein with antioxidant effects [2, 21]. Vitamin A levels are decreased in preterm newborns, proportionally to the degree of prematurity. The benefits of vitamin A in limiting the incidence of bronchopulmonary dysplasia have been described in many studies. Its beneficial effect in reducing the incidence of the disease could not be demonstrated. Also, the fact that it requires intramuscular administration and relatively high doses to exert its antioxidant effects is a major disadvantage [15, 22].

Regarding vitamins E and C, their beneficial effect in preventing the teratogenic effect of maternal diabetes has been studied by a number of authors [19].

In the category of water-soluble vitamins, other vitamins besides vitamin C have an antioxidant role: riboflavin, pyridoxine, and niacin, which maintain GSH activity.

Vitamin E is the antioxidant that is present in the highest amount in the human body. It is a lipophilic vitamin, which accumulates in lipid-rich cell membranes. It is an important lipid peroxyl scavenger [15].

Carotenoids are also lipid-soluble and have a characteristic color. Lutein plays a role in ROS elimination. In umbilical cord blood, studies have evidenced higher lutein levels in preterm compared to term newborns [29].

Ceruloplasmin is an extracellular antioxidant that acts like a ferroxidase enzyme, catalyzing the oxidation reaction of Fe^{2+} to Fe^{3+}, thus limiting Haber-Weiss and Fenton reaction.

$$LOH + Fe^{2+} \rightarrow L{-}O^{\bullet} + OH^{\bullet} + Fe^{3+} \qquad (2)$$

Uric acid is a non-enzymatic antioxidant resulting from purine metabolism. It is a scavenger of many ROS, but in certain situations, in excessive amounts, it has a cytokine-mediated pro-inflammatory effect, playing a role in the pathogenesis of diseases such as diabetes [15, 30].

4. Evaluation of antioxidants in neonates

Antioxidant defense in neonates can be evaluated by measuring enzymatic and non-enzymatic systems. Among enzymatic systems, glutathione reductase, peroxidase, transferase, the oxidized/reduced glutathione ratio, superoxide dismutase, as well as other antioxidants such as ceruloplasmin, transferring are the most frequently measured.

The non-enzymatic antioxidant systems that can be measured in newborns are vitamins A, E, and C. Vitamin A and E values measured in newborns are presented in many studies. Shah et al. describe a correlation between hepatic vitamin A reserves and gestational age, as well as between nutritional status and maternal vitamin A levels. Vitamin A has an important role in the development of visual acuity, and also in lung development and surfactant synthesis [1]. Vitamin A levels are significantly lower in preterm compared to term neonates. Antenatal corticoid administration has a beneficial effect on vitamin A levels in premature babies. Thus, in preterm newborns benefiting from antenatal corticosteroids, the levels of these vitamins with antioxidant effect are higher than in preterm babies without antenatal treatment. The mechanism of corticosteroids in increasing vitamin synthesis is unknown. It seems that these act by increasing the plasma levels of retinol-binding proteins, stimulating the hepatic synthesis of these proteins [2].

Vitamin E, another important non-enzymatic antioxidant, with a role in stabilizing cell membranes, also has lower values in preterm compared to term neonates. Vitamin E has been used in many studies for its antioxidant effect in preventing retinopathy and bronchopulmonary dysplasia. However, in a 2003 Cochrane analysis, Brion et al. demonstrated that vitamin E plays a role in reducing the incidence of ROP and IVH, but increases the incidence of neonatal sepsis [3]. Allopurinol, melatonin, and acetylcysteine have been used in studies for their antioxidant effect, mainly as neuroprotective agents. Melatonin and acetylcysteine were used in the studies of Gitto, and subsequently Barceló, to reduce the incidence of NEC in premature neonates [4, 5]. However, there is no consensus regarding their use for the treatment of NEC in neonates or for the treatment of other conditions associated with hypoxia-ischemia. Nevertheless, it should be taken into consideration that exogenous antioxidant therapy with high doses of vitamin C and beta-carotene in particular will have a pro-oxidant effect.

For the evaluation of antioxidant defense in newborns, the levels of ceruloplasmin were measured in our service. This non-enzymatic antioxidant defense marker proved to be deficient in preterm compared to term neonates. Ceruloplasmin is a peroxyl radical scavenger. Free oxygen radical excess caused by certain oxidative stress-inducing situations will put a strain on the impaired defense mechanisms of the premature newborn. Antioxidant values will be lower compared to those of full-term newborns. Ceruloplasmin determined by spectrophotometry had lower values in preterm neonates with respiratory distress. Also, ceruloplasmin levels decreased with the decrease in gestational age. Determinations evidenced lower ceruloplasmin values on the first day compared to the third day of life (**Table 1**).

Exposure to asphyxia at birth results in decreased ceruloplasmin levels. Under these oxidative stress-inducing conditions, the measurements performed evidenced lower ceruloplasmin values in preterm newborns with asphyxia compared to term newborns with asphyxia. Asphyxia is followed by a diminution of antioxidant levels and an increase in transferrin saturation. Current data confirm the fact that in

	N	T	Z	p-Level
FiO_2—DOL_1 & FiO_2—DOL_3	59	52,5000	6,149,591	0.000000
pH—DOL_1 & pH—DOL_3	60	175,5000	4,346,968	0.000014
pCO_2—DOL_1 & pCO_2—DOL_3	60	412,5000	3,429,860	0.000604
pO_2—DOL_1 & pO_2—DOL_3	60	573,0000	2,014,110	0.043999
SaO_2—DOL_1 & SaO_2—DOL_3	60	208,5000	3,761,957	0.000169
CP—DOL_1 & CP—DOL_3	60	492,0000	2,814,343	0.004888

FiO_2-oxygen concentration; pH-value.

pCO_2-CO_2 partial pressure; pO_2-oxygen partial pressure.

SaO_2-oxygen saturation; CP-ceruloplasmin.
p-test significance; Z = test parameter.

Table 1.
Evolution of ceruloplasmin on 1st vs 3rd day of life (DOL).

neonatal asphyxia and in the post-asphyxic period, ROS are generated particularly during the re-oxygenation phase after perinatal asphyxia [10]. The brain is the most susceptible to oxidative injury, for the following reasons:

- Neuronal membranes are rich in polyunsaturated fatty acids, an important source of free oxygen radicals.

- The activity of antioxidant enzymes (catalase and SOD) is significantly diminished in the brain.

- Some brain areas are rich in iron [10]. The increase in CP in mild and severe asphyxia cases can represent a form of adaptation of the organism to the action of oxidative stress [15].

Ceruloplasmin was measured by Lindeman [23], who evidenced the fact that in premature newborns, its levels are constantly low until the age of 3–6 weeks. Its deficiency in premature newborns increases the risk of oxidative stress under conditions of exposure to the oxidative attack of ROS.

Another marker of antioxidant defense is represented by hydrogen donors. Like total antioxidant activity, these assess several natural non-enzymatic antioxidants: cysteine, glutathione, ascorbic acid, tocopherol, polyphenols, aromatic amines, and sulfhydryl protein groups. In the case of measurements performed with 1,1-diphenyl-picrylhydrazyl in neonates admitted to our service, we found a correlation of hydrogen donor values with the severity of respiratory distress. The presence of respiratory distress was a triggering factor for hydrogen donors, stimulating their antioxidant activity in a group of patients with impaired enzymatic antioxidant defense (**Table 2**).

Hydrogen donor levels in healthy, late preterm newborns are higher compared to those of preterm newborns with oxidative stress-inducing conditions such as respiratory distress or asphyxia at birth. Non-enzymatic antioxidant defense assessed by hydrogen donor values improves with time; our determinations showed significantly higher values on the third day compared to the first day ($p < 0.05$) (**Table 3**).

The enzymatic antioxidants studied in neonates are: catalase (CAT), superoxide dismutase (SOD), and glutathione peroxidase (GSH-Px). These are endogenous antioxidants and have the following antioxidant action mechanisms: superoxide dismutase catalyzes superoxide radical dismutation, resulting in hydrogen peroxide.

	1st day	3rd day	Stat (p-value)
Mild Stat (p-value)*b	42.20 (39.80-45.30) −3.11 (0.0019)	46.65 (41.53-52.05) −2.09 (0.0369)	2.42 (0.0157)
Moderate Stat (p-value)*b	62.70 (59.40-64.20) 1.55 (0.1218)	61.50 (60.43-64.35) 1.68 (0.0926)	0.00 (0.9999)
Severe Stat (p-value)*b	48.30 (46.48-51.31) −1.02 (0.3082)	49.60 (45.30-54.00) −0.91 (0.3650)	0.0 (0.9999)

[b]median (Q1-Q3), Q = quartile, Wilcoxon Matched Test
[*]as compared to control

Table 2.
Hydrogen donors by severity of respiratory distress and comparisons with the controls.

	Group	n	Mean±Stdev	Std. Error Mean	t-value (p-value)
HD 1	Case	24	45.82 ± 10.36	2.12	−2.64 (0.0124)
	Control	13	54.38 ± 7.33	2.03	
HD 2	Case	24	49.03 ± 11.97	2.44	−1.47 (0.1514)
	Control	13	54.38 ± 7.33	2.03	

Table 3.
Hydrogen donors (HD) by groups.

Glutathione peroxidase and catalase catalyze hydrogen peroxide reduction to water and oxygen. Thus, they exert a protective effect against oxidative injury (**Figure 1**).

The levels of these enzymes decrease with the decrease in gestational age. Another factor that influences enzymatic antioxidant mechanisms is neonatal development. In neonates with intrauterine growth restriction, the antioxidant enzymes SOD, CAT, and GSH-Px have lower values than in term AGA neonates [12, 13].

In our study, for the assessment of enzymatic antioxidant defense capacity, erythrocyte SOD was measured using the Winterbourn method. Hemoglobin concentration was determined in K3 EDTA samples by the Drabkin method.

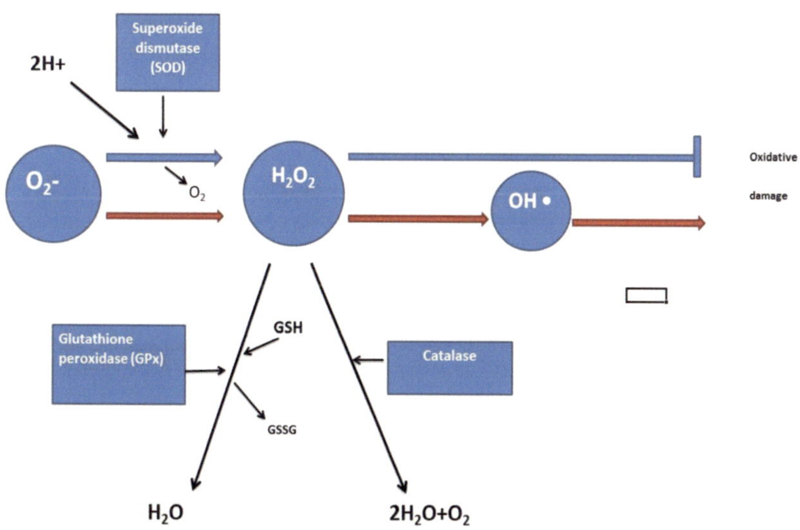

Figure 1.
Enzymatic antioxidant mechanism.

Determinations in the study group of preterm neonates compared to the values of the control group including full-term newborns evidenced a statistically significant difference, SOD values being higher in term newborns compared to the group of premature babies [6]. The same results were obtained in the case of SOD measurement using Ransod kits (Cat. No. SD 125, Randox Labs, UK). SOD activity was expressed as the amount of proteins leading to inhibition of 90% formazan (505 nm) using xanthine oxidase to generate superoxide radicals [7].

Other studies, as well as our findings show the fact that antioxidant defense is impaired in neonates. This impairment increases with the decrease in gestational age, but is also influenced by the association of oxidative stress-inducing factors that put a strain on the defective defense mechanisms of the newborn.

5. Antioxidant treatment

5.1 Enzymatic therapies

Animal studies have demonstrated the beneficial effects of SOD on ROS. SOD administration as aerosols in animals improved alveolar development in the case of bronchopulmonary dysplasia induced by the common action of multiple factors: prematurity, hyperoxia, and mechanical ventilation.

Cysteine, which has glutathione stimulating effects, was studied in premature babies. Glutathione is an important antioxidant and a cofactor for GPx. However, studies failed to demonstrate its beneficial effect in reducing oxidative stress, since the harmful effects of ROS could not be prevented by cysteine administration. Glutathione levels were significantly higher after cysteine administration. Administration of recombinant CuZnSOD to preterm babies during the intubation period led to a decrease in the incidence of wheezing episodes, but did not reduce the incidence of BPD compared to preterm babies who received placebo during the same period [20]. The incidence of ROP in preterm babies receiving this treatment also decreased [11].

5.2 Non-enzymatic therapies

The beneficial effects of vitamin E have been studied by different authors. Randomized controlled trials could not demonstrate the effect of vitamin E in preventing BPD. There are studies that evidence the beneficial effects of vitamin E in reducing the incidence of cerebral hemorrhage, while increasing the risk of neonatal sepsis; consequently, the risk exceeds the benefits provided by the antioxidant effect.

A Cochrane analysis of vitamin A describes its role in preventing BPD, but neurological and respiratory development at 18–22 months is not superior in babies receiving vitamin A [15, 21].

Regarding vitamin C, studies have demonstrated that in addition to its antioxidant effect, in certain situations, after a significant oxidative attack, vitamin C can act as a pro-oxidant and will cause additional injuries [13, 15].

High vitamin C concentrations will inhibit ceruloplasmin and will induce oxidation of Fe^{2+}, which will have a catalytic action in lipid peroxidation and thus will generate new free radicals [23].

Excess of protein-unbound iron has a pro-oxidant effect, resulting in the production of free radicals with harmful effects. Lactoferrin has a key role in limiting the pro-oxidant action of free iron, its presence in milk formulas being particularly important [22, 28].

5.3 Other antioxidant therapies

Resveratrol is known for its antioxidant effect in astrocytes. Its role is important after asphyxia episodes. It acts by stimulating glutamate synthase activity and increases GSH levels in hippocampal astrocytes. The increase in glutamate synthase activity counters the toxic effect of glutamate.

Melatonin is a substance studied for its antioxidant effect. It has a role in repairing leukomalacia lesions, but its beneficial action has been described when it is administered early, in the first 2 hours after injury. Animal studies have demonstrated beneficial effects of enteral arginine and glutamine in preventing NEC [4, 5, 28].

Human milk feeding has a number of benefits over formulas. Studies demonstrate the antioxidant effect of breast milk, which contributes to ROS elimination. Higher amounts of oxidative stress metabolites are eliminated in the urine of preterm babies fed with formula compared to those fed with breast milk. Oxidative stress is increased in premature neonates fed with formula. The antioxidant capacity of breast milk is higher than that of neonatal blood [24].

Author details

Melinda Matyas* and Gabriela Zaharie
University of Medicine and Pharmacy, Cluj-Napoca, Romania

*Address all correspondence to: melimatyas@yahoo.com

References

[1] Saugstad OD. Optimal oxygenation at birth and in the neonatal period. Neonatology. 2007;**91**:319-322

[2] Biesalski HK, Nohr I. Importance of vitamin-A for lung function and development. Molecular Aspects of Medicine. 2003;**24**:431-440

[3] Brion LP, Bell EF, Raghuveer TS. Vitamin E supplementation for prevention of morbidity and mortality in preterm infants. Cochrane Database of Systematic Reviews. 2003;**4**: CD003665

[4] Gitto E, Karbownik M, Reiter RJ, et al. Effects of melatonin treatment in septic newborns. Pediatric Research. 2001;**50**(6):756-760

[5] Sánchez-Barceló EJ, Mediavilla MD, Tan DX, Reiter RJ. Clinical uses of melatonin: Evaluation of human trials. Current Medicinal Chemistry. 2010;**17**(19):2070-2095

[6] Matyas M, Zaharie G, Craciun C, Blaga L. Evaluation of superoxide dismutase in preterm newborns. Obsterica Ginecologia. 2012;**LX**:267-271

[7] Matyas M, Craciun C, Popescu A, Popa M. The activity of erythrocytes superoxide dismutase in premature and mature infants-the relationship with gestational age. Physiology. 2007;**17, 1**(53):25-28

[8] Gitto E, Reiter RJ, Xian-Tan D, Barberi I. Respiratory distress syndrome in the newborn: Role of oxidative stress. Intensive Care Medicine. 2001;**27**:1116-1123

[9] Allen RG, Tresini M. Oxidative stress and gene regulation. Free Radical Biology & Medicine. 2000;**28**:463-499

[10] Sola A, Rodigo MR, Deulofeut R. Oxygen as a neonatal health hazard: Call for détente in clinical practice. Acta Paediatrica. 2007;**96**(6):801-812

[11] Ozsurekci Y, Aykac K. Oxidative stress related diseases in newborns. Oxidative Medicine and Cellular Longevity. 2016;**15**:1-9

[12] Gupta BP, Narang S, Banerjee BD. Oxidative stress in term small for gestational age neonates born to undernourished mothers: A case control study. BMC Pediatrics. 2004;**4**:14. DOI: 10.1186/1471-2431-4-14

[13] Shoji H, Koletzko B. Oxidative stress and antioxidant protection in the perinatal period. Current Opinion in Clinical Nutrition and Metabolic Care. 2007;**10**(3):324-328

[14] Martin A, Camille F, Debevec T, Rytz C, Millet G, Pialoux V. Preterm birth and oxidative stress: Effects of acute physical exercise and hypoxia physiological responses. Redox Biology. 2018;**17**:315-322

[15] Buonocore G, Groenendaal F. Anti-oxidant strategies. Seminars in Fetal & Neonatal Medicine. 2007;**12**:287e295

[16] Muresan A. Reactive Oxygen Species in Clinical Pathology. Romania: Editura Dacia; 1997:24-30. ISBN: 35-0703-2

[17] Matyas M, Zaharie G. Particularities of oxidative stress in newborns in Novel Propsects in Oxidative and Nitrosative Stress by Pinar Atukeren, IntechOpen: Rijeka 2018; 93-109

[18] Quango S, Mukherjea M. Ontogenic profile of some antioxidants and lipid peroxidation in human placental and fetal tissue. Molecular and Cellular Biochemistry. 2000;**215**(1-2):11-19

[19] Dheen ST, Tay SS, Boran J, et al. Recemnt studies on neural tube defects in embryos of diabetic pregnancy: An

overview. Current Medicinal Chemistry. 2009;**16**:2345-2354

[20] Davis JM, Parad R, Michele T, Allred E, Price A, Rosenfeld W. Pulmonary outcome at 1 year corrected age in premature infants treated at birth with recombinant human CuZn SOD dismutase. Pediatrics. 2003;**111**:469-476

[21] Ambalavanan N, Tyson JE, Kennedy KA, et al. Vitamin A supplementation for extremely low birth weight infants: Outcome at 18-22 months. Pediatrics. 2005;**115**:249-254

[22] Collard KJ. Iron homeostasis in the neonate. Pediatrics. 2009;**123**:1208-1216

[23] Lindeman JH, Lentjes EG, van Zoeren-Grobben D, Berger HM. Postnatal changes in plasma ceruloplasmin and transferrin antioxidant activities in preterm babies. Biology of the Neonate. 2000;**78**:73-76

[24] Ledo A, Arduini A, Asensi MA, et al. Human milk enhances antioxidant defenses against hydroxyl radical aggression in preterm infants. The American Journal of Clinical Nutrition. 2009;**89**:210-215

[25] Sahni PV, Zhang J, Sosunov S, Galkin A, Niatsetskaya Z, Starkov A, et al. Krebs cycle metabolites and preferential succinate oxidation following neonatal hypoxic-ischemic brain injury in mice. Pediatric Research. 2018;**83**:491-497

[26] Perlman JM, Wyllie J, Kattwinkel J, Wyckoff MH, Aziz K, Guinsburg R, et al. Part 7: Neonatal resuscitation: 2015 International consensus on cardiopulmonary resuscitation and emergency cardiovascular care science with treatment recommendations. Pediatrics; **2015**(Suppl 2):136, S120-S166

[27] Kuligowski J, Aguar M, Rook D, Lliso I, Torres-Cuevas I, Escobar J, et al. Urinary lipid peroxidation byproducts: Are they relevant for redicting neonatal morbidity in preterm infants? Antioxidants & Redox Signaling. 2015;**23**:178-184

[28] Sánchez-Illana Á, Thayyil S, Montaldo P, Jenkins D, Quintás G, Oger C, et al. Novel free-radical mediated lipid peroxidation biomarkers in newborn plasma. Analytica Chimica Acta. 2017;**996**:88-97

[29] Picone S, Ritieni A, Fabiano A, Troise AD, Graziani G, Paolillo P, et al. Arterial cord blood lutein levels in preterm and term healthy newborns are sex and gestational age dependent. Clinical Biochemistry. 2012;**45**:1558-1563. DOI: 10.1016/j.clinbiochem.2012.07.109

[30] Davis JM, Auten RL. Maturation of the antioxidant system and effects on preterm birth. Seminars in Fetal & Neonatal Medicine. 2010;**15**:191-195

Chapter 11

Prevention of Oxidative Injury Associated with Thrombolysis for Ischemic Stroke

Darryl R. Peterson and Ernest J. Sukowski

Abstract

Although treatment of ischemic stroke focuses on re-establishing blood flow to the brain (e.g., thrombolysis), delayed reperfusion may be associated with oxidative damage to brain capillary endothelial cells, resulting in cerebral bleeding and death (hemorrhagic transformation). The goal of this study was to define cellular mechanisms responsible for reperfusion injury to brain capillaries, and to provide a rationale for more effective treatment of stroke. Mechanisms of oxidative injury to cerebral capillary endothelial cells were measured in the presence and absence of experimental inhibitors to define the roles of transport and metabolic pathways. *In vitro* experiments provided evidence that: (1) intracellular calcium is elevated in brain capillary endothelial cells following simulated transient ischemia and reperfusion, due to reverse movement of Na/Ca exchange; (2) a simultaneous increase of calcium and reactive oxygen species (ROS) during re-oxygenation causes mitochondrial dysfunction, thus initiating apoptosis and loss of brain capillary integrity. *In vivo* studies showed that γ-glutamylcysteine (an antioxidant precursor of glutathione) and the experimental compound KB-R7943 (inhibits reverse movement of Na/Ca exchange) protect brain capillary endothelial cells when co-administered just before reperfusion following transient ischemia. The data indicate that these agents may be useful in preventing oxidative injury associated with thrombolysis for ischemic stroke.

Keywords: glutathione, gamma-glutamylcysteine, antioxidant, stroke, thrombolysis, hemorrhagic transformation

1. Introduction

Cerebrovascular stroke is a leading cause of death and disability in the world [1, 2]. Strokes may be ischemic or hemorrhagic, but most (ca. 85%) are due to interrupted blood flow to the brain, resulting in hypoxia [2]. Thus, the treatment for cerebral ischemia accompanying stroke includes therapies to re-establish blood flow using a thrombolytic agent [3–8]. Delayed reperfusion following cerebral ischemia (>3–4.5 hours) may cause damage to brain capillary endothelial cells [9–11] that can lead to cerebral bleeding and death [12, 13], a process called *reperfusion injury* leading to *hemorrhagic transformation* [14, 15]. Recent evidence has verified that using tissue plasminogen activator (tPA) to dissolve clots is an effective treatment for ischemic stroke, if administered prior to the 3–4.5 hour interval [11, 16, 17]. However, only about 5% of patients with cerebral ischemia arrive at the hospital in time to be treated without causing vascular damage and cerebral hemorrhage, and

IntechOpen

a significant number of eligible patients bleed anyway [18]. Thus, preventing injury to the cerebral vasculature when using a thrombolytic agent to induce reperfusion is of great importance. In this study, we provide evidence that reperfusion injury is associated with *oxidative* damage to brain capillary endothelial cells in the presence of elevated calcium. Furthermore, we show that the antioxidant γ-glutamylcysteine [19, 20] (a precursor of glutathione) together with an agent to prevent calcium sequestration inhibit oxidative injury to brain capillaries when co-administered immediately prior to inducing reperfusion for ischemic stroke.

2. Materials and methods

To understand the mechanisms responsible for reperfusion injury to cerebral blood vessels, pertinent transport properties were first defined in isolated plasma membranes derived from brain capillary endothelial cells (i.e., the blood-brain barrier). This was followed by examining the effects of simulated ischemia and reperfusion on cultured blood-brain barrier endothelial cells, and testing the utility of experimental drugs in preventing cellular damage. Finally, the experimental therapeutic approach was tested *in vivo*, using the middle cerebral artery occlusion technique in rats to simulate ischemic stroke.

2.1 *In vitro* studies

2.1.1 Preparation of brain capillary endothelial membrane vesicles

Brain capillary endothelial cells are polarized and possess tight junctions (i.e., zonula occludens) [21]. Luminal (blood-facing) and abluminal (brain-facing) membrane vesicles were isolated from bovine brain capillary endothelial cells by methods that we have described in detail [10–12, 22, 23]. Briefly, cerebral capillaries were isolated from cow brains by homogenization, differential centrifugation, and separation on a column of glass beads. Following mild treatment with collagenase, the capillaries were further homogenized, and the endothelial membranes were separated in a discontinuous Ficoll gradient.

2.1.2 Transport measurements in membrane vesicles

The methods for quantifying transport measurements using membrane vesicles from brain capillary endothelial cells have been published by us [8, 9, 24–26]. Rates of substrate uptake by luminal and abluminal membrane vesicles were determined using radiolabeled tracers and a rapid filtration technique [27, 28].

2.1.3 Western blot analysis of membrane vesicles

NHE1 (Na/H antiporter, isoform 1) and NCX1 (Na/Ca exchanger, isoform 1) were identified in isolated plasma membranes from bovine brain capillary endothelial cells using immunoblotting with mouse monoclonal antibodies (Chemicon) and horseradish peroxidase-conjugated goat anti-mouse antibody, as previously described [29, 30]. The bands were analyzed by laser scanning densitometry.

2.1.4 Polymerase chain reaction analysis of cerebral capillaries

After mRNA was isolated from bovine cerebral capillaries [31], first-strand cDNA was synthesized using oligo-dT and AMV reverse transcriptase (Promega or

Invitrogen), and sense and antisense primers (Sigma) were used to generate PCR products for NHE1, Na/K ATPase α2, and Na/K ATPase α3, as previously described [31, 32]. Sequencing was performed on both strands, using a commercial service. Quantitative Western blotting was done as previously described [30]. The bands were scanned and quantified using NIH Image software.

2.1.5 Culturing cerebral capillary endothelial cells

Cultured cerebral capillary endothelial cells were used as an *in vitro* model to measure the effects of simulated ischemia and reperfusion on blood-brain barrier function [33–37]. The capillary endothelial cells were isolated from bovine brain using the method of Meresse *et al.* [33], or purchased from Cell Systems Corporation (Kirkland, Washington). Cells were grown, maintained, seeded, and incubated in the presence of an astrocyte conditioned medium supplemented with cAMP, as previously described [33–37].

2.1.6 Simulating ischemia and reperfusion using cultured cells

Cultured brain capillary endothelial cells were exposed to conditions simulating ischemia and reperfusion by incubating first at 37°C in an ischemic medium (without glucose, pH 6.8) equilibrated with an atmosphere of 95% N_2 and 5% CO_2, followed by simulated reperfusion in a control medium (5.6 mM glucose, pH 7.4) equilibrated with room air and 5% CO_2 [38, 39]. To provide a constant environment, the cells were maintained in sealed chambers (Billups-Rothenberg, CA) pre-equilibrated to the desired atmospheric conditions [39].

2.1.7 Measuring intracellular calcium and sodium concentrations

Intracellular calcium was quantified in cultured cerebral capillary endothelial cells by using a fluorescent probe and confocal laser microscopy, as previously described by us [39]. Cells were preloaded with 5 μM Fluo-4 [39] and treated under conditions of ischemia and reperfusion as described above. Calcium concentration was quantified by measuring emitted fluorescence [39, 40] at a wavelength of 494 nm in 50 randomly chosen (computer-assisted) cells, representing each treatment.

Intracellular sodium in cultured cerebral capillary endothelial cells was measured as previously described by us [39]. Cells were pre-treated with Sodium Green (5 μM), and the fluorescent signal was quantified by fluorescence microscopy. Measurements were made from 50 randomly chosen cells representing each treatment.

2.1.8 Measuring actin stress fibers in cultured cells

Cerebral capillary endothelial cells were grown on coverslips and exposed to conditions simulating normoxia, ischemia, and reperfusion as described above. Following treatment, the monolayers were washed in phosphate buffered saline (pH 7.4), fixed for 5 minutes in 3.7% buffered formaldehyde at room temperature, and rinsed again with the buffer [41]. A mixture of phalloidin (0.05 mg/ml buffer) and 1% dimethyl sulfoxide was added to the cells for 40 minutes at room temperature, in a humidified chamber. Following staining, the coverslips were washed with buffer and mounted in a mixture of 30% glycerol in 70% buffer (vol/vol). To determine the effects of calcium-mediated cytoskeletal activation, the cells were incubated in the presence of a myosin light chain kinase inhibitor (0.1 μM, Sigma).

The tissue was observed and evaluated using laser confocal microscopy, at a thickness of 4 microns.

2.1.9 *Measuring permeability of cultured cells*

To quantify functional injury to brain capillaries, ^{14}C-sucrose permeability was measured across a monolayer of cerebral capillary endothelial cells [42], under conditions simulating ischemia and reperfusion as described above. Cyclosporin A (1 μM) was used as an inhibitor of the mitochondrial permeability transition [43, 44], to determine if this process is associated with reperfusion injury to the endothelium.

2.1.10 *Measuring caspase activity of cultured cells*

Caspase 3 activity was measured fluorometrically using an oncogene caspase-3 activity kit, as previously described [39]. Cultured blood-brain barrier cells were lysed, and the lysate was added to the caspase substrate: L-aspartyl-L-glutamyl-L-valyl-L-aspartic acid amide (DEVD) tagged with the fluorescent molecule 7-amino-4-trifluoromethyl coumarin (AFC). Cleaved AFC was fluorescent, and was quantified at an excitation wavelength of 390 nm, and an emission wavelength of 510 nm.

2.1.11 *Measuring lysis/death of cultured cells*

Lactate dehydrogenase (LDH) release was used to determine cell lysis, and was measured colorimetrically at a wave-length of 490 nm with a commercial kit (Promega). The effectiveness of various antioxidants [19, 20, 45] in preventing cell death was tested by incubating the cells in the presence (1 mM) and absence of glutathione (GSH), N-acetylcysteine (NAC), and gamma-glutamylcysteine (γGlu-Cys).

2.2 *In vivo* studies

2.2.1 *Middle cerebral artery occlusion*

Ischemia and reperfusion were simulated in rats using the middle cerebral artery occlusion (MCAO) technique [46], by placing a thread in the left cerebral artery to reduce blood flow in the left hemisphere, and withdrawing it to re-establish circulation. Briefly, adult female Long-Evans rats (250–300 g) were anesthetized with isoflurane (5% induction and 2% for maintenance). The pterygopalatine artery and branches of the carotid artery were cauterized on the left side, after which a 3 centimeter length of 3.0 Dermalon suture (blunt tip) was introduced in a retrograde direction into the external carotid artery. It was advanced cranially in the internal carotid artery for 23 mm, as measured from the bifurcation of the common carotid artery. This model reduced cerebral blood flow to about 10% of control in the core of the ischemic area. Reperfusion was achieved by withdrawing the thread into the external carotid artery.

2.2.2 *Measuring brain capillary mitochondrial morphology*

Mitochondrial damage indicative of reperfusion injury was measured in cerebral capillary endothelial cells of rats exposed for 1 hour to cerebral ischemia, followed by 24 hours of reperfusion. Cerebral ischemia and reperfusion was accomplished using the MCAO model of ischemic stroke. Stroked animals not treated with drugs were infused intravascularly (IV, femoral vein) with 1 ml of physiological saline approximately 1 minute prior to initiating reperfusion. Treated animals were co-administered γGlu-Cys (400 mg/kg) and KB-R7943 (10 mg/kg) IV in 1 ml of physiological saline 1 minute before reperfusion. The mitochondrial permeability transition was assessed by measuring a typical change in ultrastructural morphology characterized by swelling [47]. Following 60 minutes of transient ischemia and 24 hours of reperfusion, the animals were killed, and brain cortical tissue adjacent to the putamen was sampled and treated with a fixative and prepared for electron microscopy. Fixation involved 2% paraformaldehyde and 2.5% glutaraldehyde in phosphate buffer, and tissue blocks were osmicated, dehydrated in an ethanol series, cleared in propylene oxide, and embedded in Epon. Ultra-thin sections were stained with uranyl acetate and lead citrate, and examined on a Jeol JEM-1230 (HC) electron microscope. Measurements of mitochondrial cross sectional area in cerebral capillary endothelial cells were determined by examining electron micrographs and using computer-assisted morphometry. Briefly, random samples including blood-vessels from the outer cerebral cortical zones of the ipsilateral and contralateral sides were photographed for each animal. Five random samples included 3 blood vessels, 9 endothelial cells, and 45 mitochondria from each of 4 animals per treatment. These samples were measured by outlining the mitochondria with an electronic pen, and compiling the data with commercial stereological software (Neurolucida).

2.2.3 Measuring brain apoptosis

Evidence of apoptosis in the cerebral cortex of the above animals exposed to ischemia/reperfusion (1 hour/24 hours) was determined by using the Apop-Tag Kit (Oncor). Tissue sections were randomly sampled from the cortex, and prepared for immunocytochemistry using the Tunnel assay [48]. The number of stained nuclei were quantified per unit area, as determined with the Neurolucida program.

2.2.4 Measuring neurological behavior

After 1 hour of ischemia and 24 hours of reperfusion, the above animals were observed for obvious neurological deficits indicated by behavioral changes. Attention was focused on motor deficits, torticollis, and obvious paresis.

2.3 Analysis of the data

For the measurements collectively described in this study, values were expressed as an average ± SD or SE. Means were compared by Student's t test, a paired t test, or an ANOVA, depending upon the conditions. Mean values were considered significantly different if the probability of their being the same was 0.05 or less.

2.4 Vertebrate animals

Plasma membrane vesicles derived from cerebral capillary endothelial cells were isolated from cow brains obtained at a local slaughterhouse immediately after death. The cows were killed for food according to Federal and State laws, and not for the purposes of these experiments. Cultured cerebral capillary endothelial cells originated either from the fresh cow brains described above, or were purchased commercially (Cell Systems Corporation). The middle cerebral artery occlusion procedure *in vivo* was done using rats in the Blood–Brain Barrier Lab at Oregon

Health and Science University (OHSU), Portland, OR. OHSU is in full compliance with Federal and State statutes regarding the use and care of vertebrate animals in research. The animal care facility is AAALAC accredited, and all rat maintenance, treatment, recovery, and euthanasia procedures were approved for the reported middle cerebral artery occlusion studies.

To achieve middle cerebral artery occlusion, female Long Evans rats (250–300 grams) were anesthetized with isoflurane inhalant (5% induction, 2% maintenance). Analgesia was provided by administering butorphanol (0.05–2.0 mg/kg SQ) as needed, and seizures were controlled with diazepam (5 mg/kg) if necessary. Animals were monitored daily by staff veterinarians. Upon completion of the experiments, the rats were euthanized after inhalant anesthetic induction with an intracardiac overdose of sodium pentobarbital, or if symptoms necessitated earlier sacrifice. This method of euthanasia is consistent with requirements of the Panel of Euthanasia of the American Veterinary Medical Association.

3. Results

3.1 Evidence for the presence of NHE1, NCX1, and Na/K ATPase

3.1.1 Sodium flux studies

^{22}Na uptake was measured in membrane vesicles from brain capillary endothelial cells, and revealed both saturable and unsaturable components (**Figure 1**). In the presence of specific inhibitors, three transport pathways were found, including: (a) a low affinity (Km = 52 mM), high capacity, dimethyl amiloride (DMA, 100 μM) sensitive sodium carrier, indicative of Na/H antiport; (b) a high affinity (Km = 4.6 mM), low capacity, DMA resistant carrier; and (c) a non-specific phenamil inhibitable cationic channel (Kd = 1.7 μl/mg/min).

3.1.2 Immunoblotting

Immunoblotting using specific antibodies (Chemicon) to NHE1 (Na/H antiporter, isoform 1) and NCX1 (Na/Ca exchanger, isoform 1) revealed that both proteins are present in isolated luminal and abluminal membranes derived from

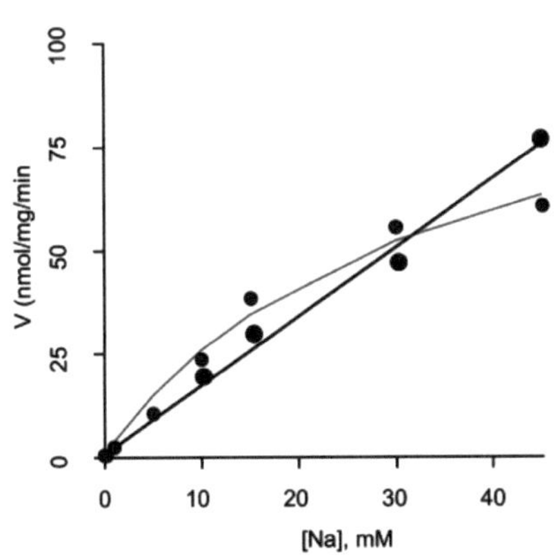

Figure 1.
Both saturable and unsaturable ^{22}Na uptake was measured in plasma membrane vesicles derived from bovine brain capillary endothelial cells. A saturable component (Km = 52 mM) was dimethyl amiloride (DMA) sensitive (100 μM), indicative of a sodium-hydrogen ion exchanger.

brain capillary endothelial cells. NHE1 appeared as a single band with a molecular weight of 106 kD. NCX1 displayed the usual two bands at 43 kD and 150 kD.

3.1.3 PCR studies

Messenger RNA was prepared from isolated bovine brain capillaries, and RT-PCR was performed with specific primers identifying NHE1, Na/K ATPase α_2, and Na/K ATPase α_3. The expected PCR products were found for NHE1 (**Figure 2**) and Na/K ATPase α_3, and sequencing demonstrated a high level of homology to the human transporters (>90%). Na/K ATPase activity was previously measured by us in luminal and abluminal membrane vesicles derived from endothelial cells forming the blood-brain barrier [25]. Activity was found to be present predominantly at the abluminal membrane domain, and was characterized by a ouabain binding constant (Kd = 25 ± 3 nM) typical of either the α_2 or α_3 isoform [49]. The PCR studies reported in the current study confirmed that it is the α_3 isoform.

3.2 Evidence that Na/H exchange elevates intracellular sodium

Intracellular sodium concentration was measured in cultured bovine brain capillary endothelial cells exposed to conditions simulating ischemia and reperfusion. **Figure 3A** shows that intracellular sodium was elevated ($P < 0.05$) during ischemia (120 minutes), and remained elevated during ischemia followed by reperfusion (90/30 minutes). Inhibiting the Na/H antiporter with 100 μM dimethyl amiloride (DMA) completely prevented the elevation of intracellular sodium observed during ischemia/reperfusion (90/30 minutes), indicating that its activity was responsible for the sustained increase in intracellular sodium observed during ischemia and reperfusion.

3.3 Evidence that Na/Ca exchange elevates intracellular calcium

Intracellular calcium was measured in cultured bovine blood-brain barrier cells exposed to conditions simulating ischemia and reperfusion. **Figure 3B** shows that calcium was significantly ($P < 0.05$) elevated during ischemia (120 minutes), and remained elevated during ischemia followed by reperfusion (90/30 minutes). Inhibition of the reverse mode of Na/Ca exchange (20 μM KB-R7943) reduced ($P < 0.05$) the level of intracellular calcium observed following reperfusion. Calcium uptake was also significantly inhibited with DMA (100 μM, not shown), indicating that both activation of Na/H antiport and reverse movement of Na/Ca exchange contributed to the sustained elevation of calcium.

NHE-1
SLPAERILPALSKDKEEEIRKILRNNLQKTRQ (Cow)
SLPSERILPALSKDKEEEIRKILRNNLQKTRQ (Human)

RLRSYNRHTLVADPYEEAWNQMLLRRQKARQL (Cow)
RLRSYNRHTLVADPYEEAWNQMLLRRQKARQI (Human)

EQKISNYLTVPAHKLDSPTMSRARIGSDPLAYEP (Cow)
EQKINNYLTVPANKLDSPTMSRARIGSDPLAYEP (Human)

KADLPVITIDPASPQSPESVDLVNEELKG (Cow)
KEDLPVITIDPASPQSPESVDLVNEELKG (Human)
96.8% Homologous

Figure 2.
The RT-PCR product for NHE1 was derived from bovine brain capillary endothelial cells, with a high homology (96.8%) for the respective isoform in human tissue.

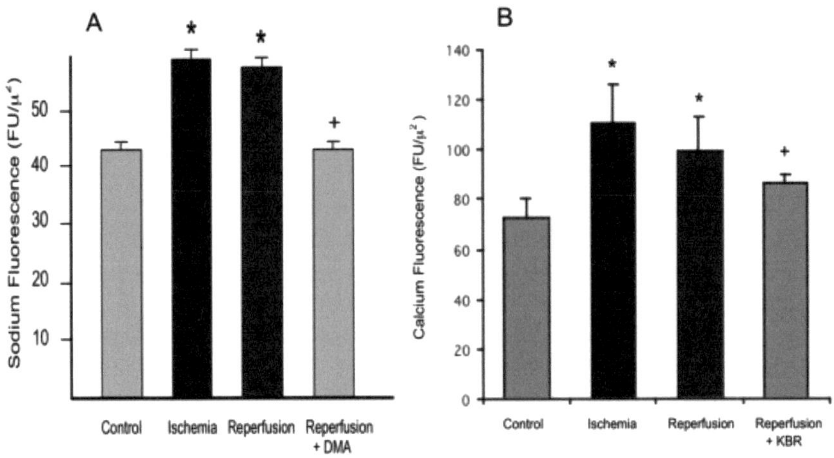

Figure 3.
*Simulating ischemia-reperfusion in cultured brain capillary endothelial cells resulted in a significant increase in intracellular sodium (panel a) during ischemia (120 minutes), that was maintained during ischemia followed by reperfusion (90/30 minutes). The rise observed during ischemia/reperfusion was prevented by inhibiting Na/H exchange (100 μM DMA). The same results were observed when measuring intracellular calcium (panel B). The rise in calcium during ischemia/reperfusion was significantly reduced with a specific inhibitor of the reverse movement of Na/Ca exchange (20 μM KB-R 7943). Intracellular calcium was also significantly reduced by DMA (100 μM (not shown). *P < 0.05, different from control; + P < 0.05, different from ischemia/reperfusion. Values are mean ± SD. Measurements are made from 50 cells randomly chosen to represent each treatment.*

3.4 Evidence for calcium-mediated alteration of the cytoskeleton

Cultured blood-brain barrier endothelial cells were exposed to conditions simulating ischemia and reperfusion, as described above. Following treatment, the cytoskeletal component actin was stained with phalloidin (0.05 mg/ml) [41] and examined using confocal laser microscopy. Incubating cells for 120 minutes under control conditions revealed the usual configuration of actin, which forms an organized ring of fibrils just inside the plasma membrane. Incubating under ischemic conditions either did not alter this configuration at all, or had a relatively minor effect on cytoskeletal arrangement. However, exposing the cells to ischemic conditions for 90 minutes, followed by 30 minutes of control treatment (reperfusion) caused a remarkable reorganization of the actin (**Figure 4**), which assumed the usual stress fiber configuration associated with damage and increased permeability characteristics [44]. An inhibitor of calcium activated myosin light chain kinase [50] (Sigma, 0.1 μM) prevented the appearance of stress fibers observed during reperfusion (**Figure 4**).

3.5 Evidence for alterations of permeability characteristics

Cultured cerebral capillary endothelial cells were incubated in transwells under conditions simulating ischemia (90 minutes) and reperfusion (30 minutes), and permeability properties of the endothelial barrier were measured by quantifying unidirectional flux of ^{14}C-sucrose across the endothelium [42]. **Figure 5** shows that selective inhibition of Na/H exchange, a brain capillary endothelial carrier shown earlier to contribute to calcium uptake (**Figure 3**) and structural damage (**Figure 4**) during reperfusion, caused a significant reduction in the observed permeability to sucrose.

3.6 Evidence for mitochondrial dysfunction

Figure 6 shows that 1 μM Cyclosporin A (CsA), an inhibitor of mitochondrial damage and apoptosis [42, 43, 51], significantly reduced sucrose permeability across

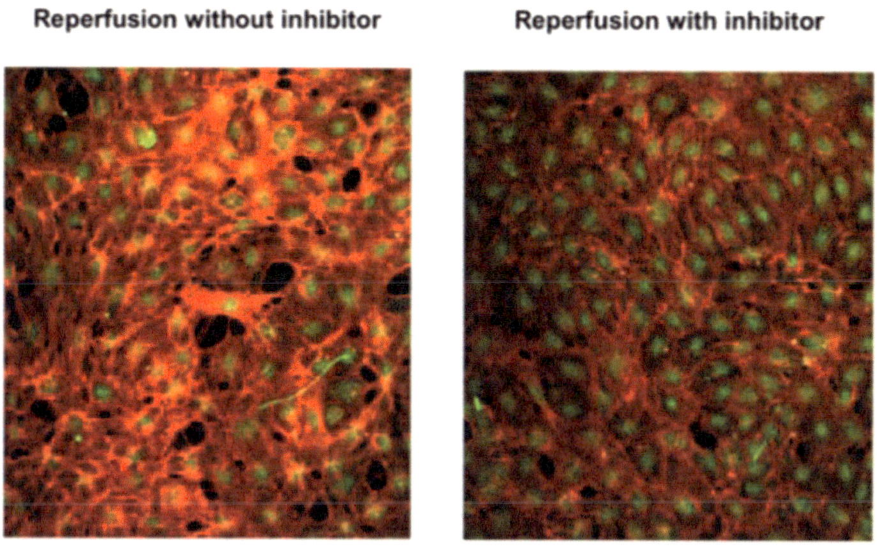

Figure 4.
Cultured blood-brain barrier cells were stained for actin with phalloidin following incubation under conditions of ischemia and reperfusion. Normally the actin forms a concentrated ribbon inside the plasma membrane, and ischemia alone causes only minor changes, if any. Simulated reperfusion (30 minutes) following ischemia (90 minutes), however, causes a random and diffuse rearrangement of actin, termed stress fibers (reperfusion without inhibitor). This pattern is typical of cell damage and enhanced permeability of passive solute markers through tight junctions. An inhibitor of calcium-activated myosin light chain kinase (sigma, 0.1 μM) completely prevented the appearance of stress fibers (reperfusion with inhibitor). These are representative fields from 4 sets of monolayers for each treatment.

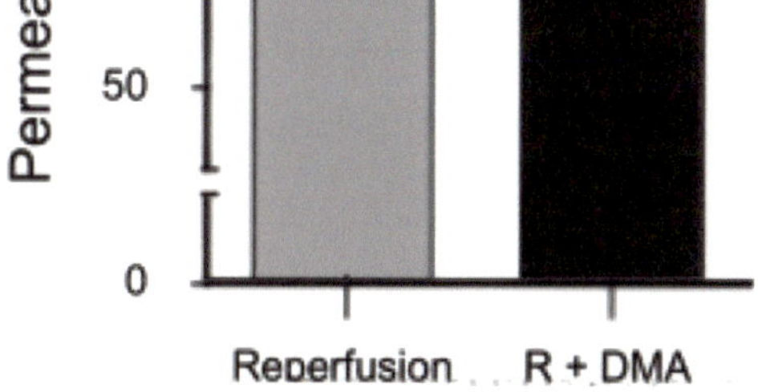

Figure 5.
*An inhibitor of Na/H antiport (100 μM DMA, R + DMA) significantly reduced the permeability (% of control) to ^{14}C-sucrose across cultured brain capillary endothelial cells observed during 90 minutes ischemia/30 minutes reperfusion (reperfusion). *P = 0.05. Values are mean ± SD, n = 4 observations.*

brain capillary endothelial cell monolayers associated with simulated ischemia (90 minutes) and reperfusion (30 minutes). In addition, **Figure 7** confirms that ischemia (30 minutes) followed by reperfusion (24 hours) greatly increased caspase 3 activity that is typically associated with apoptosis [51], and that this was significantly reduced with DMA (100 μM), an inhibitor of Na/H antiport and calcium loading (**Figure 3**). A specific inhibitor of caspase 3 activity (z-VAD-FMK, 10 μM)

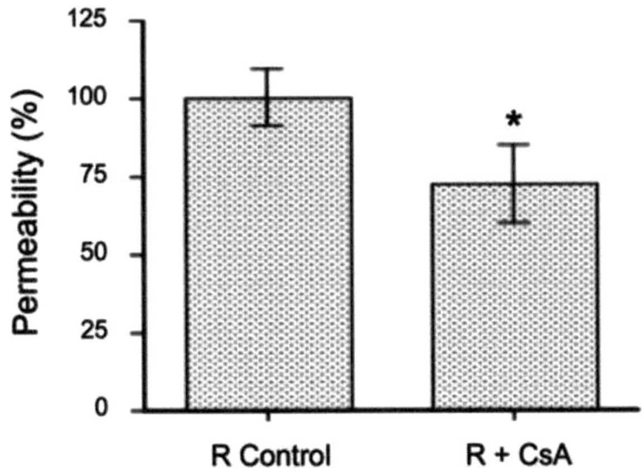

Figure 6.
*Inhibiting the mitochondrial permeability transition with Cyclosporin A (1 μM, R + CsA) significantly inhibited the sucrose permeability (% of control) observed during 30 minutes of reperfusion (R control), following 90 minutes of ischemia. *P < 0.05. Values are mean ± SD, n = 3 observations.*

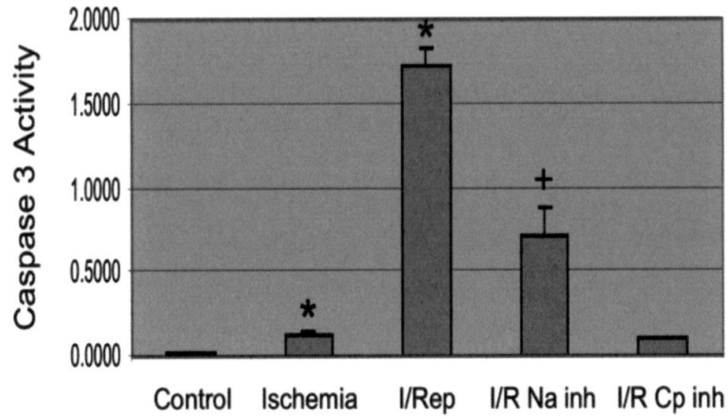

Figure 7.
*Caspase 3 activity was expressed in cultured blood-brain barrier cells exposed to conditions simulating ischemia-reperfusion. Twenty-four hours of reperfusion following 30 minutes of ischemia resulted in a large increase in caspase 3 activity that was inhibited with DMA (100 μM). *P < 0.05 from control; +P < 0.05 from I/rep. I/rep is ischemia plus reperfusion; I/R Na inh is ischemia-reperfusion with DMA inhibition; I/R Cp inh is ischemia-reperfusion with a specific caspase inhibitor. Values are mean ± SD, n = 3 observations.*

served as an internal control. The non-mitochondrial caspase 8 pathway for apoptosis showed no significant response in these cells.

3.7 Evidence for the protective role of antioxidants

We have previously shown that the antioxidant γ-glutamylcysteine reduces injury to cultured brain capillary endothelial cells [58] under conditions of simulated ischemia/reperfusion. Cells were incubated for 1.5 hours under ischemic conditions, followed by 3 hours of simulated reperfusion. The presence of 1 mM γ-glutamylcysteine significantly inhibited release of lactate dehydrogenase (LDH) into the incubation medium, thus reducing cell lysis. Additional new studies in our laboratory confirm that the antioxidants glutathione and *N*-acetylcysteine significantly ($P<0.05$) inhibit LDH release from cultured brain capillary endothelial cells under the same circumstances. Compared to cultured cells incubated under conditions simulating ischemia (1.5 hours) and reperfusion (3 hours) in the *absence* of these antioxidants, 1 mM glutathione and 1 mM *N*-acetylcysteine inhibited mean LDH release by factors of 0.51 and 0.45, respectively. Collectively, the data indicate that injury to cultured brain capillary endothelial cells exposed to ischemia/reperfusion is significantly reduced in the presence of known antioxidants [19, 20, 45] including native glutathione, and its precursors *N*-acetylcysteine, and γ-glutamylcysteine.

3.8 *In vivo* evidence for a strategy to prevent reperfusion injury

The purpose of the following experiments was to confirm that the mechanisms revealed by our cellular and molecular studies could be used to design a therapeutic approach in whole animals for the treatment of reperfusion injury to the brain capillaries, following transient ischemic stroke. The *in vitro* data suggested that two key factors are responsible for cellular injury and disruption of brain capillaries: (1) a rise in intracellular calcium due to reverse movement of the Na/Ca exchanger during reperfusion, and (2) depletion of endogenous antioxidant activity during the prolonged ischemia, resulting in an elevation of reactive oxygen species upon reperfusion. This led to our conclusion that a reasonable treatment for damage to brain capillary endothelial cells following transient ischemia would be to administer an inhibitor of reverse movement of Na/Ca exchange to prevent the rise in intracellular calcium, and to buffer reactive oxygen species by restoring antioxidant activity within the cells.

To test this hypothesis, middle cerebral artery occlusion (MCAO) was performed on Long-Evans female rats, involving 1 hour of ischemia to the left cerebral hemisphere, and 24 hours of reperfusion. One group of animals received KB-R7943 (10 mg/kg) and γ-glutamylcysteine (400 mg/kg) in 1 ml of isotonic saline solution 1 minute prior to reperfusion (IV, femoral vein), while the other group was administered a placebo (isotonic saline). Following treatment, tissue from the lateral cortex was prepared for electron microscopy, and the cross-sectional area of mitochondria in blood-brain barrier endothelial cells was quantified using morphometric techniques. The contralateral (right) hemisphere served as an internal control for non-ischemic tissue. The data is represented by electron micrographs in **Figure 8** from 2 of 4 animals in each group. As observed in the left panels of **Figure 8** depicting tissue exposed to ischemia/reperfusion without the drugs, mitochondria of blood-brain barrier endothelial cells (solid arrows) are noticeably swollen and abnormal in appearance, indicative of the mitochondrial permeability transition associated with apoptosis [43, 51]. In some instances, mitochondria have actually been extruded into the lumen (dashed arrows) of the capillary, indicating extensive cell damage. In the right panels showing tissue from 2 of 4 stroked animals administered the drugs, the mitochondria are normal, and the blood-brain barrier endothelial cells look healthy. When comparing the groups of animals, morphometric measurements of endothelial mitochondrial size revealed a highly significant ($P = 0.0015$) increase in swelling in stroked animals without the drugs vs. those with the drugs, expressed as a percent change in cross-sectional area from the control contralateral hemisphere (67 ± 15 vs. 13 ± 12, mean ± SD, $n = 4$ animals per group).

3.9 *In vivo* evidence for inhibition of apoptosis

Cerebral cortical tissue was randomly sampled from the animals above (1 hour ischemia/24 hours reperfusion), and the TUNEL assay was performed to determine if apoptosis was occurring. Representative tissue from 2 of 4 animals in each group is shown in **Figure 9**. The left panels show cerebral tissue from stroked animals without the drugs. Comparable regions are shown in the right panels, representing tissue from stroked animals that also received the drugs just prior to reperfusion. The cerebral tissue from stroked animals without the drugs showed prominent

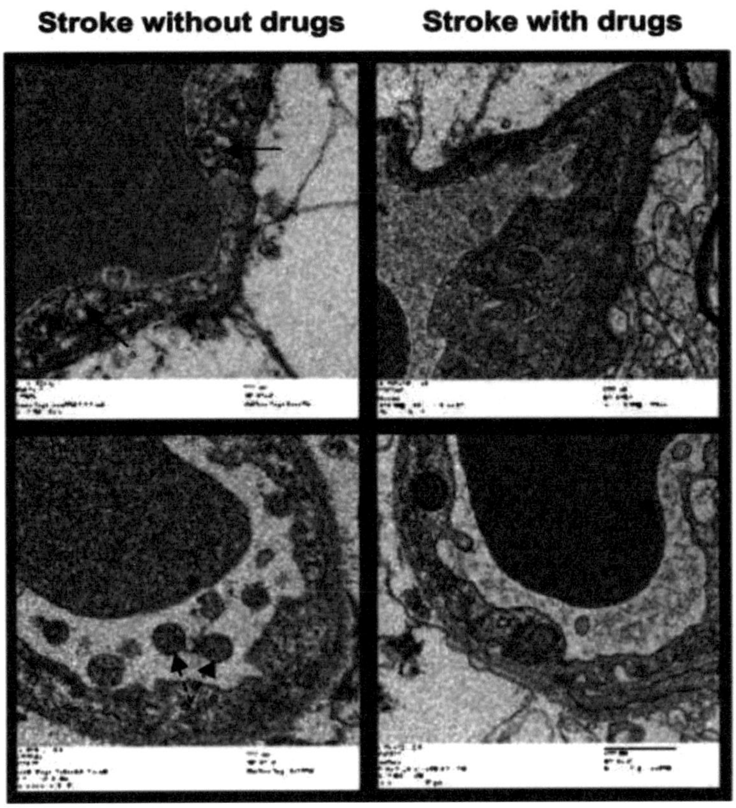

Figure 8.
Rats were subjected to conditions of transient ischemic stroke using middle cerebral artery occlusion for1 hour, followed by 24 hours of reperfusion. One group of stroked animals received cytoprotective drugs (i.e., KB-R 7943 [10 mg/kg] and γ-glutamylcysteine [400 mg/kg]) 1 minute prior to reperfusion, and a second group of stroked animals were administered a placebo. Lateral cerebral cortical tissue was prepared for electron microscopy, and the cross-sectional area of mitochondria in cerebral capillary endothelial cells was measured morphometrically. Two of four stroked animals without the drugs areshown in the left panels of the figure, and two of four stroked animals receiving the drugs are shown in the right panels. It is apparent that mitochondria are swollen in cerebral capillary endothelial cells of stroked animals without the drugs (left panels, solid arrows), suggesting the mitochondrial permeability transition [43] associated with apoptosis [51]. In some cases, damaged mitochondria have been extruded into the capillary lumen (left panels, dashed arrows). By contrast, the mitochondria of stroked animals given the drugs appear normal (right panels). When compared to mitochondria of the unstroked contralateral hemisphere (internal control), the percent increase in cross-sectional area was significantly (P = 0.0015) greater for the stroked animals not given the drugs (67 ± 15 vs. 13 ± 12, mean ± SD, n = 4 animals per group).

nuclear staining indicative of apoptosis, both in cerebral capillaries (arrows) and neural tissue. A morphometric analysis of the number of stained nuclei per unit area for 4 animals in each group (without drugs vs. with drugs) showed a significant difference (3.16 ± 2.00 grains/mm^2 vs. 0.39 ± 0.47 grains/mm^2, P = 0.036). No staining was observed in tissue from the contralateral, unstroked cerebral hemispheres.

3.10 *In vivo* evidence for inhibition of neurological dysfunction

To examine the effects of the drugs on neurological behavior following ischemic stroke, the animals for each group above were observed following 1 hour of ischemia and 24 hours of reperfusion. **Table 1** indicates that all 4 of the stroked animals without the drugs showed neurological deficits. Two additional stroked animals not receiving the drugs died. By contrast, 3 of 4 stroked animals that were given the drugs at the time of reperfusion showed no signs of neurological deficit. Furthermore, none of the animals receiving the drugs died.

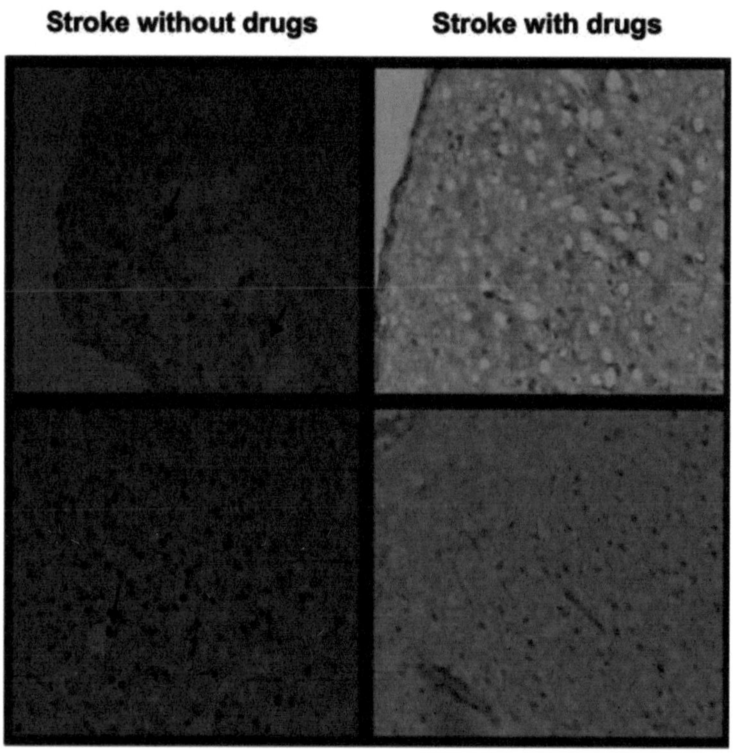

Figure 9.
Brain tissue from the above rats subjected to transient ischemic stroke (1 hour ischemia/24 hours reperfusion) was probed for evidence of apoptosis, using the TUNEL assay. Two of four stroke animals without and with the cytoprotective drugs (left and right panels, respectively) are depicted. In this figure, immunocytochemical nuclear reactions indicative of apoptosis are clearly visible in the animals without the drugs (left panels), but are not observed in the animals that were given the drugs (right panels). All four stroked animals without the drugs demonstrated apoptosis in blood-brain barrier endothelial cells (arrows) and neural tissue. Quantifying the number of stained nuclei per unit area showed a significant difference between animals without and with the drugs (3.1 6 ± 2.00 grains/mm^2 vs. 0.39 ± 0.47 grains/mm^2, mean ± SD, n = 4 animals per group, P = 0.036).

Stroked animals **without** drugs:	*Stroked* animals **with** drugs:
1. Right front paw deficit	1. No observable deficits
2. Slow moving, with some torticolis	2. No observable deficits
3. Obvious paresis	3. No observable deficits
4. Obvious paresis	4. Displays some motor deficits
Two additional animals died following stroke.	No deaths following stroke.

Table 1.
Neurological behavior following transient ischemic stroke.

4. Discussion

The purpose of this study was to define cellular mechanisms that contribute to reperfusion injury of blood vessels within the brain following thrombolysis for ischemic stroke, and to identify pharmacological agents that may be used to prevent cerebral bleeding associated with thrombolytic treatment for stroke. It is known that administering the thrombolytic agent tPA after approximately 3–4.5 hours of ischemia may cause reperfusion injury to brain capillaries [9–11] that can result in cerebral hemorrhage and death [12, 13]. Since approximately 95% of patients with ischemic strokes do not reach the hospital in time to be properly evaluated and safely administered a thrombolytic agent [18], the possibility of cerebral hemorrhage severely limits the treatment of stroke with tPA.

Cerebral capillary endothelial cells represent the fundamental structure of the blood-brain barrier [52]. These cells are polarized, containing both luminal (blood-facing) and abluminal (brain-facing) plasma membranes with distinct properties [21–23, 25, 26, 53–56]. The cells are held together by tight junctions that effectively inhibit paracellular transport [21], implying that the properties of the respective luminal and abluminal plasma membranes regulate transport across the blood-brain barrier. Based upon observations in other tissues [40, 57], we hypothesized that ischemia-reperfusion injury to cerebral capillary endothelial cells is due to oxidative injury associated with the formation of reactive oxygen species in the presence of elevated intracellular calcium during reperfusion [58–62]. This would require loss of intracellular antioxidant (e.g., glutathione) during prolonged ischemia, formation of free reactive oxygen species and uptake of calcium during re-oxygenation, and damage to mitochondria causing programmed cell death (apoptosis).

To test this hypothesis, we began by determining if the cellular processes required for these mechanisms are functional in blood-brain barrier endothelial cells. We reasoned that intracellular glutathione, an endogenous antioxidant, would diffuse out of the cells during ischemia, utilizing passive carriers we had previously described on both plasma membranes [58]. We next provided evidence that both Na/H (NHE1) and Na/Ca (NCX 1) exchangers are present on the plasma membrane domains of these cells, and that conditions simulating ischemia and reperfusion result in elevated intracellular calcium due to activation of sodium-hydrogen ion antiport and reverse movement of sodium-calcium exchange (**Figure 3**). Cellular lysis following these events was significantly inhibited by adding the antioxidant γGlu-Cys [19, 20, 58], which is consistent with the formation of reactive oxygen species expected upon re-oxygenation in glutathione depleted cells. These findings reinforced our interpretation that a combination of elevated intracellular calcium and reactive oxygen species are involved in injury to cerebral capillary endothelial cells, under conditions of ischemia and reperfusion.

Our studies further indicated that injury to brain capillaries involves two phases. An early increase in permeability to sucrose (**Figure 5**), a marker of paracellular transport, was associated with the formation of actin stress fibers inside the endothelial cells (**Figure 4**). This was, in turn, accompanied by the appearance of large intercellular holes (**Figure 4**), apparently due to the opening of tight junctions [63]. We reasoned that such a change could be due to activation of myosin light chain kinase in the presence of the elevated intracellular calcium that we previously observed (**Figure 3**). Since it has been shown that ischemia causes actin filaments to conjugate with ZO-1 [64], a tight junctional protein, force generated by contraction of the cytoskeleton could weaken the tight junctions and result in the formation of stress fibers. Indeed, treatment with a myosin light chain kinase inhibitor effectively reversed the effects of simulated ischemia and reperfusion on the formation of actin stress fibers, and the appearance of large intercellular holes (**Figure 4**). These morphological and functional changes in cerebral capillary endothelial cells occurred within a few hours of exposure to conditions simulating ischemia and reperfusion, and generally correlated with an early and reversible phase of altered permeability to the cerebral vasculature when exposed to conditions of ischemia and reperfusion *in vivo* [64].

A second phase of injury to cerebral capillaries following transient ischemia and reperfusion involved apoptosis and endothelial cell death. In an initial set of experiments, sucrose permeability was measured across monolayers of cultured blood-brain barrier endothelial cells exposed to conditions simulating ischemia and reperfusion. Permeability was significantly reduced by co-incubating with cyclosporin A (**Figure 6**), an inhibitor of the mitochondrial permeability transition associated with the early stages of apoptosis [42, 43, 51]. Under similar conditions, cultured blood-brain barrier endothelial cells expressed a large increase in caspase 3 activity after 24 hours of simulated reperfusion following ischemia (**Figure 7**), indicating activation of the apoptotic pathway [51].

These *in vitro* findings were consistent with our working hypothesis which predicted that elevated intracellular calcium and reactive oxygen species would activate apoptosis in cerebral capillary endothelial cells exposed to conditions of ischemia and reperfusion. Furthermore, the results suggested that: (1) inhibiting reverse movement of Na/Ca exchange with KB-R7943 [65], and (2) replenishing lost antioxidant with γGlu-Cys [19, 20] would prevent reperfusion (oxidative) injury to brain capillaries. Since γGlu-Cys is a precursor of the antioxidant glutathione [59] lost during ischemia, and γGlu-Cys itself possesses antioxidant properties [19, 20], it represents a reasonable antioxidant therapeutic in this setting.

The next logical step was to determine if drugs that prevent increased levels of intracellular calcium and reactive oxygen species in brain capillary endothelial cells would inhibit damage to cerebral capillaries *in vivo*. Thus, rats were exposed to middle cerebral artery occlusion to simulate ischemic stroke, after which the animals were either treated with a placebo (isotonic saline), or administered a combination of γGlu-Cys (400 mg/kg) and KB-R7943 (10 mg/kg) in isotonic saline that was infused intravenously approximately 1 minute prior to initiating reperfusion of cerebral blood flow. The rationale was that administering the combination of drugs immediately before re-establishing cerebral blood flow would protect the endothelial cells of cerebral capillaries from oxidative injury upon reperfusion. **Figure 8** indeed illustrates that such a therapeutic approach significantly inhibited morphological damage to cerebral capillary endothelial cells, including swelling of the mitochondria that is indicative of oxidative injury and the permeability transition that precedes apoptosis [51, 61, 62]. Furthermore, the Tunnel assay revealed that co-infusion of the drugs immediately before reperfusion inhibited the appearance of apoptosis in representative cerebral cortical tissue 24 hours after re-establishing blood flow to the brain (**Figure 9**). Finally, an assessment of neurological behavior confirmed that use of the drugs inhibited functional damage due to ischemia and reperfusion (**Table 1**).

5. Conclusions

Together these studies support the interpretation that prolonged cerebral ischemia followed by reperfusion of oxygenated blood may cause oxidative damage to cerebral capillary endothelial cells consistent with loss of vascular integrity and hemorrhage. The mechanisms involve mitochondrial injury and apoptosis due to the formation of reactive oxygen species in the presence of elevated cellular calcium. This condition may be treated by using the antioxidant γGlu-Cys to buffer reactive oxygen species, and a Na/Ca inhibitor (reverse mode) to prevent calcium loading in cerebral capillary endothelial cells. The *in vivo* studies indicate that co-administering both drugs intravascularly 1 minute prior to reperfusion provides cytoprotection that reduces reperfusion injury to the cerebral vasculature. Thus, this may represent a means of prolonging the window of opportunity to use a thrombolytic agent for treatment of ischemic stroke, and reduce the occurrence of hemorrhagic transformation in a clinical setting.

Acknowledgements

This study was supported by grants from the American Heart Association, a grant from the Medical Research and Development Fund, Christ Hospital and Medical Center, Oak Lawn, IL, and a Federal Work Study Program Award. We wish to thank Drs. P. Kosari, T. Lyu, E. Neuwelt, M. Pagel, A. Shoushtari, and Ms. J. Rambow for professional assistance during the conduct of this project.

Conflict of interest

Dr. Peterson (inventor) and Rosalind Franklin University of Medicine and Science (assignee) have been awarded patents that are related to research done in this study. They both may benefit financially upon commercialization of the patents. Dr. Peterson is a Professor at Rosalind Franklin University of Medicine and Science and owns Harbor Biotechnology, LLC, a company that seeks to commercialize the patents referenced above. Further details may be obtained from Dr. Peterson upon request.

Author details

Darryl R. Peterson[1,2*] and Ernest J. Sukowski[1]

1 Discipline of Physiology and Biophysics, Chicago Medical School, Rosalind Franklin University of Medicine and Science, North Chicago, IL, USA

2 Discipline of Medicine, Chicago Medical School, Rosalind Franklin University of Medicine and Science, North Chicago, IL, USA

*Address all correspondence to: darryl.peterson@rosalindfranklin.edu

References

[1] Thrift AG, Thayabaranathan T, Howard G, et al. Global stroke statistics. International Journal of Stroke. 2017;**12**:13-32. DOI: 10.1177/1747493016676285

[2] Mozaffarian D, Benjamin EJ, Go AS, et al. Heart disease and stroke statistics—2016 update: A report from the American Heart Association. Circulation. 2016;**133**:e38-e60. DOI: 10.1161/CIR.0000000000000350

[3] Emberson J, KR L, Lyden P, et al. Effect of treatment delay, age, and stroke severity on the effects of intravenous thrombolysis with alteplase for acute ischaemic stroke: A meta-analysis of individual patient data from randomized trials. Lancet. 2014;**384**:1929-1935. DOI: 10.1016/S0140-6736(14)60584-5

[4] Nasr DM, Brinjikji W, Cloft HJ, et al. Utilization of intravenous thrombolysis is increasing in the United States. International Journal of Stroke. 2013;**8**:681-688. DOI: 10.1111/j.1747-4949.2012.00844.x

[5] Musuka TD, Wilton SB, Traboulsi M, et al. Diagnosis and management of acute ischemic stroke: Speed is critical. CMAJ. 2015;**187**:887-893. DOI: 10.1503/cmaj.140355

[6] Demaerschalk BM, Kleindorfer DO, Adeoye OM, et al. Scientific rationale for the inclusion and exclusion for intravenous alteplase in acute ischemic stroke. Stroke. 2016;**47**:581-641. DOI: 10.1161/STR.0000000000000086

[7] Catanese L, Tarsia J, Fisher M. Acute ischemic stroke therapy overview. Circulation Research. 2017;**120**:541-558. DOI: 10.1161/CIRCRESAHA.116.309278

[8] Haldal S, Beary J, Nattanmai PC, et al. Acute ischemic stroke management review for the hospitalist. American Journal of Hospital Medicine. 2018;**2**:1-16. DOI: 10.24150/ajhm/2018.001

[9] Todd NV, Picozzi P, Crockard A, Russell RW. Duration of ischemia influences the development and resolution of ischemic brain edema. Stroke. 1986;**17**:466-471

[10] Warach S, Latour LL. Evidence of reperfusion injury, exacerbated by thrombolytic therapy, in human focal brain ischemia using a novel imaging maker of early blood-brain barrier disruption. Stroke. 2004;**35**:2659-2661. DOI: 1161/01.STR.0000144051.32131.09

[11] Hacke W, Kaste M, Bluhmki E, et al. Thrombolysis with alteplase 3 to 4.5 hours after acute ischemic stroke. The New England Journal of Medicine. 2008;**359**:1317-1329. DOI: 10.1056/NEJMoa0804656

[12] Gartshore G, Patterson J, Macrae IM. Influence of ischemia and reperfusion on the course of brain tissue swelling and blood–brain barrier permeability in a rodent model of transient focal cerebral ischemia. Experimental Neurology. 1997;**147**:353-360. DOI: 10.1006/exnr.1997.6635

[13] Wang X, Tsuji K, Lee SR, et al. Mechanisms of hemorrhagic transformation after tissue plasminogen activator reperfusion therapy for ischemic stroke. Stroke. 2004;**35**:2726-2730. DOI: 1161/01.STR.0000143219.16695.af

[14] Khatri R, McKinney AM, Swenson B, et al. Blood-brain barrier, reperfusion injury, and hemorrhagic transformation in acute ischemic stroke. Neurology. 2012;**79**:S52-S57. DOI: 10.1212/WNL.0b013e3182697e70

[15] Nour M, Scalzo F, Liebeskind DS. Ischemia-reperfusion injury in stroke. Interventional Neurology. 2012;**1**:185-199. DOI: 10.1159/000353125

[16] The National Institute of Neurological Disorders and Stroke rt-PA Stroke Study Group. Tissue plasminogen activator for acute ischemic stroke. The New England Journal of Medicine. 1995;**333**:1581-1587. DOI: 10.1056/NEJM199512143332401

[17] Gensicke H, Seiffge DJ, Polasek AE, et al. Long-term outcome in stroke patients treated with IV thrombolysis. Neurology. 2013;**80**:919-925. DOI: 10.1212/WNL.0b013e3182840c35

[18] Miller DJ, Simpson JR, Silver B. Safety of thrombolysis in acute ischemic stroke: A review of complications, risk factors, and newer technologies. The Neurohospitalist. 2011;**1**:138-147. DOI: 10.1177/1941875211408731

[19] Quintana-Cabrera R, Bolanos JP. Glutathione and γ-glutamylcysteine in the antioxidant and survival functions of mitochondria. Biochemical Society Transactions. 2013;**41**:106-110. DOI: 10.1041/BST20120252

[20] Peterson DR, Huang H, Peresada D, et al. A glutathione precursor reduces oxidative injury to cultured embryonic cardiocyocytes. American Journal of Therapeutics. 2018. DOI: 1097/MJT.0000000000000854 [Epub ahead of print]

[21] Peterson DR. Blood-brain barrier. In: Encyclopedia of Life Sciences. London: John Wiley & Sons, Ltd.; 2012. DOI: 10.1002/9780470015902.a0000023.pub/pdf

[22] Peterson DR, Hawkins RA. Isolation and behavior of plasma membrane vesicles made from cerebral capillary endothelial cells. In: Pardridge W, editor. Introduction to the Blood-Brain Barrier. London: Cambridge University Press; 1998. pp. 62-70. DOI: 10.1017/CBO9780511570216

[23] Peterson DR, Hawkins RA. Transport studies using membrane vesicles. In: Nag S, editor. The Blood-Brain Barrier: Biology and Research Protocols. Totowa: Humana Press; 2003. pp. 233-247

[24] Sanchez del Pino MM, Hawkins RA, Peterson DR. Neutral amino acid transport by the blood-brain barrier: Membrane vesicle studies. The Journal of Biological Chemistry. 1992;**267**:25951-25957

[25] Sanchez del Pino MM, Hawkins RA, Peterson DR. Biochemical discrimination between luminal and abluminal enzyme and transport activities of the blood-brain barrier. The Journal of Biological Chemistry. 1995a;**270**:14907-14912. DOI: 10.1074/jbc.270.25.14907

[26] Sanchez del Pino MM, Peterson DR, Hawkins RA. Neutral amino acid transport characterization of isolated luminal and abluminal membranes of the blood-brain barrier. The Journal of Biological Chemistry. 1995b;**270**:14913-14918. DOI: 10.1074/jbc.270.25.14913

[27] Skopicki HA, Fisher K, Zikos D, Flouret G, Bloch R, Kubillus S, et al. Carrier-mediated transport of pyroglutamyl-histidine in renal brush border membrane vesicles. The American Journal of Physiology. 1988;**255**:C822-C827. DOI: 10.1152/ajpcell.1988.255.6.C822

[28] Skopicki HA, Fisher K, Zikos D, Flouret G, Peterson DR. Low-affinity transport of pyroglutamyl-histidine in renal brush-border membrane vesicles. The American Journal of Physiology. 1989;**257**:C971-C975. DOI: 10.1152/ajpcell.1998.257.5.C971

[29] Cook SA, Sugden PH, Clerk A. Regulation of bcl-2 family proteins during development and in response to oxidative stress in cardiac myocytes: Association with changes in

mitochondrial membrane potential. Circulation Research. 1999;**85**:940-949

[30] Pignataro G et al. Two sodium/calcium exchanger gene products, NCX1 and NCX3, play a major role in the development of permanent focal cerebral ischemia. Stroke. 2004;**35**:2566-2570. DOI: 10.1161/01.STR.0000143730.29964.93

[31] Boado RJ, Pardridge WM. A one-step procedure for isolation of poly(a)+ mRNA from isolated brain capillaries and endothelial cells in culture. The Journal of Neuroscience. 1991;**57**: 2136-2139. DOI: 10.1111/j.1471-4159.1991.tb06433.x

[32] Morales A, Lachuer J, Bilbaut A, Georges B, Andrieu J-L, Diez J. Characterization of a Na-Ca exchanger NCX1 isoform in bovine fasiculata cells of adrenal gland. Molecular and Cellular Biochemistry. 2001;**218**:41-45. DOI: 10.1023/A:1007289902405

[33] Meresse S, Dehouck M-P, Delmore P, Bensaid M, Tauber J-P, Delbart C, et al. Bovine brain endothelial cells express tight junctions and monoamine oxidase activity in long-term culture. Journal of Neurochemistry. 1989;**53**:1363-1371. DOI: 10.1111/j.1471-4159.1989.tb08526.x

[34] Rubin LL, Hall DE, Porter S, Barbu K, Cannon C, Horner HC, et al. A cell culture model of the blood-brain barrier. The Journal of Cell Biology. 1991;**115**:1725-1735. DOI: 10.1083/jbc.115.6.1725

[35] Sun D, Lytle C, O'Donnell M. Astroglial cell-induced expression of Na-K-Cl cotransporter in brain microvascular endothelial cells. The American Journal of Physiology. 1995;**269**:C1506-C1512. DOI: 10.1152/ajpcell.1995.269.6.C1506

[36] Audus KL, Rose JM, Wang W, Borchardt R. Brain microvessel endothelial cell culture systems. In: Pardridge WM, editor. Introduction to the Blood-Brain Barrier. Cambridge: Cambridge University Press; 1998. pp. 86-93. DOI: 10.1017/CBO9780511570216

[37] Beuckmann CT, Galla H-J. Tissue culture of brain endothelial cells-induction of blood-brain barrier properties by brain factors. In: Pardridge WM, editor. Introduction to the Blood-Brain Barrier. Cambridge: Cambridge University Press; 1998. pp. 79-85. DOI: 10.1017/CBO9780511570216

[38] Ikeda K, Nagashima T, Wu S, Yamaguchi M, Tamaki N. The role of calcium ion in anoxia/reoxygenation damage of cultured brain capillary endothelial cells. Acta Neurochirurgica. Supplement. 1997;**70**:4-7

[39] Peterson D. Cytoprotective Therapeutic Agents for the Prevention of Reperfusion Injury Following Ischemic Stroke. US Patent US7956037B2; 2011

[40] Greene EL, Paller MS. Calcium and free radicals in hypoxia/reoxygenation injury of renal epithelial cells. The American Journal of Physiology. 1994;**266**:F13-F20. DOI: 10.1152/ajprenal.1994.266.1.F13

[41] Wulf E, Deboben A, Bautz FA, Faulstich H, Wieland T. Fluorescent phallotoxin, a tool for the visualization of cellular actin. Proceedings of the National Academy of Sciences of the United States of America. 1979;**76**:4498-4502

[42] Abbruscato TJ, Davis TP. Combination of hypoxia/aglycemia compromises in vitro blood-brain barrier integrity. The Journal of Pharmacology and Experimental Therapeutics. 1999;**289**:668-675

[43] Halestrap AP. The mitochondrial permeability transition: Its molecular mechanism and role in reperfusion

injury. Biochemical Society Symposium. 1999;**66**:181-203. DOI: 10.1042/bss0660181

[44] Griffiths EJ, Ocampo CJ, Savage JS, Stern MD, Silverman HS. Protective effects of low and high doses of cyclosporin a against reoxygenation injury in isolated rat cardiomyocytes are associated with differential effects on mitochondrial calcium levels. Cell Calcium. 2000;**27**:87-95. DOI: 10.1054/ceca.1999.0094

[45] Kersick C, Willoughby D. The antioxidant role of glutathione and N-acetylcysteine supplements and exercise-induced oxidative stress. Journal of the International Society of Sports Nutrition. 2005;**2**:38-44. DOI: 10.1186/1550-2783-2-2-38

[46] Masada T, Hua Y, Xi G, Ennis SR, Keep R. Attenuation of ischemic brain edema and cerebrovascular injury after ischemic preconditioning in the rat. Journal of Cerebral Blood Flow and Metabolism. 2001;**21**:22-33. DOI: 10.1097/00004647-200101000-00004

[47] Halestrap AP, Woodfield K-Y, Connern CP. Oxidative stress, thiol reagents, and membrane potential modulate the mitochondrial permeability transition by affecting nucleotide binding to the adenine nucleotide translocase. The Journal of Biological Chemistry. 1997;**272**: 3346-3354. DOI: 10.1074/jbc.272.6.3346

[48] O'Brien MA, Moravec RA, and Reiss. Poly(ADP-ribose)polymerase cleavage monitored in situ in apoptotic cells. BioTechniques. 2001;**30**:886-891. DOI: 10.2144/01304pf01

[49] Matsui H, Homareda H, Inoue N. Increase in Na pump activity of brain-type isoforms via increased turnover rate after glutamate excitation of cerebral neurons. In: Schoner W, editor. The Sodium Pump: Structure Mechanism, Hormonal Control and its Role in Disease. New York: Springer; 1994. pp. 710-713. DOI: 10.1007/978-3-642-72511-1

[50] Karaki H, Ozaki H, Hori M, Mitsui-Saito M, Amano K-I, Harda K-I, et al. Calcium movement, distribution, and functions in smooth muscle. Pharmacological Reviews. 1997;**49**:157-230

[51] Mayer B, Oberbauer R. Mitochondrial regulation of apoptosis. News in Physiological Sciences. 2003;**18**:89-94. DOI: 10.1152/nips.01433.2002

[52] Bradbury MWB. The blood-brain barrier. Transport across the cerebral endothelium. Circulation Research. 1985;**57**:213-222

[53] Hawkins RA, Viña JR, Peterson DR, O'Kane R, Mokashi A, Simpson IA. Amino acid transport across each side of the blood-brain barrier. In: D'Mello JPF, editor. Amino Acids in Nutrition and Health. Oxford: CABI; 2011. pp. 191-214

[54] Lee W-J, Hawkins RA, Peterson DR, Vina J. Role of oxoproline in the regulation of neutral amino acid transport across the blood-brain barrier. The Journal of Biological Chemistry. 1996;**271**:19129-19133. DOI: 10.1074/jbc.271.32.19129

[55] Lee W-J, Hawkins RA, Vina JR, Peterson DR. Glutamine transport by the blood-brain barrier: A possible mechanism for nitrogen removal. The American Journal of Physiology. 1998;**274**:C1101-C1107. DOI: 10.1152/ajpcell.1998.274.4.C1101

[56] Lee W-J, Peterson DR, Sukowski EJ, Hawkins RA. Glucose transport by isolated plasma membranes of the blood-brain barrier. The American Journal of Physiology. 1997;**272**:C1552-C1557. DOI: 10.1152/apjcell.1997.272.5.C1552

[57] Kalogeris T, Baines CP, Krenz M, et al. Cell biology of ischemia/reperfusion injury. International Review of Cell and Molecular Biology. 2012;**298**:229-317. DOI: 10.1016/B978-0-12-394309-5.00006-7

[58] Peterson DR, Sukowski EJ, Zikos D. Blood-brain barrier transport pathways for cytoprotective thiols. American Journal of Therapeutics. 2013;**20**(5):469-479. DOI: 10.1097/MJT.0b013e31829e8b7f. Available from: https://journals.lww.com/americantherapeutics/Abstract/2013/09000/Blood_Brain_Barrier_Transport_Pathways_for.4.aspx

[59] Meister A, Anderson ME. Glutathione. Annual Review of Biochemistry. 1983;**52**:711-760. DOI: 10.1146/annurev.bi.52.070183.003431

[60] Bridge JHB. The physiology of the Na-Ca exchange. In: Morad M, Ebashi S, Trautwein W, Kurachi Y, editors. Molecular Physiology and Pharmacology of Cardiac Ion Channels and Transporters. Vol. 182. Dordrecht: Springer; 1996. pp. 469-480

[61] Zoratti M, Szabo I. The mitochondrial permeability transition. Biochimica et Biophysica Acta. 1995;**1241**:138-176

[62] Kowaltowski AJ, Castilho RF, Vercesi AE. Mitochondrial permeability transition and oxidative stress. FEBS Letters. 2001;**495**:12-15. DOI: 10.1016/S0014-5793(01)02316-X

[63] Tsukamoto T, Nigam SK. Tight junction proteins form large complexes and associate with the cytoskeleton in an ATP depletion model for reversible junction assembly. The Journal of Biological Chemistry. 1997;**272**:16133-16139. DOI: 10.1074/jbc.272.26.16133

[64] Rosenberg GA, Estrada EY, Dencoff JE. Matrix metalloproteinases and TIMPs are associated with blood-brain barrier opening after reperfusion in rat brain. Stroke. 1998;**29**:2189-2195. DOI: 10.1161/01.STR.29.10.2189

[65] Brustovetsky T, Brittain MK, Sheets PL, et al. KB-R7943, an inhibitor of the reverse Na^+/Ca^{2+} exchanger, blocks N-methyl-D-aspartate receptor and inhibits mitochondrial complex I. British Journal of Pharmacology. 2011;**162**:255-270. DOI: 10.1111/j.1476-5381.2010.01054.x

Chapter 12

Dietary Antioxidants in the Chemoprevention of Prostate Cancer

Dwayne Tucker, Melisa Anderson, Fabian Miller, Kurt Vaz, Lennox Anderson-Jackson and Donovan McGrowder

Abstract

Prostate cancer is the second most common cancer and the fifth leading cause of cancer death. The incidence of prostate cancer is rising due to increased screening and awareness, and there is epidemiological evidence suggesting an interaction among biological and environmental risk factors in the development and progression of prostate cancer. Vegetables and fruits provide a wide range of antioxidants and phytochemicals that have been demonstrated to have a negative, positive, or no association with prostate cancer risk. Therefore, it is evident that the effect of dietary antioxidants on risk of prostate cancer remains undecided and inconclusive. The main focus of this review was to examine recent and past literature of the chemoprotective properties of five major groups of phytochemicals against prostate cancer development including both *in vivo* and *in vitro* findings.

Keywords: antioxidants, prostate, cancer, risk, association

1. Introduction

Among men worldwide, prostate cancer is the second most common cancer and the fifth leading cause of cancer death, with an estimated recorded amount of 1.3 million cases and 359,000 deaths in 2018 [1]. The incidence of prostate cancer is rising due to increased awareness and screening, and it is estimated that 42% of prostate cancer cases occur in men over 50 years old [2]. There is epidemiological proof that suggests an interaction among several known biological and environmental risk factors in the development and progression of prostate cancer [3]. These include age, race, family history, genetic risk, socioeconomic status, and modifiable risk factors such as physical activity, obesity, and possibly dietary factors [4].

Oxidative stress defined as an imbalance between prooxidant and antioxidant processes, and interference of the oxidation-reduction circuitry is one of the many proposed underlying mechanisms of prostate carcinogenesis [5, 6]. There is increasing epidemiological data that diet plays a key role in the biology and tumorigenesis of prostate cancer, and higher intake of the main phytochemical-containing diets lowers the risk of the disease [7]. Vegetables and fruits provide a wide range of phytochemicals and antioxidants that have been demonstrated to have a positive effect on decreasing the incidence or averting the occurrence of prostate cancer [8]. Several of these antioxidants may attenuate prostate cancer development, given that

IntechOpen

oxidative stress from reactive oxygen species and loss of antioxidant enzymes may contribute to genomic instability prior to prostate cancer [9].

This paper will review information in the literature on the relationship between nutrients with antioxidant properties from the diet, and the risk of prostate cancer.

2. Method of article selection

A literature search was conducted for all English language literature published before December 2018. The search was conducted using the electronic databases, including PubMed, Embase, Web of Science, and Cochrane Library. The search strategy included keywords such as prostate cancer, epidemiology, incidence, mortality, risk factor, selenium, vitamin E, vitamin C, carotenoids, and polyphenols.

The authors include many interventional and observational studies that have reported findings of dietary antioxidants, prostate cancer incidence, and progression. The majority of these studies focused on vitamins E and C, carotenoids, specifically beta- and alpha-carotene and lycopene, phenols including tea and coffee, and the flavonoids, as well as selenium.

3. Vitamin E and prostate cancer

Vitamin E is a potent lipid-soluble antioxidant, which is well recognized for safeguarding the body against free radical-mediated peroxidative damage. It is a naturally occurring essential vitamin mainly found in foods such as nuts, oils, fruits, and vegetables and is available as a dietary supplement. Vitamin E scavenges highly reactive free radical species such as hydroxyls, superoxides, lipid peroxyls, hydroperoxyls, and nitrogen radicals; and prevents lipid peroxidation related to carcinogen-induced DNA damage [10].

It is known that a deficient antioxidant defense system can result in oxidative stress. As such, increased levels of reactive oxygen species over time may have an etiological role in the development of malignancies such as prostate cancer [11]. Vitamin E may therefore be considered as adjuvant therapy for the prevention of prostate cancer [12]. However, despite emerging evidence supporting vitamin E as a powerful antioxidant, its effect on prostate cancer risk remains poorly understood.

Two categories of vitamin E compounds exist: tocopherols (α, β, γ, and δ-Toc) and tocotrienols (α, β, γ, and δ-T3) [12]. Despite structural differences between both categories, tocopherols and tocotrienols each have sufficient antioxidant properties [12].

3.1 Alpha-, gamma-, and delta-tocopherols

Alpha-tocopherol accounts for the most abundant and active isoform of vitamin E in human tissues and is the most widely used in dietary supplements [10]. Alpha-tocopherol terminates free radical chain reactions by transferring hydrogen protons to free radicals yielding nonradical products [13]. Fairly stable alpha-tocopheroxyl radicals are generated, which do not react with polyunsaturated fatty acids but with each other or couples with other free radicals to form nonradical products [13]. The generation of nonradical products by vitamin E may therefore provide a protective effect against free radical-mediated cell membrane damage and consequently reduces mutagenesis and carcinogenesis.

A number of studies have reported findings on vitamin E supplementation (alpha-, gamma-, and delta-tocopherols) and risk of prostate cancer [14–18].

Notably, in the Alpha-Tocopherol, Beta-Carotene Cancer Prevention Study (ATBC), daily supplementation of alpha-tocopherol (50 mg) reduced the risk of prostate cancer [17] and moderate dose decreased posttrial mortality [15]. However, a follow-up of the Physicians Health Study II, a large-scale randomized trial, suggested that vitamin E supplementation had no immediate or long-term effect on the incidence of prostate cancer (HR 0.99; 95% CI: 0.89–1.10) [14]. Conversely, findings from the large-scale selenium and vitamin E cancer prevention trial (SELECT) demonstrated that the risk of prostate cancer was significantly increased with dietary vitamin E supplementation containing alpha-tocopherol [16]. However, it was found that the incidence of prostate cancer did not increase in men who received combination therapy of vitamin E and selenium [19]. As such, it can be speculated that there may be a synergistic effect between both antioxidants which attenuates prostate cancer risk [19]. The increased risk of the disease associated with vitamin E therapy could be attributed to the disturbance of the normal physiological balance of vitamin E isomers by the high dosage of alpha-tocopherol, which may result in depletion of other important isomers such as gamma-tocopherol [20].

Studies have supported that gamma-tocopherol may have more superior chemopreventive effects than alpha-tocopherol, considering its stronger anti-inflammatory and antinitrative effects [12]. However, it is important to note that analysis of 15 prospective studies involving data for prostate cancer cases and controls and using risk estimation by multivariable-adjusted conditional logistic regression found that gamma-tocopherol was not associated with risk of aggressive prostate cancer, and the latter was inversely associated with alpha-tocopherol [21]. As such, it was suggested that the protective effect against prostate cancer may be lost with impaired balance of vitamin E isomers [20]. Findings from the SELECT trial were later recapitulated, as alpha-tocopherol was found to upregulate prostate cancer cell proliferation in the early stages of the disease [22]. It was found that premalignant rather than benign or malignant prostate cells had increased proliferation in response to vitamin E [22]. These data indicate that the effect of vitamin E antioxidant activity may be dependent on the stage of the prostate cells in the tumor development process [22]. Conversely, it was later found that combination therapy of delta-tocotrienol and gamma-tocopherol was efficacious in inhibiting the proliferation of prostate cancer cells by apoptosis and cell cycle arrest in the G1 and G2/M phases of the cell cycle [12].

A recent study conducted on mice revealed that delta-tocopherol and not alpha-tocopherol blocks the activation of the Akt pathway which drives tumorigenesis, inhibiting the survival of prostate cancer cells [23]. Another study which supports the chemopreventative activity of delta-tocopherol is that of Wang et al. which reported a novel mechanism by which this antioxidant inhibits prostate cancer cell growth by the attenuation of EGF/IGF-induced activation of Akt on T308 [24]. In examining the efficacy of other tocopherol, gamma-tocopherol (0.3% in diet) supplementation was found to significantly reduce the development of mouse prostatic intraepithelial neoplasia lesions and 2-amino-1-methyl-6-phenylimidazo [4,5-b] pyridine-induced elevation of nitrotyrosine, 8-oxo-deoxyguanosine, p-Akt, Ki-67 and COX-2, and the loss of Nrf2 and PTEN [25].

There is supporting evidence that gamma-tocopherol significantly inhibits the growth of human prostate PC-3 tumor cell line by decreasing progression into the S-phase, upregulation of transglutaminase 2 and downregulation of (TG2), and downregulation of cyclin D1 and cyclin E levels [26]. These findings suggest that different isoforms of vitamin E may differ in their influence on prostate cancer risk and that alpha-tocopherol supplementation alone may increase the risk of the disease.

It was reported that the association between vitamin E and prostate cancer risk may be linked to genetic variation in genes that regulate antioxidant and vitamin E metabolism [18, 27]. Furthermore, it was found that genetic variation in SOD genes responsible for detoxifying superoxide free radicals and protecting cells from oxidative stress may be associated with an increased risk of high-grade prostate cancer and disease recurrence [18]. Similarly, it was shown that single nucleotide polymorphisms (SNPS) in genes associated with vitamin E metabolism such as SEC14L2, SOD1, and TTPA may influence an individual's response to vitamin E supplementation and associated prostate cancer risk [28]. As such, inherited genotypes may confer prostate cancer risk.

It is therefore anticipated that clinical trials will be undertaken with vitamin E isomers combination therapy for further assessment of prostate cancer risk. It may be useful to conduct more studies including isomers other than alpha-tocopherol. Men with a strong family history of prostate cancer should undergo genetic testing, to identify antioxidant gene mutations that may be implicated in prostate cancer.

4. Carotenoids and prostate cancer

Fruits and vegetables supply dietary carotenoids, which are potent antioxidants as they modify cell growth and induce apoptosis [8]. Epidemiological studies indicate that consuming more fruits and vegetables containing plant carotenoids such as beta-carotene and lycopene may decrease the risk of prostate cancer as indicated by an inverse association [21, 29–31]. In addition to these two carotenoids, alpha-carotene, beta-cryptoxanthin, zeaxanthin, and lutein are commonly studied because of their potential protective benefit, although lycopene and, to some extent, beta-carotene have demonstrated so far the strongest evidence while that of the others have proven inconclusive [32, 33].

Carotenoids possess distinctive antioxidative properties including the protection of important biomolecules such as DNA from free radicals [34]. Peto et al. in 1981 hypothesized that β-carotene from vegetables and fruits could possibly decrease incidence rates of human cancers [35], and subsequently, there have been a number of epidemiological studies addressing this topic [7, 36, 37]. For many years, carotenes such as alpha-carotene and beta-carotene have been investigated relating to prostate cancer risk, but the results have proved mostly inconclusive.

4.1 Beta-carotene

Several epidemiological studies have investigated the relationship between beta-carotene and prostate cancer risk [38–48]. In the Alpha-Tocopherol, Beta-Carotene Cancer Prevention Study, subjects receiving beta-carotene supplementation had a 23% increase in prostate cancer incidence and 15% higher mortality from the disease [17]. However, during the postintervention follow-up, the effect of supplemental beta-carotene was no longer evident (RR 1.01, 95% CI: 0.96–1.05) [44]. In a case-control study involving men with primary histologically confirmed prostate cancer and population-based controls, beta-carotene (OR 0.60, 95% CI: 0.47–0.97) and alpha-carotene (OR 0.67, 95% CI: 0.47–0.97) were inversely associated with the risk of prostate cancer. Similarly, dietary beta-carotene intake had a protective effect for prostate cancer (RR 0.30, 95% CI: 0.13–0.66) among subjects younger than 68 years of age in a case control study conducted in the United States [47] (**Table 1**) and another in Japan [43]. In a recent study, circulating beta-carotene (RR 0.55, 95% CI: 0.28–1.08) and alpha-carotene (RR 0.31, 95% CI: 0.15–0.63) were inversely associated with risk of high-grade prostate cancer, especially among those with specific somatic variations [39] (**Table 1**).

Method	Name of author(s)	Year of study	Carotenoids	Risk	95% CI	P.R.E outcome
Case-control						
	Mettlin et al. [47]	1989	β-carotene (sup.)	RR = 0.60	0.47–0.97	40%
	Nordstrom et al. [43]	2016	β-carotene (diet) α-carotene (diet) Lycopene (diet)	RR = 0.31 RR = 0.34 RR = 0.55	0.15–0.63 0.18–0.66 0.28–1.08	69% 66% 45%
	Van Hoang et al. [45]	2018	Lycopene (diet)	OR = 0.46	0.27–0.77	54%
	McCann et al. [66]	2005	β-carotene (diet) α-carotene (diet) Lycopene (diet)	OR = 0.53 OR = 0.67 OR = 0.62	0.36–0.79 0.47–0.97 0.37–0.81	47% 33% 38%
Cohort						
	Umesawa et al. [46]	2014	α-carotene (diet)	OR = 0.50	0.26–0.98	50%
	Karppi et al. [50]	2012	β-carotene (serum)	RR = 2.29	1.12–4.66	129%
	Zu et al. [54]	2014	Lycopene (diet)	HR = 0.72	0.56–0.94	28%
	Giovanucci et al. [53]	2002	β-carotene (diet)	0.84	0.73–0.96	16%
Randomized control trial						
	Virtamo et al. [44]	2003	β-carotene (diet)	RR = 1.07	1.02–1.12	7%
Meta-analysis						
	Catano et al. [56]	2018	β-carotene (diet)	OR = 0.94	0.89–1.00	6%
	Rowles et al. [58]	2017	β-carotene (serum)	RR = 0.88	0.79–0.98	12%
	Key et al. [21]	2015	β-carotene	RR = 0.65	0.46–0.91	35%
	Wang et al. [33]	2015	α-carotene (diet) Lycopene (diet)	RR = 0.87 RR = 0.86	0.76–0.99 0.75–0.98	13% 14%

RR = relative risk, CI = confidence interval, P.R.E = percentage relative effect, Sel. Sup = selenium supplement.

Table 1.
Showing studies on the effect of carotenoids on prostate cancer.

There are epidemiological studies that have found no protective effect of carotenes on prostate cancer risk [7, 21, 44–50]. In a recent case-control study involving incident prostate cancer patients, no statistically significant was observed for dietary beta-carotene intake as well as for alpha-carotene and beta-cryptoxanthin [45]. In the Japan Collaborative Cohort study, beta-carotene had no protective effect as there was no association with prostate cancer risk [46]. However, there are studies that have reported an adverse rather than a protective effect of beta-carotene on prostate cancer. In the Kuopio Ischaemic Heart Disease Risk Factor (KIHD) cohort study conducted in Japan among middle-aged men, the highest levels of serum beta-carotene resulted in a 2.29-fold (RR 2.29, 95% CI: 1.12–4.6; P = 0.023) higher risk of prostate cancer compared to participants with lowest levels of the antioxidant [50]. In the 18-year postintervention follow-up of the Alpha-Tocopherol, Beta-Carotene Cancer Prevention Study, beta-carotene increased the posttrial prostate cancer mortality (RR 1.20, 95% CI: 1.01–1.42) [15] (**Table 1**). Thus, the effect of beta-carotene remains inconclusive and may involve an adverse effect where high serum concentrations may elevate prostate cancer risk and mortality.

4.2 Lycopene

Lycopene has been reported to possess more effective antioxidant properties compared to the carotenes and alpha-tocopherol [51]. Lycopene in the form of tomato-based products and to a lesser extent as a supplement is extensively studied with regards to risk of prostate cancer; however, the clinical evidence is inconclusive. In the prostate, lung, colorectal, and ovarian cancer screening trials, lycopene consumption decreased the risk of prostate cancer particularly in men with family history [52]. Similarly, in the Health Professionals Follow-Up Study, lycopene consumption was significantly associated with decreased prostate cancer risk (RR for high vs. low quintiles 0.84, 95% CI: 0.73–0.96; P = 0.003), and tomato sauce consumption had a greater reduction [53] (**Table 1**). Other prospective studies have reported that circulating levels of lycopene were inversely associated with high-grade prostate cancer (RR 0.55, 95% CI: 0.28–1.08) [39]; dietary intake of lycopene decreased the risk of lethal prostate cancer by lowering the degree of angiogenesis in the tumor [54], and lycopene consumption was associated with lower prostate cancer-specific mortality among men high-risk disease [55].

A number of meta-analysis sought to examine the efficacy of lycopene intake in primary prevention of prostate cancer. In a recent meta-analysis of 27 studies (22 were case studies), a statistically significant, though weak inverse association, was found between prostate cancer and lycopene [56]. In another systemic review and meta-analysis, circulating lycopene levels between 2.17 and 85 μg/dL were inversely associated with risk of prostate cancer; however, there was no linear association with levels greater than 85 μg/dL [57]. Further supporting evidence of the protective effect of lycopene intake was demonstrated in a recent meta-analysis of 42 studies where higher circulating and dietary lycopene levels were inversely associated with a 12% risk of prostate cancer but not with the advanced disease [58]. Other supporting evidence involves meta-analysis by Key et al. where lycopene though not associated with overall prostate cancer risk results in a 36% significantly lower risk with aggressive disease [21]; and a meta-analysis of 34 studies showed an association between reduced prostate cancer risk and dietary and blood lycopene levels [33]. Furthermore, Mariani et al. reported no overall benefit of decreasing the rate of high-grade prostatic intraepithelial neoplasia (HGPIN) progression from a 6-month lycopene supplementation [59].

Possible pathways involving multiple mechanisms exist through which lycopene intake may reduce prostate cancer risk. Lycopene attenuates prostate cancer risk by modulating the expression of genes such as EGFR, CDK7, BCL2, and IGF-1R which are related to growth and survival [60]. Another study showed that lycopene increases the expression of BCO2, a tumor suppressor which mediates the inhibition of NF-κB signaling [61]. There is also evidence that lycopene can inhibit the proliferation of prostate cancer cell via PPARγLXRα-ABCA1 pathway [62]. Additionally, lycopene decreases prostate cancer cell proliferation partly by normal inhibition of cell cycle progression [63] and promotes cell cycle arrest in the G0/G1 phase [64]. The chemoprevention mechanism of lycopene could be the regulation of proteins involved in apoptosis, cytoprotection, growth inhibition, antioxidant responses, the Akt/mTOR cascade, and androgen receptor signaling [65].

4.3 Alpha-carotene and beta-cryptoxanthin

Other carotenoids such as alpha-carotene and that beta-cryptoxanthin have been investigated for possible association with prostate cancer risk. In a case control study, there was reduced risk of prostate cancer with lutein (OR 0.55, 95% CI: 0.37–0.81) and alpha-carotene (OR 0.67, 95% CI: 0.47–0.97) [66]. Nordström et al. found that circulating levels of alpha-carotene (RR 0.31, 95% CI: 0.15–0.63) were associated with decreased risk of prostate cancer [39]. Similarly, alpha-carotene intake was associated with decreased risk of prostate cancer (RR 0.87, 95% CI: 0.76–0.99) [33]. Further, a meta-analysis of 34 studies suggests that dietary alpha-carotene intake was associated with reduced risk of prostate cancer [14], and a study by Schuurman et al. showed similar findings for beta-cryptoxanthin [7].

However, in a case-control study conducted in Vietnam, there was no statistically significant association between prostate cancer risk and intake of alpha-carotene, beta-cryptoxanthin, zeaxanthin, and lutein [44]. Similarly, in the Japan Collaborative Cohort study, dietary alpha-carotene intake was not associated with risk of prostate cancer [46]. The absence of the association of dietary intakes of lutein, beta-cryptoxanthin, and zeaxanthin with prostate cancer risk requires confirmation in future studies.

5. Polyphenols and prostate cancer

Dietary polyphenols (PPs) have gained much traction over the last years for their potential as reliable chemopreventive and antitumor agents. This was partly due to their presence in a range of foods and beverages commonly consumed by humans including fruits, vegetables, coffee, tea, and wine [67, 68]. In terms of chemical structure, polyphenols are compounds with at least one aromatic ring with one or more hydroxyl group attached [68]. They are grouped into four different classes based on their chemical structure and orientation of the number of phenolic rings bound to each other. These four classes are as follows: phenolic acids, flavonoids, stilbenes, and curcuminoids [67]. Phenolic acids are found in all plant materials and account for 30% of all polyphenols consumed. They are found mainly in acidic-tasting fruits, coffee, and green tea. As the most abundant group of polyphenols, flavonoids account for 60% of all polyphenols consumed by humans. Good sources of flavonoids include berries, black tea, all citrus fruits, and wine. Together, phenolic acids and flavonoids are the most abundant dietary polyphenols consumed by humans and, consequently, are the most studied with regard to their health benefits to conditions including cancer.

5.1 Coffee

There are studies that have investigated the relationship between coffee consumption and risk of prostate cancer [55, 69–75]. There are those which have found an inverse relationship between coffee consumption and risk of prostate cancer [73–75]. The "Coffee Consumption and Prostate Cancer Risk Progression in Health Professionals Follow Up" report shows that there is a lower risk for prostate cancer and significant association for reduced lethal and advanced cancer diagnosis in participants who consumed six or more cups of coffee per day. There was an inverse association for regular (each one cup per day increment: RR 0.94, P = 0.08) and decaffeinated coffee (RR 0.91, P = 0.05) [71].

In the Collaborative Prospective Cohort study conducted in the United Kingdom between 1970 and 1973 and followed up after 34 years, there was an inverse association between coffee consumption and risk of high-grade prostate cancer, but not the overall risk of the disease [70]. Notably, adjusting for social class and age, higher coffee consumption (three or more cups of coffee) was associated with significantly reduced risk of high Gleason grade prostate cancer compared with noncoffee drinkers [70]. Similarly, in a population cohort study, men with highest coffee consumption (>3 cups per day) had a 53% lower risk of prostate cancer compared with those with lower consumption (<2 cups per day) [72]. Another study supporting the potential beneficial effect of coffee consumption is a population-based case-control study reported by Russnes et al. where high coffee consumption (>6 cups per day) was associated with reduced risk of high grade (OR 0.45, 95% CI: 0.22–0.90; P < 0.05) and fatal prostate cancer [76]. In a recent population-based case-control study in a single institution in Italy, multivariate logistic regression demonstrated that both ferulic acid (OR 0.30, P < 0.05) and caffeic acid (OR 0.32, P < 0.05) were associated with decreased risk of prostate cancer, and higher dietary intake of the latter may be associated with reduced risk of the disease [67].

However, population-based study reported by Arab et al. using data from the North Carolina-Louisiana Prostate Cancer Project showed no association between decaffeinated or caffeinated coffee (4 cups per day) and highly aggressive prostate cancer (OR 0.92, 95% CI 0.61–1.39) [69] (**Table 2**). Similarly, in a most recent European study, there was no evidence of association for risk of total prostate cancer or cancer by grade, grade or fatality, and consumption of total, decaffeinated, or caffeinated coffee [77]. The findings of these studies bring attention to potential anticancer effect of polyphenols in coffee in reducing progression and metastasis of prostate cancer. However, some studies show no association with reduced nonlethal or advanced prostate cancer.

5.2 Green tea

Green tea (GT) is one of the most widely studied source of phenolic acids such epigallocatechin-3-gallate (EGCG), epicatechin-3-gallate (ECG), and epicatechin (EC). There are a number of studies that have investigated the relationship between risk of prostate cancer and green tea [78–82], and preclinical, clinical, and epidemiological data suggest that green tea catechins may reduce prostate cancer risk [83]. In a recent case-control study of Chinese men, epigallocatechin 3-gallate and green tea reduced the risk of prostate cancer; however, the authors indicated that these results should be replicated in larger cohort or case-control studies [84]. In a systematic review conducted by Cui et al., green tea catechins significantly decreased prostate cancer in high-grade prostatic intraepithelial patients (7.60 vs. 23.1%, RR 0.39, P = 0.044) [82]. In another systematic review and meta-analysis study involving three randomized controlled trials and seven observational studies, there was a linear association between green tea catechins consumption (>7 cups per day) and risk of prostate cancer [78].

There is further evidence of the chemopreventative effect of green tea. In a recent case-control involving Vietnamese men, increasing tea consumption (>500 ml/day) was found to be associated with decreased risk of prostate cancer [84]. Similar findings were reported in a case-control study of Algerian men, although the results were borderline statistically [80]. In one of the first clinical

Method	Name of author(s)	Year of study	Sample	RR	95% CI	P.R.E outcome
Cohort						
	Shafique et al. [70]	2012	Tea (>7 cups/day)	HR = 1.50	1.06–2.12	50%
	Wilson et al. [71]	2011	Coffee (>6 cups/day)	RR = 0.82	0.68–0.98	18%
	Sen et al. [77]	2019	Coffee (375 ml/day) Green tea (106 ml/day)	HR = 1.02 HR = 0.98	0.93–1.27 0.90–1.07	2% 2%
Case-control						
	Russnes et al. [76]	2016	Coffee (6 cups/day)	OR = 0.45	0.22–0.90	55%
	Lee et al. [81]	2017	Green tea	OR = 0.60	0.37–0.98	40%
	Kikuchi et al. [88]	2006	Green tea (> 5 cups/day)	HR = 0.85	0.50–1.43	15%
Observational						
	Arab et al. [69]	2012	Coffee (>4 cups/day)	OR = 0.92	0.61–1.39	8%
Meta-analysis						
	Zong et al. [74]	2014	Coffee (moderate)	RR = 0.92	0.85–1.00	8%

RR = relative risk, CI = confidence interval, P.R.E = percentage relative effect, Sel. Sup = selenium supplement.

Table 2.
Showing studies on the effect of coffee and green tea on prostate cancer.

studies to examine the effect of polyphenols (from green tea) on prostate cancer, Betuzzi and colleagues showed that green tea consumption reduces the incidence of prostate cancer in men with high-grade prostate intraepithelial neoplasia (HGPIN). HGPIN is the most likely precursor to prostate cancer, and this study demonstrated that 30% of men with HGPIN would develop prostate cancer 1 year after biopsy [85]. In this double-blind placebo-control study, the green tea consumption group had a 3% incidence rate, while the placebo-treated group had 30% [85]. In a follow-up study by the same authors 2 years later, men in the green tea consumption group had lower incidence of prostate cancer compared with those in the nontreatment group [86].

There have being inconsistent results that do exist with regards to the chemopreventive capacity of green tea. For instance, one study showed a decreased risk of prostate cancer in a multisite case-control study in which participants consumed two cups or more of tea per day [87]. In another study, no association between tea consumption and prostate cancer risk was found [88]. In both studies, there was no association with prostate cancer and coffee consumption. In a large cohort European Study reported by Sen and colleagues, no association was observed for tea consumption and risk of prostate cancer by grade, stage, or fatality [77].

Initially, polyphenols were thought to eliminate cancer cells only through direct radical scavenging in a random manner. However, they were found to have moderate efficiency in this function, inferring that more complex action must be at work in eliminating cancer cells. Further investigations proved that polyphenols employ biological methods in providing cancer prevention and even elimination, such as binding to multiple cellular proteins and regulating signal transduction. Alterations in signal pathways affect multiple processes that hinder cancer initiation, progression, and metastasis [89]. Among green tea catechins, epigallocatechin-3-gallate (EGCG) is widely investigated for its cancer preventive properties. In a recent study, the difluoro analog, called (-)-5,7-difluoro-epicatechin-3-O-gallate and (-)-epicatechin-3-O-gallate from green tea dose-dependently, inhibits tumorigenesis during initiation, promotion, and progression in low-metastatic LNCaP and high-metastatic PC-3 prostate cancer cells [90]. There is also recent evidence that green tea catechins contribute to the inhibition of prostate carcinogenesis by modifying miRNA expression and their target mRNAs, as well as acting as epigenetic modulators [91]. Epicatechin-3-O-gallate and theaflavins have been found to reduce the rate of cell growth in DU 145 human prostate cancer cells [92]. The inhibition of proliferation in the human prostate cancer DU145 cells by tea polyphenols may be associated with reduction in the expression of the surviving gene [93].

The extensive methylation of green tea polyphenols and low bioavailability limits their chemopreventive activity. A combination of green tea polyphenols and a methylation inhibitor quercetin inhibit growth and proliferation in androgen-sensitive LAPC-4 prostate cancer cells. There was also evidence of stimulation of apoptosis and inhibition of phosphatidylinositol 3-kinase/Akt signaling [14]. More in-depth studies have demonstrated that green tea polyphenols induced p53-dependent and p53-independent apoptosis in human prostate cancer LNCaP cells by two distinct pathways. One pathway involved the inhibition of the survival pathway where there is Akt deactivation and loss of BAD phosphorylation, while in the other, there is FAS upregulation via activation of c-jun-N-terminal kinase resulted in caspase-8 activation, FADD phosphorylation, and truncation of BID [94]. There is documentation of other molecular mechanisms by which green tea polyphenols trigger death and apoptosis of human prostate cancer cells via inhibition histone deacetylase, irrespective of their p53 status [6].

6. Selenium and prostate cancer

Selenium (Se) is a natural nutrient which can be found in different types of food. The human body utilizes a trace amount of this mineral in order to function optimally. It is reported to have powerful antioxidant properties which prevent and reduce oxidative stress. Selenium is an essential micronutrient that functions as a redox gatekeeper through its incorporation into proteins to alleviate oxidative stress in cells [95]. It also plays a crucial role in development and a wide variety of other physiological processes including effect immune responses, metabolism, and thyroid function [96, 97]. This has been attributed to selenium's ability to reduce DNA damage and oxidative stress, boost the immune system, and destroy cancer cells. The nutritional status of this metalloid has been difficult to assess via food intake data alone because many factors influence its presence in the food chain [98]. Regular adult intakes of at least 40 μg/day are required to support the maximal expression of the selenium enzymes, and perhaps as much as 300 μg/day to reduce risks of cancer is needed [99].

A number of randomized intervention trials and epidemiological studies suggest that prostate cancer risk may be decreased by selenium intake [100–105]. Studies from 2008 to 2014 (**Table 3**) have shown that selenium supplementation may have some level of a protective role against prostate cancer. In the Nutritional Prevention Cancer Study (a multicenter, double-blind, randomized, placebo-controlled cancer

Method	Name of author(s)	Year of study	Sample	RR	95% CI	P.R.E outcome
Random control trials						
	Lippman et al. [132]	2009	Sel. Sup	1.04	0.90–1.18	4%
	Dunn et al. [133]	2010	Sel. Sup	1.04	0.87–1.24	4%
	Marshall et al. [134]	2011	Sel. Sup	1.09	0.93–1.27	9%
	Klein et al. [16]	2011	Sel. Sup	0.90	0.93–1.27	10%
	Algatar et al. [135]	2013	Sel. Sup	0.90	0.48–1.70	10%
	Kristal et al. [42]	2014	Sel. Sup	1.25	0.79–1.98	25%
Cohort						
	Peters et al. [104]	2008	Sel. Sup	0.90	0.62–1.30	10%
	Chan et al. [105]	2009	Plasma	1.35	0.99–1.84	35%
	Geybels et al. [112]	2013	Nail	0.37	0.27–0.51	63%
Case-control						
	Allen et al. [136]	2008	Plasma	0.96	0.07–1.31	4%
	Pourmand et al. [137]	2008	Serum	0.16	0.06–0.49	84%
	Gill et al. [138]	2009	Serum	0.82	0.59–1.14	18%
	Zhang et al. [139]	2009	Diet	1.30	0.30–5.70	30%
	Outzen et al. [108]	2016	Plasma	1.01	0.94–1.08	1%

RR = relative risk, CI = confidence interval, P.R.E = percentage relative effect, Sel. Sup = selenium supplement.

Table 3.
Showing studies on the effect of selenium on prostate cancer.

prevention trial), oral selenium supplementation (200 μg of selenium per day) lowers the incidence of prostate cancer (RR 0.37, 95% CI: 0.18–0.71, P = 0.02) [106]. Follow-up from this study reported 2 years later found that selenium supplementation reduced the incidence of localized and also advanced prostate cancer disease [106].

In the selenium and vitamin E cancer prevention trial (SELECT), there was decrease in prostate cancer risk with either vitamin E or selenium supplements [107]. In a follow-up from this study, there was an absolute elevation of the risk of prostate cancer (per 1000 person-years) that was 0.8 for selenium, 1.6 for vitamin E, and 0.4 for the combination [16]. Chan and colleagues conducted a case-cohort study of participants in SELECT, randomized to placebo, vitamin E and selenium. They reported that selenium- or vitamin E variants may influence the overall and high-grade risk of prostate cancer and could possibly modify the patient's response to either selenium or vitamin E supplementation [28]. Furthermore, from the SELECT trial involving a stratified case-cohort sample of incident prostate cancer cases, elevated high-grade prostate cancer risk was observed in men supplemented with high-dose alpha-tocopherol and selenium, possibly due to interaction between selenium (or selenomethionine) and alpha-tocopherol [41]. The results of the SELECT study showed that it failed to demonstrate any significant decrease in prostate cancer ascribable vitamin E and selenium supplementations.

Researchers found it useful to investigate any possible association between plasma selenium levels and prostate cancer risk. In the case-control study by Brooks et al., low plasma selenium levels were associated with a four- to fivefold elevated risk of prostate cancer [101]. In a retrospective cohort study, higher levels of selenium were associated with decreased risk of aggressive prostate cancer (RR 0.60, 95% CI: 0.32–1.12), and the relationship at diagnosis may be modified by the manganese superoxide dismutase (SOD2) gene [105]. Furthermore, in a study involving the Within the Danish "Diet, Cancer and Health" cohort, higher levels of plasma selenium were not associated with lower risk of high-grade prostate cancer disease or prostate cancer-specific mortality [108]. A systematic review and meta-analysis of case-control studies, randomized controlled trials, and prospective cohort studies showed decreased prostate cancer risk with increasing serum/plasma selenium levels (up to 170 ng/ml) when 12 studies were analyzed and also lower risk of disease with toenail selenium levels between 0.85 and 0.94 μg/g (estimated RR 0.29, 95% CI: 0.14–0.61) in three high-quality studies [109]. Therefore, although there is evidence of a potential protective effect of selenium in terms of its status and supplementation, further studies are required especially in low-selenium status populations.

In the last 10 years, a number of systematic and meta-analysis have been conducted to examine the relationship between selenium status and prostate cancer. In one study reported by Sayehmirj and colleagues, the relative risks for prostate cancer (based on case-control, cohort, and randomized control trials) on serum and nail samples were 0.85 (95% CI: 0.61–1.17) and 0.66 (95% CI: 0.41–1.05), respectively. They also reported a relative risk of 0.67 (95% CI: 0.52–0.87) between selenium levels and advanced prostate cancer [110]. The authors concluded that selenium supplementation could have a protective role against the initiation and progression to advanced stages [110]. A MOOSE-compliant meta-analysis of 17 studies showed a significant inverse association between prostate cancer risk and serum selenium levels (RR 0.76, 95% CI: 0.64–0.76) [82].

Even though these studies suggest that higher levels of selenium are associated with decreased risk of prostate cancer; there are others that have demonstrated otherwise. An analysis of 15 prospective studies by Allen et al. failed to show any association between blood selenium levels and risk of prostate cancer (OR, 1.01, 95% CI: 0.83–1.23). However, high blood selenium levels were not associated with nonaggressive disease, but with aggressive disease (OR 0.43, 95% CI: 0.21–0.87) [111]. Another key finding in this study was that nail selenium levels were significantly inversely associated with prostate cancer risk (OR 0.29, 95% CI: 0.22–0.40, $P < 0.001$) and also with both aggressive and nonaggressive disease [111]. Similarly, in the prospective Netherlands cohort study, toenail selenium levels were associated with a significant reduction in the risk of advanced prostate cancer (RR 0.37, 95% CI: 0.27–0.51; $P < 0.001$) [112]. However, in a case-control study, selenium levels in toenail were not associated with prostate cancer risk, and its supplementation while not having any effect among participants with low selenium status elevates the risk (by 91%, $P = 0.07$) among those with higher selenium status [42]. The authors suggest that men with low selenium status did not benefit from its supplementation which increased the risk of high-grade prostate cancer among those participants with high selenium status [42].

The effects of selenium on prostate cancer remain uncertain. In a prospective cohort study in the United States, reported by Peter et al., showed that long-term selenium supplementation did not lower the overall risk of prostate cancer (HR 0.90, 95% CI: 0.62–1.3) with participants having an average intake of >50 μg/day over a 10-year period [104]. In a Cochrane review including randomized controlled trials and longitudinal observational studies, there was no association between selenium supplementation and the risk of prostate cancer [113], nor in a Mendelian randomization analysis by Yarmolinsky et al. where the authors suggested that selenium supplementation could have unfavorable effects on risks of advanced disease

[114]. There is further supporting evidence in the follow-up of the Procomb trial where there was no association between selenium supplementation and prostate cancer risk [115]. Conversely, there are studies that suggest caution with selenium supplement usage among males with prostate cancer. In the Health Professionals Follow-Up Study (over a 22-year period) of men diagnosed with nonmetastatic prostate cancer, supplementation of 140 or more μg/day of selenium had a 2.6-fold risk of prostate cancer mortality (95% CI: 1.44–4.70, P = 0.001) compared with nonusers [116].

The mechanism of action of selenium in the inhibition of cancer development could include reduction in DNA damage. Waters et al. reported that dietary supplementation of selenium increases epithelial cell apoptosis in prostate and DNA damage in prostate tissue [117].

7. Vitamin C and prostate cancer

Vitamin C is mainly obtained from vegetables and fruit sources and is considered to be a very important water-soluble antioxidant [118]. Foods and supplements are sources, which provide vitamin C intake while that from foods only is referred to as dietary vitamin C. There is evidence that the mechanisms by which vitamin C prevents the harmful effects of carcinogens include decreasing oxidative DNA damage [119, 120]. Vitamin C functions as a scavenger of free radicals and, therefore, has a potential role in the chemoprevention of prostate cancer [121]. Animal and *in vitro* studies have demonstrated that it could inhibit the cell growth and viability [8]. Menon and colleagues suggested that vitamin C may be a potent anticancer agent as it inhibits tumor growth by producing reactive oxygen species [122]. In another study, vitamin C inhibits cell growth and division via the generation of hydrogen peroxide, which eventually damages the cell [123].

A number of epidemiological studies have documented the relationship between risk of prostate cancer and vitamin C intake; however, the findings have been inconclusive [48, 66, 124, 125]. In a case-control study conducted in Italy involving men with incident, histologically confirmed prostate cancer, there was a significant inverse association (OR 0.78, 95% CI: 0.58–0.96; P = 0.02), especially among men with the highest vitamin C intake [125]. Similar findings were reported in another case-control study where vitamin C decreased prostate cancer risks among men in the highest quartile of intake of the antioxidant (OR 0.49, 95% CI: 0.33–0.74) [66]. There are two other case control studies that have reported reduced prostate cancer risk due to vitamin C intake [48, 126]. There is also evidence in prospective studies such as the North Carolina-Louisiana Prostate Cancer Project where >1500 mg (compared with <500 mg vitamin C equivalent/day) reduced prostate cancer risk (RR 0.31, 95% CI: 0.15–0.67; P < 0.01) [127] (**Table 4**). In meta-analysis conducted by Bai and colleagues involving 103,658 subjects, dietary vitamin C intake (150 mg/day) reduced risk among case-control studies (RR 0.79, 95% CI: 0.69–0.91, P = 0.001) and 0.95 (95% CI: 0.90–0.99, P = 0.039) in cohort studies [125].

However, a number of studies have reported no association between prostate cancer risk and vitamin C [14, 128]. In The Prostate Cancer and Environment Study (PROtEuS), a recent population-based case-control study conducted in Montreal, there was the absence of an association between overall or grade of prostate cancer incidence and either recent dietary or supplemented vitamin C uptake [129]. Key evidence also comes from the posttrial follow-up in the Physicians' Health Study II randomized trial where no effect was observed of vitamin C on incidence of prostate cancer (HR 0.99, 95% CI: 0.89–1.10) [14]. Earlier in the Physicians' Health Study II randomized controlled trial, vitamin C supplement (500 mg daily) had

Method	Name of author(s)	Year of study	Sample	Risk	95% CI	P.R.E outcome
Case-control						
	Bidoli et al. [124]	2009	Diet	OR = 0.86	0.65–1.08	14%
	McCann et al. [66]	2005	Diet	OR = 0.49	0.33–0.74	51%
	Deneo-Pellegrini et al. [126]	1999	Diet	OR = 0.40	0.0.20–0.80	60%
	Vance et al. [127]	2016	Sup.	OR = 0.31	0.15–0.67	69%
	Parent et al. [129]	2018	Diet	OR = 0.95	0.77–1.18	5%
Cohort						
	Gaziano et al. [128]	2009	Sup.	HR = 1.02	0.90–1.15	2%
	Wang et al. [14]	2014	Sup.	OR = 1.03	0.93–1.15	2%
Meta-analysis						
	Bai et al. [125]	2015	Sup.	RR = 0.91	0.84–0.98	9%
	Jiang et al. [130]	2010	Sup.	RR = 0.98	0.91–1.06	2%

RR = relative risk, OR = odds ratio, CI = confidence interval, P.R.E = percentage relative effect, Sup. = supplement.

Table 4.
Showing studies on the effect of vitamin C on prostate cancer.

no effect on prostate cancer (HR 1.02, 95% CI: 0.90–1.15; P = 0.80), a finding that remained even after stratification by various cancer risk factors [128]. Further, a systematic review of nine randomized controlled trials found no significant effects of vitamin C supplementation (RR 0.98, 95% CI: 0.91–1.06) on prostate cancer incidence [130] (**Table 4**).

Studies involving the use of supplements might favor results that are bias as the period of use may be relatively short term, associated health problems in persons who use vitamin C supplements, and the different biological activity or absorption contributing to the possibly different effects of dietary compared with supplemental use of vitamin C [121, 131].

The studies cited above on vitamin C and prostate cancer risk provide inconclusive evidence. While some case-control studies demonstrate a protective effect, randomized trials and meta-analysis fail to clearly demonstrate any beneficial effect of vitamin C on the risk of prostate cancer.

8. Conclusion

The effect of dietary and supplemental antioxidants on risk of prostate cancer remains undecided and inconclusive. More epidemiological and human clinical trials as well as animal studies are needed to give an improved understanding on the biology of prostate cancer and how antioxidants at supranutritional and nutritional levels influence the risk of prostate cancer.

Nothing to disclose

The authors have no funding and conflicts of interest to disclose regarding the content of this chapter.

Author details

Dwayne Tucker[1], Melisa Anderson[1], Fabian Miller[2,3], Kurt Vaz[1], Lennox Anderson-Jackson[1] and Donovan McGrowder[1*]

1 Department of Pathology, Faculty of Medical Sciences, The University of the West Indies, Kingston, Jamaica, West Indies

2 Department of Physical Education, Faculty of Science and Technology, The Mico University College, Kingston, Jamaica, West Indies

3 Biotechnology Centre, Faculty of Science and Technology, The University of the West Indies, Kingston, Jamaica, West Indies

*Address all correspondence to: dmcgrowd@yahoo.com; donovan.mcgrowder@uwimona.edu.jm

References

[1] Bray F, Ferlay J, Soerjomataram I, Siegel RL, Torre LA, Jemal A. Global cancer statistics 2018:GLOBOCAN estimates of incidence and mortality worldwide for 36 cancers in 185 countries. CA: A Cancer Journal for Clinicians. 2018;**68**(6):394-424

[2] Patel AR, Klein EA. Risk factors for prostate cancer. Nature Clinical Practice. Urology. 2009;**6**(2):87-95

[3] Dunn MW, Kazer MW. Prostate cancer overview. Seminars in Oncology Nursing. 2011;**27**(4):241-250

[4] Hori S, Butler E, McLoughlin J. Prostate cancer and diet: Food for thought? BJU International. 2001;**107**(9):1348-1359

[5] Gupta-Elera G, Garrett AR, Robison RA, O'Neill KL. The role of oxidative stress in prostate cancer. European Journal of Cancer Prevention. 2012;**21**:155-162

[6] Thapa D, Ghosh R. Antioxidants for prostate cancer chemoprevention: challenges and opportunities. Biochemical Pharmacology. 2012;**83**:1319-1330

[7] Schuurman AG, Goldbohm RA, Brants HA, Van den Brandt PA. A prospective cohort study on intake of retinol, vitamins C and E, and carotenoids and prostate cancer risk (Netherlands). Cancer Causes & Control. 2002;**13**:573-582

[8] Willis MS, Wians FH. The role of nutrition in preventing prostate cancer: A review of the proposed mechanism of action of various dietary substances. Clinica Chimica Acta. 2003;**330**(1-2):57-83

[9] Nelson WG, De Marzo AM, Isaacs WB. Prostate cancer. The New England Journal of Medicine. 2003;**349**(4):366-381

[10] Klein EA, Thompson IN, Lippman SM, Goodman PJ, Albanes D, Taylor PR, et al. SELECT: The selenium and vitamin E cancer prevention trial. Urologic Oncology. 2009;**321**:51-65

[11] Lakshmipathi K, Binod K, Sweaty K, Paul M, Hari KK. Role of oxidative stress in prostate cancer. Cancer Letters. 2010;**282**:125-136

[12] Sato C, Kaneko S, Sato A, Virgona N, Namiki K, Yano T. Combination effect of δ-tocotrienol and γ-tocopherol on prostate cancer cell growth. Journal of Nutritional Science and Vitaminology. 2017;**63**:349-354

[13] Bramley PM, Elmadfa I, Kafatos A, Kelly FJ, Manios Y, Roxborough HE. Vitamin E. Journal of the Science of Food and Agriculture. 2000;**80**:913-938

[14] Wang L, Sesso HD, Glynn RJ, Christen WG, Bubes V, Manson JE. Vitamin E and C supplementation and risk of cancer in men: Posttrial follow-up in the Physicians' Health Study II randomized trial. The American Journal of Clinical Nutrition. 2014;**100**(3):915-923

[15] Virtamo J, Taylor PR, Kontto J, Männistö S, Utriainen M, Weinstein SJ. Effects of α-tocopherol and β-carotene supplementation on cancer incidence and mortality: 18-year post-intervention follow-up of the Alpha-Tocopherol, Beta-Carotene Cancer Prevention Study. International Journal of Cancer. 2014;**135**(1):178-185

[16] Klein EA, Thompson IM Jr, Tangen CM, Crowley JJ, Lucia MS, Goodman PJ, et al. Vitamin E and the risk of prostate cancer: The selenium and vitamin E cancer prevention trial (SELECT).

Journal of the American Medical Association. 2011;**306**:1549-1556

[17] Heinonen OP, Albanes D, Virtamo J, Taylor PR, Huttunen JK, Hartman AM, et al. Prostate cancer and supplementation with alpha-tocopherol and beta-carotene: Incidence and mortality in a controlled trial. Journal of the National Cancer Institute. 1998;**90**(6):440-446

[18] Bauer SR, Richman EL, Sosa E, Weinberg V, Song X, Witte JS, et al. Antioxidant and vitamin E transport genes and risk of high-grade prostate cancer and prostate cancer recurrence. Prostate. 2013;**73**:1786-1795

[19] Vance TM, Su J, Fontham ETH, Koo SI, Chun OK. Dietary antioxidants and prostate cancer: A Review. Nutritional Cancer. 2013;**65**(6):793-801. DOI: 10.1080/01635581.2013.806672

[20] Gaby AR. Prostate cancer risk and vitamin E. Journal of the American Medical Association. 2012;**307**(5):453-454

[21] Key TJ, Appleby PN, Travis RC, Albanes D, Alberg AJ, Barricarte A, et al. Carotenoids, retinol, tocopherols, and prostate cancer risk: Pooled analysis of 15 studies. The American Journal of Clinical Nutrition. 2015;**102**:1142-1157

[22] Njoroge RN, Unno K, Zhao JC, Naseem AF, Anker JF, WA MG. Organoids model distinct Vitamin E effects at different stages of prostate cancer evolution. Scientific Reports. 2017;7(1). DOI: 10.1038/s41598-017-16459-2

[23] Wang H, Yang X, Liu A, Wang G, Bosland MC, Chung SY. δ-Tocopherol inhibits the development of prostate adenocarcinoma in prostate specific Pten$^{-/-}$ mice. Carcinogenesis. 2018;**39**:158-169

[24] Wang Y, Jacobs EJ, Newton CC, McCullough ML. Lycopene, tomato products and prostate cancer-specific mortality among men diagnosed with nonmetastatic prostate cancer in the Cancer Prevention Study II Nutrition Cohort. International Journal of Cancer. 2016;**138**(12):2846-2855

[25] Chen JX, Li G, Wang H, Liu A, Lee MJ, Reuhl K, et al. Dietary tocopherols inhibit PhIP-induced prostate carcinogenesis in CYP1A-humanized mice. Cancer Letters. 2016;**371**(1):71-78

[26] Torricelli P, Caraglia M, Abbruzzese A, Beninati S. γ-Tocopherol inhibits human prostate cancer cell proliferation by up-regulation of transglutaminase 2 and down-regulation of cyclins. Amino Acids. 2013;**44**(1):45-51

[27] Major JM, Yu K, Weinstein SJ, Berndt SI, Hyland PL, Yeager M. Genetic variants reflecting higher vitamin E status in men are associated with reduced risk of prostate cancer. The Journal of Nutrition. 2014;**144**(5):729-733

[28] Chan JM, Darke AK, Penney KL, Tangen CM, Goodman PJ, Lee GM, et al. Selenium- or vitamin E-related gene variants, interaction with supplementation, and risk of high-grade prostate cancer in SELECT. Cancer Epidemiology Biomarkers and Prevention. 2016;**25**(7):1050-1058. DOI: 10.1158/1055-9965

[29] Perez-Cornago A, Travis RC, Appleby PN, Tsilidis KK, Tjonneland A, Olsen A, et al. Fruit and vegetable intake and prostate cancer risk in the European Prospective Investigation into Cancer and Nutrition (EPIC). International Journal of Cancer. 2017;**141**:287-297

[30] Chan JM, Giovannucci EL. Vegetables, fruits, associated micronutrients, and risk of prostate cancer. Epidemiologic Reviews. 2001;**23**:82-86

[31] Young CY, Yuan HQ, He ML, Zhang JY. Carotenoids and prostate cancer risk. Mini Reviews in Medicinal Chemistry. 2008;**8**:529-537

[32] Lewis JE, Soler-Vila H, Clark PE, Kresty LA, Allen GO, Hu JJ. Intake of plant foods and associated nutrients in prostate cancer risk. Nutrition and Cancer. 2009;**61**:216-224

[33] Wang Y, Cui R, Xiao Y, Fang J, Xu Q. Effect of carotene and lycopene on the risk of prostate cancer: A systematic review and dose-response meta-analysis of observational studies. PLoS One. 2015;**10**(9):e0137-e0427

[34] Krinsky NI. The antioxidant and biological properties of the carotenoids. Annals of the New York Academy of Sciences. 1998;**854**:443-447

[35] Peto R, Doll R, Buckley JD, Sporn MB. Can dietary beta-carotene materially reduce human cancer rates? Nature. 1981;**290**:201-208

[36] Shibata A, Paganini-Hill A, Ross RK, Henderson BE. Intake of vegetables, fruits, beta-carotene, vitamin C and vitamin supplements and cancer incidence among the elderly: A prospective study. British Journal of Cancer. 1992;**66**:673-679

[37] Andersson SO, Wolk A, Bergstrom R, Giovannucci E, Lindgren C, Baron J, et al. Energy, nutrient intake and prostate cancer risk: A population-based case-control study in Sweden. International Journal of Cancer. 1996;**68**:716-722

[38] Bonn SE, Barnett MJ, Thornquist M, Goodman G, Neuhouser ML. Body mass index and prostate cancer risk in the carotene and retinol efficacy trial. European Journal of Cancer Prevention. 2019;**28**(3):212-219. DOI: 10.1097/CEJ.0000000000000438

[39] Nordström T, Van Blarigan EL, Ngo V, Roy R, Weinberg V, Song X, et al. Associations between circulating carotenoids, genomic instability and the risk of high-grade prostate cancer. Prostate. 2016;**76**(4):339-348

[40] Antwi SO, Steck SE, Su LJ, Hébert JR, Zhang H, Fontham ET. Dietary, supplement, and adipose tissue tocopherol levels in relation to prostate cancer aggressiveness among African and European Americans: The North Carolina-Louisiana Prostate Cancer Project (PCaP). Prostate. 2015;**75**(13):1419-1435

[41] Albanes D, Till C, Klein EA, Goodman PJ, Mondul AM, Weinstein SJ. Plasma tocopherols and risk of prostate cancer in the selenium and vitamin E cancer prevention trial (SELECT). Cancer Prevention Research (Phila). 2014;**7**(9):886-895

[42] Kristal AR, Darke AK, Morris JS, Tangen CM, Goodman PJ, Thompson IM. Baseline selenium status and effects of selenium and vitamin E supplementation on prostate cancer risk. Journal of the National Cancer Institute. 2014;**106**(3):djt456

[43] Ohno Y, Yoshida O, Oishi K, Okada K, Yamabe H, Schroeder FH. Dietary beta-carotene and cancer of the prostate: A case-control study in Kyoto. Japanese Journal of Cancer Research. 1988;**48**(5):1331-1336

[44] Virtamo J, Pietinen P, Huttunen JK, Korhonen P, Malila N, Virtanen MJ. Incidence of cancer and mortality following alpha-tocopherol and beta-carotene supplementation: A post-intervention follow-up. Journal of the American Medical Association. 2003;**290**(4):476-485

[45] Van Hoang D, Pham NM, Lee AH, Tran DN, Binns CW. Dietary carotenoid intakes and prostate cancer risk: A case-control study from Vietnam. Nutrients. 2018;**10**(1):E70

[46] Umesawa M, Iso H, Mikami K, Kubo T, Suzuki K, Watanabe Y, et al. Relationship between vegetable and carotene intake and risk of prostate cancer: The JACC study. British Journal of Cancer. 2014;**110**(3):792-796

[47] Mettlin CI, Selenskas S, Natarajan N, Huben R. Beta-carotene and animal fats and their relationship to prostate cancer risk. A case-control study. Cancer. 1989;**64**(3):605-612

[48] Hodge AM, English DR, McCredie MR, Severi G, Boyle P, Hopper JL. Foods, nutrients and prostate cancer. Cancer Causes & Control. 2004;**15**(1):11-20

[49] Norrish AE, Jackson RT, Sharpe SJ, Skeaff CM. Prostate cancer and dietary carotenoids. American Journal of Epidemiology. 2000;**151**(2):119-123

[50] Karppi J, Kurl S, Laukkanen JA, Kauhanen J. Serum β-carotene in relation to risk of prostate cancer: The Kuopio Ischaemic Heart Disease Risk Factor study. Nutrition and Cancer. 2012;**64**(3):361-367

[51] Di Mascio P, Kaiser S, Sies H. Lycopene as the most efficient biological carotenoid singlet oxygen quencher. Archives of Biochemistry and Biophysics. 1989;**274**:532-538

[52] Kirsh VA, Mayne ST, Peters U, Chatterjee N, Leitzmann MF, Dixon LB, et al. A prospective study of lycopene and tomato product intake and risk of prostate cancer. Cancer Epidemiology, Biomarkers & Prevention. 2006;**15**(1):92-98

[53] Giovannucci E, Rimm EB, Liu Y, Stampfer MJ, Willett WC. A prospective study of tomato products, lycopene, and prostate cancer risk. Journal of the National Cancer Institute. 2002;**94**(5):391-398

[54] Zu K, Mucci L, Rosner BA, Clinton SK, Loda M, Stampfer MJ, et al. Dietary lycopene, angiogenesis, and prostate cancer: A prospective study in the prostate-specific antigen era. Journal of the National Cancer Institute. 2014;**106**(2). DOI: 10.1093/jnci/djt430

[55] Wang H, Hong J, Yang CS. δ-Tocopherol inhibits receptor tyrosine kinase-induced AKT activation in prostate cancer cells. Molecular Carcinogenesis. 2016;**55**(11):1728-1738

[56] Cataño JG, Trujillo CG, Caicedo J, Bravo-Balado A, Robledo D, Mariño-Alvarez AM, et al. Efficacy of lycopene intake in primary prevention of prostate cancer: A systematic review of the literature and meta-analysis. Archivos Españoles de Urología. 2018;**71**(2):187-197

[57] Chen P, Zhang W, Wang X, Zhao K, Negi DS, Zhuo L, et al. Lycopene and risk of prostate cancer: A systematic review and meta-analysis. Medicine (Baltimore). 2015;**94**(33):e1260

[58] Rowles JLIII, Ranard KM, Smith JW, An R, Erdman JW Jr. Increased dietary and circulating lycopene are associated with reduced prostate cancer risk: A systematic review and meta-analysis. Prostate Cancer and Prostatic Diseases. 2017;**20**:361-377

[59] Mariani S, Lionetto L, Cavallari M, Tubaro A, Rasio D, De Nunzio C, et al. Low prostate concentration of lycopene is associated with development of prostate cancer in patients with high-grade prostatic intraepithelial neoplasia. International Journal of Molecular Sciences. 2014;**15**(1):1433-1440

[60] Rafi MM, Kanakasabai S, Reyes MD, Bright JJ. Lycopene modulates growth and survival associated genes in prostate cancer. The Journal of Nutritional Biochemistry. 2013;**24**(10):1724-1734

[61] Gong X, Marisiddaiah R, Zaripheh S, Wiener D, Rubin LP. Mitochondrial

beta-carotene 90,100 oxygenase modulates prostate cancer growth via NF-kappaB inhibition: A lycopene-independent function. Molecular Cancer Research. 2016;**14**:966-975

[62] Yang CM, Lu YL, Chen HY, Hu ML. Lycopene and the LXR agonist T0901317 synergistically inhibit the proliferation of androgen-independent prostate cancer cells via the PPAR-LXR-ABCA1 pathway. The Journal of Nutritional Biochemistry. 2012;**23**:1155-1162

[63] Ford NA, Elsen AC, Zuniga K, Lindshield BL, Erdman JW Jr. Lycopene and apo-12′-lycopenal reduce cell proliferation and alter cell cycle progression in human prostate cancer cells. Nutrition and Cancer. 2011;**63**(2):256-263

[64] Soares NC, Teodoro AJ, Oliveira FL, Santos CA, Takiya CM, Junior OS. Influence of lycopene on cell viability, cell cycle, and apoptosis of human prostate cancer and benign hyperplastic cells. Nutrition and Cancer. 2013;**65**(7):1076-1085

[65] Qiu X, Yuan Y, Vaishnav A, Tessel MA, Nonn L, van Breemen RB. Effects of lycopene on protein expression in human primary prostatic epithelial cells. Cancer Prevention Research (Phila). 2013;**6**(5):419-427

[66] McCann SE, Ambrosone CB, Moysich KB, Brasure J, Marshall JR, Freudenheim JL. Intakes of selected nutrients, foods, and phytochemicals and prostate cancer risk in western New York. Nutrition and Cancer. 2005;**53**(1):33-41

[67] Russo G, Campisi D, Di Mauro M, Regis F, Reale G, Marranzano M, et al. Dietary consumption of phenolic acids and prostate cancer: A case-control study in sicily, Southern Italy. Molecules. 2017;**22**(12):1-9

[68] Zhou Y, Zheng J, Li Y, Xu DP, Li S, Chen YM, et al. Natural polyphenols for prevention and treatment of cancer. Nutrients. 2016;**8**(8):E515. DOI: 10.3390/nu8080515

[69] Arab L, Su LJ, Steck SE, Ang A, Fontham ET, Bensen JT, et al. Coffee consumption and prostate cancer aggressiveness among African and Caucasian Americans in a population-based study. Nutrition and Cancer. 2012;**64**(5):637-642

[70] Shafique K, McLoone P, Qureshi K, Leung H, Hart C, Morrison DS. Tea consumption and the risk of overall and grade specific prostate cancer: A large prospective cohort study of Scottish men. Nutrition and Cancer. 2012;**64**(6):790-797

[71] Wilson KM, Kasperzyk JL, Rider JR, Kenfield S, van Dam RM, Stampfer MJ, et al. Coffee consumption and prostate cancer risk and progression in the health professionals follow-up study. Journal of the National Cancer Institute. 2011;**103**(11):876-884

[72] Pounis G, Tabolacci C, Costanzo S, Cordella M, Bonaccio M, Rago L, et al. Reduction by coffee consumption of prostate cancer risk: Evidence from the Moli-sani cohort and cellular models. International Journal of Cancer. 2017;**141**(1):72-82

[73] Lu QY, Hung JC, Heber D, Go VL, Reuter VE, Cordon-Cardo C, et al. Inverse associations between plasma lycopene and other carotenoids and prostate cancer. Cancer Epidemiology, Biomarkers & Prevention. 2001;**10**:749-756

[74] Zhong S, Chen W, Yu X, Chen Z, Hu Q, Zhao J. Coffee consumption and risk of prostate cancer: An up-to-date meta-analysis. European Journal of Clinical Nutrition. 2014;**68**(3):330-337

[75] Discacciati A, Wolk A. Lifestyle and dietary factors in prostate cancer prevention. Recent Results in Cancer Research. 2014;**202**:27-37

[76] Russnes KM, Möller E, Wilson KM, Carlsen M, Blomhoff R, Smeland S, et al. Total antioxidant intake and prostate cancer in the Cancer of the Prostate in Sweden (CAPS) study. A case control study. BMC Cancer. 2016;**16**:438

[77] Sen A, Papadimitriou N, Lagiou P, Perez-Cornago A, Travis RC, Key TJ, et al. Coffee and tea consumption and risk of prostate cancer in the European Prospective Investigation into Cancer and Nutrition. International Journal of Cancer. 2016;**144**(20):240-250

[78] Guo Y, Zhi F, Chen P, Zhao K, Xiang H, Mao Q, et al. Green tea and the risk of prostate cancer: A systematic review and meta-analysis. Medicine (Baltimore). 2017;**96**(13):e6426. DOI: 10.1097/MD.0000000000006426

[79] Lane JA, Er V, Avery KNL, Horwood J, Cantwell M, Caro GP, et al. ProDiet: A phase II randomized placebo-controlled trial of green tea catechins and lycopene in men at increased risk of prostate cancer. Cancer Prevention Research (Phila.). 2018;**11**(11):687-696

[80] Lassed S, Deus CM, Djebbari R, Zama D, Oliveira PJ, Rizvanov AA, et al. Protective effect of green tea (*Camellia sinensis* L. Kuntze) against prostate cancer: From in vitro data to Algerian patients. Evidence-Based Complementary and Alternative Medicine. 2017:1691568. DOI: 10.1155/2017/1691568

[81] Lee PMY, Ng CF, Liu ZM, Ho WM, Lee MK, Wang F, et al. Reduced prostate cancer risk with green tea and epigallocatechin 3-gallate intake among Hong Kong Chinese men. Prostate Cancer and Prostatic Diseases. 2017;**20**(3):318-322

[82] Cui Z, Liu D, Liu C, Liu G. Serum selenium levels and prostate cancer risk: A MOOSE-compliant meta-analysis. Medicine (Baltimore). 2017;**96**(5):e5944

[83] Hashibe M, Galeone C, Buys SS, Gren L, Boffetta P, Zhang ZF, et al. Coffee, tea, caffeine intake, and the risk of cancer in the PLCO cohort. British Journal of Cancer. 2015;**113**(5):809-816

[84] Lee VD, Pham NM, Xu D, Binns CW. Habitual tea consumption reduces prostate cancer risk in Vietnamese men: A case-control study. Asian Pacific Journal of Cancer Prevention. 2016;**17**(11):4939-4944

[85] Bettuzzi S, Brausi M, Rizzi F, Castagnetti G, Peracchia G, Corti A. Chemoprevention of human prostate cancer by oral administration of green tea catechins in volunteers with high-grade prostate intraepithelial neoplasia: A preliminary report from a one-year proof-of-principle study. Cancer Research. 2006;**66**(2):1234-1240

[86] Brausi M, Rizzi F, Bettuzzi S. Chemoprevention of human prostate cancer by green tea catechins: Two years later. A Follow-up Update (2008). European Urology. 2008;**54**(2):472-473

[87] Jain MG, Hislop GT, Howe GR, Burch JD, Ghadirian P. Alcohol and other beverage use and prostate cancer risk among Canadian men. International Journal of Cancer. 1998;**78**(6):707-711

[88] Kikuchi N, Ohmori K, Shimazu T, Nakaya N, Kuriyama S, Nishino Y, et al. No association between green tea and prostate cancer risk in Japanese men: The Ohsaki Cohort Study. British Journal of Cancer. 2006;**95**:371-373

[89] Lewandowska H, Kalinowska M, Lewandowski W, Stepkowski TM, Brzóska K. The role of natural polyphenols in cell signaling and cytoprotection against cancer

development. The Journal of Nutritional Biochemistry. 2016;**32**:1-19

[90] Stadlbauer S, Steinborn C, Klemd A, Hattori F, Ohmori K, Suzuki K, et al. Impact of green tea catechin ECG and its synthesized fluorinated analogue on prostate cancer cells and stimulated immunocompetent cells. Planta Medica. 2018;**84**(11):813-819

[91] Giudice A, Montella M, Boccellino M, Crispo A, D'Arena G, Bimonte S, et al. Epigenetic changes induced by green tea catechins are associated with prostate cancer. Current Molecular Medicine. 2017;**17**(6):405-420

[92] Kobalka AJ, Keck RW, Jankun J. Synergistic anticancer activity of biologicals from green and black tea on DU 145 human prostate cancer cells. Central-European Journal of Immunology. 2015;**40**(1):1-4

[93] Liang X, Gao JG, Sun XQ, Zhu LY, Jia Y, Gu YC, et al. Tea polyphenols inhibits the proliferation of prostate cancer DU145 cells. Zhonghua Nan Ke Xue. 2013;**19**(6):495-500

[94] Gupta K, Thakur VS, Bhaskaran N, Nawab A, Babcook MA, Jackson MW, et al. Green tea polyphenols induce p53-dependent and p53-independent apoptosis in prostate cancer cells through two distinct mechanisms. PLoS One. 2012;7(12):e52572

[95] Chen YC, Prabhu KS, Mastro AM. Is selenium a potential treatment for cancer metastasis? Nutrients. 2013;**5**(4):1149-1168

[96] Avery JC, Hoffmann PR. Selenium, selenoproteins, and immunity. Nutrients. 2018;**10**(9):1203

[97] Rayman MP. The argument for increasing selenium intake. The Proceedings of the Nutrition Society. 2002;**61**:203-215

[98] Stoffaneller R, Morse NL. A review of dietary selenium intake and selenium status in Europe and the Middle East. Nutrients. 2015;**7**(3):1494-1537

[99] Combs GF. Selenium in global food systems. The British Journal of Nutrition. 2001;**85**:517-547

[100] Ledesma MC, Jung-Hynes B, Schmit TL, Kumar R, Mukhtar H, Ahmad N. Selenium and vitamin E for prostate cancer: Post-SELECT (selenium and vitamin E cancer prevention trial) status. Molecular Medicine. 2011;**17**(1-2):134-143

[101] Brooks JD, Metter EJ, Chan DW, Sokoll LJ, Landis P, Nelson WG, et al. Plasma selenium level before diagnosis and the risk of prostate cancer development. The Journal of Urology. 2001;**166**(6):2034-2038

[102] Clark LC, Dalkin B, Krongrad A, Combs GF Jr, Turnbull BW, Slate EH. Decreased incidence of prostate cancer with selenium supplementation: Results of a double-blind cancer prevention trial. British Journal of Urology. 1998;**81**(5):730-734

[103] Rayman MP, Combs GF Jr, Waters DJ. Selenium and vitamin E supplementation for cancer prevention. Journal of the American Medical Association. 2009;**301**(18):1876

[104] Peters U, Littman AJ, Kristal AR, Patterson RE, Potter JD, White E. Vitamin E and selenium supplementation and risk of prostate cancer in the Vitamins and lifestyle (VITAL) study cohort. Cancer Causes & Control. 2008;**19**(1):75-87

[105] Chan JM, Oh WK, Xie W, Regan MM, Stampfer MJ, King IB, et al. Plasma selenium, manganese superoxide dismutase, and intermediate-or high-risk prostate cancer. Journal of Clinical Oncology. 2009;**27**(22):3577-3583

[106] Clark L, Combs GF Jr, Turnbull BW, Slate EH, Chalker DK, Chow J, et al. Effects of selenium supplementation for cancer prevention in patients with carcinoma of the skin. A randomized controlled trial. Nutritional Prevention of Cancer Study Group. Journal of the American Medical Association. 1996;**276**(24):1957-1963

[107] Dunn BK, Ryan A, Ford LG. Selenium and vitamin E cancer prevention trial: A nutrient approach to prostate cancer prevention. Recent Results in Cancer Research. 2009;**181**:183-193

[108] Outzen M, Tjønneland A, Larsen EH, Friis S, Larsen SB, Christensen J. Selenium status and risk of prostate cancer in a Danish population. The British Journal of Nutrition. 2016;**115**(9):1669-1677

[109] Hurst R, Hooper L, Norat T, Lau R, Aune D, Greenwood DC. Selenium and prostate cancer: Systematic review and meta-analysis. The American Journal of Clinical Nutrition. 2012;**96**(1):111-122

[110] Sayehmiri K, Azami M, Mohammadi Y, Soleymani A, Tardeh Z. The association between selenium and prostate cancer: A systematic review and meta-analysis. Asian Pacific Journal of Cancer Prevention. 2018;**19**(6):1431-1437

[111] Allen NE, Travis RC, Appleby PN, Albanes D, Barnett MJ, Black A, et al. Selenium and prostate cancer: Analysis of individual participant data from fifteen prospective studies. Journal of the National Cancer Institute. 2016;**108**(11). DOI: 10.1093/jnci/djw153

[112] Geybels MS, Verhage BA, van Schooten FJ, Goldbohm RA, van den Brandt PA. Advanced prostate cancer risk in relation to toenail selenium levels. Journal of the National Cancer Institute. 2013;**105**(18):1394-1401

[113] Vinceti M, Filippini T, Del Giovane C, Dennert G, Zwahlen M, Brinkman M, et al. Selenium for preventing cancer. Cochrane Database of Systematic Reviews. 2018:CD005195. DOI: 10.1002/14651858

[114] Yarmolinsky J, Bonilla C, Haycock PC, Langdon RJQ, Lotta LA, Langenberg C, et al. Circulating selenium and prostate cancer risk: A Mendelian randomization analysis. Journal of the National Cancer Institute. 2018;**110**(9):1035-1038

[115] Morgia G, Voce S, Palmieri F, Gentile M, Lapicca G, Giannantoni A, et al. Association between selenium and lycopene supplementation and incidence of prostate cancer: Results from the post-hoc analysis of the procomb trial. Phytomedicine. 2017;**34**(1-5). DOI: 10.1016/j.phymed.2017.06.008

[116] Kenfield SA, Van Blarigan EL, DuPre N, Stampfer MJ, Giovannucci E, Chan JM. Selenium supplementation and prostate cancer mortality. Journal of the National Cancer Institute. 2014;**107**(1):360

[117] Waters D, Shen S, Cooley DM, Bostwick DG, Qian J, Combs GF Jr. Effects of dietary selenium supplementation on DNA damage and apoptosis in canine prostate. Journal of the National Cancer Institute. 2003;**95**(3):237-241

[118] Putchala MC, Ramani P, Sherlin HJ, Premkumar P, Natesan A. Ascorbic acid and its pro-oxidant activity as a therapy for tumours of oral cavity—A systematic review. Archives of Oral Biology. 2013;**58**:563-574

[119] Lee KW, Lee HJ, Surh YJ, Lee CY. Vitamin C and cancer chemoprevention: Reappraisal. The American Journal of Clinical Nutrition. 2003;**78**:1074-1078

[120] Han X, Li J, Brasky TM, Xun P, Stevens J, White E, et al. Antioxidant intake and pancreatic cancer risk: The vitamins and lifestyle (VITAL) Study. Cancer. 2013;**119**:1314-1320

[121] Bender MM, Levy AS, Schucker RE, Yetley EA. Trends in prevalence and magnitude of vitamin and mineral supplement usage and correlation with health status. Journal of the American Dietetic Association. 1992;**92**:1096-1101

[122] Menon M, Maramag C, Malhotra RK, Seethalakshmi L. Effect of vitamin C on androgen independent prostate cancer cells (PC3 and Mat-Ly-Lu) in vitro: Involvement of reactive oxygen species-effect on cell number, viability and DNA synthesis. Cancer Biochemistry Biophysics. 1998;**16**(1-2):17-30

[123] Maramag C, Menon M, Balaji KC, Reddy PG, Laxmanan S. Effect of vitamin C on prostate cancer cells in vitro: Effect on cell number, viability, and DNA synthesis. Prostate. 1997;**32**(3):188-195

[124] Bidoli E, Talamini R, Zucchetto A, Bosetti C, Negri E, Lenardon O. Dietary vitamins E and C and prostate cancer risk. Acta Oncologica. 2009;**48**(6):890-894

[125] Bai XY, Qu X, Jiang X, Xu Z, Yang Y, Su Q. Association between dietary vitamin C intake and risk of prostate cancer: A meta-analysis involving 103,658 subjects. Journal of Cancer. 2015;**6**(9):913-921

[126] Deneo-Pellegrini H, De Stefani E, Ronco A, Mendilaharsu M. Foods, nutrients and prostate cancer: A case-control study in Uruguay. British Journal of Cancer. 1999;**80**(3-4):591-597

[127] Vance TM, Wang Y, Su LJ, Fontham ET, Steck SE, Arab L. Dietary total antioxidant capacity is inversely associated with prostate cancer aggressiveness in a population-based study. Nutrition and Cancer. 2016;**68**(2):214-224

[128] Gaziano JM, Glynn RJ, Christen WG, Kurth T, Belanger C, MacFadyen J. Vitamins E and C in the prevention of prostate and total cancer in men: The Physicians' Health Study II randomized controlled trial. Journal of the American Medical Association. 2009;**301**(1):52-62

[129] Parent ME, Richard H, Rousseau MC, Trudeau K. Vitamin C intake and risk of prostate cancer: The Montreal PROtEuS Study. Frontiers in Physiology. 2018;**1218**. DOI: 10.3389/fphys.2018.01218

[130] Jiang L, Yang KH, Tian JH, Guan QL, Yao N, Cao N. Efficacy of antioxidant vitamins and selenium supplement in prostate cancer prevention: A meta-analysis of randomized controlled trials. Nutrition and Cancer. 2010;**62**(6):719-727

[131] Ferrucci LM, McCorkle R, Smith T, Stein KD, Cartmel B. Factors related to the use of dietary supplements by cancer survivors. Journal of Alternative and Complementary Medicine. 2009;**15**:673-680

[132] Lippman SM, Klein EA, Goodman PJ, Lucia MS, Thompson IM, Ford LG, et al. Effect of selenium and vitamin E on risk of prostate cancer and other cancers: The selenium and vitamin E cancer prevention trial (SELECT). Journal of the American Medical Association. 2009;**301**:39-51

[133] Dunn BK, Richmond ES, Minasian LM, Ryan AM, Ford LG. A nutrient approach to prostate cancer prevention: The selenium and vitamin E cancer prevention trial (SELECT). Nutrition and Cancer. 2010;**62**:896-918

[134] Marshall JR, Tangen CM, Sakr WA, Wood DP, Berry DL, Klein EA, et al. Phase III trial of selenium to prevent

prostate cancer in men with high-grade prostatic intraepithelial neoplasia: SWOG S9917. Cancer Prevention Research. 2011;**4**:1761-1769

[135] Algotar AM, Stratton MS, Ahmann F, Ranger-Moore J, Nagle RB, Thompson BA, et al. Phase 3 clinical trial investigating the effect of selenium supplementation in men at high-risk for prostate cancer. The Prostate. 2013;**73**:328-335

[136] Allen NE, Appleby PN, Roddam AW, Tjønneland A, Johnsen NF, Overvad K, et al. Plasma selenium concentration and prostate cancer risk: Results from the European prospective investigation into cancer and nutrition (EPIC). The American Journal of Clinical Nutrition. 2008;**88**:1567-1575

[137] Pourmand G, Salem S, Moradi K, Nikoobakht MR, Tajik P, Mehrsai A, et al. Serum selenium level and prostate cancer: A case-control study. Nutrition and Cancer. 2008;**60**:171-176

[138] Gill JK, Franke AA. Association of selenium, tocopherols, carotenoids, retinol, and 15-isoprostane F2t in serum or urine with prostate cancer risk: The multi-ethnic cohort. Cancer Causes & Control. 2009;**20**:1161-1171

[139] Zhang Y, Coogan P, Palmer JR, Strom BL, Rosenberg L, et al. Vitamin and mineral use and risk of prostate cancer: The case-control surveillance study. Cancer Causes & Control. 2009;**20**:691-698

Chapter 13

Condensed Benzimidazoles Are a Novel Scaffold for Antioxidant Agents' Search and Development

Vadim A. Kosolapov, Alexander A. Spasov, Vera A. Anisimova and Olga N. Zhukovskaya

Abstract

Taking into account that the imidazole ring has π-electron redundancy, condensed benzimidazole derivatives have attracted our attention as a promising class for the search for antioxidant substances. Synthesis was carried out, and information on the antioxidant activity of imidazo- and tetrahydropyrimido benzimidazoles was provided. Highly active antioxidant substance enoxifol has been revealed. The data on the synthesis and study of the pharmacodynamic, pharmacokinetic, and toxicological properties of the new antioxidant compound enoxifol are presented. The antioxidant activity of the compound is due to its ability to inactivate superoxide, hydroxyl, and peroxyl radicals, thereby reducing the overall oxidation rate due to a decrease in the total initiation rate. It has been shown that enoxifol has hepatoprotector, antihypoxic, cerebroprotective, nootropic, stress-protective, neuropsychotropic, actoprotective, cardioprotective, antiaggregant, and antithrombogenic properties and is able to prevent rheological disorders in diabetes mellitus.

Keywords: benzimidazoles, antioxidant, free radicals, enoxifol

1. Introduction

Currently, the fact that considered the leading role of free radical processes in the pathogenesis of more than 200 diseases has been established. Special attention is paid to damage to the brain tissue due to their particular sensitivity to disruption of oxygen balance and redox balance. The chain character of the reactions of lipid peroxidation (LPO) causes the appearance of a whole cascade of reactive oxygen forms, including superoxide, hydroxyl, and perhydroxyl radicals, singlet oxygen, hydrogen peroxide, and their active metabolites (nitrogen oxide, hypochlorite, etc.). The result is a violation of the integrity and permeability of the cell membrane and the destruction of proteins, lipids, carbohydrates, and nucleic acids, the cell genome suffers, and degenerative changes and neuron death develop. The processes of lipid peroxidation underlie most of the diseases of the central nervous system, which include acute and chronic disorders of cerebral blood circulation, degenerative diseases of the brain and spinal cord, cancer pathology, etc. [1, 2].

Antioxidants, both endogenous and exogenous substances, limit LPO processes. Today, in practical health care, antioxidant preparations of natural origin and synthetic compounds are used [3]. It should be noted that the group of drugs related to natural antioxidants has found quite wide application in clinical practice. At the same time, there is a clear shortage of synthetic antioxidant drugs. In view of the abovementioned, the emergence of a new effective antioxidant compound should arouse the interest of qualified specialists.

2. The results

A computer prediction of the antioxidant activity of new compounds was carried out in the "Microcosm" software [4], and the high predictive ability of the "Microcosm" information technology regarding the antioxidant activity of imidazo-benzimidazole derivatives has been demonstrated.

Condensed benzimidazole derivatives were synthesized, and experimental screening of the antioxidant activity of new chemical compounds was carried out among the derivatives of 2-(hetaryl) imidazo[1,2-a]benzimidazoles (IMBI) [5], 3-aroyl- and 3-hetaroyl-IMBI [6], 2-methoxyphenyl-substituted 9-dialkylaminoethyl-IMBI [7], 2-methoxy- phenyl- and 2-oxyphenyl-substituted 1-dialkylaminoalkyl-IMBI [8], N-acylmethyl derivatives of 9H-2,3-dihydro-IMBI and 10H-2,3,4,10-tetrahydropyrimido[1,2-a]benzimidazoles [9], 9-dialkylaminoethyl-2-oxy(dioxy)phenyl-IMBI [10], aroylmethyl derivatives of tricyclic benzimidazole systems containing hydroxy groups in aroyl radicals [11], 3-(2,2,2-trichloro-1-hydroxyethyl)-IMBI [12], 3-acetyl-2-R-9-dialkylaminoethyl-IMBI [13], 1-dialkyl(alkyl)aminoethyl-2,3-dihydro-IMBI [14], 9-R-2-halogenophenyl-IMBI [15], 10-alkylaminoethyl-2,3,4,10-tetrahydropyrimido[1,2-a]benzimidazoles [16], 3-(n,n-disubstituted)acetamide-1-r-2-aminobenzimidazolium [17], amides of 2,3-dihydroimidazo- and 2,3,4,10-tetrahydropyrimido[1,2-a]benzimidazolyl-acetic acids [18], phenyl- and alkylthiocarbamides of 2,9-disubstituted IMBI [19], and 1-substituted 2-benzylaminobenzimidazoles with phenyl methoxyls [20]. Butylated hydroxytoluene (BHT, CAS Number 128-37-0), also known as dibunol, was chosen as a comparative drug.

It was found that among the derivatives of 2-(hetaryl)-IMBI, high antioxidant activity superior to dibunol was shown by compounds containing in the second position of the tricycle such substituents as 1-methylbenzimidazolyl and 5-bromothienyl. The remaining substances of this series showed an average level of activity, similar to or inferior to dibunol [5]. Among the 3-aroyl- and 3-hetaroyl-IMBI, no substances with antioxidant activity were found [6]. Among 2-methoxyphenyl-substituted 9-dialkylaminoethyl-IMBI, 4-methoxy- and 3 methoxyphenyl-IMBI showed the greatest antioxidant effect, which was comparable to or exceeded dibunol [7]. Salts of the compounds 9-dialkylaminoethyl-IMBI with 3,4-dioxyphenyl substitute exhibited the greatest antioxidant activity that was twofold active than reference drug BHT. Compounds with 4- and 3-oxyphenyl substitutes or 2,4- and 2,5-dioxyphenyl substitutes, as a rule, lacked 3,4-dioxyphenyl-IMBI in activity; however they were similar in it to BHT [10]. Most of aroylmethyl derivatives of tricyclic benzimidazole systems containing hydroxy groups in aroyl radicals also proved to be highly active antioxidant substances that were superior to dibunol [11]. Derivatives of 9-R-2-halogenophenyl-IMBI had a pronounced inhibitory effect on the processes of lipid peroxidation comparable to dibunol [15]. The compounds from the series of 1-substituted 2-benzylaminobenzimidazoles with phenyl methoxyls acted similarly [20]. Amides of 2,3-dihydroimidazo- and 2,3,4,10-tetrahydropyrimido[1,2-a]benzimidazolyl-acetic acids showed moderate AO activity compared to dibunol [18]. It was revealed that 2-methoxy-phenyl- and 2-oxyphenyl-substituted 1-dialkylaminoalkyl-IMBI [8], N-acylmethyl derivatives of 9H-2,3-dihydro-IMBI and 10H-2,3,4,10-tetrahydropyrimido[1,2-a]benzimidazoles [9], most of 3-(2,2,2-trichloro-1-hydroxyethyl)-IMBI [12] и 3-acetyl-2-R-9-dialkylaminoethyl-IMBI [13], 1-dialkyl(alkyl)aminoethyl-2,3-dihydro-IMBI [14], and 3-(n,n-disubstituted)acetamide-1-r-2-aminobenzimidazolium [17] showed the weak antioxidant activity compared to the reference drug. Among 10-alkylaminoethyl-2,3,4,10-tetrahydropyrimido[1,2-a]benzimidazoles [16] and phenyl- and alkylthiocarbamides of 2,9-disubstituted IMBI [19], antioxidant action has not been found.

As a result of previous investigations, the 2-(3,4-dihydroxyphenyl)-9-diethylaminoethyl-imidazo [1,2-a]benzimidazole derivative of dihydrobromide (RU-185, enoxifol) was identified as an antioxidant compound with antiradical and membrane-protective properties [21, 22], having multicomponent mechanisms of action and a wide range of pharmacodynamic effects. For enoxifol, a cardioprotective effect and a positive effect on the microcirculation of blood vessels are characteristic. Antioxidant compound reduces platelet aggregation [23–25], reduces increased blood viscosity, and increases red blood cell deformability [26]. Preclinical toxicology studies have been carried out, and the pharmacokinetics of the compound has been studied [27].

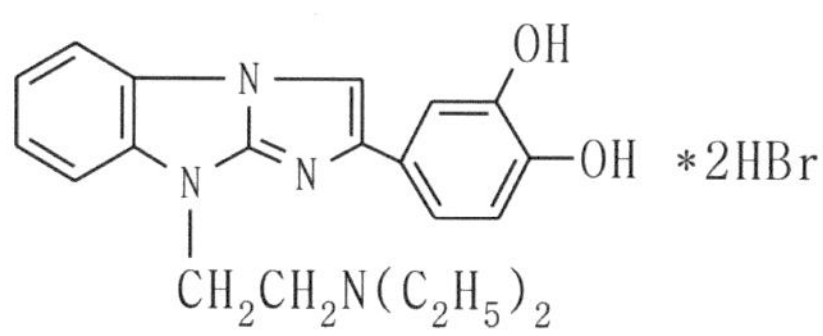

2.1 Synthesis

Synthesis of 2-(3,4-dihydroxyphenyl)-9-diethylamino-ethylimidazo[1,2-a] benzimidazole dihydrobromide (RU-185) starts from saponification of benzimidazole-2-carbamic acid methyl ester under alkaline conditions to obtain 2-aminobenzimidazole. Subsequent alkylation in acetone in the presence of alkali with *N,N*-diethylaminoethyl chloride formed by the action of thionyl chloride on *N,N*-diethylaminoethanol and condensation with a 3,4-dimetoxiphenacylbromide or or 3,4-dioxiphenacyl chloride, followed by intermolecular cyclization in 48% hydrobromic acid (boiling temperature 127°C) under reflux, afforded target compound RU-185.

2.1.1 Stage 1: preparation of 2-aminobenzimidazole

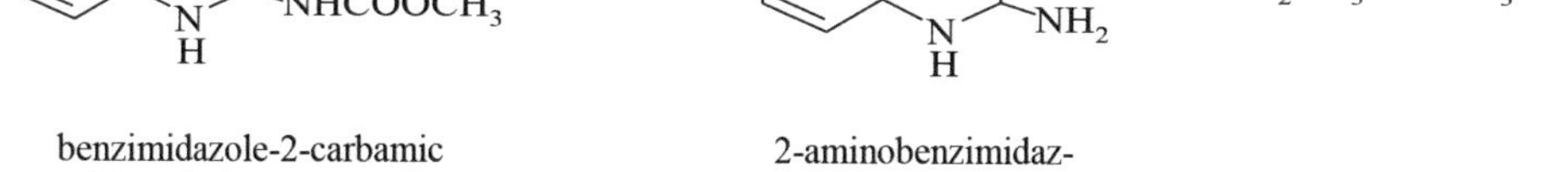

benzimidazole-2-carbamic acid methyl ester

2-aminobenzimidazole

2-Aminobenzimidazole is obtained by saponification of benzimidazole-2-carbamic acid methyl ester (BMC-2) in aqueous solution of sodium hydroxide. The yield of 2-aminobenzimidazole is 65–75%. At the next stage, 2-aminobenzimidazole is used with a melting point of 223–232°C (within 2 degrees). If necessary, the amine is purified by crystallization from water and acetone or by precipitation from an aqueous hydrochloric acid solution.

2.1.2 Stage 2: preparation of diethylaminoethyl chloride hydrochloride

$$(C_2H_5)_2NCH_2CH_2OH \xrightarrow{SOCl_2} (C_2H_5)_2NCH_2CH_2Cl \cdot HCl + SO_2\uparrow$$

diethylaminoethanol → diethylaminoethylchloride hydrochloride

Diethylaminoethyl chloride hydrochloride is obtained by chlorination of diethylaminoethanol with thionyl chloride in toluene or benzene. Purification can be performed by distillation at atmospheric pressure, collecting the fraction with 161–162°C boiling point.

Diethylaminoethanol was distilled in case of poor quality and dried over anhydrous potassium carbonate (1:10 w/v) prior to use. After standing for 6–8 hours with periodic stirring, the desiccant was filtered off. Thionyl chloride (technical) was also distilled at atmospheric pressure before use (boiling point 74–75°C).

2.1.3 Stage 3: synthesis of 2-amino-1-diethylaminoethylbenzimidazole

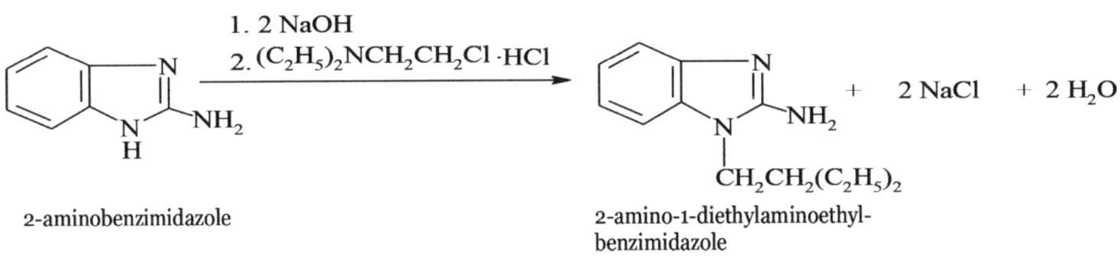

2-Amino-1-diethylaminoethylbenzimidazole is obtained by alkylation of 2-aminobenzimidazole with N,N-diethylaminoethyl chloride in acetone in a presence of a concentrated alkali solution. Upon completion of the reaction, the acetone is distilled off at atmospheric pressure and can be used at the same stage without further purification. Water is added to the residue, and the precipitate of the alkylated amine is filtered off to give 82–88% yield.

2.1.4 Stage 4: 2-(3,4-dihydroxyphenyl)-9-diethylaminoethyl-imidazo[1,2-a]benzimidazole dihydrobromide (RU-185)

Synthesis of compound RU-185 is achieved by treatment of 2-amino-1-diethylaminoethylbenzimidazole with α-chloro-3,4-dihydroxyacetophenone [28] (Method A) or with 3,4-dimethoxyphenacyl bromide. Subsequent cyclization of the formed quaternary 2-aminobenzimidazole salts is achieved in concentrated HBr (Method B).

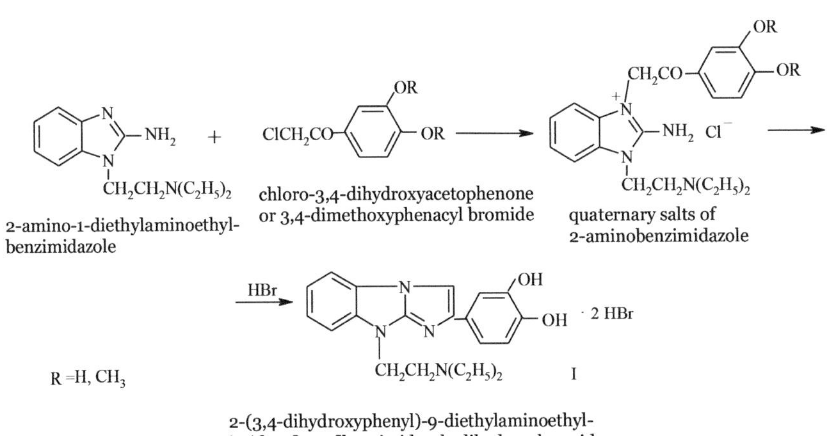

Method A The method consists of boiling of 1-diethylaminoethyl-2-aminobenzimidazole and α-chloroacetopyrocatechol in dry acetonitrile until the quaternization reaction is complete (2–3 hours with TLC control). Then the solvent is evaporated to dryness, and concentrated HBr is added followed by reflux for 1–2 hours. Reaction mixture is left overnight in the refrigerator. The next day, the precipitate formed (large needles) is filtered off. The yield of dihydrobromide (I) is 97%. Recrystallization of the crude product from 80% aqueous ethanol with addition of activated charcoal affords white crystals with a yield of 85%. The product should be protected from direct sunlight. After drying at 110–120°C, the melting point of dihydrobromide is 289–290°C (decomposition).

Method B 3,4-Dimethoxyphenacyl bromide is added to a hot solution of 2-amino-1-diethylaminoethylbenzimidazole in acetone (molar ratio 1:1). Next, the mixture is kept for 6–8 hours at room temperature. The precipitate of 2-amino-(3,4-dimethoxyphenacyl)-1-diethylaminoethylbenzimidazolium bromide is filtered off. The output is 93.5% and melting point 182°C (decomposition, from ethanol).

Next, the resulting bromide is refluxed in conc. HBr (127°C) for 6–8 hours, while as the boiling of the initially formed solution precipitates. After cooling, it is filtered off, washed with acetone, and air dried. The yield is 96%. Crystallization from 80% aqueous ethanol gives (3,4-dihydroxyphenyl)-9-diethylaminoethyl-imidazo[1,2-a] benzimidazole dihydrobromide (I) identical to the product described in method A.

2.2 Pharmacological properties

2.2.1 Antioxidant activity

For several years, the ability of compounds to inhibit oxidative processes in the cells of various tissues, organs, and biological fluids has been thoroughly investigated. The study of the antioxidant properties of enoxifol was carried out by several methods: ascorbate-induced LPO according to the method [29], Fe^{2+}-induced chemiluminescence (CL) of lipids [30], and NADPH-dependent LPO [31]. Superoxide dismutase-like activity has been studied in a quercetin oxidation model [32], interaction with the free radical of 2,2-diphenyl-1-picrylhydrazyl (DPPH*) according to the method [33], and interaction with reactive oxygen species on the luminol-dependent CL model [34], the ability to inactivate the superoxide anion radical was estimated by the xanthine-xanthine oxidase-induced lucigenin-dependent CL method [2], and the ability of substances to intercept and inactivate the peroxyl radical was determined by the ABAP-induced CL method [35]. The spectrum of antioxidant activity of enoxifol and the reference compound trolox is shown on **Figure 1**. It was found that enoxifol can react with lipid peroxyl radicals

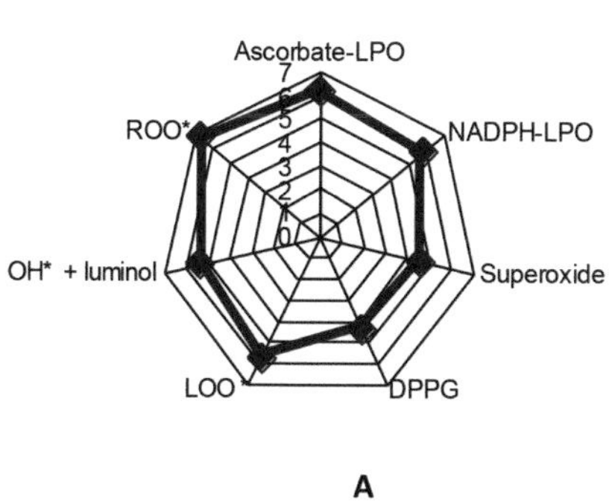

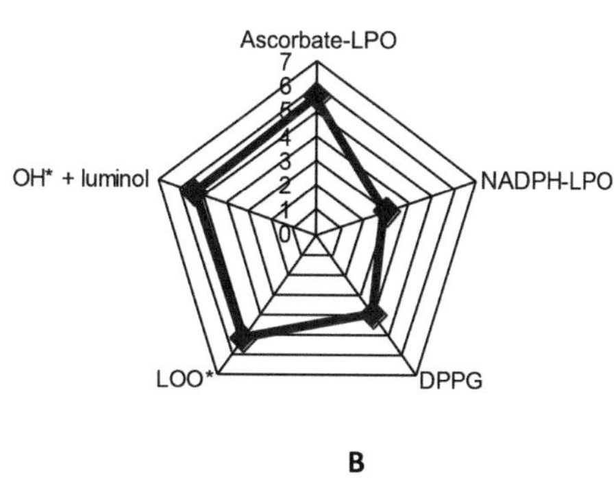

Figure 1.
Antioxidant activity spectrum of enoxifol (A) and trolox (B) ($-Lg\ IC_{50}$ (M)).

at the chain termination stage, as indirectly evidenced by its high inhibitory activity during ascorbate, NADPH-induced lipid peroxidation, and CL of lipids, as well as directly inactivate superoxide, hydroxyl, and peroxyl radicals that initiate oxidation, as demonstrated in reactions with the free radical DPPH, quercetin oxidation, Fe^{2+}-induced CL in the presence of luminol, xanthine-xanthine oxidase induced by lucigenin-dependent CL, as well as thermal decomposition of the water-soluble compound 2,2-azobis (2-methylpropionamidine) dihydrochloride (ABAP) with the release of peroxyl radicals, inactivating free radicals and enoxifol, thereby reducing the overall oxidation rate by reducing the total initiation rate [35, 36].

As a result of the analysis of the chemical structure of enoxifol, the structural descriptors were determined, allowing the compound to exhibit antioxidant and antiradical activities. The molecule of enoxifol can manifest these properties due to a fragment of 3,4-dihydroxyphenyl and π-electronic redundancy of the imidazole ring in the structure of imidazobenzimidazoles [37]. Given the relatively low toxicity and high antioxidant potential, the compound was selected for in-depth study on pathological models.

2.2.2 Membranoprotective properties

Membranoprotective activity of enoxifol was studied using the model [38], determining the mechanical strength and resistance of erythrocyte membranes to the hypoosmotic HCl solution. The membrane-stabilizing activity of the compound (inhibition of slow and fast incoming transmembrane ion currents) has been revealed. An effective dose of a compound of 20.5 mg/kg has been established [39].

2.2.3 Hepatoprotective effects

When studying the hepatoprotective properties of enoxifol with a 3-day prophylactic administration in dose 2.25 mg/kg on a model of acute tetrachloromethane hepatitis, it was found that enoxifol significantly improved the absorption and excretory function of the liver and its detoxification abilities Under its influence the development of signs of the cytolytic, hepatodepressive, mesenchymal-inflammatory, and cholestatic syndrome was significantly inhibited, surpassing tocopherol acetate in effectiveness [40].

2.2.4 Antihypoxic action

The antihypoxic properties of enoxifol have been studied in several models of hypobaric, hemic, and tissue hypoxia. In particular, the activity of the compound was established during intrauterine hypoxia and during recovery after acute hypobaric hypoxia. The potential protective effect of the antioxidant compound in hypobaric hypoxia was determined in high- and low-resistant to hypoxia animals in a flow-type pressure chamber at the “height” of 12,500 and 11,000 m, respectively [41]. The most effective doses in these models were 3 and 5 mg/kg [42]. Enoxifol showed a protective effect in modeling intrauterine hypoxia in dose 10 mg/kg during course administration [42].

The activity of the compound in the recovery period after acute hypobaric hypoxia was determined by the change in behavioral reactions, cognitive functions, and the physical condition of the animals. The protective dose of enoxifol was 5 mg/kg. Tissue and hemic hypoxias were created by injecting potassium cyanide and sodium nitrite, respectively [43]. The protective action of enoxifol was judged by the degree of survival of the animals. The range of effective doses was determined from 0.5 to 5 mg/kg [44].

2.2.5 Cerebroprotective properties

The cerebroprotective effect of enoxifol was established on two models of cerebral ischemia of two and four vascular ligature of the carotid and paravertebral arteries, respectively, as well as during the reperfusion period [25, 44]. Antioxidant compound significantly increased the survival rate of animals, decreased blood viscosity by reducing platelet and red blood cell (RBC) aggregation and improving the mechanical properties of RBC, and corrected the behavioral deficit in the postischemic period. Doses of enoxifol in which the cerebroprotective activity was established were 5 and 10 mg/kg.

2.2.6 Nootropic activity

Nootropic activity of enoxifol was established in the model of the conditioned passive avoidance reaction, which allows to evaluate the effect of a studied compounds on learning and memory. As a result, it was found that enoxifol influenced the ability of animals to consolidate information, reduced the deficit in the reproduction of a memorable trace, and intensified the input and initial processing of information in dose 10 mg/kg. The study of the enoxifol effect on the research behavior and emotionality of animals was carried out in the open-field modified test that allows to evaluate the nonassociative behavior of animals in familiar surroundings. Against the background of a 3-day course of administration of the antioxidant compound in dose of 10 mg/kg, psycho-emotional reactivity and anxiety in animals were decreased. With repeated testing, the memories of the arena research were better preserved. Experiments conducted in a Morris maze test confirmed the potential ability of enoxifol in a similar dose to increase mnestic abilities and improve the spatial orientation of animals [45].

2.2.7 Stress-protective effects

The stress-protective effect of enoxifol was studied on models of short-term (1 hour) and prolonged (48 hours) hypokinetic stress [46] and hyperkinetic stress with the paradoxical sleep phase deprivation in rats, in the test of slowly rotating rod [47]. Enoxifol was administered to animals in doses 5 and 10 mg/kg. An antioxidant compound showed an ambiguous therapeutic effect depending on the experimental model used. The antioxidant was not effective in the short-term hypokinetic stress technique. Enoxifol reduced post-stress injuries of internal organs and corrected the targeted behavior of animals in prolonged hypokinetic stress. Enoxifol did not affect the behavioral activity of rats but protected internal organs from pathological abnormalities in hyperkinetic stress [37].

2.2.8 Actoprotective activity

The effect of enoxifol on physical performance and recovery period after physical exertion was studied under normal and complicated conditions in several experimental models. We used the swim to the limit test [48], fatigue development test [49], and efficiency test in anti-orthostatic condition [50]; the model allows to study the recovery process after exercises [51] and the method of research of animals' endurance to training and exhausting loads [49]. Actoprotective properties were studied in models associated with limiting physical loads (swimming to failure), with the rate of fatigue development, and in the test of swimming in complicated anti-orthostatic condition. Enoxifol increased the duration of physical performance under normal and complicated conditions, stabilized some indicators of energy metabolism (the level of lactate, glycogen, tryptophan, the ratio of pyruvate and lactate), normalized indicators of lipid peroxidation, and had a protective effect on the myocardium of animals during the period of exhaustive physical activity. A number of effective doses amounted to 1, 3, 5, 10, 20, 25, and 50 mg/kg in various physical activity tests [52].

2.2.9 Cardioprotective properties

Cardioprotective activity was studied in isolated atrial rhythm disturbances induced by hydrogen peroxide oxidation [53], in postischemic reperfusion fibrillations of the heart ventricles [54], in the technique of rhythm disturbances caused by calcium chloride and adrenaline intoxication [55], and in the myocardial ischemia provoked by coronary occlusion [31] and the experimental myocardial infarction method [56]. As a result it was found that enoxifol exerted an antiarrhythmic effect, increasing the resistance of cardiomyocyte membranes to LPO products. The compound increased the stability of the myocardium of animals having a non-antioxidant diet to calcium chloride cardiac arrhythmias and increased myocardial tolerance to ischemia. Enoxifol completely prevented ventricular fibrillation of the heart in postischemic myocardial reperfusion. It reduced the extrasystole severity and ventricular fibrillation and reduced the death of animals in the model of coronary artery occlusion and systemic peroxidation syndrome. The novel compound limited area of necrosis in experimental myocardial infarction. It showed activity in doses 7.9, 14, and 20.5 mg/kg [39, 55].

2.2.10 Antithrombotic and antiaggregant effects

Enoxifol had a pronounced antithrombotic effect in arterial thrombosis models induced by application of ferric chloride and electric current on the rat carotid artery and blocked platelet aggregation caused by ADP, collagen, adrenaline, arachidonic acid, thrombin, and an agonist of thromboxane receptors U46619 [24]. The antioxidant compound reduced levels of proaggregant and vasoconstrictor TXA_2, which was confirmed by a decreased level of MDA in the ex vivo pathology caused by thrombin, and decreased the level of total and membrane-bound calcium in platelets, inhibiting calmodulin-dependent PDE cAMP.

2.2.11 Action on hemorheology

The study of the enoxifol action on hemorheology was carried out in the model of “increased viscosity syndrome” according to the method [57]. An improvement in blood flow, membrane plasticity, and inhibition of erythrocyte aggregation under the influence of enoxifol administration in dose 5 mg/kg was found [18]. An increase in the rate of local cerebral blood flow and a direct effect on the tone of cerebral vessels in a similar dose were determined in the method of tissue microcirculation [58]. The study of the enoxifol effect on hemorheology in models of severe forms of streptozotocin diabetes was also performed. Antioxidant compound corrected hemobiological parameters (aggregation, deformability, mechanical properties of erythrocytes), almost normalized indicators of lipid peroxidation, reducing the products of peroxidation, and increased the activity of antioxidant enzymes. The effective dose was 5 mg/kg for the course of the 3-day administration preliminary to diabetes modeling [58].

2.2.12 Pharmacokinetic profile

In the study of the pharmacokinetic properties of enoxifol [27], determination was carried out for 12 hours in the blood and internal organs and in the urine and feces within 48 hours. It was found that the absolute bioavailability of unchanged enoxifol was 30% and for the total amount of enoxifol and its active metabolites, 99%. When administered orally, enoxifol was well absorbed from the gastrointestinal tract, the maximum concentration in the blood was observed after 1 hour, and after 7 hours the compound was not detected. The excretion of the compound occurs mainly through the intestines, and only one-fifth is excreted unchanged; a small amount of enoxifol is excreted through the kidneys. The half-life for enoxifol was 1.43 hours. After the intravenous administration, the maximum concentration of the compound in the blood is determined in 10 minutes; after 7 hours the antioxidant in the blood was not recorded. The excretion of the infusion form of enoxifol occurs mainly through the kidneys in the unchanged form. In a much smaller amount, enoxifol was eliminated with feces. The half-life was 0.78 hours [27].

2.2.13 Toxicological properties

A study of the drug safety of enoxifol [59] found that the antioxidant compound can be attributed to low-toxic substances. The acute toxicity of enoxifol after oral administration was 1792.56 mg/kg for male and 2260.28 mg/kg for female rats. When administered intravenously, the LD50 was determined for male in dose 109.20 mg/kg and for female rats in dose 126.04 mg/kg. Chronic administration in therapeutic doses (5–25 mg/kg) showed that toxic effects in the central nervous system, liver function, kidney function, and the generative system were not observed. In the high dose (200 mg/kg), slight deviations in the behavioral responses of animals and a slight decrease in the detoxification function of the liver were observed. The accumulation ability of enoxifol wasn't found [59].

3. Conclusion

Summarizing the data obtained, we can conclude that condensed benzimidazole derivatives with π-electron redundancy are a new scaffold for searching antioxidant substances. The highest amount of compounds with high antioxidant activity was found in derivatives of 2-(hetaryl)-aroylmethyl-, and 9-dialkylaminoethyl-IMBI, with oxy- and dioxyphenyl substitutes especially.

The revealed compound enoxifol from the 9-dialkylaminoethyl-IMBI series exhibits pronounced antioxidant, hepatoprotective, antihypoxic, cerebroprotective, nootropic, stress-protective, neuropsychotropic, actoprotective, cardioprotective, antithrombogenic and hemorheological properties. Pharmacokinetic parameters of enoxifol were established, and general and specific toxicities were studied. All mentioned above allows us to consider enoxifol to be the basis of a new effective drug.

Author details

Vadim A. Kosolapov[1*], Alexander A. Spasov[1], Vera A. Anisimova[2] and Olga N. Zhukovskaya[2]

1 Volgograd State Medical University, Volgograd, Russia

2 Research Institute for Physical and Organic Chemistry, South Federal University, Rostov-on-Don, Russia

*Address all correspondence to: vad-ak@mail.ru

References

[1] Barrera G, Pizzimenti S, Daga M, Dianzani C, Arcaro A, Cetrangolo GP, et al. Lipid peroxidation-derived aldehydes, 4-hydroxynonenal and malondialdehyde in aging-related disorders. Antioxidants (Basel). 2018;7(8):E102. DOI: 10.3390/antiox7080102

[2] Rahal A, Kumar A, Singh V, Yadav B, Tiwari R, Chakraborty S, et al. Oxidative stress, prooxidants, and antioxidants: The interplay. BioMed Research International. 2014;**2014**:761264. DOI: 10.1155/2014/761264

[3] Kurutas EB. The importance of antioxidants which play the role in cellular response against oxidative/nitrosative stress: Current state. Nutrition Journal. 2016;**15**(1):71. DOI: 10.1186/s12937-016-0186-5

[4] Vasiliev PM, Spasov AA, Kosolapov VA, Anisimova VA. Computer forecast and experimental verification of the antioxidant activity of new chemical compounds using QSAR-relationships. Bulletin of Volgograd State Medical University. 2005;**2**(14):16-19. [Russian]

[5] Anisimova VA, Spasov AA, Kucheryavenko AF, Panchenko TI, Ostrovskii OV, Kosolapov VA, et al. Synthesis and pharmacological activity of 2-(hetaryl) imidazo[1,2-a] benzimidazoles. Pharmaceutical Chemistry Journal. 2002;**36**(10):528-533. DOI: 10.1023/A:1022498224975

[6] Anisimova VA, Spasov AA, Ostrovskii OV, Dudchenko GP, Kosolapov VA, Kucheryavenko AF, et al. Synthesis and pharmacological activity of 3-aroyl- and 3-hetaroylimidazo[1,2-a] benzimidazoles. Pharmaceutical Chemistry Journal. 2002;**36**(12):637-641. DOI: 10.1023/A:1023421709976

[7] Anisimova VA, Spasov AA, Kosolapov VA, Ostrovskii OV, Larionov NP, Libinzon RE. Synthesis and pharmacological activity of 2-methoxyphenyl-substituted 9-dialkylaminoethylimidazo[1,2-a] benzimidazoles. Pharmaceutical Chemistry Journal. 2005;**39**(9):476-482. DOI: 10.1007/s11094-006-0005-y

[8] Anisimova VA, Tolpygin IE, Spasov AA, Kosolapov VA, Chernikov MV, Stepanov AV, et al. Synthesis and pharmacological activity of 2-methoxy-phenyl- and 2-oxyphenyl-substituted 1-dialkylaminoalkylimidazo[1,2-a] benzimidazoles. Pharmaceutical Chemistry Journal. 2005;**39**(11):579-585. DOI: 10.1007/s11094-006-0024-8

[9] Anisimova VA, Tolpygin IE, Spasov AA, Kosolapov VA, Stepanov AV, Kucheryavenko AF. Synthesis and biological activity of N-acylmethyl derivatives of 9H-2,3-dihydroimidazo- and 10H-2,3,4,10-tetrahydropyrimido[1,2-a] benzimidazoles and their reduction products. Pharmaceutical Chemistry Journal. 2006;**40**(5):261-267. DOI: 10.1007/s11094-006-0105-8

[10] Anisimova VA, Spasov AA, Kosolapov VA, Chernikov MV, Stukovina AY, El'tsova LV, et al. Synthesis and biological activity of 9-dialkylaminoethyl-2-oxy(dioxy) phenylimidazo[1,2-a]benzimidazoles. Pharmaceutical Chemistry Journal. 2006;**40**(10):521-528. DOI: 10.1007/s11094-006-0185-5

[11] Anisimova VA, Tolpygin IE, Spasov AA, Kosolapov VA, Stepanov AV, Orlova AA, et al. Synthesis and pharmacological activity of aroylmethyl derivatives of tricyclic benzimidazole systems containing hydroxy groups in aroyl radicals. Pharmaceutical Chemistry Journal. 2007;**41**(3):126-130. DOI: 10.1007/s11094-007-0028-z

[12] Anisimova VA, Spasov AA, Kosolapov VA, Tolpygin IE, Porotikov VI, Kucheryavenko AF, et al. Synthesis and pharmacological activity of 3-(2,2,2-trichloro-1-hydroxyethyl) imidazo[1,2-a]benzimidazole dihydrochlorides. Pharmaceutical Chemistry Journal. 2009;**43**(9):491-494. DOI: 10.1007/s11094-009-0340-x

[13] Anisimova VA, Spasov AA, Tolpygin IE, Kosolapov VA, Kucheryavenko AF, Gurova NA, et al. Synthesis and pharmacological activity of salts of 3-acetyl-2-R-9-dialkylaminoethyl-imidazo[1,2-a] benzimidazoles. Pharmaceutical Chemistry Journal. 2010;**44**(3):117-122. DOI: 10.1007/s11094-010-0411-z

[14] Anisimova VA, Tolpygin IE, Chernikov MV, Yakovlev DS, Goryagin II, Gurova NA, et al. Synthesis and pharmacological activity of 1-dialkyl(alkyl)aminoethyl-2,3-dihydroimidazo[1,2-a]benzimidazoles. Pharmaceutical Chemistry Journal. 2010;**44**(5):241-244. DOI: 10.1007/s11094-010-0439-0

[15] Anisimova VA, Tolpygin IE, Minkin VI, Chernikov MV, Yakovlev DS, Stukovina AY, et al. Synthesis and pharmacological activity of 9-R-2-halogenophenylimidazo[1,2-a] benzimidazoles. Pharmaceutical Chemistry Journal. 2010;**44**(7):345-351. DOI: 10.1007/s11094-010-0465-y

[16] Anisimova VA, Tolpygin IE, Spasov AA, Yakovlev DS, Kolobrodova NA, Gurova NA, et al. Synthesis and pharmacological activity of 10-alkylaminoethyl-2,3,4,10-tetrahydropyrimido[1,2-a] benzimidazoles. Pharmaceutical Chemistry Journal. 2012;**46**(6):325-330. DOI: 10.1007/s11094-012-0791-3

[17] Anisimova VA, Spasov AA, Kosolapov VA, Tolpygin IE, El'tsova LV, Kucheryavenko AF, et al. Synthesis and pharmacological activity of 3-(n,n-disubstituted)acetamide-1-r-2-aminobenzimidazolium chlorides. Pharmaceutical Chemistry Journal. 2012;**46**(9):526-530. DOI: 10.1007/s11094-012-0839-4

[18] Anisimova VA, Spasov AA, Kosolapov VA, Tolpygin IE, Tibir'kova EV, Salaznikova OA, et al. Synthesis and pharmacological activity of amides of 2,3-dihydroimidazo- and 2,3,4,10-tetrahydropyrimido[1,2-a] benzimidazolyl-acetic acids. Pharmaceutical Chemistry Journal. 2013;**46**(11):647-652. DOI: 10.1007/s11094-013-0862-0

[19] Anisimova VA, Anisimova VA, Spasov AA, Kuznetsova VA, Kosolapov VA, Yakovlev DS, et al. Synthesis and pharmacological activity of 2,9-disubstituted imidazo[1,2-a]benzimidazole phenyl- and alkylthiocarbamides. Pharmaceutical Chemistry Journal. 2016;**49**(10):653-656

[20] Zhukovskaya ON, Anisimova VA, Spasov AA, Vasil'ev PM, Kosolapov VA, Kucheryavenko AF, et al. 1-Substituted 2-benzylaminobenzimidazoles with phenyl methoxyls: Synthesis, computer prediction, and pharmacological activity. Pharmaceutical Chemistry Journal. 2016;**49**(11):735-742. DOI: 10.1007/s11094-016-1362-9

[21] Anisimova VA, Kosolapov VA, Minkin VI, Petrov VI, Spasov AA. Dihydrobromide 9-(3,4-dihydroxyphenyl)-9-diethylaminoethyl-imidazo[1,2-a] benzimidazole and a pharmaceutical composition based on it. Patent RU 2391979, priority from 12.05.2008. [Russian]

[22] Kosolapov VA. Antioxidant selection strategy, application prospects [abstract of thesis for the secondary doctorate degree]. Volgograd; 2005. p.40 [Russian]

[23] Spasov AA, Ostrovskiĭ OV, Ivakhnenko IV, Kosolapov VA, Anisimova VA. The effect of compounds with antioxidant properties on thrombocyte functional activity. Eksperimental'naia i Klinicheskaia Farmakologiia. 1999;**62**(1):38-40. [Russian]

[24] Spasov AA, Anisimova VA, Kucheryavenko AF, Minkin VI. The agent possessing antithrombogenic activity. Patent RU 2440814, priority from 10.11.2010 [Russian]

[25] Spasov AA, Kosolapov VA, Ostrovskiĭ OV, Drozd VV, Vereshchagin VK, Sen'chukov ID, et al. Anti-ischemic properties of the novel antioxidant enoxifol. Eksperimental'naia i Klinicheskaia Farmakologiia. 2003;**66**(4):17-20. [Russian]

[26] Spasov AA, Stepanov AV, Samokhina MP, Kosolapov VA. The effect of enoxifol on blood viscosity and erythrocyte aggregation in vitro. Bulletin of Volgograd State Medical University. 2003;**59**(9):43-46. [Russian]

[27] Smirnova LA, Kosolapov VA, Lekomtsev AS, Spasov AA, Ozerov AA. Pharmaco-kinetic properties of cerebroprotective and antioxidant drug enoxifol. Bulletin of Volgograd State Medical University. 2002;**58**(8):32. [Russian]

[28] Rubtsov MV, Baychikov AG. Synthetic chemical and pharmaceutical preparations. Moscow: Medicine; 1971. 54 p. [Russian]

[29] Lankin VZ, Gurevich SM, Burlakova EB. The study of ascorbate-dependent lipid peroxidation of tissues using the test with 2-thiobarbituric acid. Proceedings of the Moscow Society of Nature Testers. 1975;**52**:73-78. [Russian]

[30] Farhutdinov RR, Likhovskikh VA. Chemiluminescent methods for the study of free-radical oxidation in biology and medicine. Ufa; 1995. 54 p. [Russian]

[31] Kubatiev AA, Andreev SV. On the ratio of the processes of generation and detoxification of lipid peroxides in normal and hypertrophied hearts. Myocardial Metabolism. M.: Medicine. 1981:251-262. [Russian]

[32] Kostyuk VA, Potapovich AI, Kovaleva ZV. A simple and sensitive method for determining the activity of superoxide dismutase, based on the reaction of oxidation of quercetin. Questions of medical chemistry. 1990;**36**(2):88-91. [Russian]

[33] Glavind G. Antioxidants in animal tissue. Acta Chemica Scandinavica. 1963;**17**(6):1635-1640

[34] Semeshko SG, Farhutdinov RR. Total antioxidant activity of the tear fluid. Clinical and Laboratory Diagnostics. 2002;**24**:33-34. [Russian]

[35] Kosolapov VA, Spasov AA, Anisimova VA. Study of antiradical activity of new compounds by chemiluminescence. Biomeditsinskaya Khimiya. 2005;**51**(3):287-294. [Russian]

[36] Kosolapov VA. Criteria for the use of luminol and lucigenin in chemiluminescence to study the mechanisms of action of antioxidant substances. Bulletin of Volgograd State Medical University. 2003;**9**:54-57. [Russian]

[37] Ostrovsky OV. Pharmacology of antioxidants—Condensed benzimidazole derivatives [abstract of thesis for the secondary doctorate degree]. Volgograd; 1996. p. 38 [Russian]

[38] Godin DV, Al T, Garnott MK. Membrane perturbational effects of antiarrhythmic drugs. Journal of Molecular and Cellular Cardiology. 1979;**2**(3):261-274

[39] Panchenko TI. Antiarrhythmic properties of new antioxidant substances—Condensed benzimidazole derivatives [abstract of thesis for the PhD degree]. Rostov-on-Don; 1990. p. 31 [Russian]

[40] Spasov AA, Anisimova VA, Kosolapov VA, Minkin VI, Petrov VI. Agent with antiarrhythmic and hepatoprotective properties. Patent RU 246972, priority from 13.07.2011 [Russian]

[41] Lukyanova LD, Malyshev AY, Krapivin SV. Antihypoxic effect of succinate-containing oxypyridine derivative on EEG power spectra in rats with different resistance to oxygen deficiency. Bulletin of Experimental Biology and Medicine. 1997;**124**(7): 57-61. [Russian]

[42] Tregubova IA. Effect of antioxidant substances on the mother-fetus system in hypoxic states (experimental study) [abstract of thesis for the PhD degree]. Volgograd; 2000. p. 31 [Russian]

[43] Korablev MV, Lukienko PI. Antihypoxic Drugs. Minsk: Belarus; 1976. p. 126. [Russian]

[44] Spasov AA, Anisimova VA, Kosolapov VA, Tregubova IA, Minkin VI, Petrov VI. An agent with anti-hypoxic, actoprotective, nootropic effect and affecting physical performance. Patent RU 2462245, priority of 07/12/2011 [Russian]

[45] Tregubova IA, Kosolapov VA, Spasov AA, Anisimova VA. Experimental study of the effect of a new antioxidant agent on learning and memory. Bulletin of Experimental Biology and Medicine. 2014;**156**(6):793-795. DOI: 10.1007/s10517-014-2452-x

[46] Malikova LA, Arefolov VA. Protective effect of phenazepam and sodium oxybutyrate on somatic manifestations in immobilization stress. Bulletin of Experimental Biology and Medicine. 1983;**96**(12):60-62 [Russian]

[47] Van Hulsen ZJM, Coenen AML. The pendulum technique for paradoxical sleep deprivation in rats. Physiology & Behavior. 1980;**25**:807-811

[48] Rylova MA. Methods for studying the chronic effects of harmful environmental factors in the experiment. Leningrad: Medicine; 1964. 324 p. [Russian]

[49] Kiplinger GF. The effects of drugs on the rate of development of fatigue in mice. Texas Reports on Biology and Medicine. 1967;**25**:531-540

[50] Avakian OM, Shirinian EA. New model of dynamic work in small laboratory animals. Biulleten' Eksperimental'noĭ Biologii i Meditsiny. 1977;**84**(9):375 [Russian]

[51] Dawson CA, Horvath SA. Swimming in small laboratory animals. Medicine and Science in Sports. 1970;**2**:51-78

[52] Tsibanev AV. Search for a means of increasing physical performance and recovery processes among imidazo (1,2-a) benzimidazole derivatives, which show antioxidant activity [abstract of thesis for the PhD degree]. Volgograd; 1991. p. 29 [Russian]

[53] Didenko VV. Arrhythmias caused by the induction of lipid peroxidation in an isolated atrium. Moscow; 1985. 15 p. [Russian]

[54] Penkoske PA, Sobel BC, Corr PB. Disparate electrophysiological alterations accompanying dysrhythmia due to coronary occlusion and reperfusion in the cat. Circulation. 1978;**58**:1023-1035

[55] Spasov AA, Anisimova VA, Kosolapov VA, Minkin VI, Petrov VI. The agent with antiarrhythmic and

hepatoprotective properties. Patent RU 2469720, priority from 13.07.11

[56] Harris AS. Circulation. 1950;**1**:1318 [Russian]

[57] Plotnikov MB, Aliev OI, Koltunov AA, Maslov MI. Increased blood viscosity syndrome in SHR rats: Analysis of the model adequacy. Bulletin of Experimental Biology and Medicine. 1998;**126**(8):150-151 [Russian]

[58] Samokhina MP. Hemorheological properties of condensed imidazobenzimidazole derivatives exhibiting an antioxidant effect [abstract of thesis for the PhD degree]. Volgograd; 2003. p. 27. [Russian]

[59] Bugaeva LI, Kuzubova EA, Bukatin MV, Rebrova DN. The effect of enoxifol on the gonadotropic function of male rats. Successes of Modern Natural Science. 2006;**8**:56 [Russian]

Chapter 14

Importance of the Nutrition with Antioxidants in the Treatment of Cancer and Others Damages

Eva María Molina Trinidad, Marco Antonio Becerril Flores, José Luis Imbert Palafox and Laura Vargas Servín

Abstract

The antioxidants are molecules capable of retarding or anticipating the oxidation of other molecules. Epidemiological results have shown that the persons who consume a rich diet of fruits and vegetables present a minor risk of suffering different types of cancer, cardiovascular and neurological diseases, and a minor mortality than the persons who consume few fruits and vegetables. Others studies suggests that the vitamins are antioxidants like can to decrease hurt oxidative in the physiopathology of many chronic diseases and cancer.

Nevertheless, evidence of new studies in mice shows that vitamins can promote the growth of tumors and metastasis and the expression of the gene p53. Current studies indicate that patients with cancer and people who have a major risk of cancer will have to avoid taking complements of antioxidants, due to the fact that it was thought that antioxidants might protect cells against cancer since they neutralize reactive oxygen species (ROS) that can damage the DNA, but in studies of animals, it has been indicated that the presence of major concentrations of antirust exogenous prevents the type of hurt of free radical that has been associated with the formation of cancer.

Keywords: nutrition, antioxidants, treatment, cancer, diseases

1. Introduction

Antioxidants are molecules that act disabling the reactions of oxidation in chain that they produce cellular hurt withdrawing radical free and disabling other reactions of oxidation.

Production of free radicals is regulated by different metabolic routes, and they are considered as the first line of defense in the human body.

Currently, consumption of foods rich in antioxidants such as functional foods as omega-3 and glutamine [1] plays an important role in the nutrition of the population. As functional foods that contain fiber, vitamins, minerals and which decrease saturated fats or sugars are considered [2].

The advantages of the consumption of antioxidants have been reported, but currently a research has discovered the disadvantages in their consumption; for example,

IntechOpen

vitamin A and N-acetyl-cysteine dosed to mice induced with lung cancer increase the size of the tumors, and these substances can eliminate the expression of the gene *p53* (suppressing gene of tumors) activated when hurt exists in the DNA [3].

On the other hand, a functional food is according to the ESPEN guidelines a "food fortified with additional ingredients or with nutrients or compounds intended to yield specific beneficial health effects." Functional foods can be prepared with vitamins and minerals or other compounds of nutritional or physiological effects, and their dose form can be different [4].

In Europe and USA the consumption of dietetic supplements more commonly are antirust vitamins and mineral supplements.

This paper explains the importance of the consumption of antioxidants in the human nutrition and in patients with cancer, who have been treated with chemotherapy and radiotherapy, and their use to other diseases has been mentioned.

2. Functional foods

A functional food is a nutritional food with vitamins and minerals and other compounds functional in the body; they are also known as antioxidants. In the **Table 2** we show some antioxidants report in the literature.

2.1 Glutamic acid

Glutamic acid is a nonessential amino acid and has functions that allow it to interact with other biological biomolecules in order to maintain energy between tissues for the synthesis of molecules and lead to cell growth [1].

This amino acid is considered for its function as a neurotransmitter in its molecular form as glutamate neurons because it stimulates the central nervous system and the latter is the substrate resulting in glutamine, and by this the biomolecular gamma-aminobutyric acid (inhibitory neurotransmitter at the synapse level) is formed by the glutamic carboxylase enzyme. This neurotransmitter opens the chlorine channels, hyperpolarizes the postsynaptic membrane, and decreases neuronal activity.

It has been reported that only 1.8 kg of glutamate is found in the muscle tissue, brain, and kidneys. Due to its physicochemical characteristics, its degree of acidity (2.17 and 9.13) crosses the blood-brain barrier.

Glutamine can be produced from ammonia (NH_3) in the brain and is part of the detoxification process. For this reason, this biomolecule is part of the best-known antioxidants to maintain the function of various organic systems such as the immune system, the digestive system, and the muscular system.

Given the characteristics of this compound, it is included in the human diet in the form of a food supplement and in nutritional foods in the form of glutamine, since it allows the recovery of patients who have undergone surgery treatments and in cases of electrolyte loss in patients who have decreased their immunological system, for example, patients with AIDS or cancer.

This substance is also known as the chemical messenger, for its ability to interact with neurons and allow cell communication, as well as an energy source in oxidation processes of cancer cells [5].

This compound also participates in the metabolism of carbohydrates and in the cellular respiration process of the Krebs cycle [1].

This amino acid can cause alterations in patients who are treated with antiepileptic drugs or who suffer from kidney or liver disease, for which reason the dose of this amino acid must be controlled.

It is recommended to ingest glutamic acid by supplements. The nutrient presentations range from 200 to 500 mg, and for its intake, it is presented in solid pharmaceutical forms as tablets. The dose in pediatric patients from 6 to 12 years is 200 mg every 12 hour.

In patients with cancer who have been treated with chemotherapy and radiotherapy, the intake of glutamic acid benefits their recovery.

2.2 Omega-3 fatty acids

The omega-3 fatty acids include alpha-linolenic acid (ALA), eicosapentaenoic acid (EPA), and docosahexaenoic acid (DHA). The first is found in vegetable oils (flaxseed, soybeans, and canola), and the second and third are found in seafood and fish.

The fatty acids known as omega-3 refer to the position of the carbon atoms with respect to the carboxyl functional group (COOH). They are polyunsaturated fatty acids. The term omega is derived from the position of the terminal methyl functional group of the fatty acid as the main carbon atom identifying the double bond.

EPA and DHA are structural components of the phospholipids that are part of the membranes and are the substrates that give rise to eicosanoid lipids (derived from 20 carbon atoms such as EPA) and docosanoid lipids (derived from 22 carbon atoms such as DHA). The importance of these compounds lies in several functions of cellular metabolism. It has been reported that these fatty acids have anti-inflammatory properties that have a cytoprotective function.

In the men, the intake of this type of fatty acids increases in cell membranes, specifically in lymphocytes, decreasing the amount of arachidonic acid in cell membranes and decreasing the proinflammatory products of omega-6 fatty acids.

EPA is a substrate of the enzyme cyclooxygenase (COX-1–COX-2) and lipooxygenase-5 in the plasma membrane, competes with arachidonic acid (AA) in the production of eicosanoids, and maintains the levels of prostaglandins I_2 (inhibitor of platelet aggregation).

Dietary supplements based on EPA and DHA have the property of decreasing the production of proinflammatory cytokines such as interleukin-1, interleukin-6, interleukin-8, and pulmonary necrosis factor-alpha (TNF-alpha) released by activation of macrophages and monocytes. Although cytokines are activators of the immune response, the hyperactivity of the same can cause inflammation in the intestine, rheumatoid arthritis, and other inflammatory diseases. Therefore, dietary supplements based on EPA and DHA can decrease the production of inflammatory cytokines and the effects of TNF-alpha [6–8].

The documented mechanisms for the modulation of cytokines are based on the decrease of proinflammatory gene expression through changes in the activity of genetic transcription factors such as in the hyperactivation of receptors activated by PPAR-gamma peroxisomes and by inhibition in the release of the transcription nuclear factor-kB (NF-kB). Modification in the cell membrane related to cell signaling is also included.

Chemically, it is a carboxylic acid. It is found in fish oil and some seaweed. DHA is a polyunsaturated essential fatty acid of the omega-3 series [8]. The oil of unicellular algae is known as *Crypthecodinium cohnii* [9]. The omega fatty acid it is use for coronary disease and depression [7, 10] (**Figure 1**).

Also, DHA lowers blood pressure and prevents the development of hypertension and cardiovascular pathologies like atherosclerosis [11]. This substance has a strong positive relationship between dietary fat in the treatment of cancer. DHA inhibits cyclooxygenase, thereby decrementing the amount of prostaglandins and increasing the lipoxygenase activity. This in turn results in higher production of hydroxyeicosatetraenoic acids (HETE) and leukotriene B4 (LTB4), which have

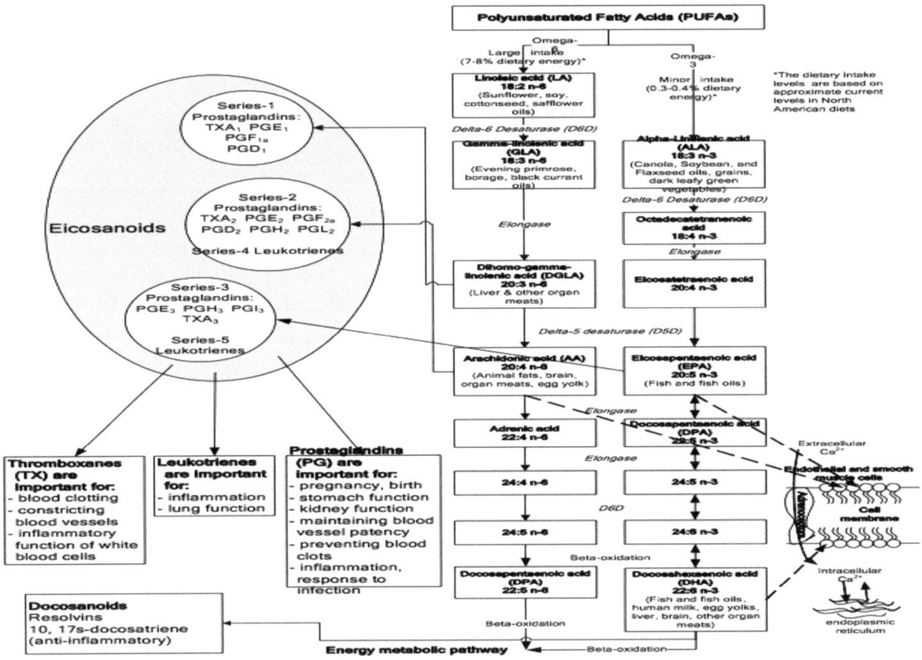

Figure 1.
Function of omega-3 fatty acid in regulating health markers and omega-3 and omega-6 fatty acid synthesis [7].

Names		Abbreviations		
Trivial	**IUPAC***	**Carboxyl-reference**	**Omega-reference**	**Other**
Linolenic acid	9,12,15-octadecenoic acid alpha-linolenic acid	$18{:}3\Delta^{9\ 12\ 15}$	18:3n-3 18:3 (ω-3)	ALA α-LA LNA α-LNA
Docosahexaenoic acid	4,8,12,15,19-docosahexaenoic acid cervonic acid	$22{:}6\Delta^{4\ 8\ 12\ 15\ 19}$	22:6n-3 22:6 (ω-3)	DHA
Docosapentaenoic acid	7,10,13,16,19-docosapentaenoic acid	$22{:}5\Delta^{7\ 10\ 13\ 16\ 19}$	22:5n-3 22:5 (ω-3)	DPA
Eicosapentaenoic acid Icosapentaenoic acid Timnodonic acid	5,8,11,14,17-eicosapentaenoic acid	$20{:}5\Delta^{5\ 8\ 11\ 14\ 17}$	20:5n-3 20:5 (ω-3)	

IUPAC, International Union of Pure and Applied Chemistry. Trivial names, chemical names and abbreviations for the omega-3 fatty acids. Categorize according to their chain length of the polyunsaturated fatty acids (PUFAs) [7].

Table 1.
Nomenclature of omega-3 fatty acids.

been suggested as retarding the process of cancerous cells taking over a tissue. In an experimental animal model, DHA act inhibiting transcription factor activator protein 1 (AP-1), which has been implicated in the development of cancer [12]. DHA could decrement the risk of neuropsychiatric disorders and could be attribute to their effect on neurotransmitter receptor and G-proteins via effects on the biophysical properties of cell membranes and secondary messengers, and on protein kinases [11, 13, 14]. The consumption of DHA can positively influence to avoid the deterioration caused by Alzheimer's (AD), associated with the production of amyloid beta protein that make up hyperphosphorylated tau protein and ubiquitin. The disease is also related to the E4 allele of the apolipoprotein E (ApoE) gene found on the chromosome 19. The treatment for this disease is multiple and drug therapy is based on the stabilization of cognitive impairment and the behavior of the individual. As this disease is related to cholinergic function, the treatment is based on the intake of acetylcholinesterase inhibitor drugs. Therefore, the intake of omega-3 fatty acids is associated with the treatment of Alzheimer's due to its neuronal function [15]. **Table 1** shows the nomenclature of different omega-3 fatty acids [7].

3. Antioxidants

Antioxidants include vitamins A, C, and E and selenium.

3.1 Vitamin A

Carotene is a pigment that animals can turn into vitamin A in their body. C The intestine is the organ that is responsible for transforming carotene into vitamin A for storage in the liver and is rarely stored in fat tissue. Its common form is found as beta-carotene. Due to its chemical structure, it is part of the terpenes, formed by isoprene units (40 carbon atoms). The biosynthesis of these compounds is initially from isopentenyl pyrophosphate.

Beta-carotene was the first purified carotene (*Daucus carota*). Vitamin A is the active form of retinol. Milk and carrots, green vegetables, and some fruits are dietary sources of vitamin A. Isomerization reactions affect the vitamin A content.

Among its functions it is said that it protects the skin from the ultraviolet rays derived from the sun; it also keeps the immune system in optimal conditions, as well as the cardiac system, and is used as an antioxidant.

It is known that the oxidation process of low-density lipoprotein (LDL) decreases the risk of manifesting coronary diseases and arteriosclerosis.

With regard to cancer, it is said that vitamin A allows good cellular functioning by decreasing the development of cancer cells. The intake of this vitamin prevents colon, breast, lung, and oral cavity cancers.

Consumption of vitamin A allows the brain to function in good condition because it has been proven to delay cognitive aging and decrease the oxidative stress derived from the production of free radicals that can generate cell damage generating dementia.

With respect to respiratory diseases, the intake of carotenoids reduces the manifestation of respiratory disorders such as pulmonary emphysema, bronchitis, and asthma to keep the lungs in good condition.

These compounds prevent macular degeneration or loss of sight in adults. Among other things, it prevents skin aging due to its antioxidant properties, since it diminishes the effect of the ultraviolet light generated by the sun's rays and by environmental contamination.

One of the disadvantages due to the excessive use of this vitamin lies in the malformation of the fetus in pregnant women by high doses of carotene continuously.

The reactions that are carried out in the organism are oxidation, reduction, and esterification that give rise to different metabolic processes [16].

3.1.1 Oxidation

Retinol is the main form of vitamin A; it is a derivative of alcohols. In the eyes, vitamin A plays a fundamental role because it is part of the visual purple of the retina, and if the amount of vitamin A decreases, the ability to see is reduced.

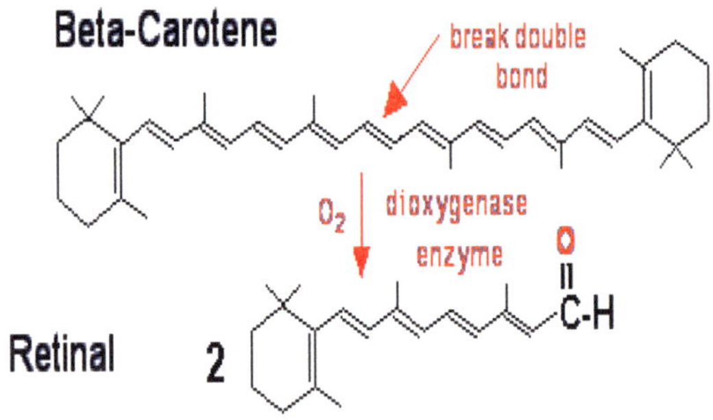

Figure 2.
Synthesis of retinal from beta carotene.

Beta-carotene is denatured in the walls of the intestinal mucosa where it interacts with the enzyme β-carotene desoxygenase to produce retinal (see **Figure 2**) [16].

3.1.2 Reduction reaction

The reduction reaction that vitamin A presents involves the passage from retinal to retinol in the presence of the enzyme retinaldehyde reductase in the intestine. The chemical reaction includes the reduction of an aldehyde by accepting hydrogen atoms to produce an alcohol known as retinol.

3.1.3 Esterification reaction

Retinoids are found in nature in the form of retinol (alcohol) and retinal (aldehyde). The three active forms of vitamin A in the body are retinol, the compound retinal, and retinoic acid. The compound retinal is metabolized in the body, producing retinoic acid and, by esterification reactions, retinol palmitate is produced which is part of the storage in the body.

The digestion of vitamin A is carried out as the degradation of fatty acids, that is, the retinol esters are hydrolyzed by the pancreatic lipase enzymes when they bind to the bile salts forming micelles where the free retinol is absorbed in the intestine specifically in the duodenum and jejunum. The absorption of retinoids is 80–90% and that of carotenoids is 30–40%.

In enterocytes or epithelial cells of the intestine, carotenoids and beta-carotene are attached to the chylomicrons and transported to the liver where they are stored as retinol palmitate. In hepatic cells, retinol binds to the retinol transporter protein (RBP) forming a conjugate by binding to prealbumin in order to travel over the bloodstream where it is transferred to other tissues. On the other hand, carotenoids travel to the bloodstream as part of very-low-density lipoproteins (VLDL) and are stored in adipose tissue.

In dietary supplements vitamin A reduces cancer risk [17].

3.2 Vitamin C

In 1920, Albert Szent-Györgyi, un bioquímico húngaro, identificó la vitamina C. Después, fue llamado ácido hexurónico por un médico llamado Joseph Svibely, Szent-Györgyi. Más tarde fue nombrado ácido ascórbico por Szent-Györgyi y Norman Haworth, un científico que también estudió la vitamina C [18]. Fue conocido desde su descubrimiento como factor de escorbuto. La vitamina C es un compuesto soluble en agua [19].

It is known as ascorbic acid; its chemical name is (R)-3,4,-dihydroxy-5-((S)-1,2-dihydroxyethyl) furan-2(%H)-one. In its oxidized form, it is known as dehydro-ascorbic acid ($C_6H_8O_6$).

As part of its functions, this compound is considered necessary for the organism since it participates in the growth and repair of tissues in the human body. It is important for the function of the skin, tendons, ligaments, and blood vessels. It is also important to heal wounds and tissues. It also participates in the repair and maintenance of the cartilage, bones, and teeth. Finally, it is important in the iron absorption process.

It presents oxidation and reduction reactions in the organism, since it gives hydronium ions to form L-dehydroascorbic acid.

Vitamin C is excreted in the small intestine (duodenum) and is passed into the bloodstream through a process of active transport of sodium ions. The process is saturable and dose-dependent. At high concentrations a part of the ascorbic acid is diffused by a simple diffusion process.

Its functions depend on the redox processes that is manifested in the interaction with other molecules [19]. Vitamin C functions as a cofactor in various hydroxylation and amination reactions by transferring electrons to enzyme complexes that produce reducing equivalents that facilitate the conversion of proline and lysine, which are amino acids that are part of procollagen in the form of hydroxyproline and hydroxylysine during synthesis of collagen. It also participates in the oxidation of the lysine side chains to form hydroxytrimethylisin in the synthesis of carnitine and in the conversion of folic acid into folinic acid. It is also an essential compound in the oxidation of amino acids such as phenylalanine and tyrosine and is important in the metabolism of tryptophan, and participates in the synthesis of noradrenaline [20].

It is considered an antioxidant agent because of its ability to capture free radicals such as H_2O_2, O_2^-, and hypochlorous acid [21].

Vitamin C prevents the oxidation of low-density lipoproteins (LDL) facilitating the absorption of iron [22]. In foods rich in vitamin C such as broccoli and cauliflower, it was shown that it has a correlation of phytochemicals (phenol, flavonoid, and glucosinolate) [23]. Another study highlighted the antioxidant capacity of vitamin C in fruits [24].

The physiological importance of vitamin C is its role as a cofactor and its participation in enzyme reduction reactions [22].

Vitamin C protects cell membranes, DNA [25], cellulose proteins and lipids against the oxidative effects of free radicals (ROS) [26, 27] and reactive oxygen species. At the immunological level, it stimulates phagocytosis and the formation of antibodies.

Adverse reactions to the consumption of this vitamin are rare, but care should be taken when dosing pregnant women. It can cause nausea, vomiting, acidity, abdominal cramps, fatigue, headache, insomnia, and drowsiness. Inappropriate consumption of vitamin C can cause arthritis [28].

In heroin addicts who present with oxidative stress, vitamin C levels [29, 30] can damage their health. Foods rich in potassium tend to be high in vitamin C; therefore, a decrease in potassium causes a decrease in vitamin C [31–34].

3.3 Alpha-tocopherol

Vitamin E is a substance with liposoluble characteristics and has been reported to have antioxidant properties. It is chemically presented with eight isoforms of vitamin E: four tocopherols (α, β, and δ) and four tocotrienols (α, β, and δ). It is found in foods such as wheat germ and sunflower, safflower, corn, and soybean oils.

It is absorbed in the small intestine and is passed into the bloodstream by transporting plasma lipoproteins. The serum vitamin E levels reported are from 11.6 to 46.4 μmol/L.

Vitamin E group includes all of the tocol and tocotrienol derivatives which qualitatively exhibit the biological activity of d-alpha-tocopherol. There are eight natural forms of vitamin E and they are divided into 2 fundamental groups: the 4 tocopherols (TF) and the 4 tocotrienols (TT) that differ in the saturation of the side chain; the tocopherols have a saturated chain and the tocotrienols an unsaturated with 3 double bonds. They are classified into alpha, beta, gamma and delta classes and derivatives of tocopherol and tocotrienol, which are synthesized by plants from homogentisic acid. Alpha and gamma-tocopherols are the two main forms of vitamin E. Vitamin E is known as alpha-tocopherol because it is the most abundant isoform in nature. It is absorbed in greater proportion in the gastrointestinal tract and is responsible for the activity in many metabolic processes.

The beneficial properties of alpha-tocopherol are manifested when the hydronium H^+ phenolic ion is transferred to a radical derived from polyunsaturated fatty acids.

It is the first line of defense against DNA oxidative damage and the peroxidation of polyunsaturated fatty acids in cell membranes.

It is found in many foods of vegetable origin such as nuts, hazelnuts, almonds, and pistachios and also in different food supplements. It has been proven that adverse reactions are minimal. Therefore, it is an excellent preventive compound of diseases and is part of the diet of man [35].

Currently it has been reported that tocopherols inhibit platelet aggregation by inhibiting protein kinase C (PKC) [36, 37] and increase the activity of nitric oxide synthase enzymes, the catalytic enzyme N-arginine and L-citrulline [38].

Alpha-tocopherol is used in inflammatory processes, in its inhibition of platelet aggregation, in the activity of the immune system, and in the reduction of cardiovascular complications (gamma-tocopherol) [39, 40].

In Alzheimer's disease (AD), amyloid beta protein is a substance involved in the cytotoxic processes due to peroxidation and the production of free radicals that produces cell death in the brain producing the symptoms of this disease. This is why vitamin E can act by blocking peroxide production and decreasing cytotoxic effects.

Alpha-tocopherol as an anti-inflammatory can decrease the discomfort caused in patients positive for the human immunodeficiency virus (HIV). Doses of 400 IU of alpha-tocopherol restore cutaneous hypersensitivity and interleukin-2 production, as well as increased proliferation of helper T cells (CD4 T cells) [41–45].

In the immune system, alpha-tocopherol increases the conditions of biological immunity in humans, the humoral and cellular immune response, and the phagocytosis process [46–49].

It is said that the antioxidant effect of vitamin E in combination with alpha-lipoic acid (AAL) enhances its antioxidant effect in cardiovascular and brain diseases [50].

3.4 Selenium

The selenium atom can be presented in different allotropic forms, in its vitreous and black form. When reduced it appears red. It has various uses, for example, for the treatment of seborrheic arthritis.

This element is found in foods like bread, cereals, fish, meat, lentils, potato peel, and eggs. It is found in conjugated amino acid molecules such as selenocysteine and selenomethionine, glutathione peroxidase enzymes (GSHPx), and thioredoxin reductase that have selenium in their chemical structure.

As an antioxidant it participates in the neutralization of free radicals in the process of the production of peroxides; it also induces apoptosis and is an agent

Antioxidant	Chemist structure	Function	Treatment
Glutamic ácid $[C_5H_9NO_4]$ or glutamine	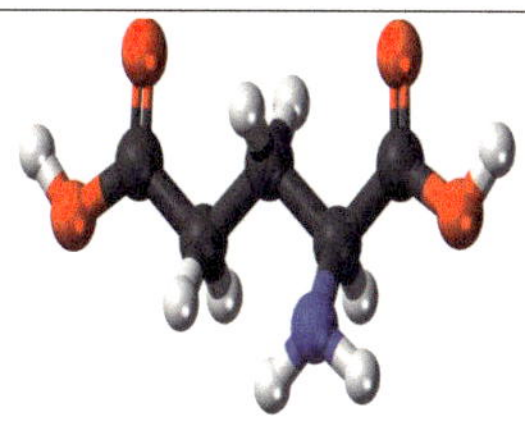	Is critical for cellular function and is not an essential nutrient because humans can synthesize it from other compounds. It is an acidic amino acids, or negatively charged at physiological pH, because it has a second carboxyl group in its secondary chain.	Contributes to trophism, since the small intestine is the body's main glutamine consumer, is the precursor of glutathione, a key molecule in the antioxidant chain, modulates the inflammatory response in different cells of the immune system and regulates cytokine production; protects cells from diverse insults, including heat shock proteins and apoptosis.
Docohexanoic acid $[C_{22}H_{32}O_2]$	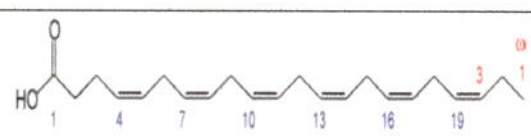	The DHA is found at high concentrations in the phospholipids of neural cell membranes, where it serves several physiologic functions, including the regulation of membrane fluidity, the release of neurotransmitters, genetic expression, myelination, and cellular differentiation, and growth.	The consumption of DHA could prevent the deterioration caused by Alzheimer's.
Vitamin C	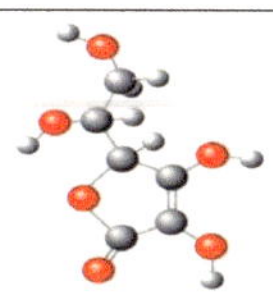	Relation as a cofactor and reduces certain enzymes by providing them with electrons.	Vitamin C decreases more quickly with increased oxidative stress, therefore, vitamin C is used to control oxidative stress.
Vitamin E	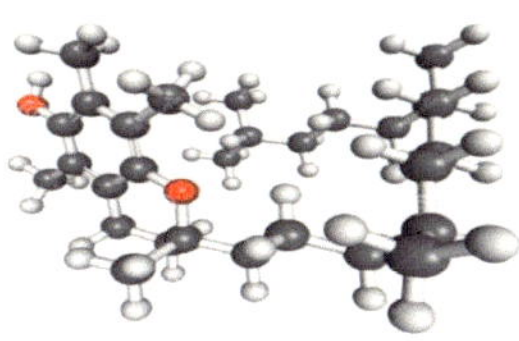	Vitamin E promotes membrane repair by preventing the formation of oxidized phospholipids that theoretically might interfere with the membrane fusion events.	Regulation of platelet, aggregation and protein kinase C activation, in disease prevention, cardiovascular diseases, cancer, cataracts, Alzheimer´s disease, human immunodeficiency virus and acquired immunodeficiency syndrome and the immunity.
β-carotene	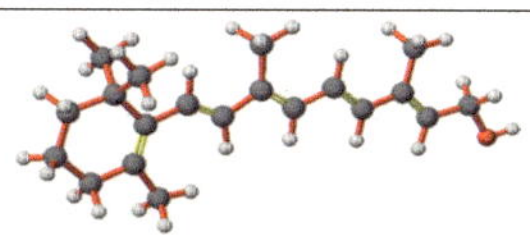	Vitamin A has several functions in the body as the role in vision.	Decrement the risk of breast or lung cancer.
Selenium	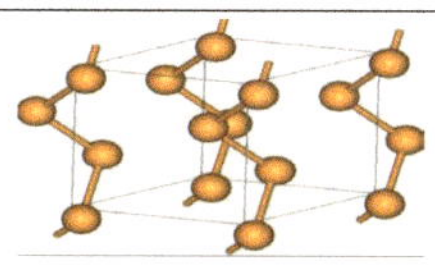	Associated with an increase in glutathione peroxidase (GSHPx) activity.	Se, may inhibit lipid peroxidation in higher plants through GSH-Px and no enzymatic reactions.

Table 2.
Description of some antioxidants, chemist, structure, function and treatment.

that stimulates the immune system and participates in the proper functioning of the thyroid gland. Studies of this element indicate that it can prevent cancer by the chemoprotective action against oxidative stress. It is found in the form of selenite and selenate or as a conjugate derived from amino acids; the latter is beneficial for humans. It can be toxic at high doses causing the disease known as selenosis [51].

It is important in genetic engineering since the UGA termination codon serves as a codon for Se-cysteine and can be decoded by Se-cysteyl-tRNAs in herbs; so, this chemical element has specific biological functions. In **Table 2**, we show some antioxidants.

4. Polyphenols

Polyphenols are substances derived from plants with good absorption properties and bioavailability and are bioactive. They are classified into flavonoids, phenolic acids, stilbenes, lignans, and other derivatives.

According to the World Health Organization (WHO), diseases such as depression, diabetes, cardiovascular diseases, and cancer are caused by genetic inheritance, environment, and socioeconomic factors as causal agents in the development of these diseases.

Oxidative stress associated with certain diseases is part of epidemiological studies associated with a diet rich in antioxidants to reduce the effects caused by free radicals (ROS).

Antioxidants can be obtained from a diet rich in fruits and vegetables that include cocoa, coffee, and tea.

Studies related to polyphenols indicate beneficial effects on human health, since their consumption modifies absorption, bioavailability, and metabolism. Its antioxidant effect lies in the way of extracting plants and obtaining in some foods how potatoes improve microbial digestion in the colon due to the phenolic metabolites that are formed.

The antioxidant effects of polyphenols in the diet are attributed to the enzymatic regulation that reduce free radicals and modulate the enzymatic process during the development of cell reduction reactions.

Marmouzi et al. demonstrated that antioxidants form hybrids that prevent hyperglycemia via enzymatic modulation in phase II. The anticancer effect is also attributed to the signaling of cancer cells and to the progression of the cell cycle and modulation of apoptosis.

Derived polyphenols have antitumor effects in breast cancer with estrogen-mediated receptor activity (ERc) and with receptor 2 or epidermal growth factor (HER2) and in proliferation and chronic inflammation [50].

Degenerative disorder with Alzheimer's disease is related to human aging, and it has been observed that patients suffering from this disease have high levels of free radicals. The phenolic derivative resveratrol can inhibit the aggregation of the amyloid beta peptide, present in these patients. It is a phenol with antioxidant properties and anti-inflammatory that is involved with neuronal differentiation through activation as a silent regulator of cellular information.

Substances with important phytochemical properties used as antioxidants are curcumin, resveratrol, propolis, polyunsaturated fatty acids (PUFAS), and ginseng derivatives. They are used to decrease cerebral neuroinflammation. Avenanthramide is a substance that can serve as a therapeutic agent for the treatment of brain disorders.

The extracts of ethanol of *Diospyros kaki* rich in flavonoids diminish the oxidative stress and are mediators in the processes of inflammation and are related to the memory in synaptic processes in the communication of proteins.

On the other hand, the action of sulfhydryl (SH) and thiol groups in antistress processes is related to the enzymatic process of the carbonic anhydrase enzymes III and VII and the reactivity with amino acids such as cysteine and its residues in S-glutathionylation processes [52].

In Mediterranean countries diet rich in antioxidants including polyphenols has decreased coronary heart disease and cancer. The consumption of a diet rich in vegetables, fish oil, and olive oil and the consumption of wine and the reduction of saturated fats of the trans type have allowed to decrease cellular aging [53].

The diet based on polyphenols is included in the continents of Europe, Asia, and South America. The adherence and origin of polyphenols depend on the place of production [54].

5. Other causes of cancer

The presence of free radicals (ROS) can induce cell death in tissues and organs. The liver as an organ that metabolizes many substances as nutrients and drugs is the place most damaged by free radicals in parenchymal cells, mitochondria, and perixomes. ROS are related to fatty acid oxidation and gene expression.

The TNF-alpha cytokines can produce in Kupffer cells oxidative stress that give rise to inflammatory processes and apoptosis, which can cause liver damage and affect hemostasis, leading to irreversible damage to the synthesis of lipids, proteins, and DNA by the effect of modulators that control different biological functions.

The presence of ROS affects genetic regulation in the transcription process, in the expression of proteins, in apoptosis, and in cell activation, causing severe damage to metabolic processes leading to liver diseases such as chronic viral hepatitis and fatty liver caused by excess consumption of alcohol.

The clinical treatment derives from the consumption of antioxidants as adjuvants that can be synthetic products or derivatives of vitamins C and E and other substances such as mitoquinone, N-acetylcysteine, and silibinin for the treatment of chronic hepatitis C and for patients with cirrhosis [55].

Antioxidants such as zinc, coenzyme Q10, sylimarin, metadoxine, N-acetylcysteine, propofol and mitoquinone mesylate, selenium, methionine, and lipoic acid can be used in patients suffering from fatty liver and steatohepatitis. Methionine can also be used for liver treatment.

On the other hand, some foods induce the inhibition or inactivation of the P53 gene, which was known as the guardian of the genome, because of his function to identify and prevent the multiplication of cells with modified DNA in its structure due to carcinogenic people.

P53 is a transcription factor whose gene is located on the short arm of chromosome 17. P53 is a DNA repair sensor; if the damage is severe, P53 induces programmed cell death or apoptosis. If P53 has mutations, its functions are not carried out. If mutations occur in the germ line (gametic cells), it can lead to Li-Fraumeni syndrome, characterized by breast cancer and other neoplasms, which leads to a pattern of autosomal dominant transmission [56].

6. Conclusions

Therapy with antioxidants of synthetic origin and of natural origin is important for the treatment of different diseases including those derived from liver diseases. In the case of the use of plants, it is necessary to have knowledge of the pharmacological studies of dosage effect, pharmacokinetics, and bioavailability of the compounds with antioxidant properties.

The inflammatory processes present in various pathologies such as cancer, intestinal inflammation, neurodegenerative diseases, cardiovascular diseases, asthma, and rheumatoid arthritis can be treated with omega-3 fatty acids in terms of prevention and treatment and with treatment of other antioxidants as selenium, polyphenols, and vitamins E and C.

In general for the treatment of cancer and other diseases that lead to the study of this disease, foods and supplements rich in antioxidants are a positive option that can be of preventive nature and can be used during the treatment of some anomaly derived from cancer and after the treatment with drugs and the application of radiations, since they favor the recovery of the patients.

Proper nutrition is very important to prevent certain diseases; for this reason, right consumption of nutrients and antioxidants and other substances such as probiotics and probiotics favors recovery in patients whose medical treatments have been aggressive, such as chemotherapies and radiotherapies in the treatment of cancer, diabetes, and hypertension, among others.

Author details

Eva María Molina Trinidad*, Marco Antonio Becerril Flores,
José Luis Imbert Palafox and Laura Vargas Servín
Área Académica de Medicina, Instituto de Ciencias de la Salud, Universidad Autónoma del Estado de Hidalgo, Hidalgo, México

*Address all correspondence to: emolinatrinidad@gmail.com

References

[1] Serna-Thomé G, Castro-Eguiluz D, Fuchs-Tarlovsky V, Sánchez-López M, Delgado-Olivares L, Coronel-Martínez J, et al. Use of functional foods and oral supplements as adjuvants in cancer treatment. Revista de Investigación Clínica. 2018;**70**:136-146

[2] Coronado HM, Vega y León S, Gutiérrez TR, Vázquez FM, Radilla VC. Antioxidants: Present perspective for the human health. Revista Chilena de Nutricion. 2015, 2015;**42**(2):206-212

[3] Ríos Hernández MA, Hernández Menéndez M. Los genes supresores de tumores y el cáncer. Revista Cubana de Oncología. 2001;**17**(1):65-71

[4] Cederholm T, Barazzoni R, Austin P, et al. ESPEN guidelines on definitions and terminology of clinical nutrition. Clinical Nutrition. 2017;**36**:49-64

[5] Kucuktulu E, Guner A, Kahraman I, Topbas M, Kucuktulu U. The protective effects of glutamine on radiation-induced diarrhea. Supportive Care in Cancer. 2013;**21**:1071-1075

[6] Meydani M. Protective role of dietary vitamin E on oxidative stress in aging. Age. 1992;**15**(3):89-93

[7] MacLean CH, Issa AM, Newberry SJ, Mojica WA, Morton SC, Garland RH, et al. Effects of omega-3 fatty acids on cognitive function with aging, dementia, and neurological diseases. Evidence report/technology assessment. Agency for Healthcare Research and Quality. 2005;**114**:1-88

[8] Valenzuela BR, Tapía OG, González EM, Valenzuela BA. Omega-3 fatty acids (EPA and DHA) and its application in diverse clinical situations. Revista Chilena de Nutricion. 2011;**38**(3):356-367

[9] Calder R. Docosahexaenoic acid. Advances in Nutrition. 2016;7:1139-1141

[10] Mendes A, Reis A, Vasconcelos R, Guerra P, Lopes da Silva T. Crypthecodinium cohnii with emphasis on DHA production: A review. Journal of Applied Phycology. 2009;**21**:199-214. DOI: 10.1007/s10811-008-9351-3

[11] Joordens JCA, Kuipers RS, Muskief FAJ. Performed dietary DHA: The answer to a scientific question may in practice become translated to its opposite. American Journal of Human Biology. 2007;**19**:582-584. DOI: 10.1002/ajhb.20675

[12] Narayan B, Miyashita K, Hosakawa M. Physiological effects of eicosapentaenoic acid (EPA) and docosahexaenoic acid (DHA): A review. Food Review International. 2006;**22**:291-307. DOI: 10.1080/87559120600694622

[13] Liu G, Bibus DM, Bode AM, Ma WY, Holman RT, Dong Z. ω-3 but not polyunsaturated fat content of canned meats commonly available in Australia. Food Australia. 2001;**54**:311-315

[14] Hibbeln JR, Salem JN. Dietary polyunsaturated fatty acids and depression: When cholesterol does not satisfy. The American Journal of Clinical Nutrition. 1995;**62**:1-9

[15] Edwards RH, Peet M. Essential fatty acid intake in relation to depression. In: Peet M, Glennm I, Horrobin DF, editors. Phospholipid Spectrum Disorder in Psychiatry. Lancashire: Marius Press; 1999. p 211

[16] Waitzberg DL, Garla P. Contribución delos ácidosgrasosomega-3 para la memoriay la función cognitiva. Nutrición Hospitalaria. 2014;**30**(3):467-477

[17] Engel P, Wyss A. Vitamin A. 2017. Available from: http://www.nutri-facts.org/content/dam/nutrifacts/

pdf/Nutrients-pdf/Vitamin-A-v2.pdf [Accessed: December 19, 2018]

[18] Grzybowski A, Pietrzak K. Albert Szent-Györgyi (1893-1986). The scientist who discovered vitamin C. Clinics in Dermatology. 2013;**31**(3):327-331

[19] Gallie DR. Increasing vitamin C content in plant foods to improve their nutritional value successes and challenges. Nutrients. 2013;**5**:3424-3446

[20] Mandl J, Szarka A, Bánhegyi G. Vitamin C: Update on physiology and pharmacology. British Journal of Pharmacology. 2009;**157**:1097-1110

[21] Chatterjee IB. Evolution and the biosynthesis of ascorbic acid. Science. 1973;**182**:1271-1272

[22] Doll S, Ricou B. Severe vitamin C deficiency in a critically ill adult: A case report. European Journal of Clinical Nutrition. 2013;**67**:881-882

[23] Young IS, Woodside JV. Antioxidants in heath and disease. Journal of Clinical Pathology. 2001;**54**:176-186

[24] Padayatty SJ, Levine M. New insights into the physiology and pharmacology of vitamin C. Canadian Medical Association Journal. 2001;**164**(3):353-355

[25] Bhandari SR, Kwak JH. Chemical composition and antioxidant activity in different tissues of brassica vegetables. Molecules. 2015;**20**(1):1228-1243

[26] Kou X, Chen Q, Li X, Li M, Kan C, Chen B, et al. Quantitative assessment of bioactive compounds and the antioxidant activity of 15 jujube cultivars. Food Chemistry. 2015;**173**:1037-1044

[27] Padayatty SJ, Katz A, Wang Y, Eck P, Kwon O, Lee JH, et al. Vitamin C as an antioxidant: Evaluation of its role in disease prevention. Journal of the American College of Nutrition. 2003;**22**(1):18-35

[28] Wang Y, Russo TA, Kwon O, Chanock S, Rumsey SC, Levine M. Ascorbate recycling in human neutrophils: Induction by bacteria. Proceedings of the National Academy of Sciences of the United States of America. 1997;**94**(25):13816-13819

[29] Traber MG, Stevens JF. Vitamins C and E: Beneficial effects from a mechanistic perspective. Free Radical Biology & Medicine. 2011;**51**(5):1000-1013

[30] Sharkey JR, Branch LG, Zohoori N, Giuliani C, Busby-Whitehead J, Haines PS. Inadequate nutrient intakes among homebound elderly and their correlation with individual characteristics and health-related factors. The American Journal of Clinical Nutrition. 2002;**76**(6):1435-1445

[31] Hsiao PY, Mitchell DC, Coffman DL, Allman RM, Locher JL, Sawyer P, et al. Dietary patterns and diet quality among diverse older adults: The University of Alabama at Birmingham Study of Aging. The Journal of Nutrition, Health & Aging. 2013;**17**(1):19-25

[32] Zhou JF, Yan XF, Ruan ZR, Peng FY, Cai D, Yuan H, et al. Heroin abuse and nitric oxide, oxidation, peroxidation, lipoperoxidation. Biomedical and Environmental Sciences. 2000;**13**(2):131-139

[33] Morena M, Cristol J-P, Bosc J-Y, Tetta C, Forret G, Leger C-L, et al. Convective and diffusive losses of vitamin C during haemodiafiltration session: A contributive factor to oxidative stress in haemodialysis patients. Nephrology, Dialysis, Transplantation. 2002;**17**(3):422-427

[34] Pacier C, Martirosyan DM. Vitamin C: Optimal dosages, supplementation

and use in use in disease prevention. Functional Foods in Health and Disease. 2015;**5**(3):89-107

[35] Di Mascio P, Murphy ME, Sies H. Antioxidant defense systems: The role of carotenoids, tocopherols, and thiols. The American Journal of Clinical Nutrition. 1991;**53**:194S-200S

[36] Freedman JE, Farhat JH, Loscalzo J, Keaney JF Jr. Alpha-tocopherol inhibits aggregation of human platelets by a protein kinase C-dependent mechanism. Circulation. 1996;**94**:2434-2440

[37] Li D, Saldeen T, Romeo F, Mehta JL. Different isoforms of tocopherols enhance nitric oxide synthase phosphorylation and inhibit human platelet aggregation and lipid peroxidation: Implications in therapy with vitamin E. Journal of Cardiovascular Pharmacology and Therapeutics. 2001;**6**:155-161

[38] Brigelius-Flohé R, Traber MG. Vitamin E: Function and metabolism. The FASEB Journa. 1999;**13**:1145-1155

[39] Liu M, Wallmon A, Olsson-Mortlock C, Wallin R, Saldeen T. Mixed tocopherols inhibit platelet aggregation in humans: Potential mechanisms. The American Journal of Clinical Nutrition. 2003;**77**:700-706

[40] Steinberg D, Parthasarathy S, Carew TE, Khoo JC, Witztum JL. Beyond cholesterol: Modifications of low-density lipoprotein that increase its artherogenicity. The New England Journal of Medicine. 1989;**320**:915-924

[41] McAnally JA, Gupta J, Sodhani S, Bravo L, Mo H. Tocotrienols potentiate lovastatin-mediated growth suppression in vitro and in vivo. Experimental Biology and Medicine (Maywood, N.J.). 2007;**232**:523-531

[42] Sesso HD, Buring JE, Christen WG, Kurth T, Belanger C, MacFadyen J, et al. Vitamins E and C in the prevention of cardiovascular disease in men: The Physicians' Health Study II randomized controlled trial. Journal of the American Medical Association. 2008;**300**:2123-2133

[43] Stone WL, Krishnan K, Campbell SE, Qui M, Whaley SG, Yang H. Tocopherols and the treatment of colon cancer. Annals of the New York Academy of Sciences. 2004;**1031**:223-233

[44] Wells SR, Jennings MH, Rome C, Hadjivassiliou V, Papas KA, Alexander JS. Alpha-, gamma- and delta-tocopherols reduce inflammatory angiogenesis in human microvascular endothelial cells. The Journal of Nutritional Biochemistry. 2010;**21**:589-597

[45] Wada S. Chemoprevention of tocotrienols: The mechanism of antiproliferative effects. Forum of Nutrition. 2009;**61**:204-216

[46] Jiang Q, Wong J, Fyrst H, Saba JD, Ames BN. Gamma-tocopherol or combinations of vitamin E forms induce cell death in human prostate cancer cells by interrupting sphingolipid synthesis. Proceedings of the National Academy of Sciences of the United States of America. 2004;**101**:17825-17830

[47] Ganser A, Greher J, Volkers B, Staszewski A, Hoelzer D. Azidothymidine in the treatment of ATDS. The New England Journal of Medicine. 1988;**318**:250-251

[48] Kono N, Ohto U, Hiramatsu T, Urabe M, Uchida Y, Satow Y, et al. Impaired a TTP-PIPs interaction underlies familial vitamin E deficiency. Science. 2013;**340**:1106-1110

[49] Saliha R, Syed TR, Faizal A, Absar A, Shania A, Farzana M. The role of vitamin E in human and some diseases. SQU Medical Journal. 2014;**14**(2):e157-e165

[50] González PO, Moy NA, Gúzman MJ. El alfa tocoferol y el ácido alfa-lipoico. Una sinergía antioxidante con potencial en medicina preventiva. Revista de investigación clínica. 2008;**60**(1):5867

[51] Hartikainen H, Xue T, Piironen V. Selenium as an anti-oxidant and pro-oxidant in ryegrass. Plant and Soil. 2000;**225**:193-200

[52] Grosso G. Dietary antioxidants and prevention of non-communicable diseases. Antioxidants. 2018;7:94. Available from: www.mdpi.com/journal/antioxidants

[53] Monti DM, Rigano M, Monti S, Peixoto HS. Role of Antioxidants in the protection from Aging-related diseases. Oxidative Medicine and Cellular Longevity. Hindawi. 2018;**2019**:1-2

[54] Godos J, Rapisarda G, Marventano S, Galvano F, Mistretta A, Grosso G. Association between polyphenol intake and adherence to the Mediterranean diet in Sicily, Southern Italy. Nepal Forum of Science Journal. 2017:1-7

[55] Li S, Tan HY, Wang N, Zhang ZJ, Lao L, Wong CHW, et al. The role of oxidative stress and antioxidants in liver diseases. International Journal of Molecular Sciences. 2015;**16**:26087-26124

[56] Salamanca GF. Células troncales, cancer y P53. Gaceta medica de Mexico. 2009;**145**(5):441-442

Chapter 15

Prospects for Using the Natural Antioxidant Compounds in the Obesity Treatment

Andriy Zagayko, Tatiana Briukhanova, Dmytro Lytkin, Anna Kravchenko and Victoria Fylymonenko

Abstract

Obesity is strongly associated with the insulin resistance development and is an integral pathogenic part of the metabolic syndrome, type 2 diabetes, atherosclerosis, and other comorbid pathologies. It is well known that the obesity causes the disorders in adipose tissue endocrine and metabolic activity, which results in the activation of free radical processes. The administration of natural origin substances with antioxidant properties could be a promising direction for obesity and overweight correction. The objective of the current study was to evaluate the usefulness of natural origin active substances with antioxidant properties' administration under the obesity and comorbid disorder treatment. This chapter presents the results of experimental studies that proved the usefulness of phenolic compounds from apple food concentrate (*Malus domestica* L.) and dry bilberry extract (*Vaccinium myrtillus* L.) application under experimental metabolic syndrome, insulin resistance syndrome, and type 2 diabetes mellitus, which are extremely associated with obesity. It has been found that due to expressive antioxidant activity, these compounds exhibit the high efficiency in carbohydrate metabolism disorders' correction (in cases of metabolic syndrome and type 2 diabetes), lipids metabolism disorders' correction (in case of metabolic syndrome), preventing of endothelial dysfunction under experimental insulin resistance, and normalization of antioxidant status in the liver (under experimental type 2 diabetes mellitus).

Keywords: obesity, apple polyphenol extract, blueberry dry extract, metabolic syndrome, insulin resistance, antioxidant activity, diabetes mellitus

1. Introduction

According to clinical and epidemiological studies, obesity refers to diseases with high medical and social significance and has a pandemic rate of expansion. Obesity is a component of the multimorbid disease pathogenesis, in particular of metabolic syndrome (MS), type 2 diabetes mellitus (DT2), also it is a predictor of atherosclerosis and cardiovascular complications [1]. It is known that an imbalance of antioxidant-prooxidant factors (with a predominance of prooxidants) is associated with obesity development due to pathological changes in metabolic activity of the adipose tissue [2].

The reactive oxygen species (ROS) production is primarily caused by the lipid accumulation, so it results in NADPH-oxidase excessive expression with the simultaneous decrease in the activity of antioxidant enzymes and nonenzyme antioxidants. Carbohydrate metabolism disorders lead to the activation of glucose metabolism polyol pathway and to protein pathological glycosylation along with metabolic end products accumulation. Oxidative stress leads to adipokines production dysregulation, in particular, adiponectin, plasminogen activator inhibitor-1, interleukin-6, and monocyte chemotactic factor. It plays a leading role in the involvement of other metabolic pathways to the pathological process and main disease pathogenesis complications [3, 4].

Free radical upbuilding is a major event involved in vascular endothelium damaging as a trigger mechanism for the endothelial dysfunction (ED) and cardiovascular complications development related to obesity and MS. As is well known, just cardiovascular events determine high premature mortality rates of these patient categories. In addition, the pathological changes of the antioxidant-prooxidant balance leads to the low-density lipoproteins (LDL) oxidative modification, which are the leading link to the proatherogenic process essential for obesity and associated pathologies [5].

The metabolic disorders' pathogenetic aspects that appear under MS are mainly based on the free radical oxidation (FRO) processes activation. Concerning the above mentioned, the antioxidant use is promising treatment strategy for correction of pathological states that developed under the insulin resistance (IR) [6].

Common therapeutic pharmacological correction strategies for obesity-associated diseases include the synthetic drug use, which are powerful microsomal oxidation processes activators that, in turn, initiates the FRO intensification and increases the ROS production. Recently, there is an increasing interest to the development and research of natural origin substances that can be used at the complex obesity-associated pathologies treatment. Plant polyphenols with expressive antioxidant activity can potentially demonstrate a therapeutic effect under MS pathogenetic manifestations and related comorbidities, including ED [7]. The mentioned metabolic disorders are mediated by chronic subclinical inflammatory process, which is intermediated by the adipocytes production of various active molecules, which, as usual, are factors of high cardiometabolic risk. That is why the evaluation of usefulness of natural origin substances with antioxidant properties administration under the obesity treatment was the aim of our work.

2. The preclinical study of phenolic compounds from apple food concentrate under experimental metabolic syndrome and insulin resistance syndrome

2.1 The effect of phenolic compounds from apple food concentrate on indices of carbohydrate and lipid metabolism under experimental metabolic syndrome

2.1.1 Materials and methods

Taking into account the significant role of reactive oxygen species (ROS) in the pathogenesis of obesity and associated diseases, the nutritional apple polyphenol food concentrate (APFC) investigation is seemed to be reasonable. Examined concentrate is rich in phenolic substances that reveal expressive antioxidant properties under the experimental MS. The investigated food concentrate was developed at the Pharmacognosy Department of the National University of Pharmacy under the supervision of Pharm. D. Koshoviy O.M. The food concentrate biological activity is primary caused by gallic acid, caffeic acid, chlorogenic acid, ursolic acid, quercetin, epicatechin, leuco-anthocyanins, and ascorbic acid. The purified compound epigallocatechin gallate (EGCG, Sigma-Aldrich) was selected as a reference preparation because of its proven strong antioxidant properties.

Experimental MS was modeled in Syrian golden hamsters (males, 20 weeks old) that were fed high-calorie diet enriched by energy sources (containing 29% fat, mostly saturated lipids) and fructose (1 g/100 g of body weight per day per) (as aqueous solution) for 5 weeks. Animals of intact control group were fed a standard balanced diet for hamsters during the experiment [8]. Basal blood glucose concentration in animal serum was determined using One touch ultra-easy glucose meter based on glucose oxidase method (manufactured by LifeScan, Johnson & Johnson, USA) [9]. The basal blood level of immunoreactive insulin (IRI) was determined using in vitro radioimmunoassay by the standard set of reagents (manufactured by Immundiagnostik, Germany). Insulin resistance index (HOMA-IR) was calculated from animal blood values of basal glucose and IRI indicators using Homeostasis Model Assessment algorithm (HOMA) [10]. The content of triacylglycerols (TAG) in serum and in the liver homogenate was determined using the standard set of reagents "KONE" (Finland) based on glycerol oxidation method. Determination of the free fatty acids (FFA) concentration in serum was carried out using a set of reagents produced by Kamiya biomedical company (USA). The concentration of total lipids was determined in liver homogenate using the standard kit produced by Eagle Diagnostics (USA) based on the reaction with a vanillin reagent. The content of high-density lipoproteins (HDL) and apo-B-containing lipoproteins (sum of low-density lipoproteins and very low-density lipoproteins—apoB-L) were determined in blood serum using turbidimetric method [11, 12].

Experimental animals were administered APFC for 2 weeks (since third week of pathology simulation) using a special iron catheter for intragastric administering. The dose of APFC was calculated as total content of polyphenols—9 mg/100 g of body weight (prophylactic treatment). The dose of reference preparation epigallocatechin gallate—EGCG (produced by Sigma-Aldrich, Germany) was 3 mg/100 g of body weight. Daily animal equivalent doses (AED) were calculated according to the latest recommendations for preclinical studies, taking into account the average daily dose for humans and interspecies difference in body weight and body surface area [13].

The results were statistically processed using the 4Pl statistical logistic method with free internet service of MyAssays® and nonparametric analysis methods (Mann-Whitney U-Test) with the standard software package STATISTICA 7.0 [14].

2.1.2 Results

The carried studies indicated expressive corrective effect of the test concentrate and EGCG on the markers of carbohydrate and lipid metabolism in the Syrian hamsters with experimental MS, which, however, had rather significant group differences (**Tables 1–3**).

Under the experimental conditions, APFC usage led to the normalization of glucose and IRI indices, in which content was significantly reduced by 19.5 and 21.02% respectively in comparison with animals of the model pathology group. The IR index significant reduction by 24.18% was a confirmation of the studied food concentrate therapeutic effect (**Table 1**).

EGCG also significantly decreased glucose and IRI levels by 10.9 and 10.1%, respectively, compared to animals with an experimental MS; index of IR also proportionally decreased (by 11.93%). It should be noted that the EGCG therapeutic effect was not so pronounced as after the apple concentrate of phenolic compounds administration. We suppose that it was mediated by complex multivector biologically active compounds effect in concentrate content.

Parameters	Intact control	Model pathology	APFC + model pathology	EGCG + model pathology
Glucose (mmol/l)	5.800 ± 0.440	11.200 ± 0.390*	9.021 ± 0.450**	9.983 ± 0.565**
IRI (pmol/l)	92.500 ± 2.305	138.280 ± 2.406*	109.220 ± 2.380	124.35 ± 2.250**
Index IR (HOMA-IR)	1.78	3.02*	2.29**	2.66**

n, number of animals in a group. *Variation is statistically significant in comparison with intact control group indices ($p \leq 0.001$).*
**Variation is statistically significant in comparison with model pathology group indices ($p \leq 0.001$).*

Table 1.
The effect of apple phenolic compounds food concentrate and epigallocatechin gallate on carbohydrate metabolism indices under experimental metabolic syndrome, n = 10.

Parameters	Intact control	Model pathology	APFC + model pathology	EGCG + model pathology
TAG (mmol/l)	1.950 ± 0.055	3.680 ± 0.146*	2.610 ± 0.017**	2.970 ± 0.012
FFA (mmol/l)	0.450 ± 0.020	1.438 ± 0.023*	1.015 ± 0.150**	1.109 ± 0.045
apoB-LP (mg/ml)	4.72 ± 0.23	6.68 ± 0.15*	5.09 ± 0.13**	5.44 ± 0.14
HDL (mg/ml)	1.11 ± 0.05	0.98 ± 0.07*	1.08 ± 0.02**	1.01 ± 0.03

n, number of animals in a group. *Variation is statistically significant in comparison with intact control group indices ($p \leq 0.001$).*
**Variation is statistically significant in comparison with model pathology group indices ($p \leq 0.001$).*

Table 2.
The effect of apple phenolic compounds food concentrate and epigallocatechin gallate on lipid metabolism indices in hamster's blood serum under experimental metabolic syndrome, n = 10.

Parameters	Intact control	Model pathology	APFC + model pathology	EGCG + model pathology
TL (mg/g)	108.25 ± 2.16	132.55 ± 2.35*	117.43 ± 1.86**	125.45 ± 1.67**
TAG (mg/g)	12.32 ± 0.75	14.24 ± 0.37*	13.18 ± 0.35**	13.47 ± 0.15**

n, number of animals in a group. *Variation is statistically significant in comparison with intact control group indices ($p \leq 0.001$).*
**Variation is statistically significant in comparison with model pathology group indices ($p \leq 0.001$).*

Table 3.
The effect of apple food concentrate of phenolic compounds and epigallocatechin gallate on lipid metabolism parameters in hamster's liver in experimental metabolic syndrome, n = 10.

Normalization in lipid metabolism disturbances was observed under the influence of the APFC as well as EGCG administration, that was confirmed by the laboratory indices favorable dynamics in both serum and liver of animals (**Tables 2** and **3**). At the same time, a more pronounced effect was found in group of animals, which were administered with the apple concentrate.

Thereby, it was determined that in animals administered with the test concentrate, the content of FFA and TAG decreased, respectively, by 29.5 and 29.1%, compared with those in the model pathology group. Additionally, it was demonstrated with more favorable lipoprotein fractions ratio in this group of animals treated by APFC. Thus, the content of the atherogenic fraction apoB-LP decreased (by 23.9%), while the level of antiatherogenic HDL was increased (content did not significantly differ from the same index in healthy animals), which indicates a reduction in the risk of proatherogenic changes and atherosclerosis development (**Table 2**).

The same tendency was observed under EGCG administration—the significant correction as for lipid metabolism pathological changes under experimental MS, which was demonstrated via decrease in TAG and FFA content by 19.3 and 22.9% respectively. In addition, under the EGCG action, the level of apoB-LP decreased (by 18.6%) and level of HDL slightly increased (by 3.06%), which is the evidence of MS-specific proatherogenic change reduction. However, the EGCG therapeutic effect was not so pronounced compared to the apple food concentrate of phenolic compounds.

Considering the fact that the studied food concentrate and EGCG showed pronounced corrective therapeutic effect as for pathological changes in blood lipid metabolism markers, it was appeared expedient to investigate the effect of these compounds on the lipid metabolism indices in the liver tissue.

There was a significant increase in the TL and TAG content in the liver in animals with a model pathology (in 1.22 and 1.16 times, respectively, in comparison with intact hamsters), which indicated the steatosis precondition formation, and primary was due to the lipid intensive flow from the bloodstream (**Table 3**).

The APFC administration caused substantial correction of the TL and TAG content in the liver, which did not significantly differ from the same indices in healthy animals (**Table 3**). This is a confirmation of the APFC beneficial effects as for preventing the fatty liver disease development, which is an MS pathogenesis integral component. This effect was probably mediated by lipid flow inhibition from the blood to the liver under the APFC action, which was evidenced by a decrease in the blood content of these compounds (**Table 2**).

The EGCG administration to animals with experimental MS also was accompanied with a significant decrease in the TL and TAG content in the liver tissue by 5.4 and 5.5%, respectively, indicating the ability of the test compounds to prevent the steatosis development under the MS. It should be noted that the TL level under EGCG administration was significantly higher than under APFC administration, in which prevention indicates about a less significant effect on liver fatty degeneration under experimental pathology. This dynamics is also a reason for EGCG's less effect on the pathological change correction in lipid metabolism in animals` blood specific to MS and for significantly higher lipid flow from the blood stream.

2.1.3 Discussion

The APFC therapeutic effectiveness is the result of the constituent substances complex synergistic effect that mediates various types of biological activity, in particular, a powerful antioxidant effect, the normalization of energy homeostasis and lipid metabolism.

It is well known that gallic acid, which amount is the main part of test concentrate quantitative content, has an ability to regulate body weight and glucose homeostasis via the way of AMP-activated protein kinase (AMPK) upregulation and modulation of mitochondrial functions through the stimulation of a gamma receptor coactivator-1α, which activates by peroxisomal proliferator (PGC1α). It is assumed that the main molecular mechanism of gallic acid action is the effect on the AMRK/Sirt1/PGC1α signaling pathway. In addition, gallic acid significantly improved homeostasis of glucose and insulin by the activation of AMPK (in the liver, muscle, and brown fat tissue) and the gene expression of uncoupling protein-1, which in general was manifested by an increase in energy expenditure and thermogenesis intensification without significant effect on appetite. There is an evidence that gallic acid inhibits the gene expression of gluconeogenesis key enzymes and as a result makes a significant impact on the blood glucose level and downregulates the FFA content that was registered in our experiments. In general, these data show the gallic acid beneficial effect on energy homeostasis, making its usage sensible in treatment of IR and associated diseases [15–18].

Several studies show that another component of concentrate—quercetin—has therapeutic effect under MS. Quercetin manifests itself in improved insulin tissue sensitivity and in glucose level reduction that can be explained by α-glucosidase activity inhibition and stimulation of glucose absorption by skeletal muscle and liver cells [19]. Glucose is actively involved in glycolysis (due to increased activity of enzymes hexokinase and pyruvate kinase) and incorporated for glycogen synthesis in skeletal muscle and liver. In addition, quercetin corrects pathological changes in the cortisol and sex steroids content, counteracts the adipose tissue metabolic activity disorders, and normalizes cytokine profile under MS. The quercetin multivector effect leads to the normalization of carbohydrate and lipid metabolism, and reduced metabolic disorders caused by IR [20–23].

Ursolic acid in *in vivo* experiments in mice with simulated IR led to the inhibition of atherosclerotic plaque formation and systolic pressure reduction; however, mechanisms of these effects developing have not studied yet [24, 25]. Caffeic, chlorogenic, and ascorbic acids are powerful antioxidants that suppress the formation of free radicals, and ROS and strongly reduce the effects of oxidative stress, which is an MS pathogenetic component. In addition, phenolic acids inhibit the activity of α-glucosidase and sodium glucose transporter (SGLT1) [26, 27]. Leucoanthocyanins are able to induce autophosphorylation of the insulin receptor, resulting in improved insulin signaling and increased affinity of cells to its action [28].

Thus, the APFC compounds administration under experimental MS significantly prevented an increase in glucose and IRI, corrected the manifestations of IR, decreased the content of FFA and TAG, probably due to the insulin counteraction on lipolysis and the modulation of the FFA metabolism under the effect of phenolic compounds, which reduced the flow of lipids to the liver (confirmed by a decrease in TL and TAG content in the animals' liver), normalized the lipoprotein blood spectrum (confirmed by a decrease in apo-LP and increased HDL contents), and improved the oxidative state in the liver. The pronounced therapeutic effect of the APFC could be mediated by the complex synergistic antioxidant effect of the constituent components—gallic, caffeic, chlorogenic and ursolic acids, quercetin, leucoanthocyanin, and ascorbic acid.

In general, observed changes indicate the ability of the studied concentrate to prevent the induction of proatherogenic disorders and the MS negative influence, such as the atherosclerosis development. These harmful factors are the main cause of the cardiovascular diseases development and their complications in patients with metabolic disorders [29].

According to the literature data, the mechanism of EGCG usage under the experimental MS is mediated by the effect on cellular mechanisms of glucose transporters translocation stimulation, in particular GLUT4 (mainly due to activation of AMPC and/or phosphoinositide-3-kinase), which is manifested by a hyperglycemia reduction due to increased glucose transport in cells of fat and muscle tissue. The activation of AMPK also correlates with a decrease in the accumulation of lipids in the liver. As for EGCG, there is also the ability to induce the activity of the glycogenesis enzymes (liver glucokinase) and suppress the expression of enzymes of gluconeogenesis. EGCG inhibits the activity of α-glucosidase to a lesser extent than chlorogenic, gallic, and caffeic acids, and it is due to a smaller length of the hydrocarbon chain of the polyphenolic molecule [7, 30].

Thus, EGCG in the experimental MS showed a therapeutic effect, which was mainly due to the normalization of glucose metabolism and inhibition of lipid accumulation in the liver, but anyway, the therapeutic effect of apple phenolic compounds food concentrate was more expressive.

2.2 The effect of apple polyphenolic food concentrate on the endothelial function under experimental insulin resistance

2.2.1 Materials and methods

The complications of cardiovascular system disorders' development are specific to the diseases associated with obesity and IR syndrome. The main pathogenetic component of cardiovascular pathologies is the progression of ED. This fact has been proved in our studies and was corresponded with the literature data. Concerning the glycemic profile positive changes under the influence of the studied APFC and EGCG, it was decided to investigate these compounds effect on the endothelium functional state under the experimental IR (**Tables 4** and **5**).

Experimental groups	Parameters		
	$NO_2^- + NO_3^-$ (mmol/l)	Arginine (mmol/l)	Citrulline (mmol/l)
Intact control	122.20 ± 1.23	64.40 ± 0.65	41.30 ± 1.05
Model pathology	164.50 ± 1.15*	42.80 ± 0.43*	54.50 ± 1.21*
APFC + model pathology	125.82 ± 1.78**	69.50 ± 0.75**	43.39 ± 1.25**
EGCG + model pathology	136.85 ± 2.02**, #	58.25 ± 0.67**,#	46.13 ± 1.43**,#

n, number of animals in a group. *Variation is statistically significant in comparison with intact control group indices ($p \leq 0.001$).*
**Variation is statistically significant in comparison with model pathology group indices ($p \leq 0.001$).*
#Variation is statistically significant in comparison with indices of animals that were on apple food concentrate of phenolic compounds ($p \leq 0.001$).*

Table 4.
The effect of test compounds on rat's NO-synthase system markers under experimental insulin resistance (the fifth week of experiment), n = 10.

Experimental groups	Parameters		
	ET-1 (pg/ml)	S-NO (mmol/l)	ET-1/S-NO
Intact control	2.29 ± 0.14	0.49 ± 0.03	4.67 ± 0.13
Model pathology	5.91 ± 0.23*	0.15 ± 0.04*	39.4 ± 1.05*
APFC + model pathology	3.60 ± 0.15**	0.32 ± 0.04**	11.25 ± 1.04**
EGCG + model pathology	3.88 ± 0.10**	0.26 ± 0.02**	14.92 ± 1.01**

n, number of animals in a group. *Variation is statistically significant in comparison with intact control group indices ($p \leq 0.001$).*
**Variation is statistically significant in comparison with model pathology group indices ($p \leq 0.001$).*

Table 5.
The effect of examined compounds on rat's specific markers of endothelial function underexperimental insulin resistance (the tenth week of experiment), n = 10.

A balance between the content of vasoconstrictor and vasodilator substances play the key role in vascular tone regulation, progression and prognosis as for the course of endothelial dysfunction (ED) [5]. The IR syndrome was modeled on male Wistar rats weighing 160–200 g, 3 months of age by continuous intraperitoneally dexamethasone administration in low doses (15 μg/kg), while feeding high calorie diet (containing 29% fat—mostly saturated lipids) enriched with fructose (daily 1/100 g of body weight as an aqueous solution) for 5 or 10 weeks [31].

Determination of arginine content in blood serum was carried out using a photometric method based on the reaction with α-naphthol and hypobromite reagent. The citrulline content was determined by reaction with diacetyl monoxime in strongly acidic conditions [32]. The content of nitrites and nitrates in blood serum was determined by spectrophotometric method using Griess test. The method is based on the determination of the total level of nitrogen (II) oxide metabolites (blood serum is incubated with a Griess reagent without vanadium chloride (III), determined spectrophotometrically). To obtain the value of the content of nitrates, it has to subtract concentrations of nitrite ions from the obtained value (the blood serum was incubated with a Griess reagent and vanadium chloride (III), spectrophotometrically determined) [33]. The serum endothelin-1 (ET-1) content was measured by the immune enzyme method using a standard set of reagents (DRG, manufactured in Germany). The content of nitrogen (II) oxide stable active metabolites S-nitrosothiols was determined by fluorimetric method [34].

Experimental animals were administered APFC for 2 weeks (since third week of pathology simulation) using a special iron catheter for intragastric administration. The dose of APFC was calculated as total content of polyphenols—9 mg/100 g of body weight (prophylactic treatment). The dose of reference preparation EGCG (produced by Sigma-Aldrich, Germany) was 3 mg/100 g of body weight. Daily animal equivalent doses (AED) were calculated according to the latest recommendations for preclinical studies, taking into account the average daily dose for humans and interspecies difference in body weight and body surface area [13].

The results were statistically processed using the 4Pl statistical logistic method with free internet service of MyAssays® and nonparametric analysis methods (Mann-Whitney U-Test) with the standard software package STATISTICA 7.0 [14].

2.2.2 Results

Under our experimental conditions, it was observed a significant simultaneous increase in glucose and IRI level, which at the IR development initial stages (fifth week of experiment) mediated the nitrogen oxide production increase; it was confirmed by the nitrate and nitrite evaluation of the (NO-2 + NO-3) content. The last fixed fact was caused by the insulin inducing effect on the endothelial cell NO-synthase (iNOS) and the arginine flow activation (NOS substrate) into the cells (**Table 4**). Since citrulline is the another product of the NO-synthase reaction in addition to nitrogen (II) oxide, in our experiments, growth of this indicator was observed, which directly correlated with the increase in the content of NO-2 + NO-3 (**Table 4**).

According to the other studies in *in vivo* experiments, it has shown that insulin in physiological concentrations mediates NO-dependent vasodilation, which is accompanied by blood pressure normalization. The insulin vasoprotective action is based on the phosphatidylinositol-3-kinase activation in endothelial cells and microvessels. It leads to the endothelial NOS gene expression and insulin-mediated vasodilatation.

Hyperglycemia that developed under our experimental conditions led to the iNOS expression up-regulation and increased ROS production with free radical processes activation. Simultaneous increase in the nitrogen oxide and ROS content resulted in the peroxynitrite formation and significantly contributed in ED pathogenesis. The synchronous free radical formation under hyperglycemia caused damage to protein and lipid cell structures, which led to the highly toxic lipoperoxide compound formation that enhanced the cell membrane destabilization. These pathological changes are accompanied by antioxidant defense dysfunction, which resulted in cell energy homeostasis disorders due to the tricarboxylic acid cycle suppressing and uncoupling of tissue respiration and oxidative phosphorylation. Furthermore, NO hyperproduction stimulated COX-2 expression, which in turn was accompanied by the vasoconstrictor factor formation intensification (thromboxane A2, an antagonist of NO). The combination of these factors creates preconditions for endothelium damage and the ED progression.

It is known that prolonged hyperglycemia stimulates the polyol pathway of glucose metabolism, leading to the depletion of glutathione reserves (potent antioxidant factor) and endothelial NOS-NADPH(H^+) cofactor in endothelial cells. The conditions of lasting hyperglycemia cause eNOS activity inhibition and, as a result, a decrease in the nitric oxide formation [35]. The above changes are corrected by increasing of diacylglycerol and protein kinase C activity. Literature data analysis indicates the prominent role of chronic hyperglycemia as a factor of the vascular complications pathogenesis under the treatment of IR and associated diseases, primarily angiopathy under diabetes mellitus. Lasting hyperglycemia is accompanied by the increase in the content of glycosylated hemoglobin and other end products of glycosylation. The last ones significantly reduce the availability of nitrogen (II) oxide, which is an important factor in endothelial function disorders. Hyperglycemia induces an increase in the lipid peroxidation products content that suppress the endothelium ability to vasodilatation [36].

At the tenth week of the experiment, under the lasting IR, we observed a significant increase in the endothelin (ET-1) content (in 2.58 times), while the concentration of stable NO metabolites (S-NO) was significantly lower (in 3.26 times) compared with indices in healthy animals. The ED development was confirmed by the calculation of the ET-1/S-NO ratio, which was 8.4 times higher in animals with IR than the similar index in healthy animals (**Table 5**).

ET-1 has a prognostic importance for cardiovascular pathologies. This vasoconstrictor factor is a marker of coronary atherosclerosis and coronary ED. The results of other authors' studies indicate a significant role of abdominal adiposity in increasing of the ET-1 production, which evidences about increased vasoconstrictor factors production under MS. The ET-1 content directly correlates with the average blood pressure. This marker is considered as an independent factor in the development and arterial hypertension progression in patients with obesity and MS [37].

2.2.3 Discussion

Under the conditions of experimental IR, the ED formation occurs gradually with the several pathological mechanisms involvement. On the one hand, there are disorders in the NO-synthase system functional activity. On the other hand, there is a marked imbalance of antioxidant-prooxidant factors in the direction of prooxidants content increasing.

According to some researchers, under the IR in the endothelium is stimulated the vasoconstrictor substances synthesis (ET-1, thromboxane A2, prostaglandin F2) and reduced the vasodilator production (prostacyclin and nitric oxide). Lasting IR syndrome is accompanied by a decrease in endothelial- and insulin-mediated vasodilation. The activation of the MAPK-passway by insulin via stimulation of the different growth factors is an important aspect of the pathogenesis of vessel damage caused by insulin under IR. Thus MAPK activation leads to stimulation of proliferative processes and the smooth muscle cell migration, strengthening of vascular remodeling, and proatherogenic changes. It is believed that one of the points of the arterial hypertension pathogenesis under MS is the ability of insulin to promote hypertrophy of smooth muscle vessels. Under IR, the endothelium becomes a target for a number of damaging factors (oxidized LDL, free radicals, etc.), which is accompanied by disorders in the endothelium functional state and creates the basis for the cardiovascular complication development [38].

Our previous studies, which correspond with literature data, indicated that experimental IR is accompanied with proatherogenic changes in the blood profile, and the ET-1 index increase is a marker of hypoxic state that is specific to atherogenesis. Oxidatively modified very low-density lipoproteins (VLDL) are some from the ET-1 synthesis inductors [31]. Thus, under the conditions of our experiments, the ED formation was evident; it was confirmed by the corresponding changes in the studied parameters. These change dynamics proved proatherogenic disorders that took place under this modeled pathology. In general, the ED development mediated by atherogenesis is a main factor in the CVD complication pathogenesis, which caused high mortality rates.

The tested APFC administration to animals deeply corrected the pathological changes that are accompanied by the ED formation at different stages of the experimental IR development. This fact was proved by significant positive changes and normalization of the endothelium function marker content.

Under the action of food concentrate in animals, which were injected by dexamethasone for 5 weeks and fed with a high-calorie diet, the nitrate/nitrite and citrulline contents were reduced to almost healthy animals' levels. Naturally, there was a significant increase in arginine level that was not used as intensively as the substrate for NOS (as was in the case with animals of model pathology).

The above changes are the result of the complex APFC component therapeutic effects. The antioxidant-prooxidative balance was shifted, and free radical processes were activated under the IR. The formation of ED under lasting IR state was mediated by the induction of NADPH(H^+) oxidase endothelial expression, in which induction correlates with the high superoxide anion production. It, in turn, reduces the nitrogen oxide bioavailability and its stable metabolite content, which occurred in the conditions of our experiments (**Table 5**). The APFC administration to rats prevents these changes: the S-NO content significantly increased while the vasoconstrictor ET-1 level and their ratio were decreased. The possible mechanism can involve both direct antioxidant activity of phenolic compounds and suppressing of the NADPH(H^+)-oxidase expression, which plays a prominent role in the oxidative stress development in the endothelium. The ability of phenolic compounds in red wine and green tea to suppress the expression of NADPH(H^+)-oxidase subunits (in particular, p22phox and nox1) and, respectively, to inhibit the endothelial production of superoxide anion was proved [39]. Polyphenols are also characterized by an increase in catalase activity. Phenolic compounds, due to the phosphoinositol pathway initiation, stimulate the NO production and the endothelial hyperpolarizing factor. Taking into account the chemical composition of these substances and the APFC are similar, it is possible that their mechanisms for the realization of biological activity, in particular vasoprotective action, can be equivalent.

The concentrate contains the highest quantity of gallic acid, which mediates a variety of biological effects. According to literary data, gallic acid has powerful anti-inflammatory properties, which are mediated by several mechanisms. It has been demonstrated that gallic acid and its esters (gallates) have ability to inhibit NF-κB activation, mainly due to suppression of IL-1 and tumor necrosis factor (TNF) (including endothelial cells) production. Thus, gallic acid and its derivatives are capable of inhibiting the cytokine-induced nuclear translocation of NF-κB. It is assumed that galactic acid blocks the activation of the NF-κB and Akt signaling pathway through the suppression of COX and ribonucleotide reductase (It is associated with the presence of anticarcinogenic properties). Some studies have shown the gallic acid antagonism against P-selectin, which, as known, mediate the blood-formed element adhesion, in particular, leukocytes and monocytes, to the endothelium, which is accompanied by the inflammation progression. Considering the fact that the inflammatory reaction in the endothelium is one of the main components in the ED formation, inhibition of this process prevents the disorders in its functional activity. Gallic acid reduces the secretion of monocyte chemotaxis protein 1 (MCP-1), intercellular adhesion molecule 1 (ICAM-1), and vascular endothelial adhesion molecule 1 (VCAM-1) in endothelial cells [40].

The therapeutic effect on hyperglycemia and hyperinsulinemia mediated the peroxynitrite production suppression (specific to quercetin), which was resulted in the NO-synthase system improvement (at the initial stages of the model pathology development) [41].

Long-term quercetin and its metabolites supplementation, which are contained in the studied concentrate, caused AMPK and eNOS activation (probably via increasing phosphorylation) in endothelium cells. This activation leads to an increase in the S-NO concentration that was observed in the conditions of our experiments (**Table 5**). In this case, quercetin was able to reduce the content of ET-1, which was also determined in our experiments (**Table 5**), and it was corresponded with the literature data. It is supposed that quercetin reduces H_2O_2-induced expression of the mRNA of ET-1, and thus, it reduced ED severity mediated by ET-1 hyperproduction. In addition, quercetin reduces the p47phox subunit of NADPN(H^+)-oxidase expression by protein kinase C inhibition, which is resulted in an oxidative stress reduction. Quercetin supplementation leads to a decrease in platelet excessive aggregation, which leads to atherosclerosis complications and stenotic arteries embolism. According to the literature, quercetin exhibits distinct anti-inflammatory effects, reducing the activation of NF-κB, TNF-α, IL-1β, IL-6, and SRP. It is known that anti-inflammatory properties of quercetin are improved by ascorbic acid (the studied concentrate contains both components that suggested more pronounced anti-inflammatory effect) [21, 22].

Long-term supplementation of caffeic, chlorogenic, and ursolic acids exhibits a potent antioxidant effect and increases the nitrogen oxide bioavailability, which was proved by S-NO increase in our experiments. According to the other authors, chlorogenic acid is characterized by ability to decrease in the malondialdehyde content in LDL, which is evidenced about their stability against oxidative modification and, accordingly, prevention of proatherogenic changes [42].

The EGCG administration also improved the pathological changes in the endothelium functional state, mediated by the experimental IR, but this effect was less pronounced at all stages of the model pathology development than the effect of APFC. It should be noted that at the experimental IR initial stage (fifth week of the experiment), the effect on nitrates and nitrites level, arginine, and citrulline content under EGCG administration was significantly less compared with the results determined in the group of animals that administered the food concentrate.

Thus, the APFC administration prevented ED formation under experimental IR. We suppose that this effect was mediated by the complex synergistic effect of its constituent components including a potent antioxidant effect and abilities to modulate the activity of nitric oxide synthase and suppress the ET-1production, resulting in a vasoprotective effect. The EGCG administration was also accompanied by an improvement of the endothelium functional state under experimental pathology; however, the EGCG therapeutic effect was less pronounced compared with complex compound—the APFC, due to multivector effects on different parts of the ED formation.

3. The study of the blueberry (*Vaccinium myrtillus* L.) extract effectiveness under experimental diabetes mellitus induced by a high-fructose diet combined with dexamethasone injections

3.1 Materials and methods

DM2 is an endocrine disorder characterized by defects in mechanism of glucose insulin-mediated transport into the cells, resulting in persistent hyperglycemia. It is well known that glucose high levels lead to the free radical overformation, which activates lipoperoxidation—one of the main pathogenetic factors in atherosclerosis development [3, 4].

Bilberry leaf chemical composition usually consists of flavonoids, proanthocyanidins, triterpenes, and also phenolic compounds, in particular, of myricetin, which revealed an effectiveness at the DM2 initial stages of according to some authors [43, 44].

The experiment was conducted on male Wistar rats weighing 160–200 g. The experimental animals were divided into groups: (1) intact animals fed a standard vivarium chow; (2) animals fed a high-fructose diet (2 g of fructose/100 g of body weight daily) combined with daily subcutaneous dexamethasone injections in the dose of 2 mg/100 g body weight for 6 weeks; and (3) animals, which administered intragastric feeding of bilberry leaf dry extract in the dose of 9 mg/100 g of body weight for 2 weeks in addition to dexamethasone administration [45].

The glycosylated hemoglobin (HbA1C) concentration was determined in blood serum by immunoturbidimetric method. The fructosamine level was measured by the spectrophotometric method using nitro-blue tetrazolium chloride [46]. The area under the glycemic curves (AUC) during IGGTT was calculated using the computer software program MATLAB [47]. The glucose content was determined using standard kit of "Filisit-Diagnostika" (Ukraine). The basal level of immunoreactive insulin (IRI) was measured in the blood of animals by the in vitro radioimmunoassay using a standard set of reagents produced by "Immundiagnostik" (Germany) [10].

The lipoperoxidation markers were determined spectrophotometrically by the measuring of diene conjugates (DC) and TBA-reactive products (TBA-RP) content using reaction with thiobarbituric acid [48]. The antioxidant system status was evaluated via determination of reduced glutathione (GSH) concentration (spectrophotometrically by reaction with alloxan) and glutathione reductase (GR) activity [49]. Glucose homeostasis in test and control animals was evaluated at different times after the model inducing (7, 14, and 21 days) by basal glycemic indexes and intraperitoneal glucose tolerance test (IPGTT, 3 g/kg body weight) [50]. Statistical processing of the experimental data was performed using the STATISTICA software program (StatSoft Inc., USA, version 6.0). The significance of intergroup differences was estimated according to the Student's t-test [14].

3.2 Results and discussion

The dexamethasone low dose administration to laboratory animals under high-fat diet caused the multiple disorder formation specific to MS and DT2. In the rats' blood serum, there was a significant increase in the glycosylated hemoglobin level, fructosamine concentration, glucose content, basal glycemia, and increased area under glycemic curves. These changes were probably developed due to a decrease in the glucose utilization by peripheral tissues caused by inhibition of the glucose transporters expression (GLUT1 and GLUT4) under the influence of dexamethasone action. Change in HbA1C level is an objective indicator of carbohydrate metabolism in diabetic patients and the effectiveness of glycemic control. An increase in

Parameters	Intact control	Model pathology	BLE + model pathology
Glycosylated hemoglobin (%)	7.5 ± 0.5	9.6 ± 0.7*	8.4 ± 0.6*,#
Fructosamine (mmol/l)	1.91 ± 0.12	3.6 ± 0.29*	2.45 ± 0.24*,#
Basal blood glucose level (mmol/l)	4.04 ± 0.11	13.42 ± 0.38*	12.08 ± 0.24*
AUC (glycemic) (mmol/l/min)	625.44 ± 16.56	2092.25 ± 60.48*	1100 ± 61.56*,#
Glucose, mmol/l	4.6 ± 0.1	11.2 ± 0.2*	8.2 ± 0.1*,#
IRI (pmol/l)	221.74 ± 20.79	317.97 ± 39.72*	302 ± 36.70*

n, number of animals in a group. *Variation is statistically significant in comparison with intact control group indices ($p \leq 0.05$).*
#Variation is statistically significant in comparison with model pathology group indices ($p \leq 0.05$).

Table 6.
The effect of bilberry leaf extract on carbohydrate metabolism indices under experimental diabetes mellitus induced by high-fructose high-calorie diet combined with dexamethasone injection, n = 10.

Parameters	Intact control	Model pathology	BLE + model pathology
TBA-AP (nmol/g)	0.96 ± 0.27	3.56 ± 0.41*	0.98 ± 0.39#
DC (nmol/l)	22.30 ± 1.42	28.5 ± 0.94*	26.9 ± 0.96
GSH (mmol/g)	0.25 ± 0.01	0.12 ± 0.02*	0.19 ± 0.03
GR (nmol/min mg) of protein	18.56 ± 0.64	14.20 ± 1.06*	17.9 ± 0.98

n, number of animals in a group. *Variation is statistically significant in comparison with intact control group indices ($p \leq 0.05$).*
#Variation is statistically significant in comparison with model pathology group indices ($p \leq 0.05$).

Table 7.
The effect of bilberry leaf extract on the specific markers of antioxidative-prooxidative status of rat's liver in experimental diabetes mellitus induced by high-fructose high-calorie diet combined with dexamethasone injection, n = 10.

the content of glycosylated hemoglobin is usually considered as an indirect marker for the retinopathy development, nephropathy, and other complications of diabetes. Due to the long-term hyperglycemia, albumin was subjected to nonenzymatic glycosylation, which was confirmed by the increase in fructosamine in our experiments (**Table 6**). The dry bilberry leaf extract (BLE) administration under model pathology was accompanied by a significant normalization of the studied indices (**Tables 6** and 7).

In particular, it was significant for the suppression of glycosylated hemoglobin (by 12.5%) and fructosamine (by 32%) concentration, hyperglycemia (by 26.8%), the area under the glycemic curves (by 47.4%), and the immunoreactive insulin level (by 5.1%) compared to untreated animals. In our opinion, it is due to the high content of different phenolic compounds in the bilberry extract, which have hypoglycemic and antioxidant effects. The mechanism of hypoglycemic effect of polyphenols is related to their impact on the process of glucose transport into the cell. The main role in hypoglycemic action of the extract of bilberry leaves belongs to myrtilline, which is a mixture of delphinidin and malvinidin esters that act as insulin synthesis activator [51].

It is proved that hyperglycemia is accompanied by free radical processes activation, which leads to complications in the main disease pathogenesis and tissue damage. Under the conditions of our experiments, the model pathology formation was accompanied by the oxidative stress development, which was confirmed by significant increase in the content of TBA-AP and DC (basic lipoperoxidation products) in the liver—by 270.8 and 27.8%, respectively, compared with healthy rats. At the same time, antioxidant defense was reduced as evidenced by the decrease in the content of GSH and GR in the liver by 52 and 23.5%, respectively, compared to intact control animals. The above changes confirmed the oxidative stress development under pathology. The BLE administration under the model pathology led to the antioxidative-prooxidative balance normalization, which was evidenced by the significant suppression of lipoperoxidation and antioxidant status improvement, which was reflected in the relevant indicator dynamics. We suggested that these changes were the result of remarkable antioxidant and antiradical properties of the investigated extract components.

Thus, the effectiveness of the BLE under the experimental DT2 primary was due to the expressive antioxidant properties of the biologically active substances that are part of its composition.

4. Conclusions

Summarizing the above, the results of these and other experiments demonstrate that natural antioxidants of polyphenolic structure have a significant corrective effect on major factors in the pathogenesis of obesity. Firstly, polyphenolic antioxidants promote lipid and carbohydrate metabolism, which is very important for directional therapy of obesity. In the other hand, these compounds prevent comorbid conditions of obesity, such as endothelial dysfunction and atherosclerosis, which greatly increases the risk of mortality. Also, polyphenolic antioxidants reverse insulin resistance and its after-effects linked with oxidative tissue damage. The main explanation of such protective effects of natural polyphenolic compounds is based on their powerful antioxidative properties, because the pathogenesis of noted disorders is usually amplified by exponential releasing reactive oxygen species and their products. Consequently, the pool of current experimental data points out that concentrates of polyphenolic compounds could be used in adjuvant therapy of obesity, diabetes, and similar conditions, complicated by metabolic disorders and free radical oxidation.

Author details

Andriy Zagayko, Tatiana Briukhanova, Dmytro Lytkin*, Anna Kravchenko and Victoria Fylymonenko
National University of Pharmacy, Kharkiv, Ukraine

*Address all correspondence to: d.v.lytkin@gmail.com

References

[1] Hruby A, Hu FB. The epidemiology of obesity: A big picture. PharmacoEconomics. 2015;**33**(7):673-689. DOI: 10.1007/s40273-014-0243-x

[2] Manna P, Jain SK. Obesity, oxidative stress, adipose tissue dysfunction, and the associated health risks: Causes and therapeutic strategies. Metabolic Syndrome and Related Disorders. 2015;**13**(10): 423-444. DOI: 10.1089/met.2015.0095

[3] Hurrle S, Hsu WH. The etiology of oxidative stress in insulin resistance. Biomedical Journal. 2017;**40**(5):257-262. DOI: 10.1016/j.bj.2017.06.007

[4] Henriksen EJ, Diamond-Stanic MK, Marchionne EM. Oxidative stress and the etiology of insulin resistance and type 2 diabetes. Free Radical Biology & Medicine. 2010;**51**(5):993-999. DOI: 10.1016/j.freeradbiomed.2010.12.005

[5] Gradinaru D, Borsa C, Ionescu C, Prada GI. Oxidized LDL and NO synthesis—Biomarkers of endothelial dysfunction and ageing. Mechanisms of Ageing and Development. 2015;**151**:101-113. DOI: 10.1016/j.mad.2015.03.003

[6] Vincent HK, Bourguignon CM, Weltman AL, Vincent KR, Barrett E, Innes KE, et al. Effects of antioxidant supplementation on insulin sensitivity, endothelial adhesion molecules, and oxidative stress in normal-weight and overweight young adults. Metabolism: Clinical and Experimental. 2009;**58**(2):254-262. DOI: 10.1016/j.metabol.2008.09.022

[7] Wang S, Moustaid-Moussa N, Chen L, Mo H, Shastri A, Sui R, et al. Novel insights of dietary polyphenols and obesity. The Journal of Nutritional Biochemistry. 2014;**25**(1):1-18. DOI: 10.1016/j.jnutbio.2013.09.001

[8] Wong SK, Chin KY, Suhaimi FH, Fairus A, Ima-Nirwana S. Animal models of metabolic syndrome: A review. Nutrition & Metabolism. 2016;**13**:65. DOI: 10.1186/s12986-016-0123-9

[9] Muktabhant B, Sanchaisuriya P, Sarakarn P, Tawityanon W, Trakulwong M, Worawat S, et al. Use of glucometer and fasting blood glucose as screening tools for diabetes mellitus type 2 and glycated haemoglobin as clinical reference in rural community primary care settings of a middle income country. BMC Public Health. 2012;**12**:349. DOI: 10.1186/1471-2458-12-349

[10] Yajnik CS, Katre PA, Joshi SM, Kumaran K, Bhat DS, Lubree HG, et al. Higher glucose, insulin and insulin resistance (HOMA-IR) in childhood predict adverse cardiovascular risk in early adulthood: The Pune Children's Study. Diabetologia. 2015;**58**(7):1626-1636. DOI: 10.1007/s00125-015-3602-z

[11] Maranhão RC, Carvalho PO, Strunz CC, Pileggi F. Lipoprotein (a): Structure, pathophysiology and clinical implications. Arquivos Brasileiros de Cardiologia. 2014;**103**(1):76-84. DOI: 10.5935/abc.20140101

[12] Schaefer EJ, Tsunoda F, Diffenderfer M, Polisecki E, Thai N, Asztalos B. The Measurement of Lipids, Lipoproteins, Apolipoproteins, Fatty Acids, and Sterols, and Next Generation Sequencing for the Diagnosis and Treatment of Lipid Disorders [Internet]. 2016. Available from: https://www.ncbi.nlm.nih.gov/books/NBK355892/ [Accessed: 2016-05-29]

[13] Nair AB, Jacob S. A simple practice guide for dose conversion between animals and human. Journal of Basic and Clinical Pharmacy. 2016;**7**(2):27-31. DOI: 10.4103/0976-0105.177703

[14] Bang H, Davidian M. Experimental statistics for biological sciences. Methods

in Molecular Biology. 2010;**620**:3-104. DOI: 10.1007/978-1-60761-580-4_1

[15] Rodriguez-Ramiro I, Vauzour D, Minihane AM. Polyphenols and non-alcoholic fatty liver disease: Impact and mechanisms. Proceedings of the Nutrition Society. 2016;**75**(1):47-60. DOI: 10.1017/S0029665115004218

[16] Doan KV, Ko CM, Kinyua AW, Yang DJ, Choi YH, Oh IY, et al. Gallic acid regulates body weight and glucose homeostasis through AMPK activation. Endocrinology. 2015;**156**(1):157-168. DOI: 10.1210/en.2014-1354

[17] Huynh MK, Kinyua AW, Yang DJ, Kim KW. Hypothalamic AMPK as a regulator of energy homeostasis. Neural Plasticity. 2016:1-12. DOI: 10.1155/2016/2754078

[18] Zagayko A, Kravchenko G, Strelchenko K, Shkapo A, Briukhanova T. Sex and age differences in lipoprotein metabolism proatherogenic changes under the experimental metabolic syndrome in hamsters. In: Kostner G, editor. Lipoproteins—From Bench to Bedside. Croatia, Rijeka: InTech; 2015. pp. 17-58. DOI: 10.5772/59331

[19] Pereira DF, Cazarolli LH, Lavado SC, Mengatto SV, Figueiredo MSRB, Guedes A, et al. Effects of flavonoids on α-glucosidase activity: Potential targets for glucose homeostasis. Nutrition. 2011;**27**(11-12):1161-1167. DOI: 10.1016/j.nut.2011.01.008

[20] Kawabata K, Kawai Y, Terao J. Suppressive effect of quercetin on acute stress-induced hypothalamic-pituitary-adrenal axis response in Wistar rats. The Journal of Nutritional Biochemistry. 2010;**21**(5):374-380. DOI: 10.1016/j.jnutbio.2009.01.008

[21] Mkhize N, Qulu L, Mabandla MV. The effect of quercetin on pro- and anti-inflammatory cytokines in a prenatally stressed rat model of febrile seizures. Journal of Experimental Neuroscience. 2017;**11**:1-11. DOI: 10.1177/1179069517704668

[22] Nair MP, Mahajan S, Reynolds JL, Aalinkeel R, Nair H, Schwartz SA, et al. The flavonoid quercetin inhibits proinflammatory cytokine (tumor necrosis factor alpha) gene expression in normal peripheral blood mononuclear cells via modulation of the NF-kappa beta system. Clinical and Vaccine Immunology. 2006;**13**(3):319-328. DOI: 10.1128/CVI.13.3.319-328.2006

[23] Seo MJ, Lee YJ, Hwang JH, Kim KJ, Lee BY. The inhibitory effects of quercetin on obesity and obesity-induced inflammation by regulation of MAPK signaling. The Journal of Nutritional Biochemistry. 2015;**26**(11):1308-1316. DOI: 10.1016/j.jnutbio.2015.06.005

[24] Li Q, Zhao W, Zeng X, Hao Z. Ursolic acid attenuates atherosclerosis in ApoE−/− mice: Role of LOX-1 mediated by ROS/NF-κB pathway. Molecules (Basel, Switzerland). 2018;**23**(5):1101. DOI: 10.3390/molecules23051101

[25] Ullevig SL, Zhao Q, Zamora D, Asmis R. Ursolic acid protects diabetic mice against monocyte dysfunction and accelerated atherosclerosis. Atherosclerosis. 2011;**219**(2):409-416. DOI: 10.1016/j.atherosclerosis.2011.06.013

[26] Manzano S, Williamson G. Polyphenols and phenolic acids from strawberry and apple decrease glucose uptake and transport by human intestinal Caco-2 cells. Molecular Nutrition & Food Research. 2010;**54**(12):1773-1780. DOI: 10.1002/mnfr.201000019

[27] Schulze C, Bangert A, Kottra G, Geillinger KE, Schwanck B, Vollert H, et al. Inhibition of the intestinal sodium-coupled glucose transporter 1

(SGLT1) by extracts and polyphenols from apple reduces postprandial blood glucose levels in mice and humans. Molecular Nutrition & Food Research. 2014;**58**:1795-1808. DOI: 10.1002/mnfr.201400016

[28] Kawser Hossain M, Abdal Dayem A, Han J, Yin Y, Kim K, Kumar Saha S, et al. Molecular mechanisms of the anti-obesity and anti-diabetic properties of flavonoids. International Journal of Molecular Sciences. 2016;**17**(4):569. DOI: 10.3390/ijms17040569

[29] Krakauer NY, Krakauer JC. Anthropometrics, metabolic syndrome, and mortality hazard. Journal of Obesity. 2018:1-7. DOI: 10.1155/2018/9241904

[30] Legeay S, Rodier M, Fillon L, Faure S, Clere N. Epigallocatechin gallate: A review of its beneficial properties to prevent metabolic syndrome. Nutrients. 2015;7(7):5443-5468. DOI: 10.3390/nu7075230

[31] Zagako AL, Briukhanova TO, Kravchenko GB, Maloshtan AV. Comparison of quercetin and epigallocatechin gallate effect on the lipid profile under experimental insulin resistance in rats. In: 9th European Conference on Biology and Medical Sciences; 5 March 2016; Vienna, Austria. Vienna: ≪East West≫ Association for Advanced Studies and Higher Education GmbH; 2016. pp. 122-125

[32] Verma N, Singh AK, Singh M. L-arginine biosensors: A comprehensive review. Biochemistry and Biophysics Reports. 2017;**12**:228-239. DOI: 10.1016/j.bbrep.2017.10.006

[33] Tsikas D. Analysis of nitrite and nitrate in biological fluids by assays based on the Griess reaction: Appraisal of the Griess reaction in the L-arginine/nitric oxide area of research. Journal of Chromatography. B, Analytical Technologies in the Biomedical and Life Sciences. 2007;**851**(1-2):51-70. DOI: 10.1016/j.jchromb.2006.07.054

[34] Gow A, Doctor A, Mannick J, Gaston B. S-Nitrosothiol measurements in biological systems. Journal of Chromatography. B, Analytical Technologies in the Biomedical and Life Sciences. 2007;**851**(1-2):140-151

[35] Du XL, Edelstein D, Dimmeler S, Ju Q, Sui C, Brownlee M. Hyperglycemia inhibits endothelial nitric oxide synthase activity by posttranslational modification at the Akt site. The Journal of Clinical Investigation. 2001;**108**(9):1341-1348. DOI: 10.1172/JCI11235

[36] Muniyappa R, Sowers JR. Role of insulin resistance in endothelial dysfunction. Reviews in Endocrine & Metabolic Disorders. 2013;**14**(1):5-12. DOI: 10.1007/s11154-012-9229-1

[37] Sandoval YH, Atef ME, Levesque LO, Li Y, Anand-Srivastava MB. Endothelin-1 signaling in vascular physiology and pathophysiology. Current Vascular Pharmacology. 2014;**12**(2):202-214. DOI: 10.2174/1570161112666140226122054

[38] Manrique C, Lastra G, Sowers JR. New insights into insulin action and resistance in the vasculature. Annals of the New York Academy of Sciences. 2014;**1311**(1):138-150. DOI: 10.1111/nyas.12395

[39] Maraldi T. Natural compounds as modulators of NADPH oxidases. Oxidative Medicine and Cellular Longevity. 2013:1-10. DOI: 10.1155/2013/271602

[40] BenSaad LA, Kim KH, Quah CC, Kim WR, Shahimi M. Anti-inflammatory potential of ellagic acid, gallic acid and punicalagin A&B isolated from Punica granatum. BMC Complementary and Alternative Medicine. 2017;**17**(1):47. DOI: 10.1186/s12906-017-1555-0

[41] Yokoyama A, Sakakibara H, Crozier A, Kawai Y, Matsui A, Terao J, et al. Quercetin metabolites and protection against peroxynitrite-induced oxidative hepatic injury in rats. Free Radical Research. 2009;**43**(10):913-921. DOI: 10.1080/10715760903137010

[42] Okutan H, Ozcelik N, Yilmaz HR, Uz E. Effects of caffeic acid phenethyl ester on lipid peroxidation and antioxidant enzymes in diabetic rat heart. Clinical Biochemistry. 2005;**38**(2):191-196. DOI: 10.1016/j.clinbiochem.2004.10.003

[43] Sarian MN, Ahmed QU, Mat So'ad SZ, Alhassan AM, Murugesu S, Perumal V, et al. Antioxidant and antidiabetic effects of flavonoids: A structure-activity relationship based study. BioMed Research International. 2017:1-14. DOI: 10.1155/2017/8386065

[44] Testa R, Bonfigli AR, Genovese S, De Nigris V, Ceriello A. The possible role of flavonoids in the prevention of diabetic complications. Nutrients. 2016;**8**(5):310. DOI: 10.3390/nu8050310

[45] Martínez BB, Pereira AC, Muzetti JH, Telles FP, Mundim FG, Teixeira MA. Experimental model of glucocorticoid-induced insulin resistance. Acta Cirúrgica Brasileira. 2016;**31**(10):645-649. DOI: 10.1590/S0102-865020160100000001

[46] Ribeiro RT, Macedo MP, Raposo JF. HbA1c, fructosamine, and glycated albumin in the detection of dysglycaemic conditions. Current Diabetes Reviews. 2016;**12**(1):14-19. DOI: 10.2174/1573399811666150701143112

[47] Ugi S, Maegawa H, Morino K, Nishio Y, Sato T, Okada S, et al. Evaluation of a novel glucose area under the curve (AUC) monitoring system: Comparison with the AUC by continuous glucose monitoring. Diabetes & Metabolism Journal. 2016;**40**(4):326-333. DOI: 10.4093/dmj.2016.40.4.326

[48] Yoshida Y, Umeno A, Shichiri M. Lipid peroxidation biomarkers for evaluating oxidative stress and assessing antioxidant capacity in vivo. Journal of Clinical Biochemistry and Nutrition. 2012;**52**(1):9-16. DOI: 10.3164/jcbn.12-112

[49] Iskusnykh IY, Popova TN, Agarkov AA, Pinheiro de Carvalho MÂ, Rjevskiy SG. Expression of glutathione peroxidase and glutathione reductase and level of free radical processes under toxic hepatitis in rats. Journal of Toxicology. 2013:1-9. DOI: 10.1155/2013/870628

[50] King AJ. The use of animal models in diabetes research. British Journal of Pharmacology. 2012;**166**(3):877-894. DOI: 10.1111/j.1476-5381.2012.01911.x

[51] Belwal T, Nabavi SF, Nabavi SM, Habtemariam S. Dietary anthocyanins and insulin resistance: When food becomes a medicine. Nutrients. 2017;**9**(10):1111. DOI: 10.3390/nu9101111

Chapter 16

Potential Antioxidative Effects of Kolaviron on Reproductive Function in Streptozotocin-Induced Diabetic Wistar Rats

Claudine Manirafasha, Omolola Rebecca Oyenihi, Nicole Lisa Brooks, Stefan S. du Plessis and Yapo Guillaume Aboua

Abstract

The present study investigated the effects of Kolaviron (KV) on the testicular and epididymal tissue antioxidant status in streptozotocin (STZ)-induced diabetic rats. Diabetes was induced by a single intraperitoneal injection of STZ at 50 mg/kg body weight. The antioxidant status was studied by evaluating epididymal and testicular levels of malondialdehyde (MDA), a lipid peroxidation (LPO) marker, and the activities of catalase (CAT) glutathione peroxidase (GPX) and superoxide dismutase (SOD) were also assessed using biochemical techniques. Diabetes induction resulted in testicular and epididymal LPO and adversely affected the activities of antioxidant enzymes evident by a noticeable decrease in enzyme activity in both tissues. The potential antioxidative effects of KV in the testicular and epididymal tissues of STZ-induced diabetes were revealed by its ability to mitigate against LPO and increase the activity of antioxidant defense enzymes in the reproductive tissues studied. KV might potentially be used as an antioxidant as well as antidiabetic treatment; however, further studies are needed.

Keywords: antioxidant, diabetes, infertility, Kolaviron, oxidative stress, streptozotocin

1. Introduction

Infertility is a reproductive health disease defined by the failure to achieve a pregnancy after 12 months or more of regular unprotected sexual intercourse [1]. Male factor infertility can contribute between 30 and 50% to this condition and may arise from several factors such as physiological, systemic pathologies, genetic abnormalities, environmental pollution, and oxidative stress (OS) [2, 3].

OS is described as an imbalance between the production of reactive oxygen species (ROS) and their removal or reducing agents called antioxidants [4]. This state of OS potentially leads to the damage of biomolecules such as proteins, nucleic acids, and lipids [4]. In recent years, OS has become more prevalent and has significantly contributed to abnormal sperm morphology [5–8] and sperm quality and quantity [6, 7, 9]. In the testes, OS is capable of disrupting the steroidogenic capacity of Leydig cells as well as the spermatogenesis process [10]. Spermatozoa contain polyunsaturated fats (PUFAs) and limited cytoplasm antioxidant enzymes [11] and are susceptible to oxidative attack. The free radical attack can induce lipid peroxidation (LPO) and DNA fragmentation, disrupting both sperm development and motility [2, 11].

Numerous disorders of the male reproductive system such as cancer, varicocele, cryptorchidism, testicular torsion of the spermatic cords, and diabetes have been associated with male infertility due to OS caused by the uncompensated hyperproduction of ROS [12]. The OS derived from diabetic mellitus (DM) may affect the male reproductive function [11]. Diabetes mellitus is a group of metabolic conditions that are characterized by high glucose levels (hyperglycemia) caused by abnormal insulin secretion/insulin deficiency, abnormal insulin action, or both. It has been demonstrated that diabetes has a direct effect on male fertility [13]. OS in diabetic patients develops from pathways including the nonenzymatic, enzymatic, and mitochondrial signaling pathways [12–14]. Although the problems arising from DM have been widely investigated, the mechanisms responsible for the male reproductive dysfunction are still poorly understood [15]. In hyperglycemic patients, glucose undergoes autoxidation and reacts with proteins leading to the development of Amadori products and advanced glycosylation end products (AGEs). In hyperglycemia, there is enhanced metabolism of glucose through the polyol (sorbitol) pathway, which also results in the enhanced production of superoxide [11, 16]. Another enzymatic generation of ROS is via the mitochondrial respiratory chain through the oxidative phosphorylative process where electrons are transferred from electron carriers NADH and $FADH_2$, through four complexes in the inner mitochondrial membrane, to oxygen, generating ATP in the process [17]. Hyperglycemic conditions disturb endothelial cells, and ROS are produced which participate in the development of diabetic complications. There are enzymatic overproductions of ROS in diabetes through NADPH oxidase that enhance O_2^- [18].

Diabetes-related OS, endocrine disorders, and neuropathy may contribute to the reproductive impairment by causing sexual function alterations including testicular function and epididymal sperm transit [19]. Moreover, under OS condition the protective effects of testicular and epididymal antioxidant enzymes decline [6, 20].

Many artificial and natural agents possessing antioxidant properties, such as dietary antioxidants, may be of great importance as additional protective measures and have been proposed to prevent and/or treat oxidative damage induced by DM [6]. The use of derivatives of plant materials might be important and effective because they are less toxic and affordable as well as minimize side effects or risks caused by other options [20]. Phytochemicals are considered strong natural antioxidants and play an important role in healthcare systems [6]. They have adaptive characteristics to respond to stress and help regulate the interconnected endocrine, immune, and nervous systems [6]. Moreover, ethnobotanical research, literature reviews, and experimental studies reported the beneficial effect of plant materials which have been used many years ago in prevention and treatment of diabetes as well as its complications [20]. More than 1200 flowering plants have been claimed to possess antidiabetic properties [22–24]. These properties have been found to be present in different parts of plants such as the aerial parts, bark, flowers, roots, seeds, leaves, bulbs, tubers, and/or the whole plant [22–24].

Garcinia kola (*G. kola*), commonly referred to as bitter kola, is one of such plants that has been widely used in ethnomedicine [25]. The therapeutic and medicinal values of *Garcinia kola* are the subject of many studies, and several researchers have described their functional health benefits [5, 26–30] *G. kola* is an angiosperm plant that belongs to the family of Guttiferae (Clusiaceae) [5, 28–30]. It adapts and grows up in moist lowland forest and subtropical or tropical region. *Garcinia kola* tree is up to 14 m high and produces brown nut-like seeds (**Figure 1**). *G. kola* is highly valued in African countries such as Nigeria, Benin, Cameroon, Democratic Republic of Congo, Ivory Coast, Gabon, Ghana, Liberia, Senegal, and Sierra Leone. These countries used *G. kola* seeds as source of food and medication [5].

Moreover, phytochemical screening of *Garcinia kola* seed showed the presence of polyphenol compound, which is a bioflavonoid Kolaviron (KV). This extract was found in a 2:2:1 ratio of bioflavonoid GB1, GB2, and kola flavanone [21] (**Figure 2**). Polyphenolic compounds are composed of three benzene rings with hydroxyl (OH) groups which preserve antioxidant activity [31, 32] (**Figure 2**).

KV, extract from *G. kola* nut, has shown great potential for use in therapeutic medicine against many health-threatening chronic diseases of the liver and reproductive system and diabetes [5, 25–30]. It is widely used in traditional medicine in southern Nigeria for the treatment of different conditions associated with increased OS [5]. KV is known to possess antihyperglycemic effects in normal and alloxan- and streptozotocin (STZ)-induced diabetic animals [21, 25]. Moreover, KV has elicited strong antioxidant activity in in vivo and in vitro models [33]. This property is due to the high flavonoid (bioflavonoids) contents which are able to terminate the free radical chain reactions in response to OS [33].

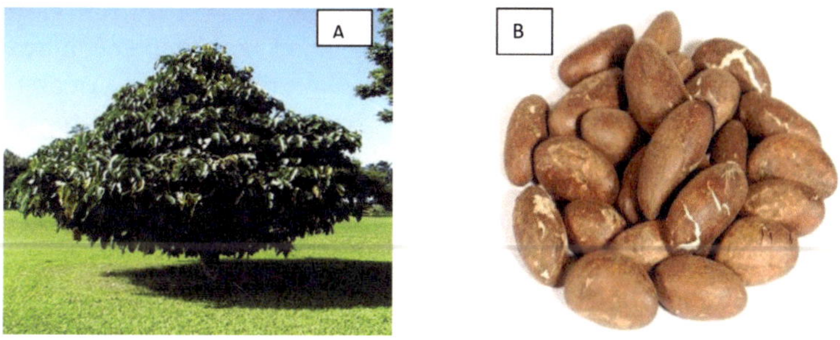

Figure 1.
Garcinia kola tree (A) and its brown seeds (B).

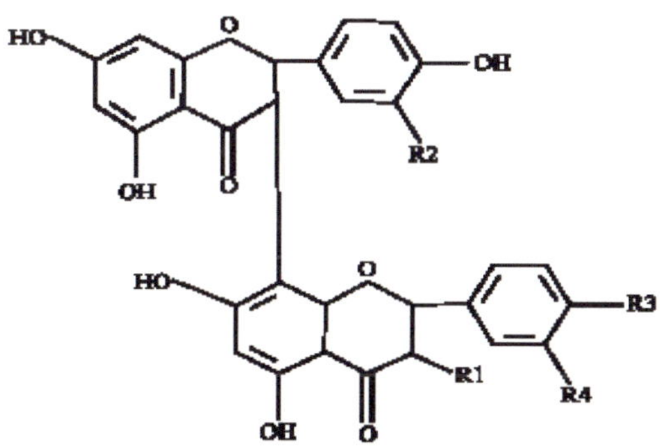

	R1	R2	R3	R4
GB1	OH	H	OH	H
GB2	OH	H	OH	OH
Kolaflavanone	OH	H	OCH_3	OH

Figure 2.
Chemical structure of KV isolated from Garcinia kola seed.

This study was therefore designed to evaluate any potential effects of KV in boosting testicular and epididymal antioxidant status in STZ-induced diabetic Wistar rats.

2. Materials and methods

2.1 Plant materials and KV extraction

Fresh seeds of *G. kola* were purchased from the Bodija market in Ibadan, Oyo State, Nigeria, and authenticated by Professor E. Ayodele at the Department of Botany, University of Ibadan. A voucher specimen (FHI-109777) is available at the University of Ibadan, at the herbarium of the Forestry Research Institute of Nigeria (FRIN), Ibadan.

KV was extracted and isolated according to the method of [34]. The seeds were peeled, sliced, and air-dried (25–28°C). Briefly, the powdered seeds were extracted with light petroleum ether (boiling point, 40–60°C) in a soxhlet for 24 h. The defatted dried product was repacked into the soxhlet and extracted with acetone. The extract was concentrated and diluted twice its volume with water and extracted with ethylacetate (6 × 300 mL). The concentrated ethylacetate yielded a golden yellow solid termed KV.

Liquid chromatography-mass spectrometry (LC-MS) analysis of the Garcinia kola seed extract was performed on a Dionex HPLC system (Dionex Softron, Germering, Germany) equipped with a binary solvent manager and autosampler coupled to a Brucker ESI Q-TOF mass spectrometer (Bruker Daltonik GmbH, Germany) as previously described [35]. KV was separated by reversed-phase chromatography on a Thermo Fischer Scientific C18 column 5 μm, 4.6 × 150 mm (Bellefonte, USA), using gradient elution with 0.1% formic acid in water (solvent A) and acetonitrile (solvent B) as solvent at a flow rate of 1.0 mL min^{-1}, an injection volume of 10 μL, and an oven temperature of 30°C. MS spectra were acquired in negative mode using the full scan and auto MS/MS (collision energy 25 eV) scan modes with dual spray for reference mass solution. Electrospray voltage was set to +3500 V. Dry gas flow was set to 9 L min^{-1} with a temperature of 300°C, and nebulizer gas pressure was set to 35 psi.

2.2 Treatment of animals and ethical clearance

Sixty adult male Wistar rats, weighing between 240 and 290 g, were purchased from the animal facility of the Medical Research Council, South Africa. The animals were accommodated individually in plastic cages. They were supplied with water and standard rat feed ad libitum. Animals were maintained under standard laboratory conditions at 22 ± 2°C with a 12-h light/dark cycles and humidity at 55 ± 5%. Body weights were measured from the onset of the study and monitored throughout the feeding period until sacrifice. All animals received care according to the principles of Laboratory Animal Care of the National Society of Medical Research and the National Institutes of Health Guide for the Care and Use of Laboratory Animals of the National Academy of Sciences (National Institutes of Health publication no. 80-23, revised 1978). The study was approved by the Ethical Committee of the Faculty of Health and Wellness Sciences, University of Cape Peninsula Technology, South Africa (Cape Town, South Africa) (NHREC: REC-230408-014).

2.3 Experimental induction of diabetes

The animals were fasted overnight, and diabetes was induced by a single intraperitoneal injection (50 mg/kg body weight) of freshly prepared STZ solution (Sigma, USA) dissolved in 0.1 M cold citrate buffer at pH 4.5 [36]. Five days after the STZ injection, blood glucose levels were measured using a portable glucometer (Accu-Chek, Roche, Germany) in blood collected from the tail, and diabetes status was confirmed when glucose level was above 18 mmol/L.

2.4 Experimental design

The overall time period for the current study was 6 weeks. Rats were randomly divided into five groups (n = 12 per group) as follows:

- Group 1 (N): control animals (healthy, nondiabetic animals); received dimethylsulfoxide (DMSO) orally.
- Group 2 (N + KV): control animals received KV dissolved in DMSO orally.
- Group 3 (D): untreated diabetic group; injected with a single dose of STZ (50 mg/kg) intraperitoneally.
- Group 4 (D + KV): received KV (100 mg/kg) orally five times weekly starting 5 days post STZ injection; this served as the KV-treated diabetic group.
- Group 5 (D + INS): received subcutaneous insulin (INS) injection (2 u/kg) every other day starting 5 days post STZ injection; this served as the insulin-treated diabetic group.

2.5 Sample collection and preparation

At completion of the treatment periods, rats were weighed and anesthetized with an intraperitoneal injection of sodium pentobarbital (60 mg/kg). Fasting blood glucose levels were measured after 4 h of fasting (usually between 10 am and 2 pm). Blood samples were collected from the abdominal aorta into glucose tubes (containing sodium fluoride/potassium oxalate) and EDTA-containing tubes. The epididymis and testes were also excised and weighed. The tissue samples were snap frozen in liquid nitrogen and stored at −80°C.

Briefly, 250 μL of phosphate buffer (50 mM $NaH_2PO_4{\cdot}2H_2O$, 0.5% (v/v) TritonX-100, pH 7.5) was added to 50 mg of testicular or epididymal tissue. The homogenates were transferred into tubes and centrifuged at 10,000 rpm for 10 min at 4°C. The supernatants were subsequently transferred to new tubes and kept at −80°C until used.

3. Biochemical assays

3.1 Determination of protein concentration

Testicular and epididymal protein levels were determined using the bicinchoninic acid (BCA) method as describe by [37]. Briefly, BCA working reagents, samples, and standards were prepared referring to the manufacturer's instructions for the assay kit supplied by Sigma Aldrich.

3.2 Lipid peroxidation

Malondialdehyde (MDA) levels were determined in the samples through a modern HPLC-based thiobarbituric acid (TBA) assay method. This method is highly specific because it quantifies the genuine MDA-(TBA)$_2$ adduct formed [38]. The quantitative analysis of MDA was performed using a modified method of Cuny et al. [39] on a Spectra SYSTEM™ HPLC (Agilent Technology, 1200 series, Germany).

Briefly, 50 μL of sample was mixed with 375 μL orthophosphoric acid 0.44 M, 125 μL thiobarbituric acid, and 225 μL distilled water. This mixture was heated at 100°C for 60 min and cooled on ice. Thereafter, 775 μL of alkaline methanol was added, and the sample was subsequently vortexed and centrifuged at 3500 rpm for 3 min at 4°C. The supernatant (1 mL) was collected; 500 μL of n-hexane was added and centrifuged at 14,000 rpm for 2 min. The supernatant (500 μL) was collected in chromatographic tubes and injected into the HPLC system. The readings were performed after 10 min, and sample concentration MDA levels were expressed in μmol/g of tissue.

3.3 Superoxide dismutase activity

Superoxide dismutase (SOD) activity was determined by a modified method from Ellerby and Bredesen [40]. Briefly, samples were run in duplicate, in a 96-well plate; 15 μL of 6-HD was added to 6 μL of supernatant. An amount of 170 μL of diethylenetriaminepentaacetic acid (DETAPAC) solution (0.1 mM) in SOD assay buffer and readings were taken immediately at 490 nm for 4 min at 1 min intervals. The activity of SOD was calculated from a linear calibration curve and expressed as μmol/mg protein.

3.4 Catalase activity

The catalase (CAT) activity was assessed according to Aebi [41]. The CAT induced decomposition of hydrogen peroxide (H_2O_2) into water and oxygen. The rate of disintegration is proportional to the concentration of CAT activity. The CAT activity was determined by measuring the change in absorbance of H_2O_2 and sample mixture. Briefly, the CAT assay was performed in duplicate; 150 μL H_2O_2 was added to 20 μL of sample. Readings were determined by using a spectrophotometer (Thermo Electron Corporation, Multiskan Spectrum, USA) at 240 nm wavelength. The CAT activity was expressed as μmol/mg of protein.

3.5 Glutathione peroxidase activity

The activity of glutathione peroxidase (GPx) is derived from the oxidation of reduced β-NADPH in a conjugated glutathione reductase (GR) system using H_2O_2 (12 mM) as a substrate. Glutathione peroxidase reacts with H_2O_2 oxidizing reduced glutathione (GSH) to oxidized glutathione (GSSG). In brief, the GPx assay was performed in duplicate in a 96-well UV Costar plate. Each well contained 215 μL assay buffer (AB: 50 mM potassium phosphate, 1 mM EDTA, pH 7.0), 5 μL GSH (30.7 mg/mL in water), 5 μL GR (0.1 U/mL in AB), and 20 μL of sample, and 5 μL NAD(P)H was added to the mixture. Two readings were recorded [38]. The first was the background of oxidation at 340 nm for 3 min in 30 s intervals for samples (A_1) and blank (A_{1b}). The second reading was performed after adding 50 μL H_2O_2. This reading monitored the decrease of H_2O_2 due to NAD(P)H oxidation at 340 nm for 2 min. The GPX activity was expressed in μmol/mg of protein.

3.6 Statistical analysis

Data are expressed as mean ± standard deviation (mean ± SEM). One-way analysis of variance (ANOVA) was used to test for significance between the groups.

The Bonferroni multiple comparison analysis was used to compare the differences between the groups. Differences were considered significant at $P < 0.05$. The GraphPad PRISM 5 software package was used for all statistical evaluations and graphical representations.

4. Results

4.1 Plasma glucose levels in diabetic and nondiabetic groups before initiation of treatments

Figure 3 shows the non-fasted plasma glucose levels in both nondiabetic (N) and diabetic (STZ) groups before the start of KV and insulin (IN) treatments. The average fasting glucose level was significantly higher in the D group than the N group (28.19 ± 2.25 mmol/L versus 9.93 ± 0.51 mmol/L, $p < 0.05$).

4.2 Evaluation of body weights after subjecting the rats to various treatments

The induction of diabetes with STZ resulted in a significant loss of body weight (**Figure 4**). KV administration to normal rats did not affect body weight compared to untreated nondiabetic rats. On the other hand, the body weights of KV-treated diabetic rats significantly increased compared to diabetic control. Injection of the standard antidiabetic drug, insulin, also improved body weight gains in diabetic rats compared to the untreated diabetic rats.

4.3 Evaluation of testicular and epididymal weights of rats subjected to various treatments

Figure 5 presents the testicular weights of rats treated with STZ, KV, and/or IN. Diabetes induction decreased testicular weight in rats, whereas KV treatment of diabetic rats reversed this alteration. This is evident by a significant increase in testicular weight in KV-treated diabetic rats in comparison to untreated diabetic rats. However, insulin treatment did affect testicular weight in diabetic rats when compared to untreated diabetic rats.

Figure 6 presents epididymal weights of rats subjected to different treatments. Diabetic rats had a lower epididymal weight compared to the nondiabetic rats (0.431 g ± 0.062 g versus 0.529 ± 0.058 g, $p < 0.05$). Treatment of diabetic rats with KV significantly increased epididymal weight in comparison to

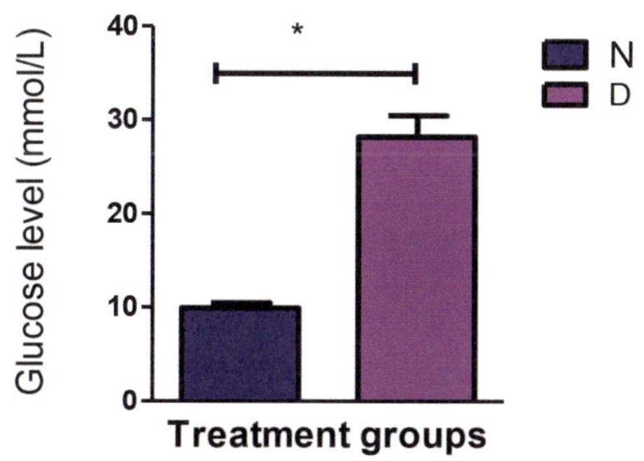

Figure 3.
Glucose levels in diabetic and nondiabetic rats before KV and IN treatments. Data are presented as mean ± SEM. (*) indicates significant difference with p < 0.05. N, nondiabetic control group; D, diabetic group.

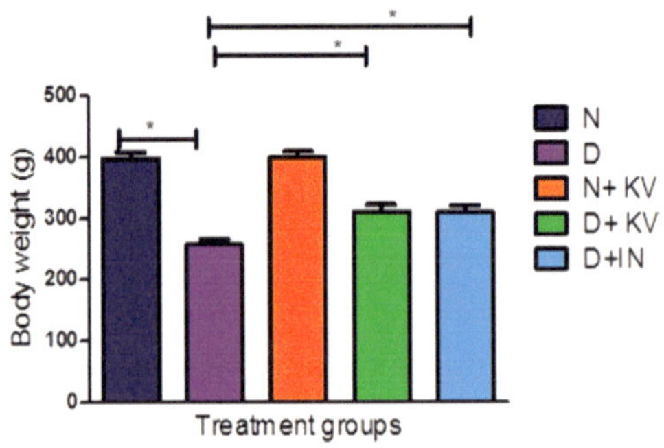

Figure 4.
Effect of KV and insulin on body weight of rats. Data are presented as mean ± SEM. (*) indicates significant difference with p < 0.05. N, nondiabetic control group; D, diabetic group; N + KV, nondiabetic group treated with KV; D + KV, diabetic group treated with KV; D + IN, diabetic group treated with insulin (standard drug).

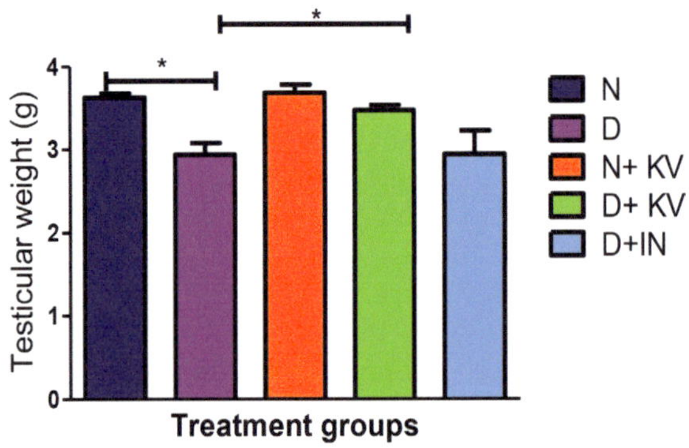

Figure 5.
Effect of KV and insulin treatment on testicular weight of rats. Data are presented as mean ± SEM. (*) indicates significant difference with p < 0.05. N, nondiabetic control group; D, diabetic group; N + KV, nondiabetic group treated with KV; D + KV, diabetic group treated with KV; D + IN, diabetic group treated with insulin (standard drug).

untreated diabetic rats. KV treatment did not affect the epididymal weight of normal rats as no apparent difference was observed between N + KV group and N group (0.529 ± 0.058 g versus 0.475 ± 0.09 g, $p > 0.05$). On the other hand, the epididymal weight of insulin-treated diabetic rats was not significantly different compared to the untreated diabetic rats (0.454 ± 0.050 g versus 0.431 ± 0.062 g, $p > 0.05$).

4.4 Assessment of lipid peroxidation of testicular and epididymal tissues of rats subjected to various treatments

MDA levels in the testis are presented in **Figure 7** for both nondiabetic and diabetic groups treated with or without KV or insulin. The testicular MDA level was significantly higher in the D group compared to the N group (0.014 ± 0.001 μmol/g versus 0.010 ± 0.002 μmol/g, $p < 0.05$). The MDA level in the testes of nondiabetic rats treated with KV (N + KV) was significantly lower than the N group. The testes of diabetic rats treated with KV (D + KV) showed significantly lower testicular MDA level than the diabetic control group. Also, insulin treatment significantly lowered MDA levels in diabetic rats compared to the diabetic control group. It is noteworthy that a significant reduction in MDA

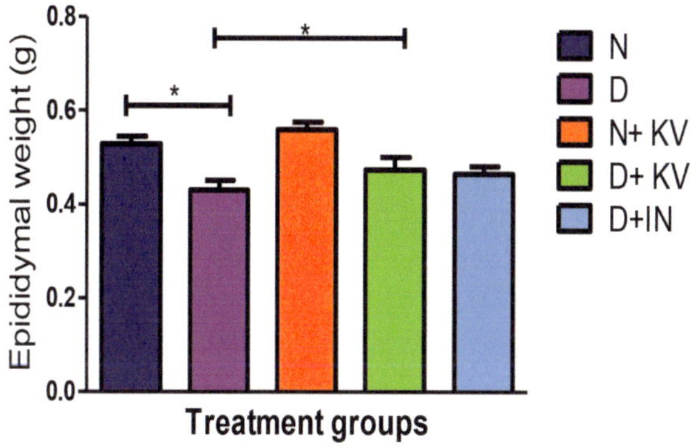

Figure 6.
Effect of KV and insulin treatment on epididymal weight of rats. Data are presented as mean ± SEM. (*) indicates significant difference with p < 0.05. N, nondiabetic control group; D, diabetic group; N + KV, nondiabetic group treated with KV; D + KV, diabetic group treated with KV; D + IN, diabetic group treated with insulin (standard drug).

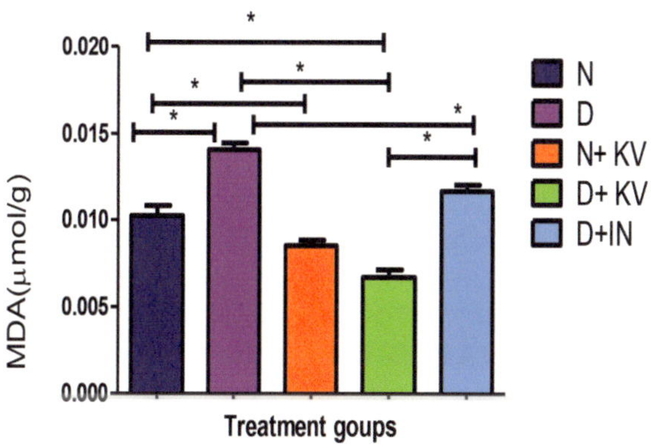

Figure 7.
Effect of KV and insulin treatment on testicular tissue LPO in rats. Data are presented as mean ± SEM. (*) indicates significant difference with p < 0.05. N, nondiabetic control group; D, diabetic group; N + KV, nondiabetic group treated with KV; D + KV, diabetic group treated with KV; D + IN, diabetic group treated with insulin (standard drug).

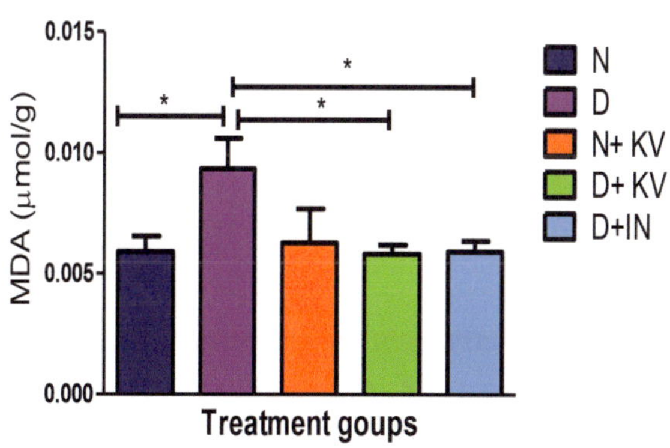

Figure 8.
Effect of KV and insulin treatment on epididymal LPO in rats. Data are presented as mean ± SEM. (*) indicates significant difference with p < 0.05. N, nondiabetic control group; D, diabetic group; N + KV, nondiabetic group treated with KV; D + KV, diabetic group treated with KV; D + IN, diabetic group treated with insulin (standard drug).

levels was observed in the testes of KV-treated diabetic rats when compared to the D + IN group (0.007 ± 0.001 μmol/g versus 0.012 ± 0.001 μmol/g, $p < 0.05$).

Figure 8 shows the MDA level in epididymis of both nondiabetic and diabetic groups treated with KV and/or insulin. The MDA level was significantly higher in epididymal tissue of the D group compared to the N group in epididymal tissue (0.009 ± 0.004 μmol/g versus 0.006 ± 0.002 μmol/g, $p < 0.05$). No significant differences in MDA levels were observed in the epididymal tissue of nondiabetic rats supplemented with KV (N + KV) compared to the untreated (N) rats. Furthermore, a significantly lower epididymal MDA level was observed in the D + KV group when compared to the D group. KV treatment normalized epididymal MDA level in diabetic rats, and this effect is comparable to that of insulin, the standard antidiabetic drug.

4.5 Assessment of SOD activity in testicular and epididymal tissues of rats subjected to various treatments

As shown in **Table 1**, no significant differences were observed in the activity of testicular superoxide dismutase (SOD) across all treatment groups. However, in the epididymal tissue, the SOD activity was significantly reduced in the diabetic (D) group when compared to the N group (0.042 ± 0.007 μmol/mg, $p < 0.05$ versus 0.556 ± 0.007 μmol/mg, $p < 0.05$). On the other hand, separate treatments of diabetic rats with KV and insulin increased SOD activity in epididymal tissue compared to untreated diabetic rats. The effects of KV on the activity of SOD in the epididymis are comparable to that of the standard drug, insulin.

4.6 Assessment of the catalase activity in testicular and epididymal tissues of male Wistar rats subjected to various treatments

A significantly lower CAT activity was observed in testicular tissue of STZ-induced diabetic rats (**Table 1**) in comparison to nondiabetic rats (12.21 ± 1.235 μmol/mg versus 18.00 ± 1.524 μmol/mg, $p < 0.05$). The supplementation of KV to nondiabetic rats (N + KV) did not significantly affect testicular CAT activity in comparison to the untreated nondiabetic group. KV treatment of diabetic rats elevated testicular CAT activity in comparison to diabetic control, and CAT activity was restored to normalcy. Likewise, a significantly higher testicular CAT activity was observed after insulin treatment in diabetic rats (D + IN) when compared to the diabetic control rats.

As shown in **Table 1**, STZ-induced diabetic rats showed significantly lower CAT activity in epididymal tissue compared to the N group (2.864 ± 0.415 μmol/mg versus 6.162 ± 0. 612 μmol/mg, $p < 0.05$). There was no significant difference in the epididymal CAT activity of rats supplemented with KV (N + KV) when compared to the N group. The separate treatment of diabetic rats with KV and insulin significantly elevated CAT activity in the epididymis compared to the diabetic controls.

4.7 Assessment of the GPX activity in the testicular and epididymal tissues of male Wistar rats subjected to various treatments

The results of testicular GPX activity of rats treated with STZ, KV, and/or IN are captured in **Table 1**. A significantly lower testicular GPx activity was observed in diabetic rats compared to the N group (3.977 ± 0.880 μmol/mg versus 12.26 ± 0.644 μmol/mg, $p < 0.05$). The nondiabetic rats treated with KV (N + KV) did not show any significant difference in testicular GPx activity compared to the N group. The testes of KV-treated diabetic rats (D + KV) showed significantly higher

Sample types and tests	Group/treatments				
	N: nondiabetic control group	**D: diabetic group**	**N + KV: nondiabetic group treated with Kolaviron**	**D + KV: diabetic group treated with Kolaviron**	**D + IN: diabetic group treated with insulin (standard drug)**
Testicular					
SOD (μmol/mg protein)	0.193 ± 0.010	0.198 ± 0.008	0.195 ± 0.019	0.169 ± 0.010	0.171 ± 0.020
CAT (μmol/mg protein)	18.00 ± 0.62*	12.95 ± 0.58	15.58 ± 1.31$^{*\#}$	13.60 ± 0.94$^{\$}$	11.86 ± 0.54$^{\&}$
GPx (μmol/mg protein)	12.28 ± 0.227$^{*\$\&}$	3.977 ± 0.280	12.06 ± 0.242$^{*\$}$	6.770 ± 0.232$^{*\#\$\&}$	8.006 ± 0.345$^{*\&}$
Epididymal					
SOD (μmol/mg protein)	0.055 ± 0.002*	0.042 ± 0.002	0.050 ± 0.003	0.052 ± 0.002*	0.053 ± 0.002*
CAT (μmol/mg protein)	2.518 ± 0.178$^{*\#\$}$	4.962 ± 0.807	4.433 ± 0.947$^{*\#}$	4.896 ± 0.385*	5.360 ± 0.369$^{\&}$
GPx (μmol/mg protein)	12.30 ± 0.225*	4.277 ± 0.279	11.81 ± 0.2476$^{*\$}$	7.056 ± 0.2484$^{*\#\$\&}$	8.006 ± 0.3624$^{*\&}$

Data are presented as mean ± SEM. N, nondiabetic control group; D, diabetic group; N + KV, nondiabetic group treated with KV; D + KV, diabetic group treated with KV; D + IN, diabetic group treated with insulin (standard drug)
**Represents a significant difference when compared to D*
$^{\#}$*Represents a significant difference when compared to N + KV*
$^{\$}$*Represents significance when compared to D + KV*
$^{\&}$*Represents a significant difference when compared to D + IN (n = 12 per group)*

Table 1.
Antioxidant (SOD, CAT, and GPx) activities in testicular and epididymal tissues of Wistar rats after a 6-week period of treatment.

GPx activity when compared to the D group. In addition, a significantly higher testicular GPx activity was observed in the D + IN group when compared to the D group.

Diabetes induction significantly lowered epididymal GPX activity in comparison to the nondiabetic rats (4.277 ± 0.884 μmol/mg versus 12.30 ± 0.636 μmol/mg, $p < 0.05$). The supplementation of KV to nondiabetic rats (N + KV) did not significantly alter GPx activity of epididymal tissue compared to the N group. However, epididymal GPX activity was significantly higher in diabetic rats treated with KV compared to the untreated diabetic group Likewise, the treatment of diabetic rats with insulin significantly increased epididymal GPx activity compared to diabetic control.

5. Discussion

Diabetes associated with OS is said to impair testicular and epididymal tissue functions which can generate male infertility [8, 11, 13, 14]. Increasingly, studies demonstrate the significant impact of phytochemicals such as flavonoids in the prevention and treatment of complications related to diabetes [20, 21]. The physiological role and properties of flavonoids in the management of OS are currently being investigated in relation to male infertility. This interest is the motivation for the current study to investigate the effects of KV (KV), a known flavonoid extract of *G. kola*, on testicular- and epididymal-induced OS using a diabetic rat model.

5.1 Evaluation of induced diabetes with STZ before KV and insulin treatment

In the current study, the single intraperitoneal administration of STZ (50 mg/kg) in adult Wistar rats was effective in causing hyperglycemia after 5 days. This was confirmed by the significantly higher plasma glucose levels (18 mmol/l, see **Figure 3**) in the STZ group of animals which is typical of type 1 diabetes mellitus. It was therefore concluded that the diabetic animal model was successfully created and the results were similar to and supported by previous findings [42, 43] where induction of DM in Wistar rats via intravenous STZ injection (of 40 and 45 mg/kg/b.w, respectively) were confirmed by hyperglycemia after 4 days and maintained for 4 weeks.

5.2 Evaluation of rat body, testicular, and epididymal weights subjected to various treatments

Blood glucose levels is an indication of proper insulin function and important energy sources [44]. Insufficient insulin secretion or dysfunction of the signaling pathway results in a disturbance of glucose homeostasis. Subsequently the body will start to use other macromolecules such as lipids and proteins as sources of energy [45]. This results in shrinking of muscle tissue accompanied by a rapid weight loss in diabetic animals [45, 46]. Data from the current study showed that the body, testes, and epididymal weights were significantly lower in STZ-induced diabetic rats than the nondiabetic control group (**Figures 3–6**). These findings are in agreement with previous studies that also demonstrated a significant decrease in body, testicular, and epididymal weights in diabetic rats [5, 18, 27, 28, 33, 45, 47]. Moreover, variations in animal body and organ weights have been reported to affect spermatogenesis, sperm quality, and sperm concentration [5, 18, 27, 28, 33, 45, 47].

In the current study, diabetic animals treated with insulin improved their body and epididymal tissue weights as there was a clear regain of body weights (**Figures 3** and **4**). Synthetic insulin is a standard drug used to treat diabetes which is different from the insulin secreted naturally by the pancreas. Pancreatic insulin promotes proper metabolism, energy balance, and the maintenance of normal body weights [48]. Though the low-dose synthetic insulin used in this study had improved the weight of diabetic animals, there was still not total recovery to their normal weights.

Supplementation with KV showed similarity to the IN treatment with a significant improvement not only of the diabetic rat's body and epididymal tissue weights but also of the rat's testicular weight. Such findings are in agreement with the results of Adaramoye and Lawal [49], who reported that the treatment with KV significantly increased the weight gained by diabetic rats when compared to the untreated diabetic counterparts. Moreover, there was no significant difference in weights of nondiabetic rats supplemented with KV (N + KV) when compared to nondiabetic control group (N) (**Figures 3–6**). These results demonstrate that KV supplementation had no adverse effects on the animal weights confirming that the decrease observed in diabetic rats supplemented with KV was only due to their diabetic condition. This also implies that the body, testes, and epididymal weight improvement observed in the diabetic animals supplemented with KV might be due to its antioxidant and hypoglycemic potential to prevent OS and diabetes. It can be argued that the ability of KV to protect against weight loss might mainly be attributed to its glucose-lowering capacity [50]. Indeed, the regulation of glucose levels as the main source of energy by KV provides a platform for less use of alternative sources of energy from body, testicular, and epididymal proteins and fats. It could therefore be postulated that KV might be considered as an antidiabetic compound in the management of weight and glucose regulation in diabetes.

5.3 Assessment of lipid peroxidation of testicular and epididymal tissues of rats subjected to various treatments

MDA is an end product of LPO, and the increased levels are an indication of oxidative damage [51, 52]. It has been shown that LPO induces disturbance of fine structures; alteration of integrity, fluidity, and permeability; and functional loss of biomembranes, modifies low density lipoprotein (LDL) to proatherogenic and proinflammatory forms, and generates potentially toxic products [52]. Thus, LPO in vivo has been implicated as the underlying mechanisms in numerous disorders and diseases such as cardiovascular diseases, cancer, neurological disorders, and aging. The mechanism of free radical-mediated LPO reactions include [46] abstraction of bisallylic hydrogen from polyunsaturated fatty acids to give carbon-centered radicals which rearranges to more stable cis, trans-pentadienyl radicals [33], addition of oxygen to the pentadienyl radical to give lipid peroxyl radicals [26], release of oxygen from the peroxyl radical to give oxygen and pentadienyl radicals, which rapidly react with oxygen to give a thermochemically more stable trans, trans form preferentially than cis, trans form, and [27] intramolecular addition of the peroxyl radical to the double bond to yield bicyclic prostaglandin-type products.

The results clearly indicate a significantly higher and increased expression of MDA in the testicular (**Figure 7**) and epididymal (**Figure 8**) tissues of the diabetic rats when compared to the nondiabetic rats. These results are in agreement with previous study also performed on diabetic experimental animal models [49]. During diabetes, hyperglycemia causes auto-oxidation of glucose and stimulates OS through excessive free radical production. The release of free radicals causes damage to biological systems by abstracting electrons from macromolecules, thereby causing instability and disintegration [53]. For instance, peroxidation of polyunsaturated lipids on sperm membrane has been reported to cause structural alterations of the biological cell membranes as well as a change in membrane stability and function [49]. The peroxidation of sperm lipids may also disturb maturation, spermatogenesis, capacitation, acrosome reaction, and eventually membrane fusion, which results in male infertility [5, 6, 28–30].

In the present study, the protective mechanism of KV and IN has been examined in the onset of LPO related to STZ-induced diabetes. The findings from the study indicate that diabetic animals treated with IN recovered from LPO in the testes and epididymal tissues. This is observed through the decrease of MDA level to values close to baseline of nondiabetic rats (**Figures 7** and **8**).

KV showed significantly healthier responses. Not only did KV supplementation significantly reduce MDA levels in the N + KV group when compared to the N group, but it also had a better effect than IN in the restoration of testicular and epididymal MDA levels of the D + KV group when compared to D only group (**Figure 7**). These findings emphasize the potentiality of KV to better restore metabolic disorders related to OS such as diabetes and male infertility [5, 6, 28, 29].

Insulin helps to control blood glucose levels, and then this reduces the amount of free radicals released. The observed protective effects of KV in this study may be due to its antioxidant properties by scavenging the effects of hydroperoxides resulting from induced OS. This is in accordance with previous studies that have reported the beneficial effects of KV against testicular damage induced by various chemicals [2, 5, 6, 28–30, 33, 35].

5.4 Assessment of antioxidant enzymes in the testicular and epididymal tissues to various treatments

Antioxidant enzymes such as SOD, CAT, and GPX play a crucial role in protecting the testes and epididymal tissues against OS associated damage and male reproductive disorders [43–45].

Physiological and pathophysiological conditions such as diabetes influence the level of production and activity of these antioxidant enzymes [2, 6]. The reduction in antioxidant enzymes has been previously reported in diabetic animals [20]. The observed reduction in antioxidant enzyme activities could be due to the oxidative inactivation of the enzyme by ROS or by the glycation of the enzymes [20, 45]. The reduced activity of SOD, CAT, and GPX in the epididymal and testicular tissues has been observed following STZ induction of diabetes, and this may result in a number of deleterious effects due to the accumulation of superoxide radicals and H_2O_2.

In epididymal tissue the SOD activity was significantly lower in STZ-induced diabetic rats when compared to nondiabetic control rats (**Table 1**). This is in agreement with a study by Adaramoye and Lawal [49] who demonstrated that a diabetogenic agent reduced SOD activity in epididymal tissue. Both catalase and GPx activities in the testes and epididymis were significantly lower in STZ-induced diabetic rats than in the nondiabetic control rats. Glutathione peroxidase shares the substrate, H_2O_2, with CAT; it alone can react effectively with lipids and other organic hydroperoxides, being the major source of protection against low levels of OS. Some authors supported the idea that GPx was essential in the protection against OS under normal conditions [54]. Others believed in a protective role for these enzymes only under OS conditions [2]. Generally, in our study, the activity of testicular and epididymal antioxidant enzymes SOD, CAT, and GPx was depleted in diabetic rats. Diabetes-induced tissue OS is further supported by the elevated levels of MDA.

Numerous compounds with antioxidant activities have been shown to improve or normalize the activities of antioxidant enzymes in nondiabetic and diabetic rats, respectively [4]. In the present study, the supplementation of KV for 6 weeks to the normal rats did not change SOD, CAT, and GPx activities compared to the nondiabetic rats. This might be due to the interference between natural antioxidants produced by the body and the antioxidant effects of KV. The treatment of STZ-induced diabetic rats with KV influenced the activity of SOD, CAT, and GPx compared to the diabetic groups (**Table 1**). Similarly, to previous studies, the supplementation of dietary antioxidants to experimental animals has shown a positive correlation between natural dietary supplementation and increased antioxidant enzyme levels in induced OS models. In other studies, KV restored antioxidant enzymes in the testes of diabetes-induced rats [5, 49]. The protective effect of KV observed in the testes and epididymis of diabetic rats might either be due to the inhibition of glycation by the antioxidant enzymes or scavenging abilities of ROS, thus decreasing the formation of LPO [5, 27–30].

Insulin has been used in the management of diabetes by restoring pancreatic insulin deficiency. From our results it is clear that synthetic insulin had improved the levels of testicular and epididymal antioxidant enzymes in STZ-induced diabetic rats. These results confirm the central role of insulin in energy homeostasis and also make it an important signaling factor in the reproductive tract [2, 7]. The observed effects of KV on the testes and epididymis of STZ-induced diabetic rats in the present study could be attributed to its hypoglycemic and antioxidant properties.

6. Conclusion

The findings of this study emphasized the protective effects of KV against diabetes-associated OS in the testicular and epididymal tissues by enhancing antioxidant defense system in STZ-induced diabetic rats. The present study showed that that KV has the potential of being used as a treatment for diabetes-related pathologies and their complications especially testicular dysfunction. We propose further investigations to elucidate the effects of KV on male reproductive organ function in order to advance the current knowledge which could also be extended to clinical research.

Author details

Claudine Manirafasha[1,2], Omolola Rebecca Oyenihi[1], Nicole Lisa Brooks[3], Stefan S. du Plessis[2] and Yapo Guillaume Aboua[4*]

1 Faculty of Health and Wellness Sciences, Cape Peninsula University of Technology, Bellville, South Africa

2 Division of Medical Physiology, Department of Biomedical Sciences, Faculty of Medicine and Health Sciences, Stellenbosch University, Cape Town, South Africa

3 Department of Wellness Sciences, Faculty of Health and Wellness Sciences, Cape Peninsula University of Technology, Cape Town, South Africa

4 Department of Health Sciences, Faculty of Health and Applied Sciences, Namibia University of Science and Technology, Windhoek, Namibia

*Address all correspondence to: yaboua@nust.na

References

[1] World Health Organization. Laboratory Manual for the Examination of Human Semen and Semen-Cervical Mucus Interaction. 5th ed. Geneva, Switzerland: Cambridge University Press; 2010. pp. 1-86

[2] Agarwal A, Virk G, Ong C, du Plessis SS. Effect of oxidative stress on male reproduction. The World Journal of Men's Health. 2014;**32**(1):1-17

[3] Trussell JC. Optimal diagnosis and medical treatment of male infertility. Seminar of Reproductive Medicine. 2013;**31**(1):235-236

[4] Ighodaro OM, Akinloye OA. First line defence antioxidants-superoxide dismutase (SOD), catalase (CAT) and glutathione peroxidase (GPX): Their fundamental role in the entire antioxidant defence grid. Alexandria Journal of Medicine. 2018;**54**(4):287-293

[5] Farombi EO, Adedara IA, Akinrinde SA, Ojo OO, Eboh AS. Protective effects of kolaviron and quercetin on cadmium-induced testicular damage and endocrine pathology in rats. Andrologia. 2012;**44**(4):273-284

[6] Gandhi J, Hernandez RJ, Chen A, Smith NL, Sheynkin YR, Joshi G, et al. Impaired hypothalamic pituitary testicular axis activity, spermatogenesis, and sperm function promote infertility in males with lead poisoning. Zygote. 2017;**25**(2):103-110

[7] Agarwal A, Roychoudhury S, Bjugstad KB, Cho CL. Oxidation-reduction potential of semen: What is its role in the treatment of male infertility? Therapeutic Advances in Urology. 2016;**8**(5):302-318

[8] Guz J, Gackowski D, Foksinski M, Rozalski R, Zarakowska E, Siomek A, et al. Comparison of oxidative stress/DNA damage in semen and blood of fertile and infertile men. PLoS One. 2013;**8**(7):68490

[9] Herwig R, Knoll C, Planyavsky M, Pourbiabany A, Greilberger J, Bennett KL. Proteomic analysis of seminal plasma from infertile patients with oligoasthenoteratozoospermia due to oxidative stress and comparison with fertile volunteers. Fertility and Sterility. 2013;**100**(2):355-366

[10] Kosan C, Heidel F, Godmann M, Bierhoff H. Epigenetic erosion in adult stem cells: Drivers and passengers of aging. Cell. 2018;**7**(12):237

[11] Inih OS, Esther YE, Adetola FO, Chinedu AA, Brenda NC, Efedaye OA. Testicular dysfunction is a common feature in men with type 2 diabetes mellitus in a nigerian tertiary hospital. Current Diabetes Reviews. 2018;**14**(3):298-306

[12] Ding GL, Liu Y, Liu ME, Pan JX, Guo MX, Sheng JZ, et al. The effects of diabetes on male fertility and epigenetic regulation during spermatogenesis. Asian Journal of Andrology. 2015;**17**(6):948

[13] Glazer CH, Bonde JP, Giwercman A, Vassard D, Pinborg A, Schmidt L, et al. Risk of diabetes according to male factor infertility: A register-based cohort study. Human Reproduction. 2017;**32**(7):1474-1481

[14] Ghasemi M, Talebi A, Rahmanyan M, Nahangi H, Ghanizadeh T. Effects of diabetes mellitus type 2 on semen parameters. SSU Journals. 2017;**25**(8):621-628

[15] Podlasek CA, Mulhall J, Davies K, Wingard CJ, Hannan JL, Bivalacqua TJ, et al. Translational perspective on the role of testosterone in sexual function and dysfunction. The Journal of Sexual Medicine. 2016;**13**(8):1183-1198

[16] Tavares RS, Portela JM, Sousa MI, Mota PC, Ramalho-Santos J, Amaral S. High glucose levels affect spermatogenesis: An in vitro approach. Reproduction, Fertility and Development. 2017;**29**(7):1369-1378

[17] Sifuentes-Franco S, Padilla-Tejeda DE, Carrillo-Ibarra S. Oxidative stress, apoptosis, and mitochondrial function in diabetic nephropathy. International Journal of Endocrinology. 2018. DOI: 10.1155/2018/1875870

[18] Artimani T, Amiri I, Soleimani Asl S, Saidijam M, Hasanvand D, Afshar S. Amelioration of diabetes-induced testicular and sperm damage in rats by cerium oxide nanoparticle treatment. Andrologia. 2018;**50**(9):e13089

[19] Kyathanahalli C, Bangalore S, Muralidhara HK. Experimental diabetes-induced testicular damage in prepubertal rats. Journal of Diabetes. 2013;**6**:48-59

[20] Mohammed A, Pandey KB, Rizvi SI. Effect of phytochemicals on diabetes-related neurological disorders. In: Farooqui T, Farooqi AA, editors. Neuroprotective Effects of Phytochemicals in Neurological Disorders. Wiley; 2017:283-298. Online ISBN: 9781119155195. Print ISBN: 9781119155140. https://doi.org/10.1002/9781119155195.ch13

[21] Tchimene MK, Anaga AO, Ugwoke CEC, Onoja OJ, Ezugwu CO, Okunji C, et al. Anti-diabetic profile of extract, kolaviron, biflavonoids and garcinoic acid from *Garcinia kola* seeds. International Journal of Current Microbiology and Applied Sciences. 2016;**5**(2):317-322

[22] Oguntibeju OO. The potential protective effects of selected medicinal plants on liver function and integrity. African Journal of Biomedical Research. 2018;**21**(3):231-236

[23] Oguntibeju OO. Medicinal plants with anti-inflammatory activities from selected countries and regions of Africa. Journal of Inflammation Research. 2018;**11**:307

[24] Wyk, Van B, Gorelik B. The history and ethnobotany of Cape herbal teas. South African Journal of Botany. 2017;**110**:18-38

[25] Ezeigbo OR, Ejike EN, Nwachukwu I, Ejike BU. Comparative antibacterial activity of methanolic, ethanolic and aqueous extract of *Garcinia kola* (Bitter kola) and *Cola nitida* (Kola nut). International Journal of Plant Research. 2016;**6**(3):53-56

[26] Oyenihi OR, Brooks NL, Oguntibeju OO. Effects of kolaviron on hepatic oxidative stress in streptozotocin induced diabetes. BMC Complementary and Alternative Medicine. 2015;**15**(1):236

[27] Kehinde A, Adefisan A, Adebayo O, Adaramoye O. Biflavonoid fraction from *Garcinia kola* seed ameliorates hormonal imbalance and testicular oxidative damage by anti-tuberculosis drugs in Wistar rats. Journal of Basic and Clinical Physiology and Pharmacology. 2016;**27**(4):393-401

[28] Farombi EO, Owoeye O. Antioxidative and chemopreventive properties of *Vernonia amygdalina* and garcinia biflavonoid. International Journal Environment Research Public Health. 2011;**8**:2533-2555

[29] Oyagbemi AA, Omobowale TO, Adedapo AA, Yakubu MA. Kolaviron, biflavonoid complex from the seed of *Garcinia kola* attenuated angiotensin II-and lypopolysaccharide-induced vascular smooth muscle cell proliferation and nitric oxide production. Pharmacognosy Research. 2016;**8**(Suppl 1):S50

[30] Oyagbemi AA, Omobowale TO, Asenuga ER, Abiola JO, Adedapo AA, Yakubu MA. Kolaviron attenuated

arsenic acid induced-cardiorenal dysfunction via regulation of ROS, C-reactive proteins (CRP), cardiac troponin I (CTnI) and BCL2. Journal of Traditional and Complementary Medicine. 2018;**8**(3):396-409

[31] Romero AC, Olvera Hernández EG, Cerón TF, Chávez AA. Oxidative stress and chronic degenerative diseases: A role for antioxidants. The Exogenous Antioxidants. 2013;**49**:52

[32] Ola MS, Nawaz MI, Alhomida AS. Effects of phytochemicals on diabetic retino-neuropathy. In: Farooqui T, Farooqi AA, editors. Neuroprotective Effects of Phytochemicals in Neurological Disorders. Wiley; 2017:199-211. Online ISBN: 9781119155195. Print ISBN: 9781119155140. https://doi.org/10.1002/9781119155195.ch13

[33] Ismail O, Adamson FM, Adeyemi OO.Ameliorative effect of kolaviron, a biflavonoid complex from *Garcinia kola* seeds against scopolamine-induced memory impairment in rats: Role of antioxidant defense system. Metabolic Brain Disease. 2017;**32**(1):235-245

[34] Iwu MM, Igboko OA, Okunji CO, Tempesta MS. Antidiabetic and aldose reductase activities of biflavanones of *Garcinia kola*. Journal of Pharmacology. 1990;**42**:290-292

[35] Ayepola OR, Chegou NN, Brooks NL, Oguntibeju OO. Kolaviron, a biflavonoid complex of *Garcinia kola* seeds modulates apoptosis by suppressing oxidative stress and inflammation in diabetes-induced nephrotoxic rats. Phytomedicine. 2014;**21**(14):1785-1793

[36] Atila S, Ayese S, Yesim S, Mahfuz E. Evaluation the anti-diabetic activity of cherry laurel (*Laurocerasus officinalis*). The Open Conference Proceedings Journal. 2012;**3**:8-12

[37] Redinbaugh MG, Turley RB. Adaptation of the bicinchoninic acid protein assay for use with microtiter plates and sucrose gradient fractions. Analytical Biochemistry. 1986;**153**(2):267-271

[38] Lykkesfeldt J. Determination of malondialdehyde as dithiobarbituric acid adduct in biological samples by HPLC with fluorescence detection: Comparison with ultraviolet-visible spectrophotometry. Clinical Chemistry. 2001;**47**(9):1725-1727

[39] Cuny D, Van Haluwyn C, Shirali P, Zerimech F, Jerome L, Haguenoer JM. Cellular impact of metal trace elements in terricolous lichen diploschistes muscorum (scop.) R. sant.—Identification of oxidative stress biomarkers. Water, Air, and Soil Pollution. 2004;**152**(1):55-69

[40] Ellerby LM, Bredesen DE. Measurement of cellular oxidation reactive oxygen species and antioxidant enzymes during apoptosis. Methods in Enzymology. 2000;**322**:413-421

[41] Aebi H. Catalase in vitro. Methods Enzymology. 1984;**105**:121-126

[42] Sadeghi A, Beigy M, Alizadeh S, Mazloom H, Vakili S, Ahmadi S, et al. Synergistic effects of ad-libitum low-dose fructose drinking and low-dose streptozotocin treatment in Wistar rats: A mild model of type 2 diabetes. Acta Medica Iranica. 2017;**55**(5):304-310

[43] Sujithra K, Srinivasan S, Indumathi D, Vinothkumar V. Allyl methyl sulfide, an organosulfur compound alleviates hyperglycemia mediated hepatic oxidative stress and inflammation in streptozotocin-induced experimental rats. Biomedicine and Pharmacotherapy. 2018;**107**:292-302

[44] Kokilavani P, Suriyakalaa U, Elumalai P, Abirami B, Ramachandran R, Sankarganesh A, et al. Antioxidant

mediated ameliorative steroidogenesis by *Commelina benghalensis L.* and *Cissus quadrangularis L.* against quinalphos induced male reproductive toxicity. Pesticide Biochemical Physiolology. 2014;**109**:18-33

[45] Asadi N, Kheradmand A, Gholami M, Moradi FH. Effect of ghrelin on the biochemical and histopathology parameters and spermatogenesis cycle following experimental varicocele in rat. Andrologia. 2018;**50**(10):e13106

[46] Benabbou A, Khaled MB, Alchalabi AS. Evaluation of the efficiency of combined and separated antioxidant supplementation of vitamin C and E on semen parameters in strepto-zotocin-induced diabetic male Wistar rats. South Asian Journal of Experimental Biology. 2018;7(4):166-172

[47] La vignera SR, Condorelli E, Vicari R, Colagero AE. Diabetes mellitus and sperm parameters. Journal of Andrology. 2012;**33**(2):145-153

[48] Blundell JE, Gibbons C, Caudwell P, Finlayson G, Hopkins M. Appetite control and energy balance: Impact of exercise. Obesity Reviews. 2015;**16**:67-76

[49] Adaramoye OA, Lawal SO. Effect of kolaviron, a biflavonoid complex from *Garcinia kola* seeds, on the antioxidant, hormonal and spermatogenic indices of diabetic male rats. Andrologia. 2013;**20**:1-9

[50] Hansen SS, Aasum E, Hafstad AD. The role of NADPH oxidases in diabetic cardiomyopathy. Biochimica et Biophysica Acta (BBA)-Molecular Basis of Disease. 2018;**1864**(5):1908-1913

[51] Avci E, Akarslan ZZ, Erten H, Coskun-Cevher S. Oxidative stress and cellular immunity in patients with recurrent aphthous ulcers. Brazilian Journal of Medical and Biological Research. 2014;**47**(5):355-360

[52] Mao H. Solution structure of an oligonucleotide containing the malondialdehyde deoxyguanosine adduct N_2-(3-oxo-1-propenyl)-dG (ring-opened M1G) positioned in a $(CpG)_3$ frameshift hotspot of the *Salmonella typhimurium* hisd3052 Gene. Biochemistry. 1999;**38**:13491-13501

[53] Atta EM, Mohamed NH, Abdelgawad AA. Antioxidants: An overview on the natural and synthetic types. European Chemical Bulletin. 2017;**6**(8):365-375

[54] Dassarma B, Nandi DK, Gangopadhyay S, Samanta S. Hepatoprotective effect of food preservatives (butylated hydroxyanisole, butylated hydroxytoluene) on carbon tetrachloride-induced hepatotoxicity in rat. Toxicology Reports. 2018;**5**:31-37

Chapter 17

Antioxidant and Biological Activity of *Cissus sicyoides and Rosmarinus officinalis* Extracts

Marielba de los Angeles Rodriguez Salazar, Glides Rafael Olivo Urbina, Priscila do Nascimento Bezerra, Vânia Maria Borges Cunha, Marcilene Paiva da Silva, Flávia Cristina Seabra Pires, Ana Paula de Souza e Silva, Sérgio Henrique Brabo de Sousa and Raul Nunes de Carvalho Jr

Abstract

This chapter will describe the antioxidant and biological activity of *Cissus sicyoides* and *Rosmarinus officinalis* leaf extracts, which represent an important natural source of antioxidants. These plants contain several bioactive compounds with high antioxidant activity, such as phenolic compounds, which are compounds that prevent or delay oxidative stress, acting as free radical scavengers (FRSs), and thus reduce the onset of cardiovascular disease, cancer, diabetes, epilepsy, stroke, among other diseases. The supercritical fluid extraction (SFE) has been studied to obtain antioxidant compounds from natural sources, without the drawbacks associated with conventional extraction processes, such as the use of organic solvents, which present toxicity and contaminate the extracts, is proposed.

Keywords: *C. sicyoides*, *R. officinalis*, antioxidant activity, biological activity, supercritical extraction

1. Introduction

The Amazonian biodiversity presents a great source of foods and medicinal plants rich in antioxidant compounds whose study and conscious exploration contribute to the region sustainable development [1, 2]. The plants have a great importance due to their medicinal and nutritional properties. About 70–90% of the world population prefers the use of medicinal plants or plant extracts to treat common diseases [3, 4]. Plants have been extensively studied in recent years for their antioxidant activity. The main classes of plant chemicals are phenolic compounds, tocopherols, carotenoids, and alkaloids. Among these compounds, phenolic compounds are the most important. They prevent or delay oxidative stress, acting as free radical scavengers (FRSs), and thus reduce the onset of different chronic diseases [5–8].

Antioxidants are a set of substances that can delay or inhibit oxidation reactions and act as a defense mechanism to neutralize the harmful effects of oxidation in biological systems and foods [6, 9, 10]. Oxidative stress is considered a state of imbalance where excessive amounts of reactive oxygen and nitrogen species (ROS/RNS, for example, superoxide anion, hydrogen peroxide, hydroxyl radical, peroxynitrite) exceed the capacity of endogenous antioxidants (uric acid, superoxide dismutase, catalase, glutathione peroxidase), leading to the oxidation of a biomacromolecule variety such as enzymes, proteins, DNA, and lipids. Exogenous antioxidants (phenolic compounds, carotenoids, tocopherols, and ascorbates) are consumed in the diet mainly of fruits, leaves, seeds, vegetables, and cereals, they have the function of increasing or protecting the antioxidant defense in biological systems and, therefore, they are important for endogenous oxidative stability [11–13].

It is conflicting that oxygen and nitrogen, considered essential for biological processes, are also cofactors for toxic and degenerative processes. In this sense, the antioxidant compounds act through different chemical mechanisms in order to minimize or maintain redox balance in vivo [9, 14]. There are several mechanisms by which oxidation can be inhibited. In general, the mechanisms involved include FRSs, ester bond enzymatic hydrolysis, transition metal ion sequestration, and enzyme-catalyzed peroxide reduction. The last three mechanisms mentioned do not cease reactive species action, but prevent the formation of molecules capable of promoting free radical chain reactions [15].

There is a growing interest in new sources of natural antioxidant compounds due to synthetic antioxidants such as butylated hydroxyanisole (BHA), butylated hydroxytoluene (BHT), and tert-butylhydroquinone (TBHQ) in the food industry being severely restricted, since they may show carcinogenic effects on living organisms [16–18]. In this sense, the scientific community and consumers are looking for new bioactive compounds of natural origin that can be used to develop new treatments against diseases. In addition, they may be employed in the food industry as functional food ingredients.

Cissus sicyoides L., which belongs to the Vitaceae family, is also known as vegetal insulin, anil-trepador, bejuco-caro, cipó-pucá, or puci. It is considered a plant from the Neotropical region and is usually found in the Amazon region [19, 20]. According to studies on *C. sicyoides* extract composition, the presence of bioactive compounds with high antioxidant activity as carotenoids and phenolic compounds (flavonoid, resveratrol, coumarins, and tannins) was found [21–23]. Therefore, it is a plant traditionally used by Brazilian popular medicine to treat rheumatism, epilepsy, stroke, abscesses, arthritis, and diabetes [23, 24].

Rosmarinus officinalis is an aromatic plant of the Lamiaceae family, native to the Mediterranean region. Today, it has been grown in many parts of the world and is known as rosemary [25, 26]. It has been recognized as one of the plants with great antioxidant activity. Among the most effective antioxidant constituents, cyclic diterpene diphenols, carnosic acid, rosmarinic acid, and carnosol have been identified. *R. officinalis* extracts have been used in the treatment and/or prevention of diseases such as cancer, Alzheimer's disease, urinary and gastrointestinal infections, diabetes, ischemia, and atherosclerosis [17, 25–32]. *R. officinalis* extract has been commercially exploited as a natural antioxidant [5, 16].

Supercritical fluid extraction (SFE) has already been studied to obtain bioactive compounds from natural sources. Salazar et al. and Carvalho et al. showed that the application of SFE technology is successful in obtaining extracts from *C. sicyoides* and *R. officinalis*, respectively, with high antioxidant capacity [24, 33]. SFE is based on the use of solvents with temperatures and pressures above their critical points, which have a high solvency power. One of the most commonly used solvents in SFE is carbon dioxide (CO_2) since its critical points are moderate, nontoxic, non-flammable, affordable, chemically inert, and apolar and has an ideal behavior for thermosensitive compound extraction. In SFE it is possible to obtain totally solvent-free extracts without compound thermal degradation due to the low operating temperatures applied [34–37].

Supercritical CO_2 (Sc-CO_2) has a limitation in dissolving polar molecules. However, this disadvantage can be solved by polar solvent addition, called modifiers or cosolvents, which modify the supercritical fluid polarity and, consequently, improve polar fraction extraction rich in bioactive substances, such as phenolic compounds related to high antioxidant activity [37, 38]. The aim of this chapter is to describe the antioxidant and biological activity of *Cissus sicyoides* and *Rosmarinus officinalis* leaf extracts that represent an important natural source of antioxidants. In addition to providing an overview of the SFE that is currently presented as a modern and environmentally safe extraction technology for antioxidant compound extraction.

2. *Cissus sicyoides*

2.1 Botanical description

Cissus sicyoides L. or *Cissus verticillata* L., which belongs to the Vitaceae family, is also known as vegetal insulin, cipó-pucá, or puci. It is considered a plant of the Neotropical region and is usually found in the Amazon region. It is a climbing plant, which can reach up to 6 m in length, and presents fleshy articulated branch, alternating leaf of ovate format, pale or yellowish-green flowers, and round fruit, with variations of color from violet to black (**Figure 1**) [19, 20].

2.2 Chemical composition

The bioactive compounds present in the leaf and stem are represented by carotenoids (α-carotene and β-carotene) [39] and phenolic compounds such as

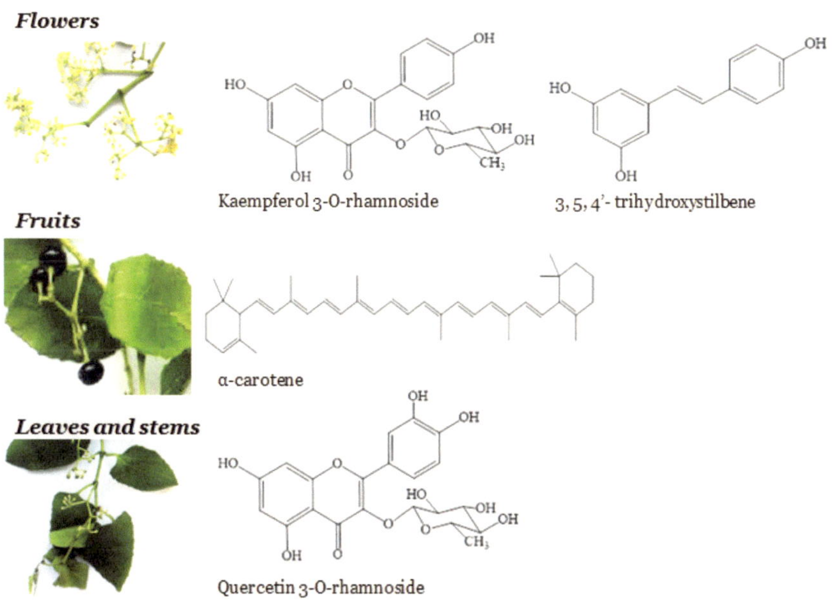

Figure 1.
Description of C. sicyoides parts and the main chemical structure of the antioxidant compounds.

flavonoids (quercetin 3-O-rhamnoside and kaempferol 3-O-rhamnoside) [21]. But also, three new flavonoid glycosides were found, denominate cissosides I, II, and III (kaempferol 3-O-α-L-(5"-O-acetyl)-arabinofuranosyl-7-O-α-L-rhamnopyranoside, quercetin 3-O-α-L-arabinofuranosyl-7-O-α-L-rhamnopyranoside, and quercetin 3-O-α-L-(5"-O-acetyl)-arabinofuranosyl-7-O-α-L-rhamnopyranoside) [22].

Recently, three different flavonoids were identified (quercetin-3-O-hexoside, quercetin-3-O-deoxyhexoside, and kaempferol-3-O-deoxyhexoside) [23]. In addition, resveratrol (3,5,4′-trihydroxystilbene) [40] and a new benzofuran-type stilbene (cissusin) [22], tannins, coumarins (glycoside 5,6,7,8-tetrahydroxycoumarin-5β-xylopyranoside and sabandin), and steroids (β-sitosterol and 3β-O-β-D-glucopyranosyl sitosterol) were found [21]. The presence of essential oils was also detected [41]. In the supercritical extracts of *C. sicyoides* phytochemical screening obtained from leaves and stems by high-performance thin-layer chromatography (HPTLC), the presence of terpenes, phenolic compounds, and flavonoids was evidenced [24]. In the fruit composition analysis, three anthocyanins were found (delphinidin-3-rutinoside, cyanidin-3-rhamnosyl-arabinoside, and delphinidin-3-rhamnoside) [42]. Therefore, the fruit of this plant may have potential use as a food coloring. **Figure 1** shows the chemical structures of the main antioxidant compounds found in *C. sicyoides*.

2.3 Antioxidant and biological activity

In *C. sicyoides* polyphenolic profile, we can find flavonoids: the quercetin and kaempferol as the majority and its various isomers. The mechanism of quercetin antioxidant action has been associated mainly with the reduction of ROS/RNS, which is a compound that prevents or retards oxidative stress, which enables the prevention of various chronic diseases [6, 43]. In the study conducted by Crespo et al., treatment with quercetin and kaempferol prevented the production of ROS such as peroxides, superoxide anion, and nitric oxide. These results confirmed the differential protective effect of these flavonoids in the diet against oxidative stress induced by pro-inflammatory stimuli in parenchymal liver cells [44]. Resveratrol plays an important antioxidant role in reducing hydroxyl radicals, superoxide, and metal-induced radicals, as well as showing antioxidant abilities in ROS-producing cells. Also, it has a protective effect against lipid peroxidation in cell membranes and DNA damage caused by ROS/RNS [45]. Benzofuran is a potent radical scavenger capable of inhibiting lipid peroxidation, its FRS capacity being greater than α-tocopherol [46].

Figure 2 shows the results of the qualitative analysis of antioxidant activity by HPTLC of C. sicyoides extracts obtained by supercritical extraction (essays 1–15), hexane extract (HE), and ethanolic extract (EE) obtained with conventional extraction by Soxhlet. The plaque was derivatized with DPPH (2,2-diphenyl-1-picrylhydrazyl), and it was possible to detect the presence of yellow spots on the plaque purple bottom resulting from the reduction of the DPPH•; in the presence of antioxidant substances, 2,2-diphenyl-picryl-hydrazine is reduced, losing its purple coloration. The study results confirmed the presence of chemical constituent characteristic of this plant, with antioxidant activity. In the same study, a quantitative determination of the antioxidant activity by the DPPH method was carried out. It was demonstrated that with the extractive methodologies (SFE and Soxhlet) used it was possible to extract with low EC_{50} values, related to a high antioxidant activity; for EE, the value of EC_{50} (325.67 g of extract/g of DPPH) is similar to the value of EC_{50} (404.81 g of extract/g of DPPH) obtained with SFE [24].

In the in vitro antioxidant activity determination by the ABTS method of the *C. sicyoides* aqueous extract obtained by decoction, it was evidenced that the extract has an antioxidant activity of $IC_{50} = 13.0 \pm 0.2$ μg/ml. These results indicate that

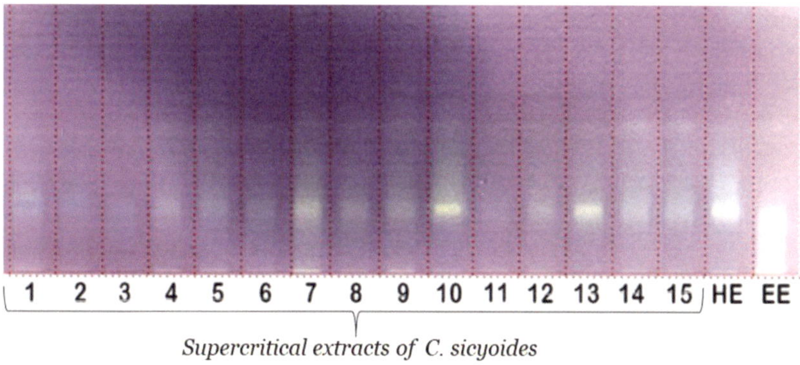

Figure 2.
Qualitative analysis of antioxidant activity by HPTLC of C. sicyoides extracts obtained by supercritical extraction and conventional extraction (Soxhlet) [29].

the extract is a potential source of natural antioxidant and may be useful in the prevention of diseases associated with oxidative stress [47]. Thus, the antioxidant activity results of *C. sicyoides* extracts are related to the extraction methods and to the solvent used.

Due to antioxidant properties, *C. sicyoides* has been used by folk medicine to treat rheumatism, epilepsy, stroke, abscesses, arthritis, and diabetes; it has also been used to treat respiratory diseases. Some biological activities are attributed to the plant as anti-inflammatory, antirheumatic, antiepileptic, antihypertensive, antimicrobial, antipyretic, antioxidant, antiallergic, anticancer, and antidiabetic activities [23, 40, 48–50].

Several studies point to the application of *C. sicyoides* in the treatment of various diseases, in order to demonstrate the cytotoxic activity of the *C. sicyoides* aqueous extract obtained by decoction against cells human epidermoid carcinoma no. 2 (HEp-2 cells), showing complete inhibition of cell division after 24 h of treatment [51]. Also, the antitumor activity of *C. sicyoides* hydroalcoholic extract obtained by maceration, in animals at doses of 300 and 600 mg/kg in weight, was investigated, being demonstrated that the extract showed an inhibition of tumor activity in sarcoma-180 of 49 and 62% and Ehrlich carcinoma of 69 and 84% [52].

Regarding the plant anti-inflammatory activity, it has been demonstrated that the oral administration of 300 and 500 mg/kg of the *C. sicyoides* stem's aqueous extract obtained by decoction in mice with induced edema has a potent anti-inflammatory activity, and administration of the extract produced an approximately 50% reduction of the induced edema [53]. Resveratrol was indicated as one of the constituents responsible for the anti-inflammatory and antiallergic properties presented by *C. sicyoides* alcoholic extract obtained by maceration [40]. However, modern ethnopharmacological use reports that the *C. sicyoides* hydroalcoholic extract by percolation has anti-inflammatory and antidiarrheal actions, due to the abundant presence of flavonol-O-glycoside derivatives of quercetin and kaempferol, which are mainly responsible for the plant pharmacological effects [23].

In addition, pharmacological effects were detected in the treatment and/or prevention of dysfunctions such as hypertension and vasoconstriction of arteries, veins, and capillaries with aqueous extract of *C. sicyoides*. These compounds act at the membrane level, increasing the calcium entry through the membrane as well as acting on the internal calcium deposits [54].

In the evaluation of the antidiabetic potential of *C. sicyoides*, the effects of leaf tea from the plant were studied; the in vivo experimental model chosen proved to be an appropriate treatment, reducing blood and urine glucose levels [48]. Later, it was demonstrated that treatment of diabetic rats with *C. sicyoides* aqueous extract obtained by decoction, for 7 days (100 and 200 mg/kg), reduced blood glucose levels by 22 and 25%, respectively [49]. However, *C. sicyoides* leaf tea was used to investigate the plant therapeutic efficacy in volunteers who are diabetic and intolerant to glucose. A single dose of tea (1 g of dried leaf powder in 150 ml of water) was used for a period of 7 days. It was observed in people intolerant to glucose that the tea had antidiabetic activity [55].

C. sicyoides has antibacterial activity, showing inhibitory capacity against bacteria that cause food poisoning [56], which causes acute effects in the gastrointestinal tract and, in some cases, a high severity that patients come to death (*Bacillus cereus*, *Bacillus subtilis*, *Bacillus megaterium*, *Staphylococcus aureus*, and *Escherichia coli*). In addition, the antifungal activity of plant leaf and stem alcoholic extracts was demonstrated, inhibiting the growth of fungi *Cladosporium sphaerospermum* and *Cladosporium cladosporioides* [57].

Recently, Salazar et al. carried out the biological activity determination of *C. sicyoides* supercritical extract; an in vivo test using a focal cerebral ischemia model was performed, and the extract had shown to have a neuroprotective and anti-inflammatory effect, justifying the use in traditional folk medicine for central nervous system diseases. These effects were associated to the presence of phenolic compounds in the extract [24]. Therefore, the results of these studies justify the traditional use of *C. sicyoides*, pointing to the plant extract potential benefit as a possible alternative medicine in disease treatment.

3. *Rosmarinus officinalis*

3.1 Botanical description

Rosmarinus officinalis is an aromatic plant of the Lamiaceae family, native to the Mediterranean region, and is also cultivated in Central Asia, India, Southeast Asia, South Africa, Australia, the United States, and Brazil. Today, it has been grown in many parts of the world and is commonly known as rosemary. The plant is a bush that reaches from 0.50 to 1.50 m in height, with very pungent aroma leaves and blue, violet, and white flowers (**Figure 3**) [25, 26, 58].

3.2 Chemical composition

R. officinalis chemical composition varies greatly, due to some factors that directly influence the quality, amount of oil, and extract produced. However, it is possible to verify, through the literature, that its main chemical constituents are flavones, diterpenes, steroids, and triterpenes [17, 26, 27, 31]. The phenolic compounds present in *R. officinalis* were grouped into three classes: (i) phenolic acids (vanillic, caffeic, ferulic, and rosmarinic acids), (ii) diterpenes (carnosol, rosmadial, carnosic acid, methyl carbonate, rosmanol, epirosmanol, epiisorosmanol, epirosmanol methyl ether, and epiisorosmanol ethyl ether), and (iii) flavonoids (hesperetin, apigenin, genkwanin, 4′-methoxytectochrysin, cirsimaritin, scutellarein, 4″,5,7,8-tetrahydroxyflavone, homoplantaginin, and 6-hydroxyluteolin 7-glucoside) [27]. Recently, a *R. officinalis* chromatographic analysis was carried out, which revealed two large groups: oxygenated monoterpenes and hydrocarbonated monoterpenes. The main constituents of these groups were 1,8-cineole followed by camphor, borneol, and α- and β-pinene. The oxygenated and hydrocarbonated sesquiterpenes were composed of caryophyllene and caryophyllene oxide [26]. In the supercritical extracts of *R. officinalis* leaves, chemical analysis confirmed the

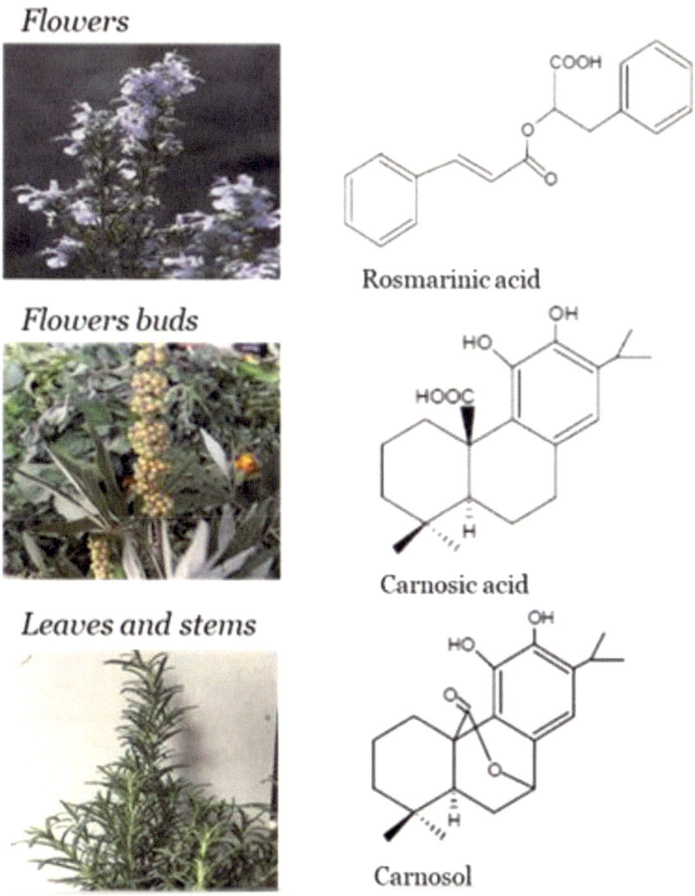

Figure 3.
Description of R. officinalis parts and the main chemical structure of the antioxidant compounds.

presence of 1,8-cineole, camphor, carnosic acid, and rosmarinic acid [17, 33, 59]. **Figure 3** shows the chemical structures of the main antioxidant compounds found in *R. officinalis*.

3.3 Antioxidant and biological activity

R. officinalis has been recognized as one of the plants with high antioxidant activity [28–30]. Its antioxidant effect is due to the phenolic compounds present in the leaves and stems [60]. Among the most effective antioxidant constituents, cyclic diterpene diphenols, carnosic acid, and carnosol were identified. In addition, its extract contains epirosmanol, rosmanol, metilcarnosato, isorosmanol, and other caffeic acid derivatives [61, 62].

The action mechanism of these compounds has been widely discussed in several studies. The carnosic acid and carnosol act as potent sequesters of peroxyl radicals and are responsible for 90% of the antioxidant properties, where both are inhibitors of lipid peroxidation in liposomal and microsomal systems, besides being good sequestrants of hydroxyl radicals. Specifically, carnosic acid removes hydrogen peroxide but may also act as a substrate for its ability to increase or maintain the superoxide dismutase and glutathione peroxidase activities. The most important elements in the *R. officinalis* structure are the diterpenes containing the aromatic ring (C_{11}–C_{12}) in the catechol group, with the conjugation of three basic rings. The catechol group is responsible for eliminating the radical electrons formed as an oxidation result. Lactone carnosol, rosmarinic acid, and hesperetin were cited in the literature as important FRSs [31, 63–65]. Rosmarinic acid has two aromatic rings, each with two OH groups that are capable of donating hydrogen and chelating metals [66]. Caffeic acid derivatives may act as metal ion chelators (Fe^{2+}), thus reducing the formation of ROS [67].

The antioxidant of *R. officinalis* extracts obtained in SFE was confirmed. Carvalho et al. analyzed the plant antioxidant activity through a coupled reaction of β-carotene and linoleic acid; the results indicated that the extracts obtained at high pressures and low temperature (300 bar/40°C) exhibited the highest antioxidant activities, in comparison to extracts obtained in low pressures (150 bar/30°C). In any case, antioxidant activities were always above the control used (β-carotene and linolenic acid) as shown in **Figure 4**. The authors state that the antioxidant action remained approximately constant for the 3-h reaction for all extracts tested. The major compounds detected in the extracts were camphor (0.6% d.b.) and 1,8-cineol (0.043% d.b.). The extract obtained by hydrodistillation showed the highest yield of camphor (1.22% d.b.) and 1,8 cineol (0.23% d.b.) compared to other extraction methods (SFE and Soxhlet) [33].

Thus, the antioxidant capacity of *R. officinalis* leaf and stem extract obtained with supercritical CO_2 was also evaluated by the ORAC method. The extract showed a high antioxidant capacity (1.9 mol Trolox/mg) similar to that of BHT and vitamin E (2.8–3.0 mol Trolox/mg). In addition, the extract presented a high percentage of lipid oxidation inhibition (88%) of fatty acids present in an analyzed cosmetic foundation. The extract volatile fraction was characterized by compounds such as camphor, 1,8-cineol, and trans-β-caryophyllene present in relative amounts of less than 25% [59].

Due to antioxidant properties, *R. officinalis* has been used in food preservation and in disease treatment. In food preservation, components such as rosmanol and carnosol prevent oxidation and microbial contamination and also can be up to four times more effective than BHA and equal to BHT as an antioxidant [27, 68, 69]. Different studies have demonstrated the potent activity of *R. officinalis* in inhibiting the formation of hydroperoxides, reducing carotenoid color loss, and retarding lipid oxidation in corn [78] and hazelnut oils [70].

The *R. officinalis* extract has been successfully commercially exploited as a natural antioxidant, for its use as synthetic antioxidants such as BHA, BHT, and TBHQ, in the food industry and is severely restricted as they may have carcinogenic effects on living organisms [5, 16, 17]. In this way, *R. officinalis* extract may be useful to

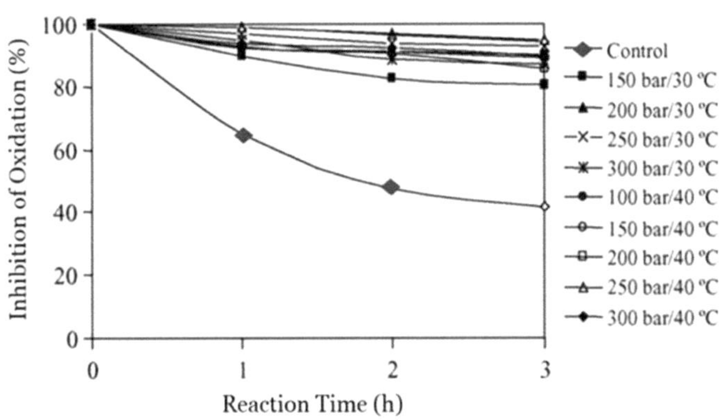

Figure 4.
Antioxidant activity of R. officinalis extracts obtained with supercritical CO_2 [38].

replace or even decrease the synthetic antioxidants in foods. As preservatives, the extracts offer several technological advantages and benefits to consumers [71].

Health problems derived from lipid oxidation have attracted consumers' and researchers' attention, since numerous diseases are linked to dietary and biological lipid oxidation products. Therefore, *R. officinalis* extracts have been related to several biological activities, such as anticancer, antidiuretic, anti-inflammatory, antibacterial, antidiabetic, antiangiogenic, antioxidant, and hepatoprotective [28, 71–74], besides allowing the use of the plant in the treatment and/or prevention of Alzheimer's disease, urinary and gastrointestinal infections, diabetes, aging, ischemia, and atherosclerosis [25, 32].

Among the most important groups of compounds isolated from the plant, phenolic diterpenes account most of their biological activity. These compounds have been indicated in recent years as inhibitors of neuronal cell-induced death by a variety of agents both in vitro and in vivo, confirming the therapeutic potential of these compounds for Alzheimer's disease, due to the compounds multifunctional nature in the neuronal protection mediated by the plant antioxidant activity [32].

Several studies show that *R. officinalis* has pharmacological activity for chemoprevention and cancer therapy. In the extract antiproliferative activity evaluation against human ovarian cancer cells, it was corroborated that the extract inhibited the proliferation of cancer cell lines, affecting the cell cycle in multiple phases. In addition, it induced apoptosis by modifying the multiple gene expression that regulates apoptosis. Thus, the extract can be considered as an adjuvant to chemotherapy [62]. Also, the antiangiogenic effect of the carnosic acid present in *R. officinalis* extract was corroborated in angiogenesis models using human umbilical vein endothelial cells in relation to the tube formation in the reconstituted basement membrane, chemotaxis, and proliferation. Carnosic acid from the extract may be useful in preventing disorders due to angiogenesis, and its antiangiogenic effect may contribute to a neuroprotective effect [72].

The actions of *R. officinalis* leaf ethanolic extract obtained with Soxhlet extraction were tested in glucose homeostasis and antioxidant defense in rabbits. Serum levels, glucose levels and insulin levels were studied in diabetic rabbits (alloxan was used to induce diabetes); it was shown that at a dose of 200 mg/kg was possible to reduce the blood glucose level and to increase the serum insulin concentration. In addition, during 1 week of animal treatment with the extract, it was demonstrated that it had an ability to inhibit lipid peroxidation and to activate the antioxidant enzymes. Due to its potent antioxidant properties, the plant extract has a remarkable antidiabetogenic effect [75]. Recently, the antidiabetic and antihypercholesterolemic action of flavonoid-rich fractions of *R. officinalis* (fractions obtained with n-butanol and diethyl ether) in diabetic mice induced by streptozotocin was evaluated. Both fractions showed a decrease in the glucose level at a dose of 400 mg/kg, especially the fraction obtained with diethyl ether; plasma glucose levels decreased up to 60.38%. The pancreas histopathological study showed that both fractions regenerated the pancreatic β cells and increased the mass of islets. *R. officinalis* fractions exhibited a potent antidiabetic effect, while the fraction obtained with n-butanol showed a high anti-hypercholesterolemic activity [76].

The anti-inflammatory activity of *R. officinalis* supercritical extracts was studied. Absorptions of extract fractions were tested on monolayers of Caco-2 cells (2–12 h of incubation). Human macrophages were treated with basolateral fractions, and TNF-α, IL-1β, IL-6, and IL-10 secretions were measured by ELISA. Fractions obtained after 8 and 12 h in absorption experiments caused a considerable reduction in the excretion of pro-inflammatory cytokines. This reduction in cytokine secretion levels was associated with the amounts of carnosol and carnosic acid. Thus, the *R. officinalis* supercritical extract can be used in formulations to inflammatory disease prevention [77].

In relation to the antibacterial activity, *R. officinalis* essential oils obtained by hydrodistillation exhibited antibacterial activity against *Escherichia coli*, *Salmonella typhi*, *S. enteritidis*, and *Shigella sonnei*; this activity was associated with the oil ability to reduce DPPH radical formation (CI_{50} = 3.82 μg/ml) [61]. However, the antibacterial and antifungal activities of *R. officinalis* leaf extracts obtained by SFE extraction were confirmed, and the extracts showed antibacterial activity against Gram-positive bacteria (*Staphylococcus aureus* and *Bacillus cereus*) and Gram-negative bacteria (*Escherichia coli* and *Pseudomonas aeruginosa*) and antifungals against *Candida albicans*. Obtaining *R. officinalis* extracts by SFE has been shown to be a promising extraction with respect to its incorporation into various foods, cosmetics, and pharmaceuticals products that a natural aroma, color, and antioxidant/antimicrobial additive are desired. These properties are also necessary for the food industry in order to find possible alternatives to synthetic preservatives [17].

4. Supercritical fluid extraction (SFE) of antioxidant compounds from plant matrices

When a new extract from a natural source is tested, the most important aspects to take into account are the extraction method and the type of solvent used, as this will affect the antioxidant properties. Several extraction methods for the selective extraction from plant matrices such as *R. officinalis* were identified in the scientific literature [71].

Thus, the bioactive compound extraction has been considered one of the most important steps in the approach of obtaining or recovering bioactive compounds. Conventional extractions have been the most used technology for these compound recovery. It is based on the extraction power of different solvents and the application of high temperatures, promoting mass transfer. However, there are drawbacks associated with conventional extraction processes such as the use of large amounts of organic solvents, toxic to human health and the environment, extraction time, and the use of high temperatures that can degrade the thermosensitive compounds [6, 8]. They motivated the search for environmentally safe extraction techniques such as microwave-assisted extraction (MAE), ultrasonic-assisted extraction (UAE), pressurized liquid extraction (PLE), and supercritical fluid extraction (SFE) [36, 78]. SFE has already been studied to obtain antioxidant compounds from natural sources [21, 33, 77, 79]. **Table 1** presents the antioxidant activity values of different plant extracts obtained with SFE, involving the plants under study (*C. sicyoides* and *R. officinalis*).

4.1 SFE procedure

A solvent is considered a supercritical fluid when the pressure and temperature of the system are above its critical point. This point is defined as the highest temperature and pressure at which a substance can exist in equilibrium between the liquid and vapor phases. Above its critical temperature (Tc) and critical pressure (Pc), the supercritical fluid can be considered as an expanded liquid or as a compressed gas, whose density (ρ) is relatively high and consequently has a high solvency power. This effect gives the solvent a certain degree of selectivity, in addition to allowing easy separation of the solvent from the solute, which can be achieved by a simple system depressurizing, resulting in products totally solvent-free and without thermal degradation of the compounds of interest, due to low operating temperatures [35, 38].

Plants	Extraction conditions	Solvents	Method of determination	Antioxidant capacity	Biological Activity	Refs.
C. sicyoides	40°C/400 bar	CO_2 + 10% of ethanol	DPPH	404.81 ± 2.78 EC_{50}: g of extract/g of DPPH	Neuroprotective and anti-inflammatory effect	[29]
R. officinalis	40°C/300 bar	CO_2	DPPH	12.85 ± 0.10 IC_{50}: µg.ml^{-1}	Antioxidant, antibacterial, and antifungal	[21]
	100°C/350 bar	CO_2	DPPH	0.23 ± 0.01 IC_{50}: mg/ml	Antioxidant	[84]
	50°C/300 bar	CO_2	ORAC	1.9 ± 0.10 µmol Trolox/mg extract	Antioxidant	[59]
Mangifera indica L.	55°C/100 bar	CO_2 + 20% of ethanol	DPPH	2.13 ± 0.24 EC_{50}: DPPH µg/µg dry extract	Antioxidant	[85]
Eugenia uniflora L.	60°C/400 bar	CO_2 + ethanol	DPPH	>200 EC_{50} (µg/ml)	Antioxidant	[86]
Raphanus sativus L.	35°C/400 bar	CO_2	DPPH	359 mg TE/100 g dry extract	Antioxidant and anti-inflammatory	[37]
Piper nigrum L	40°C/300 bar	CO_2	DPPH	103.28 EC_{50}: of µg.ml^{-1}	Antioxidant	[87]

Table 1.
Presentation of the antioxidant activity values of different plant extracts obtained with SFE, involving the plants under study (C. sicyoides and R. officinalis).

One of the most commonly used solvents in SFE is carbon dioxide (CO_2) because its critical points are moderate (Tc = 31.1°C, Pc = 73.8 bar, and critical density (ρc) = 0.468 g/cm^3), nontoxic, non-flammable, affordable, chemically inert, and apolar and has an ideal behavior for thermosensitive compound extraction [34, 37]. In addition to the supercritical CO_2 (Sc-CO_2), there are other substances that are also used as supercritical fluids, as shown in **Table 2**.

Due to its low polarity, Sc-CO_2 presents a limitation to dissolve polar molecules. However, this disadvantage can be solved by the addition of polar solvents, called modifiers or cosolvents, which modify the supercritical fluid polarity and, consequently, improve the extraction of polar fractions rich in bioactive substances, such as phenol compounds related to high antioxidant activity [37, 38]. Methanol is the solvent most used as a modifier for various plant matrices, but it is toxic and

Fluid	Tc (°C)	Pc (bar)	ρ_c (g/cm^3)
Nitrous oxide (N_2O)	36.5	71.0	0.457
Ethane (C_2H_6)	32.2	48.8	0.203
Propane (C_3H_8)	96.7	42.5	0.220
Propylene (C_3H_6)	91.9	46.2	0.230
Benzene (C_6H_6)	289.0	48.9	0.302
Toluene (C_7H_8)	318.6	41.1	0.290
Ammonia (NH_3)	132.5	112.8	0.240
Water (H_2O)	374.2	220.5	0.272

Table 2.
Critical properties of some substances used as solvents in supercritical extraction processes.

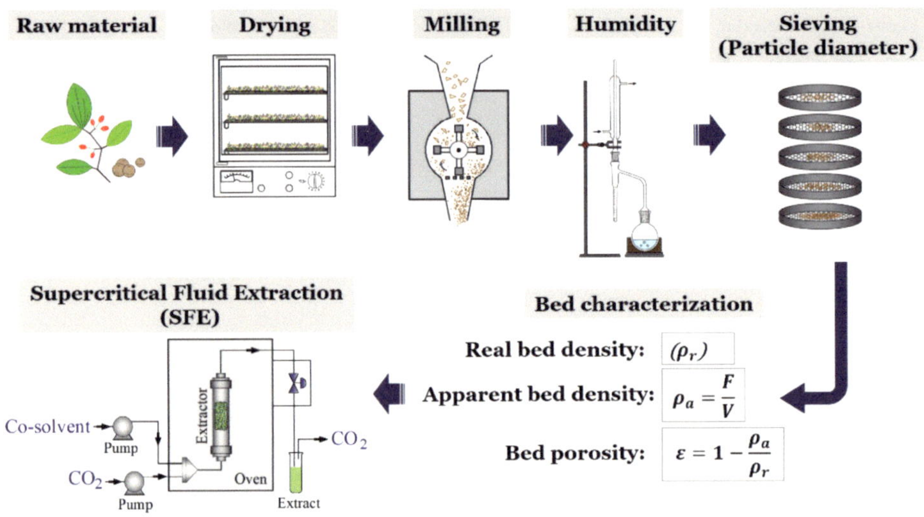

Figure 5.
Scheme of the SFE procedure of plant matrices.

different from ethanol, which is an environmentally safe solvent being a good choice for SFE processes, and can be used in the extraction of natural products [80, 81]. Water is also a very attractive cosolvent for natural product extraction due to its high polarity, which considerably increases the polarity of Sc-CO_2 [79].

For antioxidant compound extraction and recovery by SFE, several vegetable matrices were used, such as seeds, fruits, leaves, flowers, rhizomes, roots, fruit peels, and tree branches. The SFE process consists basically in the extraction of soluble compounds present in the solid matrix by a supercritical solvent and then separates these compounds from the solvent after depressurizing the system. In order to achieve an efficient and adequate extraction, several factors must be taken into account, having a careful control of the operating conditions and process step optimization [35, 36, 82].

Initially, the raw material must pass through a pretreatment stage before being fed into the fixed bed extractor; this procedure is performed to prepare the solid particles, allowing a greater efficiency to be achieved in the extraction process [83]. As shown in **Figure 5**, after the raw material is collected, one of the first stages of its pretreatment is the solid matrix moisture reduction, for example, drying leaves in an oven with air circulation. Generally, the plant matrix moisture should not exceed 14% (wet basis). Another important step is the moisture content determination by the distillation method of the Jacobs immiscible solvent, with the purpose of knowing if the quantity of water in the sample is adequate for the supercritical extraction process. The sieving stage is applied to standardize and determine the average particle size of the solid particles. The real and apparent density and bed porosity determination is also very important as they affect the particles packaging in the extraction vessel and consequently the solvent flow and the mass and heat transfer processes [35, 82].

After a suitable pretreatment, the solid matrix is placed in an extraction vessel forming a fixed bed. Depending on the compounds of interest, the supercritical solvent (Sc-CO_2) or solvent + cosolvent is fed by the solvent pump and/or cosolvent into the extraction vessel, where it continuously flows through the fixed bed and dissolves the extractable components from the solid matrix. The mixture of solutes that is removed from the solid matrix is called extract. In the separation step, the mixture formed by the solvent extraction + extract leaves the vessel and feeds the separator (collection flask) where the mixture is separated by rapid reduction of pressure (ambient pressure). The extract precipitates in the separator, and the solvent is removed from the system [38, 83].

5. Conclusion

The identification of new natural antioxidant compounds is of great interest to the food, pharmaceutical, and cosmetic industry in order to find possible alternatives to synthetic antioxidants. In this way, plants such as *C. sicyoides* and *R. officinalis* have been extensively studied for their antioxidant activity. The *C. sicyoides* extract obtained by SFE has a neuroprotective and anti-inflammatory effect; these effects are associated with the presence of phenolic compounds and the high antioxidant activity in the extract. *R. officinalis* extract is antibacterial, antifungal, anti-inflammatory, and effective, associated with the presence of carnosic acid, carnosol, rosmarinic acids, and hesperetin. It has been corroborated that these plants contain chemical compounds that exhibit the capacity of FRSs and reduce the onset of different diseases. Finally, obtaining extracts from plant matrices using environmentally safe extraction technology such as SFE represents a great opportunity to obtain bioactive compounds.

Acknowledgements

Mar Salazar (Process Number: 1777277) thanks CAPES for the doctorate scholarship.

Conflict of interest

The authors have no conflict of interest to declare and are responsible for the content and writing of the manuscript.

Author details

Marielba de los Angeles Rodriguez Salazar*, Glides Rafael Olivo Urbina, Priscila do Nascimento Bezerra, Vânia Maria Borges Cunha, Marcilene Paiva da Silva, Flávia Cristina Seabra Pires, Ana Paula de Souza e Silva, Sérgio Henrique Brabo de Sousa and Raul Nunes de Carvalho Jr
LABEX/FEA (Faculty of Food Engineering), Federal University of Para, Belém, Pará, Brazil

*Address all correspondence to: marielba434@hotmail.com

References

[1] Souza JNS, Silva EM, Loir A, Rees JF, Rogez H, Larondelle Y. Antioxidant capacity of four polyphenol-rich Amazonian plant extracts: A correlation study using chemical and biological in vitro assays. Food Chemistry. 2008;**106**(1):331-339. DOI: 10.1016/j.foodchem.2007.05.011

[2] Virgolin LB, Seixas FRF, Janzantti NS. Composition, content of bioactive compounds, and antioxidant activity of fruit pulps from the Brazilian Amazon biome. Pesquisa Agropecuaria Brasileira. 2017;**52**(10):933-941. DOI: 10.1590/S0100-204X2017001000013

[3] Ekor M. The growing use of herbal medicines: Issues relating to adverse reactions and challenges in monitoring safety. Frontiers in Neurology. 2014;**4**: 1-10. DOI: 10.3389/fphar.2013.00177

[4] Alcantara RGL, Joaquim RHVT, Sampaio SF. Plantas medicinais: O conhecimento e uso popular. Revista de APS. 2015;**18**(4):470-482

[5] Damodaran S, Parkin K, Fennema OR. Fennema's Food Chemistry. 4th ed. New York, Boca Raton: CRC Press/Taylor & Francis; 2008. 1144 p

[6] Dai J, Mumper RJ. Plant phenolics: Extraction, analysis and thcir antioxidant and anticancer properties. Molecules. 2010;**15**:7313-7352. DOI: 10.3390/molecules15107313

[7] Khoddami A, Wilkes MA, Roberts TH. Techniques for analysis of plant phenolic compounds. Molecules. 2013;**18**:2328-2375. DOI: 10.3390/molecules18022328

[8] Khaw K, Parat M, Shaw PN, Falconer JR. Solvent supercritical fluid technologies to extract bioactive compounds from natural sources: A review. Molecules. 2017;**22**:2-22. DOI: 10.3390/molecules22071186

[9] Halliwell B. The definition and measurement of antioxidants in biological systems. Free Radical Biology & Medicine. 1995;**18**(I):125-126

[10] Droge W. Free radicals in the physiological control of cell function. Physiological Reviews. 2002;**82**:47-95

[11] Sies H. Physiological society symposium: Impaired endothelial and smooth muscle cell function in oxidative stress oxidative stress: Oxidants and antioxidants. Experitnental Physiology. 1996;**82**:291-295

[12] Maleki D, Rad AH, Khalili L, Alipour B. Antioxidants and natural compounds. In: Gowder SJT, editor. Basic Principles and Clinical Significance of Oxidative Stress. London: IntechOpen; 2015. DOI: 10.5772/59293

[13] Xu D, Li Y, Meng X, Zhou T, Zhou Y, Zheng J, et al. Natural antioxidants in foods and medicinal plants: Extraction, assessment and resources. International Journal of Molecular Sciences. 2017;**18**:20-32. DOI: 10.3390/ijms18010096

[14] Halliwell B, Gutteridge JMC. The importance of free radicals and catalytic metal ions in human diseases. Molecular Aspects of Medicine. 1985;**8**:89-193

[15] Thomas MJ. The role of free radicals and antioxidants. Nutrition. 2000;**16**:716-718

[16] Gachkar L, Yadegari D, Rezaei MB, Taghizadeh M, Astaneh SA, Rasoli I. Chemical and biological characteristics of *Cuminum cyminum* and *Rosmarinus officinalis* essential oils. Food Chemistry. 2007;**102**:898-904. DOI: 10.1016/j.foodchem.2006.06.035

[17] Genena AK, Hense H, Smania Junior A, Souza SM. Rosemary

(*Rosmarinus officinalis*)—A study of the composition , antioxidant and antimicrobial activities of extracts obtained with supercritical carbon dioxide. Ciência e Tecnologia de Alimentos. 2008;**28**(2):463-469

[18] Shahidi F. Antioxidants: Principles and applications. In: Shahidi F, editor. Handbook of Antioxidants for Food Preservation. 1st ed. United Kingdom: Elsevier Ltd; 2015. p. 514. DOI: 10.1016/B978-1-78242-089-7.00001-4

[19] Drobnik J, de Oliveira AB. *Cissus verticillata* (L.) Nicolson and C.E. Jarvis (Vitaceae): Its identification and usage in the sources from 16th to 19th century. Journal of Ethnopharmacology. 2015;**171**:317-329. DOI: 10.1016/j.jep.2015.06.003

[20] Pires FCS, Almeida MM, Silva APS, Salazar MAR, Urbina GRO, Silva PS. Therapeutic potential of extracts from Amazonian plants with antimicrobial activity. In: Méndez-Vilas A, editor. Antimicrobial Research: Novel Bioknowledge and Educational Programs. 6th ed. Badajoz: Formatex Research Center; 2017. pp. 504-515

[21] Beltrame F, Ferreira A, Cortez D. Coumarin glycoside from *Cissus sicyoides*. Natural Product Letters. 2002;**16**(4):213-216. DOI: 10.1080/10.575630290015736

[22] Xu F, Matsuda H, Hata H, Sugawara K, Nakamura S, Yoshikawa M. Structures of new flavonoids and benzofuran-type stilbene and degranulation inhibitors of rat basophilic leukemia cells from the Brazilian herbal medicine *Cissus sicyoides*. Chemical and Pharmaceutical Bulletin. 2009;**57**(10):1089-1095. DOI: 10.1248/cpb.57.1089

[23] Beserra FP, de Cássia Santos R, Périco LL, Rodrigues VP, de Almeida Kiguti LR, Saldanha LL, et al. *Cissus sicyoides*: Pharmacological mechanisms involved in the anti-inflammatory and antidiarrheal activities. International Journal of Molecular Sciences. 2016;**17**(2):1-15. DOI: 10.3390/ijms17020149

[24] Salazar MAR, Costa JV, Olivo GRU, Cunha VMB, Silva MP, Bezerra PN, et al. Chemical composition, antioxidant activity, neuroprotective and anti-inflammatory effects of cipó-pucá (*Cissus sicyoides* L .) extracts obtained from supercritical extraction. The Journal of Supercritical Fluids. 2018;**138**:36-45. DOI: 10.1016/j.supflu.2018.03.022

[25] Machado DG, Cunha MP, Neis VB, Balen GO, Colla AR, Grando J, et al. *Rosmarinus officinalis* L . Hydroalcoholic extract , similar to fluoxetine , reverses depressive-like behavior without altering learning deficit in olfactory bulbectomized mice. Journal of Ethnopharmacology. 2012;**143**:158-169. DOI: 10.1016/j.jep.2012.06.017

[26] Hannour K, Boughdad A, Maataoui A, Bouchelta A. Chemical composition of Rosmarinus officinalis (Lamiaceae) essential oils and evaluation of their toxicity against Bruchus rufimanus (Coleoptera: Chrysomelidae - Bruchinae) in Morocco. International Journal of Tropical Insect Sciences. 2018;**38**:192-204. DOI: 10.1017/S1742758418000012

[27] Cuvelier M, Richard H, Berset C. Antioxidative activity and phenolic composition of pilot-plant and commercial extracts of sage and rosemary. Journal of the American Oil Chemists' Society. 1996;**73**:645-652

[28] Haloui M, Louedec L, Michel J, Lyoussi B. Experimental diuretic effects of *Rosmarinus officinalis* and *Centaurium erythraea*. Journal of Ethnopharmacology. 2000;**71**:465-472

[29] Zheng W, Wang SY. Antioxidant activity and phenolic compounds in

selected herbs antioxidant activity and phenolic compounds in selected herbs. Journal of Agricultura and Food Chemistry. 2001;**49**(11):5165-5170. DOI: 10.1021/jf010697n

[30] Moreno S, Scheyer T, Romano CS, Vojnov AA. Antioxidant and antimicrobial activities of rosemary extracts linked to their polyphenol composition. Free Radical Research. 2006;**40**:223-231. DOI: 10.1080/10715760500473834

[31] Kontogianni VG, Tomic G, Nikolic I, Nerantzaki AA, Sayyad N, Stosic-grujicic S, et al. Phytochemical profile of *Rosmarinus officinalis* and *Salvia officinalis* extracts and correlation to their antioxidant and anti-proliferative activity. Food Chemistry. 2013;**136**(1):120-129. DOI: 10.1016/j.foodchem.2012.07.091

[32] Habtemariam S. The therapeutic potential of rosemary (*Rosmarinus officinalis*) diterpenes for alzheimer's disease. Evidence-Based Complementary and Alternative Medicine. 2016;**2016**:1-14. DOI: 10.1155/2016/2680409

[33] Carvalho RN Jr, Moura LS, Rosa PTV, Meireles MAA. Supercritical fluid extraction from rosemary (*Rosmarinus officinalis*): Kinetic data, extract's global yield, composition, and antioxidant activity. The Journal of Supercritical Fluids. 2005;**35**(3):197-204. DOI: 10.1016/j.supflu.2005.01.009

[34] Brunner G. Supercritical fluids: Technology and application to food processing. Journal Food Engineering. 2005;**67**(1-2):21-33. DOI: 10.1016/j.jfoodeng.2004.05.060

[35] Pereira CG, Meireles MAA. Supercritical fluid extraction of bioactive compounds: Fundamentals, applications and economic perspectives. Food and Bioprocess Technology. 2010;**3**(3):340-372. DOI: 10.1007/s11947-009-0263-2

[36] Herrero M, Castro-Puyana M, Mendiola JA, Ibañez E. Compressed fluids for the extraction of bioactive compounds. Trends in Analytical Chemistry. 2013;**43**(2):67-83. DOI: 10.1016/j.trac.2012.12.008

[37] Goyeneche R, Fanovich A, Rodrigues CR, Nicolao MC, Discala K. Supercritical CO2 extraction of bioactive compounds from radish leaves: Yield, antioxidant capacity and cytotoxicity. The Journal of Supercritical Fluids. 2018;**135**:78-83. DOI: 10.1016/j.supflu.2018.01.004

[38] de Melo MMR, Silvestre AJD, Silva CM. Supercritical fluid extraction of vegetable matrices: Applications, trends and future perspectives of a convincing green technology. The Journal of Supercritical Fluids. 2014;**92**:115-176. DOI: 10.1016/j.supflu.2014.04.007

[39] da Silva GA, de Almeida-Muradian LB, Akisue G, Ferro VO. Padronização do extrato de *Cissus sicyoides* L. (insulina vegetal) e identificação de carotenos. Revista Brasileira de Farmacognosia. 1996;**1**:96-112

[40] Quílez AM, Saenz MT, García MD, de la Puerta R. Phytochemical analysis and anti-allergic study of *Agave intermixta* Trel. and *Cissus sicyoides* L. Journal Pharmacy Pharmacology. 2004;**56**(9):1185-1189. DOI: 10.1211/0022357044102

[41] de Oliveira AB, de Mendonça MS, Azevedo AA, Meira RMSA. Anatomy and histochemistry of the vegetative organs of *Cissus verticillata*—A native medicinal plant of the Brazilian Amazon. Brazilian Journal of Pharmacognosy. 2012;**22**(6):1201-1211. DOI: 10.1590/S0102-695X2012005000092

[42] Toledo MCF, Reyes FGR, Iaderoza M, Francis FJ, Draetta S. Anthocyanins from anil trepador (*Cissus sicyoides*, Linn.). Journal of Food Science. 1983;**48**:1368

[43] El-shafey MM, Abd-allah GM, Mohamadin AM, Harisa GI, Mariee AD. Quercetin protects against acetaminophen-induced hepatorenal toxicity by reducing reactive oxygen and nitrogen species. Pathophysiology. 2015;**22**(1):49-55. DOI: 10.1016/j.pathophys.2014.12.002

[44] Crespo I, García-Mediavilla MV, Almar M, González P, Tunón MJ, Sánchez-Campos S, et al. Differential effects of dietary flavonoids on reactive oxygen and nitrogen species generation and changes in antioxidant enzyme expression induced by proinflammatory cytokines in chang liver cells. Food and Chemical Toxicology. 2008;**46**:1555-1569. DOI: 10.1016/j.fct.2007.12.014

[45] Perrone D, Fuggetta MPIA, Ardito F, Cottarelli A, Filippis ADE, Ravagnan G, et al. Resveratrol (3,5,4′-trihydroxystilbene) and its properties in oral diseases (review). Experimental and Therapeutic Medicine. 2017;**14**:3-9. DOI: 10.3892/etm.2017.4472

[46] Bolkenius FN, Verne-mismer J, Wagner J, Grisar JM. Amphiphilic cY-tocopherol analogues as inhibitors of brain lipid peroxidation. European Journal of Pharmacology. 1996;**298**:37-43

[47] Khalil NM, Pepato MT, Brunetti IL. Free radical scavenging profile and myeloperoxidase inhibition of extracts from antidiabetic plants: *Bauhinia forficata* and *Cissus sicyoides*. Biological Research. 2008;**41**(2):165-171. DOI: 10.4067/S0716-97602008000200006

[48] Pepato MT, Baviera AM, Vendramini RC, da Silva Perez MDP, Kettelhut ID. *Cissus sicyoides* (princess vine) in the long-term treatment of streptozotocin-diabetic rats. Biotechnology and Applied Biochemistry. 2003;**37**(Part 1):15-20. DOI: 10.1042/BA20020065

[49] Viana GSB, Medeiros ACC, Lacerda AMR, Leal LKAM, Vale TG, Matos FJDA. Hypoglycemic and anti-lipemic effects of the aqueous extract from *Cissus sicyoides*. BMC Pharmacology. 2004;**4**:1-7. DOI: 10.1186/1471-2210-4-9

[50] Fernandes G, Banu J. Medicinal properties of plants from the genus Cissus: A review. Journal of Medicinal Plants Research. 2012;**6**(16):3080-3086. DOI: 10.5897/JMPR11.1637

[51] Sáenz MT, Garcia MD, Quilez A, Ahumada MC. Cytotoxic activity of *Agave intermixta* L. (Agavaceae) and *Cissus sicyoides* L. (Vitaceae). Phytotherapy Research. 2000;**14**:552-554

[52] Lucena FRS, Almeida ER, Aguiar JS, Silva TG, Souza VMO, Nascimento SC. Cytotoxic, antitumor and leukocyte migration activities of resveratrol and sitosterol present in the hidroalcoholic extract of *Cissus sicyoides* L., Vitaceae, leaves. Brazilian Journal of Pharmacognosy. 2010;**20**(5):729-733. DOI: 10.1590/S0102-695X2010005000002

[53] García MD, Quílez AM, Sáenz MT, Martínez-Domínguez ME, De La Puerta R. Anti-inflammatory activity of *Agave intermixta* Trel. and *Cissus sicyoides* L., species used in the caribbean traditional medicine. Journal of Ethnopharmacology. 2000;**71**(3):395-400. DOI: 10.1016/S0378-8741(00)00160-4

[54] García X, Cartas-Heredia L, Lorenzana-Jímenez M, Gijón E. Vasoconstrictor effect of *Cissus sicyoides* on Guinea-pig aortic rings. General Pharmacology. 1997;**29**(3):457-462. DOI: 10.1016/S0306-3623(96)00478-8

[55] Santos HB, Modesto-filho J, Diniz M de FF, Vasconcelos THC, Pereira FS de B, Ramalho J do A, et al. Artigo avaliação do efeito hipoglicemiante de *Cissus sicyoides* em estudos clínicos fase

II. Brazilian Journal of Pharmacognosy. 2008;**18**(1):70-76

[56] Garcia M, Saenz MT, Puerta R, Quilez A, Fernandez MA. Antibacterial activity of *Agave intermixta* and *Cissus sicyoides*. Fitoterapia. 1999;**70**:71-73. DOI: 10.1016/S0367-326X(98)00009-4

[57] Silva L, Carreira RC, Oniki GH, Agripino DG, Young MCM, Ladeira AM. Crescimento e análise do potencial antifúngico em plantas de *Cissus verticillata* (L.) Nicolson & Jarvis (Vitaceae). Revista Brasileira de Plantas Medicinais. 2007;**9**(1):73-79

[58] Brender T, Gruenwald J, Jaenicke C. Herbal Remedies. 2nd ed. Berlin: Schaper & Brümmer GmbH & Co., Salzgitter; 1997

[59] Rodríguez EA, Árias AJ, Vásquez EG, Martínez JR, Stashenko EE. Rendimiento y capacidad antioxidante de extractos de *Rosmarinus officinalis*, *Salvia officinalis* y *Psidium guajava* obtenidos con CO_2 supercrítico. Revista de la Academia Colombiana de Universidad del Zulia. 2012;**XXXVI**:305-315

[60] Govaris A, Florou-paneri P, Botsoglou E, Giannenas I, Amvrosiadis I, Botsoglou N. The inhibitory potential of feed supplementation with rosemary and/or a-tocopheryl acetate on microbial growth and lipid oxidation of Turkey breast during refrigerated storage. Lebensmittel-Wissenschaft & Technologie. 2007;**40**:331-337. DOI: 10.1016/j.lwt.2005.10.006

[61] Bozin B, Mimica-Dukic N, Samojlik I, Jovin E. Antimicrobial and antioxidant properties of rosemary and sage (*Rosmarinus officinalis* L. and *Salvia officinalis* L., Lamiaceae) essential oils. Journal of Agricultura and Food Chemistry. 2007;**55**:7879-7885. DOI: 10.1021/jf0715323

[62] Tai J, Cheung S, Wu M, Hasman D. Antiproliferation effect of rosemary (*Rosmarinus officinalis*) on human ovarian cancer cells in vitro. Phytomedicine. 2012;**19**(5):436-443. DOI: 10.1016/j.phymed.2011.12.012

[63] Munne-Bosch S, Alegre L. Subcellular compartmentation of the diterpene carnosic acid and its derivatives in the leaves of rosemary. Plant Physiology. 2001;**125**(2):1094-1102. DOI: 10.1104/pp.125.2.1094

[64] Wijeratne SSK, Cuppett SL. Potential of rosemary (*Rosemarinus officinalis* L.) diterpenes in preventing lipid hydroperoxide-mediated oxidative stress in Caco-2 cells. Journal of Agricultural and Food Chemistry. 2007;**55**(4):1193-1199. DOI: 10.1021/jf063089m

[65] Cui L, Kim MO, Seo JH, Kim IS, Kim NY, Lee SH, et al. Abietane diterpenoids of *Rosmarinus officinalis* and their diacylglycerol acyltransferase-inhibitory activity. Food Chemistry. 2012;**132**(4):1775-1780. DOI: 10.1016/j.foodchem.2011.11.138

[66] Hras AR, Hadolin M, Knez Z, Bauman D. Comparison of antioxidative and synergistic effects of rosemary extract with α-tocopherol, ascorbyl palmitate and citric acid in sunflower oil. Food Chemistry. 2000;**71**:229-233

[67] Fang X, Wada S. Enhancing the antioxidant effect of α-tocopherol with rosemary in inhibiting catalyzed oxidation caused by Fe^{2+} and hemoprotein. Food Research International. 1993;**26**(6):405-411. DOI: 10.1016/0963-9969(93)90086-X

[68] Nakatani N, Inatani R. Two antioxidative diterpenes from rosemary (*Rosmarinus officinalis* L .) and a revised structure for rosmanolf. Agricultural and Biological Chemistry. 1984;**48**:2081-2085

[69] Houlihan CM, Ho CT, Chang SS. The structure of rosmariquinone—A new antioxidant isolated from *Rosmarinus officinalis* L. Journal of the American Oil Chemists' Society. 1985;**62**(1):96-98. DOI: 10.1007/BF02541500

[70] Tohma S, Turan S. Rosemary plant (*Rosmarinus officinalis* L.), solvent extract and essential oil can be used to extend the usage life of hazelnut oil during deep frying. European Journal of Lipd Science and Technology. 2015;**117**:1978-1990. DOI: 10.1002/ejlt.201400382

[71] Nieto G, Ros G, Castillo J. Antioxidant and antimicrobial properties of rosemary (*Rosmarinus officinalis* L.): A review. Medicine. 2018;**5**(3):98. DOI: 10.3390/medicines5030098

[72] Kayashima TK, Matsubara KM. Antiangiogenic effect of carnosic acid and carnosol, neuroprotective compounds in rosemary leaves. Bioscience Biotechnology Biochemistry. 2012;**76**(1):115-119. DOI: 10.1271/bbb.110584

[73] Al-attar AM, Shawush NA. Influence of olive and rosemary leaves extracts on chemically induced liver cirrhosis in male rats. Saudi Journal of Biological Sciences. 2015;**22**(2):157-163. DOI: 10.1016/j.sjbs.2014.08.005

[74] Nieto G. Biological activities of three essential oils of the Lamiaceae family. Medicine. 2017;**4**(63):1-10. DOI: 10.3390/medicines4030063

[75] Bakirel T, Bakirel U, Keleş OÜ, Ülgen SG, Yardibi H. In vivo assessment of antidiabetic and antioxidant activities of rosemary (*Rosmarinus officinalis*) in alloxan-diabetic rabbits. Journal of Ethnopharmacology. 2008;**116**(1):64-73. DOI: 10.1016/j.jep.2007.10.039

[76] Belmouhoub M, Chebout I, Iguer-ouada M. Antidiabetic and anti-hypercholesterolemic effects of flavonoid-rich fractions of Rosmarinus officinalis in streptozotocin-induced diabetes in mice. Phytothérapie. 2017:1-7. DOI: 10.1007/s10298-017-1103-6

[77] Arranz E, Mes J, Wichers HJ, Jaime L, Mendiola JA, Reglero G, et al. Anti-inflammatory activity of the basolateral fraction of Caco-2 cells exposed to a rosemary supercritical extract. Journal of Functional Foods. 2015;**13**:384-390. DOI: 10.1016/j.jff.2015.01.015

[78] Garcia-Salas P, Morales-Soto A, Segura-Carretero A, Fernández-Gutiérrez A. Phenolic-compound-extraction systems for fruit and vegetable samples. Molecules. 2010;**15**(12):8813-8826. DOI: 10.3390/molecules15128813

[79] Jiao G, Pour KA. Extraction of anthocyanins from haskap berry pulp using supercritical carbon dioxide: Influence of co-solvent composition and pretreatment. LWT—Food Science and Technology. 2018;**98**:237-244. DOI: 10.1016/j.lwt.2018.08.042

[80] Moura PM, Prado GHC, Meireles MAA, Pereira CG. Supercritical fluid extraction from guava (*Psidium guajava*) leaves: Global yield, composition and kinetic data. The Journal of Supercritical Fluids. 2012;**62**:116-122. DOI: 10.1016/j.supflu.2011.11.014

[81] Solana M, Boschiero I, Acqua SD, Bertucco A. Extraction of bioactive enriched fractions from *Eruca sativa* leaves by supercritical CO_2 technology using different co-solvents. The Journal of Supercritical Fluids. 2014;**94**:245-251. DOI: 10.1016/j.supflu.2014.08.022

[82] da Silva RFF, Rocha-santos TAP, Duarte AC. Supercritical fluid extraction of bioactive compounds. Trends in Analytical Chemistry. 2016;**76**:40-51. DOI: 10.1016/j.trac.2015.11.013

[83] Jesus SP, Meireles MAA. Supercritical fluid extraction: A global perspective of the fundamental concepts of this eco-friendly extraction technique. In: Chemat F, Vian MA, editors. Alternative Solvents for Natural Products Extraction. 1st ed. London: Springer-Verlag Berlin Heidelberg; 2014. pp. 39-72. DOI: 10.1007/978-3-662-43628-8

[84] Babovic N, Djilas S, Jadranin M, Vajs V, Ivanovic J, Petrovic S, Zizovic I. Supercritical carbon dioxide extraction of antioxidant fractions from selected Lamiaceae herbs and their antioxidant capacity. Innovative Food Science and Emerging Technologies. 2010;**11**(1):98-107. DOI: 10.1016/j.ifset.2009.08.013

[85] Fernández-ponce MT, Casas L, Mantell C, Rodríguez M, De la Ossa EM. Extraction of antioxidant compounds from different varieties of Mangifera indica leaves using green technologies. The Journal of Supercritical Fluids. 2012;**72**:168-175. DOI: 10.1016/j.supflu.2012.07.016

[86] Martinez-Correa HA, Magalhães PM, Queiroga CL, Peixoto CA, Oliveira AL, Cabral FA. Extracts from pitanga (Eugenia uniflora L.) leaves: Influence of extraction process on antioxidant properties and yield of phenolic compounds. The Journal of Supercritical Fluids. 2011;**55**(3):998-1006. DOI: 10.1016/j.supflu.2010.09.001

[87] Bagheri H, Abdul Manap MY Bin, Solati Z. Antioxidant activity of Piper nigrum L. essential oil extracted by supercritical CO_2 extraction and hydro-distillation. Talanta. 2014;**121**:220-228. DOI: 10.1016/j.talanta.2014.01.007

Chapter 18

Increase of Oxidants and Antioxidant Consumption in Patients with Type 2 Diabetes Mellitus in Peritoneal Dialysis

Leonardo Pazarín-Villaseñor, Julio Alejandro Gutiérrez-Prieto, Javier Soto-Vargas, Renato Parra-Michel, Andrés García-Sanchez and Alejandra Guillermina Miranda-Diaz

Abstract

Oxidative stress (OS) is implicated as a unifying factor between chronic kidney diseases and cardiovascular diseases. The objective of the study was to compare the oxidant and antioxidant status in patients with PD according to the state of DM. Lipoperoxides (LPO), 8-isoprostanes (8-IP) and nitric oxide (NO) were determined as oxidants and the activity of superoxide dismutase (SOD) and total antioxidant capacity (TAC) as antioxidants in patients with DM and without DM (No-DM). We included 35 patients with DM, 42 No-DM patients and 10 healthy people as a control group (HC). Patients with DM were older ($p<0.0001$), had higher BMI ($p<0.0001$), high glucose levels ($p<0.0001$) and more hypertension ($p<0.0001$). It was found that LPO levels increased in patients with DM and No-DM vs. HC ($p<0.0001$). There was a decrease in the levels of 8-IP in DM and No-DM compared to HC ($p<0.0001$). The levels of NO in patients with DM and No-DM decreased significantly compared to the HC group with 197.97±34.20 μM ($p<0.0001$). The activity of the SOD enzyme in patients with DM and No-DM was found to be increased compared to the HC group ($p<0.0001$). The levels of TAC in HC were 2.62±0.17 mM and decreased in patients with DM and No-DM ($p<0.0001$).

Keywords: end-stage renal disease, chronic kidney disease, peritoneal dialysis, diabetes mellitus, oxidative stress, antioxidants

1. Introduction

Several traditional and nontraditional cardiovascular risk factors have been described in chronic kidney disease (CKD). Cardiovascular disease (CVD) still is the leading cause of death among end-stage renal disease (ESRD) patients. CVD and CKD are closely related to each other, and the disease of one of the organs causes dysfunction of the other by conditioning the failure of both organs [1]. CKD patients generally have several traditional cardiovascular risk factors like diabetes mellitus (DM), dyslipidemia, and arterial hypertension. These conditions are associated with oxidative stress (OS), and these can trigger and accelerate the progression of renal injury [2]. OS is defined as the imbalance between oxidants and the antioxidant defenses of the body. Reactive oxygen species (ROS) are generated through enzymes such as nicotinamide phosphate adenine dinucleotide (NADPH) oxidase, which reduces oxygen to superoxide anion (O^{2-}). This anion is converted to hydrogen peroxide (H_2O_2) by the enzyme superoxide dismutase (SOD). The O^{2-} anion reacts with nitric oxide (NO) by producing peroxynitrite (nitrosative stress). The H_2O_2 reacts with intracellular iron to form the hydroxyl radical. In addition, H_2O_2 is catalyzed to hypochlorous acid in the presence of the chloride ion, by myeloperoxidase activity. Uremic toxins also participate by increasing ROS generation. The excessive production of ROS is able to oxidize lipids, proteins, and nucleic acids [3].

DM is a frequent cause of the need for renal replacement therapy (RRT) [4]. In Jalisco (Mexico), nearly half of the patients in dialysis are on peritoneal dialysis (PD), and almost half of these patients have DM [5]. In 2009, it was reported that diabetic nephropathy (DN) causes ~44% of all cases of ESRD in the United States [6]. DM contributes, in large part, to the high costs of health care and the increase in mortality from the increased incidence of DN that leads to ESRD [7]. The purpose of the study was to compare the oxidants and antioxidants state in patients with PD according to DM status.

2. Patients and methods

A single-center, analytical cross-sectional study was performed with ESRD patients on PD. Patients were eligible if they were 16 years old or older and were incident or prevalent in the population of the PD program and never have had a peritoneal equilibrium test (PET) performed before or if the last PET result was older than 1 year. We exclude patients with a current or a previous peritonitis episode in the last 6 months, patients with PD catheter dysfunction, and patients with a current infectious, inflammatory, and malignant process or impaired glycemic control (serum glucose > 200 mg/dL). We collected information about PD treatment and doses, residual diuresis, ultrafiltration, and the value of D/P creatinine (creatinine ratio in the dialysis fluid and plasma), reported at 4 h at the end of the PET. The type of peritoneal transport is determined by the result obtained, modality and the dialysis glucose solution concentration [8].

2.1 Oxidative stress markers

For measurement of OS markers, 10 mL of blood samples were drawn when PET blood samples were taken, 5 mL with 0.1% of ethylenediaminetetraacetic acid (EDTA) tube and other 5 mL in dry tube. The blood was immediately centrifuged at 10,000 rpm for 10 min at room temperature; supernatants were stored in aliquots at −80°C until their final processing. We included 10 mL of extra blood from 10 blood donors (healthy control) that was used to establish the normal value of the reagents.

2.1.1 Lipoperoxides (LPO)

The levels of LPO in plasma were measured through the FR22 assay kit (Oxford Biomedical Research Inc., Oxford, MI, USA®) according to the manufacturer's instructions. The limit of detection for this test was 0.1 nmol/mL. The chromogenic reagent reacts with malondialdehyde (MDA) and 4-hydroxy-alkenals to form a stable chromophore. First, 140 μL of plasma with 455 μL of N-methyl-2-phenylindole in acetonitrile (Reagent 1) was diluted with ferric iron in methanol. Samples were agitated; after which 105 μL 37% HCl was added followed by incubation at 45°C for 60 min and centrifugation at 12,791 rpm for 10 min. Next, 150 μL of the supernatant was added, and absorbance was measured at 586 nm. The pattern curve with known concentrations of 1,1,3,3-tetramethoxypropane in Tris–HCl was used. The intra-assay CV was 8.5% [9].

2.1.2 8-Iso-prostaglandin $F_{2\alpha}$ 8-isoprostanes (8-IP)

The immunoassay reagent kit from Cayman Chemical Company® (Michigan, USA) was used according to the manufacturer's instructions. The limit of detection was 0.8 pg/mL. The 8-IP assay was based on the principle of competitive binding between samples 8-IP, 8-IP acetylcholinesterase (AChE) conjugate, and 8-IP tracer. Then, 50 μL of samples or standard was added to each well, and 50 μL of 8-IP AChE tracer was added to all wells except the total activity and blank wells; and 50 μL of 8-IP enzyme immunoassay antiserum was added to all wells except the total activity and blank wells. At once, 50 μL of 8-IP antiserum was added to all wells except total activity, non-specific binding, and blank wells. The plate was covered and incubated at 4 °C for 18 h and then washed 5 times with buffer. Absorbance was read at 420 nm. The intra-assay CV was 12.5% [10].

2.1.3 Nitric oxide (NO)

Prior to the determination of the NO levels, the serum samples were deproteinized by the addition of 6 mg of zinc sulfate to 400 μL of sample and vortexed for 1 minute and the samples were centrifuged at 10,000×*g* for 10 min at 4°C. For the determination of ON, the colorimetric method was used according to the kit (Nitric Oxide Assay Kit, NB98, Oxford Biomedical Research®). About 85 μL of the standard or sample was added to the wells of the plate, 10 μL of nitrate reductase was added to each well, and 10 μL of 2 mM NADH was added to the wells. The plate was stirred for 20 min at room temperature. Then 50 μL of dye 1 was added and stirred briefly and then 50 μL of dye 2, and again the samples were vortexed for 5 min at room temperature. Finally, the plate was read at 540 nm in a spectrophotometer within the first 20 minutes of completion of the procedure [11].

2.2 Antioxidants

2.2.1 Superoxide dismutase (SOD)

We followed the kit manufacturer's instructions (SOD No. 706002, Cayman Chemical Company®, USA) for the detection of O_2^- generated by the xanthine oxidase and hypoxanthine enzymes through the reaction of tetrazolium salts. We diluted the serum samples 1:5 in the sample buffer, 200 μL of the radicals' detector (1:400 dilution), and added 10 μL of the sample. After slow agitation, 20 μL of xanthine oxidase was then added to the wells. Then, the microplate was incubated for 20 minutes at room temperature. The absorbency was read at 440 wavelength of nm. The levels are reported in IU/mL [12].

2.2.2 Total antioxidant capacity (TAC)

The evaluations of TAC were made following the instructions of the kit manufacturer (Total Antioxidant Power Kit, No. TA02.090130, Oxford Biomedical Research®), to obtain the concentration in mM equivalents of uric acid. The detection limit was 0.075 mM. The samples and standards were diluted 1:40, and 200 μL was placed in each well. The plate was read at 450 nm as a reference value, 50 μL of copper solution was added, and the plate was incubated at room temperature for 3 minutes. Afterward, 50 μL of stop solution was added and the plate was read at 450 nm. The dilution factor was considered in the result. The intra-assay CV was 7.8% [13].

2.3 Statistical analysis

Normally distributed variables were presented as mean ± standard deviation (SD); skewed variables were exhibited as median with interquartile range (IQR). Categorical variables were expressed as frequency and percentage. All demographic and PD-related characteristics were compared between diabetics and nondiabetic patients using Chi^2, Student's *t* test, or Mann-Whitney U test accordingly to the type of data distribution. When significant differences in serum levels of oxidative stress markers were found between groups and were feasible, we conducted a multivariable analysis, to determine the interaction between DM and other factors associated with increased OS. The statistical analyses were performed using the IBM SPSS v.18 software (Chicago, IL, USA). For all the analysis, a $p \leq 0.05$ value was considered as statistically significant.

2.4 Ethics considerations

The scientific research study abides by the regulations of the internationally established guidelines of the Declaration of Helsinki 1964, revised in October 2013 at the World Medical Assembly. All procedures were performed according to regulations stipulated in the General Health Legal Guidelines for Healthcare Research in Mexico, 2nd Title, in Ethical Aspects for Research in Human Beings, Chapter 1, Article 17. The study was evaluated and approved by the Local Ethics and Research Committee at the Regional General Hospital No. 46, Mexican Institute of Social Security, Guadalajara, Jalisco, Mexico, with registration number R-2017-1303-117. All patients gave and signed the informed consent form in the presence of signed witnesses. Patients had the right to withdraw from the study at any time without representing harm to the patient-doctor relationship and without affecting their treatment. At all times, total confidentiality was maintained, and the patients were informed of the results throughout the study.

3. Results

Seventy-seven patients were included in the study, 35 with DM and 42 No-DM patients. The median age was 42 years. There was a greater prevalence of male-gendered patients, DM 62.86% and No-DM 76.19%. DM patients were older ($p < 0.0001$) and had higher body mass index ($p < 0.0001$), with significant increase in glucose ($p < 0.0001$) and more prevalence of arterial hypertension ($p < 0.0001$). A total of 63 patients used erythropoiesis-stimulating agents, with a mean dose of 140 ± 63.6 UI/kg/week, and a major dose was observed in No-DM patients. In **Table 1**, the demographic and biochemical results of the patients are shown. Significant increases in DM patients were found in triglyceride levels

	DM, n = 35	No-DM, n = 42	*p*
Gender n (%)			
Male	22 (62.86)	32 (76.19)	0.377
Female	13 (37.14)	10 (23.81)	1
Age, years	62 (54.5–66.5)	28 (25–37)	**<0.0001***
Weight, kg	73.16 ± 11.60	67.25 ± 12.52	**0.011****
Height, m	1.62 ± 0.09	1.66 ± 0.08	**0.046****
BMI, kg/m^2	27.80 ± 4.56	24.52 ± 4.29	**<0.0001****
Hypertension, n (%)	34 (97.14)	5 (11.90)	**<0.0001** '
Residual uresis, mL	500 (250–1000)	500 (57.5–1000)	0.85
Hemoglobin, g/dL	11.41 ± 1.80	10.83 ± 2.33	0.16
Urea, mg/dL	102.63 ± 30.95	124.39 ± 31.16	**<0.0001****
Creatinine, mg/dL	7.86 ± 3.07	13.89 ± 4–10	**<0.0001****
Glucose, mg/dL	131 (98–157)	95 (88.7–103)	**<0.0001***
Phosphorus, mg/dL	4.11 ± 1.42	5.63 ± 1.70	**<0.0001****
Calcium, mg/dL	8.76 ± 0.97	8.73 ± 0.92	0.35
Magnesium, mg/dL	2.13 ± 0.48	2.33 ± 0.41	**0.023****
Potassium, mEq/L	4.20 ± 0.73	4.47 ± 0.58	**0.032****
Sodium, mEq/L	138 (136–140)	140 (137–141)	0.06
Albumin, g/dL	3.17 ± 0.59	3.80 ± 0.53	**<0.0001****
Uric acid, mg/dL	6.22 ± 1.23	6.68 ± 1.39	0.08
Iron, mcg/dL	73.35 ± 26.34	77.49 ± 40.85	0.87
TSAT %	35.30 ± 17.86	32.5 ± 23.44	0.41
Cholesterol, mg/dL	171.51 ± 51.21	170.27 ± 43.38	0.91
HDL, mg/dL	41.55 ± 13.64	45.29 ± 15.34	0.28
LDL, mg/dL	93.12 ± 36.35	100.11 ± 35.46	0.45
Triglycerides, mg/dL	150 (98–219.6)	124 (88–158)	**0.046***
VLDL, mg/dL	30 (19.75–45.75)	24.5 (17.5–32.2)	**0.049***
HCO3, mEq/L	20.33 ± 3.27	21.57 ± 3.24	0.17
RCP, mg/L	3.31 (1.41–9.64)	1.98 (1–4.36)	**0.034***

Values are mean ± standard deviation (SD), percentage (%) or median (25–75th percentile), and 'Chi^2 test
**Mann-Whitney U test; **Student's t test.*
DM, diabetes mellitus; No-DM, without DM; BMI, body mass index; TSAT, transferrin saturation; HDL, high-density lipoprotein; LDL, low-density lipoprotein; VLDL, very-low-density lipoprotein; HCO_3, bicarbonate; RCP, reactive C protein.

Table 1.
Demographic and biochemical results in patients with ESRD in PD with and without diabetes mellitus

($p < 0.046$), very-low-density cholesterol (VLDL) ($p < 0.05$) and highly specific reactive C protein (RCP) ($p < 0.034$), which suggests systemic inflammation. However, phosphorus ($p < 0.0001$) and albumin ($p < 0.0001$) were found to be decreased. No-DM patients showed better biochemical results in urea ($p < 0.0001$), creatinine ($p < 0.0001$), magnesium ($p < 0.009$), and potassium ($p < 0.047$).

3.1 Dialysis characteristics

The patients had a median vintage on PD of 13 months (4–26), without differences between DM and No-DM. In addition, there were no differences in the glucose concentration used in the dialysis solutions, but DM patients were less likely to be on automated peritoneal dialysis (APD) modality (p = 0.016), and the median dwell time was 16 h (QR 16–24). There were no differences in the D/P creatinine or the history of peritonitis between patients. The median residual diuresis was 500 mL/day (250–1000), and there were no difference in the volume of urine or the number of patients with significant residual diuresis. The peritoneal ultrafiltration and the total ultrafiltration were similar in both DM and No-DM patients (p = 0.54 and 0.72, respectively) and were within guidelines and recommendations.

3.2 Oxidants

3.2.1 Lipoperoxides, 8-iso-prostaglandin $F_{2\alpha}$ (8-IP), and nitric oxide

The levels of LPO (MDA and 4-hydroxy-alkenals) in the healthy controls were 3.05 ± 0.18 μM. However, LPO levels were found to be increased in DM patients, 136.95 ± 18.17 μM ($p < 0.0001$), and 194.18 ± 54.70 μM ($p < 0.0001$) in No-DM patients. No significant difference was found between patients with and without DM.

The serum levels of 8-IP in DM patients were found to be decreased 5.36 ± 0.80 pg/mL ($p < 0.0001$) and No-DM 9.99 ± 6.41 pg/mL ($p < 0.0001$) versus the levels that were obtained in healthy controls, 22.88 ± 3.80 pg/mL ($p < 0.0001$). No significant difference was found between patients with and without DM.

The levels of the NO products (nitrites/nitrates) in healthy controls were 197.97 ± 34.20 μM. The products of NO in DM patients were found to be decreased, 18.02 ± 3.41 μM ($p < 0.0001$), and No-DM, 12.96 ± 2.78 μM ($p < 0.0001$). There was no significant difference between patients with and without DM (**Table 2** and **Figure 1**).

3.3 Antioxidants

3.3.1 Superoxide dismutase and total antioxidant capacity

An increase in the serum activity of SOD was found in patients in PD with DM, 3.36 ± 0.28 U/mL, and No-DM, 3.28 ± 0.22 U/mL ($p < 0.0001$), versus the activity

	Healthy control	No-DM	p, MW-U	DM	p, MW-U
Antioxidants					
SOD, U/mL	0.23 ± 0.015	3.28 ± 0.22	**<0.0001**	3.36 ± 0.28	**<0.0001**
Total antioxidant capacity, mM	2.62 ± 0.17	0.69 ± 0.23	**<0.0001**	0.65 ± 0.031	**<0.0001**
Oxidants					
8-Isoprostane, pg/mL	22.88 ± 3.80	9.99 ± 6.41	**<0.0001**	5.36 ± 0.80	**<0.0001**
LPO, μM	3.05 ± 0.18	194.18 ± 54.70	**<0.0001**	136.95 ± 18.17	**<0.0001**
Nitric oxide, μM	197.97 ± 34.20	12.96 ± 2.78	**<0.0001**	18.02 ± 3.41	**<0.0001**

SOD, superoxide dismutase; LPO, lipoperoxides; No-DM, without diabetes mellitus; DM, diabetes mellitus; MW-U, Mann-Whitney U test.

Table 2.
Antioxidants and oxidants with and without diabetes mellitus vs. healthy controls.

DOI: http://dx.doi.org/10.5772/intechopen.82880

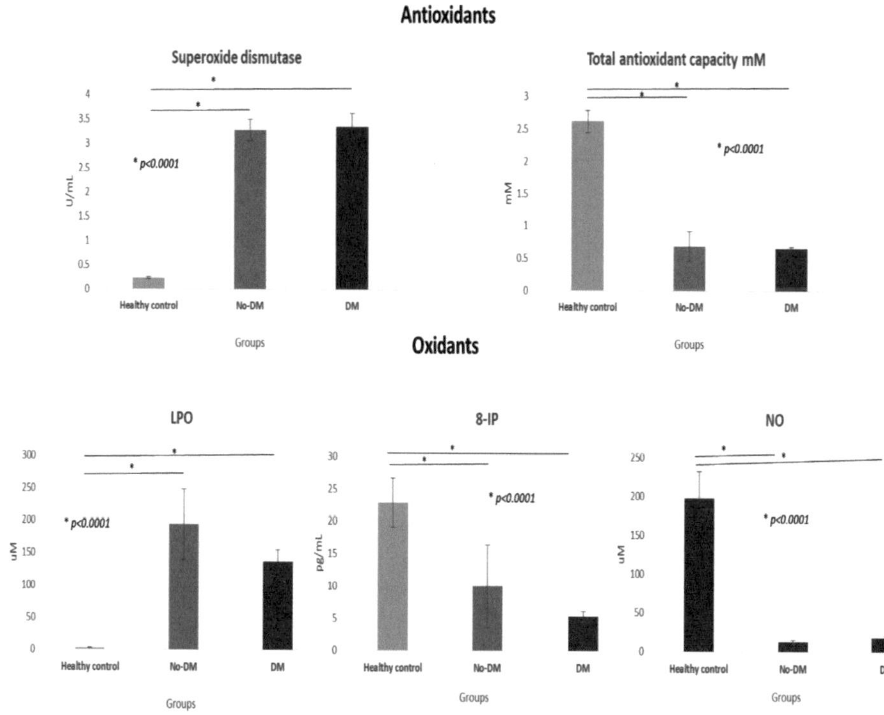

Figure 1.
Levels of antioxidant and oxidant in DM and No-DM patients.

of the enzyme in healthy controls, 0.23 ± 0.015 U/mL. There was no significant difference between patients with and without DM.

The serum levels found in healthy controls of TAC were 2.62 ± 0.17 mM; however, significantly decreased levels were found in DM patients, 0.65 ± 0.03 mM, and No-DM patients, 0.69 ± 0.23 mM ($p < 0.0001$). There was no significant difference between patients with and without DM (**Table 2** and **Figure 1**).

3.4 Correlations in all patients

When including the results of all patients, positive correlation was found between LPO with total cholesterol, LDL, triglycerides, and VLDL cholesterol. The 8-IP showed positive correlation with the reactive C protein. The NO products obtained a positive correlation with Hb, LDL, triglycerides, and VLDL cholesterol. The activity of SOD showed a positive correlation with creatinine, magnesium, and HDL cholesterol. Negative correlation was found between the products of NO and HDL cholesterol. SOD activity showed negative correlation with residual urine, Hb, triglycerides, and VLDL cholesterol (**Table 3**).

3.5 Correlations in no-DM patients

When including the results according to status in No-DM patients, there was a positive correlation between 8-IP with hemoglobin, between NO with triglycerides and LDL cholesterol, between SOD with creatinine and phosphorus, and between TAC with phosphorus and uric acid. There was negative correlation between LPO and body weight, NO and HDL cholesterol, SOD with residual diuresis, hemoglobin, triglycerides, and VLDL cholesterol (**Table 4**).

r^2	LPO	8-IP	NO	SOD	TAC
Weight	−0.12	0.05	0.02	0.06	0.03
Height	−0.10	−0.13	−0.008	−0.01	0.12
BMI	−0.05	0.15	0.04	0.08	−0.03
Residual urine	−0.007	0.04	0.061	**−0.31****	−0.09
Hemoglobin	0.07	0.09	**0.27***	**−0.38****	−0.05
Urea	−0.05	−0.01	**−0.26***	0.08	**0.36****
Creatinine	−0.14	−0.14	−0.16	**0.31****	**0.23***
Glucose	0.12	0.03	0.20	0.06	0.14
Phosphorus	−0.05	0.05	**−0.31****	0.17	**0.35****
Calcium	0.09	0.04	0.006	−0.21	0.03
Magnesium	−0.08	0.14	−0.13	**0.27***	0.07
Potassium	−0.10	0.13	−0.18	0.14	0.09
Sodium	0.16	−0.04	−0.01	−0.09	0.03
Albumin	0.06	−0.15	0.01	−0.08	0.15
Uric acid	−0.04	0.03	0.05	−0.06	**0.52****
Iron	−0.05	−0.05	−0.02	−0.04	0.07
TSAT	−0.19	0.42	−0.08	−0.14	−0.07
Cholesterol	**0.26***	0.02	0.15	−0.16	−0.08
HDL	−0.05	−0.01	**−0.44****	**0.29***	−0.21
LDL	**0.27***	0.007	**0.31***	−0.14	0.06
Triglycerides	**0.35****	0.04	**0.52****	**−0.49****	0.04
VLDL	**0.29***	0.07	**0.52****	**−0.44****	0.08
HCO_3	−0.07	−0.11	0.07	−0.03	0.03
RCP	−0.12	**0.37****	0.17	−0.19	0.08

$^*p < 0.05$, $^{**}p < 0.01$.
DM, diabetes mellitus; No-DM, without DM; BMI, body mass index; TSAT, transferrin saturation; HDL, high-density lipoprotein; LDL, low-density lipoprotein; VLDL, very-low-density lipoprotein; HCO_3, bicarbonate; RCP, reactive C protein; LPO, lipoperoxides; 8-IP, 8-isoprostanes; NO, nitric oxide; SOD, superoxide dismutase; TAC, total antioxidant capacity.

Table 3.
Correlation between demographic, biochemical, and oxidative stress markers.

3.6 Correlations in DM patients

In patients with DM, positive correlation was found between LPO, calcium, cholesterol, and triglycerides; between 8-IP with calcium and RCP; between NO and VLDL cholesterol and LDL cholesterol and triglycerides; between SOD with creatinine, magnesium, and HDL cholesterol; and between TAC with urea, uric acid, VLDL cholesterol, and PCR. There was only a negative correlation between SOD with triglycerides and VLDL cholesterol and also between total cholesterol and HDL cholesterol (**Table 4**).

r^2	LPO	8-IP	NO	SOD	TAC
No-DM patients in PD					
Weight	**−0.34***	0.07	0.15	0.041	0.03
Height	−0.22	0.01	0.28	0.043	0.06
BMI	−0.26	0.06	0.03	0.005	0.01
Residual urine	0.06	0.20	0.08	**−0.38***	−0.05
Hemoglobin	−0.09	**0.32***	0.25	**−0.49****	−0.04
Urea	−0.16	0.02	−0.26	0.22	0.28
Creatinine	−0.15	−0.16	0.04	**0.50****	0.28
Glucose	−0.07	−0.06	0.13	0.19	0.10
Phosphorus	−0.10	−0.21	−0.27	**0.30***	**0.46****
Calcium	−0.13	0.06	−0.02	−0.18	−0.09
Magnesium	−0.004	0.04	0.08	0.24	−0.10
Potassium	−0.03	0.29	−0.13	0.22	0.23
Sodium	0.03	0.02	0.08	−0.02	−0.07
Albumin	0.08	0.18	0.27	−0.24	0.05
Uric acid	−0.02	0.05	0.10	−0.17	**0.51****
Iron	−0.08	−0.15	−0.02	−0.08	0.22
TSAT	−0.09	0.57	−0.06	−0.27	−0.16
Cholesterol	0.12	−0.05	−0.06	−0.07	−0.25
HDL	0.08	0.02	**−0.44****	0.19	−0.08
LDL	0.06	−0.01	0.17	−0.07	−0.04
Triglycerides	0.22	0.04	**0.46****	**−0.53****	−0.12
VLDL	0.21	0.05	**0.43****	**−0.48****	−0.11
HCO_3	−0.06	−0.08	0.14	−0.05	0.41*
PCR	−0.15	0.27	0.23	−0.11	−0.15
Diabetic patients in PD					
Weight	0.14	−0.05	−0.27	0.03	0.12
Height	0.05	−0.22	−0.21	−0.06	0.08
BMI	0.06	0.12	−0.15	0.10	0.05
Residual urine	−0.16	−0.16	−0.02	−0.21	−0.14
Hemoglobin	0.28	−0.21	0.23	−0.25	−0.02
Urea	0.13	0.03	−0.03	−0.03	**0.36***
Creatinine	−0.09	0.09	−0.17	**0.39***	0.17
Glucose	0.23	−0.01	0.20	−0.05	0.27
Phosphorus	0.12	**0.45****	−0.17	0.07	0.19
Calcium	**0.39***	0.04	0.11	−0.23	0.14
Magnesium	−0.07	0.34	−0.25	**0.35***	0.14
Potassium	−0.19	0.05	−0.16	0.06	−0.09
Sodium	0.28	0.002	−0.06	−0.13	0.10
Albumin	0.26	−0.32	−0.02	0.07	0.13
Uric acid	0.01	0.01	0.16	0.04	**0.53****

r^2	LPO	8-IP	NO	SOD	TAC
Iron	0.003	0.05	−0.007	0.05	−0.10
TSAT	−0.65	0.21	−0.14	0.09	−0.06
Cholesterol	**0.42****	0.08	**0.42***	−0.24	0.09
HDL	−0.21	−0.03	−0.33	**0.39***	**−0.38***
LDL	**0.55****	0.05	**0.52****	−0.24	0.19
Triglycerides	**0.46****	0.003	**0.54****	**−0.46****	0.32
VLDL	0.34	0.04	**0.57****	**−0.41***	**0.35***
HCO_3	−0.03	−0.14	0.09	−0.03	−0.20
RCP	−0.03	**0.50***	0.09	−0.38	**0.44***

**$p < 0.05$, **$p < 0.01$.*
DM, diabetes mellitus; No-DM, without DM; BMI, body mass index; TSAT, transferrin saturation; HDL, high-density lipoprotein; LDL, low-density lipoprotein; VLDL, very-low-density lipoprotein; HCO_3, bicarbonate; RCP, reactive C protein; LPO, lipoperoxides; 8-IP, 8-isoprostanes; NO, nitric oxide; SOD, superoxide dismutase; TAC, total antioxidant capacity.

Table 4.
Correlation between demographic, bioquimical, and oxidative stress markers.

4. Discussion

In this cross-sectional study, we compared levels of oxidative stress markers on PD patients with and without diabetes. The DM patients were older, had higher BMI, had more prevalence of hypertension, and had higher triglycerides and VLDL levels that corresponded to the classic metabolic syndrome [14]. The prevalence of metabolic syndrome in patients with ESRD on PD is quite frequent, and its presence is reported in ~40–60% of patients with DN depending on the population studied [15].

DM is the main cause of ESRD and represents 58% of incident cases [16]. Several interventions have been suggested for the prevention and control of DM. A directed selection study is followed by a randomized controlled trial by groups, with randomization where participants were at risk for DM. The subjects received standard care or intervention. The intervention consisted of a group structured education program of 6 h with an annual update and regular telephone contact with follow up for 3 years. About 29.1% attended all the sessions; 22.6% did not attend the education. The authors found a 26% reduction in the risk of type 2 DM of those who received the intervention compared with the standard care. They found no statistical significance, which suggests that the effectiveness of all interventions is not promising [17].

When the patient already has DM, a variety of risk factors that promote the development and progression of DN have been reported: persistent high glucose levels, time of duration of DM, arterial hypertension, obesity, endothelial dysfunction, and dyslipidemia. Most of these risk factors are modifiable through antidiabetic, antihypertensive, lipid-lowering, and primarily lifestyle change [18]. It has been previously reported that patients with ESRD and DM who require dialysis have higher rates of various morbidities and worse clinical outcomes compared to non-DM patients. It has also been shown that glycemic decontrol is associated with more micro- and macrovascular complications, in addition to higher mortality [19].

In the present study, a significant increase in LPO was found in DM and No-DM patients undergoing PD *vs*. the levels found in healthy controls. It has been shown that patients in PD manifest excessive OS compared to healthy controls. OS in PD is closely related to chronic inflammation, atherogenesis, peritoneal fibrosis, and loss of residual renal function. The unfavorable serum lipid profile and the chronic exposure of peritoneal cells to super-physiological levels of glucose in patients undergoing PD could increase glycosylation and lipid oxidation, favoring the increase of LPO and consequently greater OS [20]. When there is greater permeability and biocompatibility of the peritoneal membrane, with better preserved residual renal function, it can be assumed that patients could have a lower oxidative load [21, 22]; however, reports in the literature indicate that the oxidative metabolism of peripheral and peritoneal phagocytes is activated during PD with conventional dialysate, by the products of glucose degradation, by low pH, and by high osmolarity [23]. The bio-incompatibility of DP solutions seems to play a central role in increasing ROS production [24]. Previously increased OS in patients with ESRD in RRT has been reported before undergoing kidney transplantation [25].

In the results obtained in the patients undergoing PD with DM and No-DM, the 8-IP were significantly diminished versus the healthy controls; possibly, the clearance of this marker by PD participates in the decrease of serum levels. Previous reports have shown that the residual glomerular filtration rate is independently associated with the levels of advanced glycation end products in plasma effluents and peritoneum [26]. It has been previously reported that DM is associated with increased lipid peroxidation and persistent platelet activation with increased in vivo formation of F2-isoprostane 8-iso-prostaglandin (PG) F2alfa (bioactive product of arachidonic acid peroxidation). 8-IP improves their levels in presence of DM by contributing to platelet activation related to altered glycemic control and increased lipid peroxidation by providing an important biochemical link between altered glycemic control and persistent platelet activation [27]. However, in our study this marker was found to be significantly decreased in serum in both DM and No-DM patients in inverse relation to published reports where they found increased levels in urine [18]. Kant et al. mentioned that when lipid peroxidation products were elevated in the prediabetic stage, the determination of this marker is useful in the detection of patients at risk of type 2 DM [28]. In this study, the 8-IP in residual urine was not measured.

In patients with DM and No-DM, we found significantly decreased serum levels of NO. NO is a potent biological vasodilator produced by the vascular endothelium from L-arginine. NO is synthesized by endothelial NO synthase (eNOS). Vascular NO deficiency may be involved in accelerated atherosclerosis and the dramatic cardiovascular mortality observed in patients with CKD [29]. Vascular changes can induce OS and inflammation, favoring the probability of morbidity and mortality by aggravating CVD [30]. In CKD, endothelial dysfunction is characterized by the altered capacity of the vascular endothelium to stimulate vasodilation. NO plays a key role in the development of atherosclerosis in this pathology. The decrease in the bioavailability of NO is a key factor of endothelial dysfunction. In addition, NO plays an important role in the protection of the vascular wall because it induces its own metabolic products [31].

In the present study, a significant increase in the activity of the SOD enzyme was found in DM and No-DM patients undergoing PD. The accumulated scientific evidence suggests that the main antioxidant systems are impaired in patients on PD [32]; possibly the previous finding could be explained in an attempt to compensate the oxidative state that characterized the patients included in the study. Antioxidants can be divided into intracellular and extracellular antioxidants. The intracellular enzymatic antioxidants are SOD, catalase, and glutathione peroxidase, which convert substrates (anion radicals O^{2-} and H_2O_2) into less reactive forms. The first line of defense against free radicals is SOD. Free radicals are the source of lipid peroxidation derived from oxygen, and the function of SOD is to catalyze the conversion of O^{2-} radicals into H_2O_2. Therefore, if the activity of SOD in PD had been found to be decreased, it would suggest accumulation of the O^{2-} radical anion responsible for the increase in lipid peroxidation [21]; however, in the patients included in the study, SOD was found to be significantly increased and TAC decreased in patients undergoing PD with DM and No-DM, which could suggest that peritoneal replacements could purge the systemic buffering levels of the TAC. In a recently reported study, the authors underwent to hemodialysis session in patients with ESRD; they found a significant reduction in TAC according to our findings [33]. The depletion of TAC found in patients undergoing PD is contrary to that reported by other authors in relation to increased levels of these systemic buffers in patients undergoing hemodialysis. [34]. The concentrations of bilirubin, uric acid, and plasma albumin are the main defense in the extracellular fluids generated during the normal metabolism or are ingested by the consumption of dietary products rich in antioxidants [35]. These extracellular antioxidants prevent the reaction of free radicals by sequestering transition metal ions by plasma chelation [36]; the TAC is able to determine these extracellular antioxidants. In the present study, TAC was found to be significantly consumed in all patients included.

The addition of exogenous antioxidants to the management of patients who are in PD is an incomplete and little studied subject; however, this topic is interesting that is well worth considering in these patients. In a report of the literature, the authors studied the N-acetylcysteine (NAC) which is considered as a potential antioxidant with anti-inflammatory effects for dialysis patients. Vitamin C could play an important role in helping PD patients to use iron for erythropoiesis and achieve better hemoglobin response during the treatment of anemia [37].

5. Conclusions

When comparing patients in PD according to the presence or absence of DM, we found imbalance of markers of oxidative stress characterized by increased LPO products, serum decrease of 8-PI, dysregulation of the antioxidant defense system with significant decrease in TAC, and increase in SOD possibly in an attempt to compensate for the state of oxidative stress. In this population, increased levels of triglycerides and VLDL were observed, which favors the appearance of accelerated atherosclerosis with an increase in arterial stiffness, as well as a decrease in NO levels, which favors secondary endothelial dysfunction. These factors contribute to the increase of CVD in PD patients. Supplementation with external antioxidants could be an emerging strategy to counteract OS with the potential to preserve peritoneal function.

Conflict of interests

There is no conflict of interest.

Abbreviations

OS	oxidative stress
CKD	chronic kidney diseases
PD	peritoneal dialysis
DM	diabetes mellitus
LPO	lipoperoxides
8-IP	8-isoprostanes
NO	nitric oxide
SOD	superoxide dismutase

TAC	total antioxidant capacity
No-DM	without diabetes mellitus
HC	healthy control
CVD	cardiovascular disease
ESRD	end-stage renal disease
ROS	reactive oxygen species
NADPH	nicotinamide phosphate adenine dinucleotide
D/P	creatinine ratio in the dialysis fluid and plasma (reported at 4 h at the end of the peritoneal equilibrium test)
O^{2-}	superoxide anion
H_2O_2	hydrogen peroxide
RRT	renal replacement therapy
DN	diabetic nephropathy
PET	peritoneal equilibrium test
EDTA	ethylenediaminetetraacetic
SD	standard deviation
IQR	interquartile range
TC	total cholesterol
LDL	low-density cholesterol
HDL	high-density cholesterol
VLDL	very-low-density cholesterol
RPC	reactive protein C
Hb	hemoglobin

Author details

Leonardo Pazarín-Villaseñor[1,2], Julio Alejandro Gutiérrez-Prieto[1], Javier Soto-Vargas[1], Renato Parra-Michel[1], Andrés García-Sanchez[3] and Alejandra Guillermina Miranda-Diaz[3]*

1 Universidad de Guadalajara, Centro Universitario de Ciencias de la Salud, Especialidad en Nefrologia, Hospital General Regional Instituto Mexicano del Seguro Social, Guadalajara, Jalisco, Mexico

2 Servicio de Nefrología, División de Medicina Interna, Hospital Civil de Guadalajara "Dr. Juan I Menchaca", Guadalajara, Jalisco, Mexico

3 Departamento de Fisiología, Centro Universitario de Ciencias de la Salud, Universidad de Guadalajara, Guadalajara, Jalisco, Mexico

*Address all correspondence to: kindalex1@outlook.com

References

[1] Bagshaw SM. Acute kidney injury: Diagnosis and classification of aki: Akin or rifle? Nature Reviews. Nephrology. 2010;**6**:71-73

[2] Modaresi A, Nafar M, Sahraei Z. Oxidative stress in chronic kidney disease. Iranian Journal of Kidney Diseases. 2015;**9**(3):165-179

[3] Putri AY, Thaha M. Role of oxidative stress on chronic kidney disease progression. Acta Medica Indonesiana. 2014;**46**(3):244-252

[4] Nacak H, Bolignano D, Van Diepen M, Dekker F, Van Biesen W. Timing of start of dialysis in diabetes mellitus patients: A systematic literature review. Nephrology, Dialysis, Transplantation. 2016;**31**(2):306-316

[5] Garcia-Garcia G, Briseño-Rentería G, Luquín-Arellan VH, Gao Z, Gill J, Tonelli M. Survival among patients with kidney failure in Jalisco, Mexico. Journal of the American Society of Nephrology. 2007;**18**(6):1922-1927

[6] Narres M, Claessen H, Droste S, Kvitkina T, Koch M, Kuss O, et al. The incidence of end-stage renal disease in the diabetic (compared to the non-diabetic) population: A systematic review. PLoS One. 2016;**11**(1):e0147329

[7] Packham DK, Alves TP, Dwyer JP, Atkins R, de Zeeuw D, Cooper M, et al. Relative incidence of ESRD versus cardiovascular mortality in proteinuric type 2 diabetes and nephropathy: Results from the DIAMETRIC (Diabetes Mellitus Treatment for Renal Insufficiency Consortium) database. American Journal of Kidney Diseases. 2012;**59**(1):75-83

[8] Chávez-Valencia V, Orizaga de la Cruz C, Leonardo Pazarín-Villaseñor H, Fuentes-Ramírez F, Parra-Michel R, Aragaki Y, et al. Frencuencia de los tipos de transporte peritoneal en la población del Hospital General Regional No. 46 del Instituto Mexicano del Seguro Social. Gaceta Médica de México. 2014;**150**(2):186-193

[9] Montilla-López P, Muñoz-Agueda MC, Feijóo López M, Muñoz-Castañeda JR, Bujalance-Arenas I, Túnez-Fiñana I. Comparison of melatonin versus vitamin C on oxidative stress and antioxidant enzyme activity in Alzheimer's disease induced by okadaic acid in neuroblastoma cells. European Journal of Pharmacology. 2002;**451**(3):237-243

[10] JD1 M, Frei B, Longmire AW, Gaziano JM, Lynch SM, Shyr Y, et al. Increase in circulating products of lipid peroxidation (F2-isoprostanes) in smokers. Smoking as a cause of oxidative damage. The New England Journal of Medicine. 1995;**332**(18):1198-1203

[11] Hofmann H, Schmidt HH. Thiol dependence of nitric oxide synthase. Biochemistry. 1995;**34**(41):13443-13452

[12] Mattiazzi M, D'Aurelio M, Gajewski CD, Martushova K, Kiaei M, Beal MF, et al. Mutated human SOD1 causes dysfunction of oxidative phosphorylation in mitochondria of transgenic mice. The Journal of Biological Chemistry. 2002;**277**(33):29626-29633

[13] Trachootham D, Lu W, Ogasawara MA, Nilsa RD, Huang P. Redox regulation of cell survival. Antioxidants & Redox Signaling. 2008;**10**(8):1343-1374

[14] Navaneethan SD, Schold JD, Kirwan JP, Arrigain S, Jolly SE, Poggio ED, et al. Metabolic syndrome, ESRD, and death in CKD. Clinical Journal of the American Society of Nephrology. 2013;**8**(6):945-952

[15] Lo WK. Metabolic syndrome and obesity in peritoneal dialysis. Kidney Research and Clinical Practice. 2016;**35**(1):10-14

[16] Garcia-Garcia G, Garcia-Bejarano H, Breien H, Perez-Cortes G, Pazarin-Villaseñor L, De la Torre-Campos L, et al. End stage renal disease in Mexico. In: Garcia-Garcia G, Agodoa L, Norris KC, editors. Chronic Kidney Disease in Disadvantaged Populations. London: Elsevier; 2017. pp. 17-83

[17] Davies MJ, Gray LJ, Troughton J, et al. A Community-based Primary Prevention Programme for Type 2 Diabetes Mellitus Integrating Identification and Lifestyle Intervention for Prevention: A Cluster Randomised Controlled Trial. Southampton, UK: Programme Grants for Applied Research; 2017

[18] Tziomalos K, Athyros VG. Diabetic nephropathy: New risk factors and improvements in diagnosis. The Review of Diabetic Studies. 2015;**12**(1-2):110-118

[19] Abbott KC, Bakris GL. Treatment of the diabetic patient: Focus on cardiovascular and renal risk reduction. Progress in Brain Research. 2002;**139**:289-298

[20] Ganesh SK, Hulbert-Shearon T, Port FK, Eagle K, Stack AG. Mortality differences by dialysis modality among incident ESRD patients with and without coronary artery disease. Journal of the American Society of Nephrology. 2003;**14**:415-424

[21] Ganesh SK, Hulbert-Shearon T, Port FK, Eagle K, Stack AG. Mortality differences by dialysis modality among incident ESRD patients with and without coronary artery disease. Journal of the American Society of Nephrology. 2003;**14**:415-424

[22] Ignace S, Fouque D, Arkouche W, Steghens J-P, Guebre-Egziabher F. Preserved residual renal function is associated with lower oxidative stress in peritoneal dialysis patients. Nephrology, Dialysis, Transplantation. 2009;**24**:1685-1689

[23] Müller-Krebs S, Kihm LP, Zeier B, Gross ML, Wieslander A, Haug U, et al. Glucose degradation products result in cardiovascular toxicity in a rat model of renal failure. Peritoneal Dialysis International. 2010;**30**(1):35-40

[24] Tarng DC, Wen Chen T, Huang TP, Chen CL, Liu TY, Wei YH. Increased oxidative damage to peripheral blood leukocyte DNA in chronic peritoneal dialysis patients. Journal of the American Society of Nephrology. 2002;**13**:1321-1330

[25] Cerrillos-Gutierrez JI, Miranda-Diaz AG, Preciado-Rojas P, Gomez-Navarro B, Sifuentes-Franco S, Andrade-Sierra J, et al. The beneficial effects of renal transplantation on altered oxidative status of ESRD patients. Oxidative Medicine and Cellular Longevity. 2016;**2016**:5757645

[26] van de Kerkhof J, Schalkwijk CG, Konings CJ, Cheriex EC, van der Sande FM, Scheffer PG, et al. Nε-(carboxymethyl) lysine, Nε-(carboxyethyl)lysine and vascular cell adhesion molecule-1 (VCAM-1) in relation to peritoneal glucose prescription and residual renal function; a study in peritoneal dialysis patients. Nephrology, Dialysis, Transplantation. 2004;**19**:910-916

[27] Davì G, Ciabattoni G, Consoli A, Mezzetti A, Falco A, Santarone S, et al. In vivo formation of 8-iso-prostaglandin f2alpha and platelet activation in diabetes mellitus: Effects of improved metabolic control and vitamin E supplementation. Circulation. 1999;**99**(2):224-229

[28] Kant M, Akış M, Çalan M, Arkan T, Bayraktar F, Dizdaroglu M, et al.

Elevated urinary levels of 8-oxo-2′-deoxyguanosine, (5'R)- and (5'S)-8,5′-cyclo-2′-deoxyadenosines, and 8-iso-prostaglandin F2α as potential biomarkers of oxidative stress in patients with prediabetes. DNA Repair (Amst). 2016;**48**:1-7

[29] De Deyn PP, Vanholder R, D'hooge R. Nitric oxide in uremia: Effects of several potentially toxic Guanidino compounds. Kidney International. 2003;**63**:S25-S28

[30] Brunet P, Gondouin B, Duval-Sabatier A, Dou L, Cerini C, Dignat-George F, et al. Does uremia cause vascular dysfunction? Kidney & Blood Pressure Research. 2011;**34**:284-290

[31] Zweier JL, Li H, Samouilov A, Liu X. Mechanisms of nitrite reduction to nitric oxide in the heart and vessel wall. Nitric Oxide. 2010;**22**(2):83-90

[32] Tarng DC, Chen TW, Huang T-P, Chen C-L, Liu T-Y, Wei YH. Increased oxidative damage to peripheral blood leukocyte DNA in chronic peritoneal dialysis patients. Journal of the American Society of Nephrology. 2002;**13**:1321-1330

[33] Ogunleye A, Akinbodewa AA, Adejumo OA, Oluwafemi TT, Akinfaderin DA. Changes in antioxidant status associated with haemodialysis in chronic kidney disease. Ghana Medical Journal. 2018;**52**(1):29-33

[34] Ahmadpoor P, Eftekhar E, Nourooz-Zadeh J, Servat H, Makhdoomi K, Ghafari A. Glutathione, glutathione-related enzymes, and total antioxidant capacity in patients on maintenance dialysis. Iranian Journal of Kidney Diseases. 2009;**3**(1):22-27

[35] Valko M, Rhodes CJ, Moncol J, Izakovic M, Mazur M. Free radicals, metals and antioxidants in oxidative stress induced cancer. Chemico-Biological Interactions. 2006;**160**:1-40

[36] SIES H. Oxidative stress: Oxidants and antioxidants. Experimental Physiology. 1997;**82**:291-295

[37] Finkelstein FO, Juergensen P, Wang S, Santacroce S, Levine M, Kotanko P, Levin NW, Handelman GJ. Hemoglobin and plasma vitamin C levels in patients on peritoneal dialysis. Peritoneal Dialysis International 2011;**31**(1):74-79

Chapter 19

Antioxidants: Natural Antibiotics

Syed Ali Raza Naqvi, Sana Nadeem, Sana Komal, Syed Ali Asad Naqvi, Muhammad Samee Mubarik, Sajid Yaqub Qureshi, Shahzad Ahmad, Ali Abbas, Muhammad Zahid, Naeem-Ul-Haq Khan, Syed Shujat Raza and Nosheen Aslam

Abstract

The aim of this current piece of writing is to draw the attention of readers and researchers toward the natural antioxidants that can take the place of synthetic antibiotics to avoid bacterial resistance and gastrotoxicity/nephrotoxicity. Antioxidants such as polyphenols, vitamins, and carotenoids are the organic compounds mainly extracted from natural sources and dominantly involved in boosting the defense system of organisms. The main public health-related issue over the globe is ever-growing bacterial resistance to synthetic antibiotics, which is being continuously reported during the last decade. Further, the pipeline of the development of new synthetic antibacterial agents to replace the resistant antibiotics in clinical set-up is gradually drying up. This scenario originated the concept to revive the interest toward natural antibacterial products due to their chemical diversity, which provide important therapeutic effect and make the microbes unable to copy them for creating resistance. Natural products, especially polyphenols had been seen in antioxidant, antibacterial, anticancer, anti-inflammation, and antiviral activities with encouraging results. In this chapter, we will focus over the role of natural antioxidants as antibacterial agents.

Keywords: antioxidants, antibacterial agents, infection therapy, natural antibiotics

1. Introduction

Microbes are known to human civilization due to their beneficial and lethal effects. When the symbiotic relation of microorganisms goes beyond the limit, they may cause pathogenic infections and diseases, causing damage to the body and sometimes leading to death: this is a major concerning issue especially in developing countries. The determination of exact site of infection in the body is very critical for curing the pathogenesis caused by bacteria at their early stage. Antimicrobial agents especially antibiotics, which are either obtained from natural sources or through total synthetic procedures, are practiced against pathogens. Antibiotic may be obtained naturally from living organism (e.g., fungi, actinomycete, and bacillus species), prepared synthetically and semisynthetically in the laboratory. Its mechanism of action is divided into two spectrums (narrow and broad-range spectra).

Broad-spectrum antibiotics act against both Gram-positive and Gram-negative bacteria [1]. A good antibiotic should have the following characteristics: long shelf life, nontoxic to human body, soluble in the body fluid, low cost, show long-lasting antibacterial effect, and low possibility of bacterial resistance to the agent. However, all these standard parameters for an ideal antibiotic are difficult to meet, while developing synthetic antibacterial agents that is the reason a big threat is being felt from pathogenic bacterial resistance which is the main public health-related issue, all over the globe [2]. This appeared during the last decade in a more prominent way which mainly originated either due to wrong identification of bacterial strain and prescription of antibiotic or due to imbalance use of antibacterial agents. The transmission of bacterial resistance among the individuals and across the geological border is one way of antimicrobial resistance [3]. Further, on the other way, to handle the bacterial resistance threat, the pipeline of the development of new synthetic antibacterial agents is gradually drying up. And it might be possible, on the bases of continuously increasing level of bacterial resistance; at some stage pathogenic bacteria halt antibiotic therapy—that stage will be not good in the history of human being [4].

Antioxidants such as polyphenols, vitamins, and carotenoids are the organic compounds mainly extracted from natural sources and dominantly involved in living defense system. Due to continuously increasing resistance to synthetic antibiotics, there is an urgent need to shift our focus toward natural antioxidant-based antibacterial products due to their vast chemical diversity which provide potent therapeutic effect and make the microbes unable to copy them for creating resistance. Out of many natural products and antioxidants which are showing great healthy impact on human beings, polyphenols have been reported as natural agents that fight as antioxidants, antibacterial, anticancer, anti-inflammation, and antiviral agents. We, in this chapter, tried to review the role of antioxidants as natural antibiotics. In the following section, we will discuss the inflammation and infectious process and how antioxidants play their role in fixing them. Then we will also discuss antibacterial mechanism of natural antioxidants as antibiotics in animal bodies.

2. Inflammation and infection

Pathogens like bacteria are responsible for the infection or inflammation in animals. These infections may be mild inflammation which is hardly noticeable or which appeared to human being in history as a big threat. According to one estimation, based on growing bacterial resistance, up to 2050, the death rate due to bacterial infection may increase to 390,000 in Europe and similarly all over the world as shown in **Figure 1**. Inflammation is a nonspecific immunological response by the organism's body to any trauma, neoplasm, autoimmune attack, or invading of the microbes. At the site of inflammation, several processes can be noticed such as blood supply increase and leakage of cellular fluid and small molecules, and protein penetration may take place. In the case of acute injury, body defense mechanism, i.e., leucocyte and plasma protein migration to the site of infection become activated. Neutrophils invade bacteria when seeking entrance in the body and prevent the body from further infection. The process of infection starts within a second or minute and prolongs to hours or days to heal. It causes the sequential symptoms, like inflammation, redness, warmth, and pain, which consequently affect the functions of the tissue or organ. Inflammation may be a nonspecific process, but infection consists of stepwise progress in inflammation which might be chronic if it could not be addressed timely.

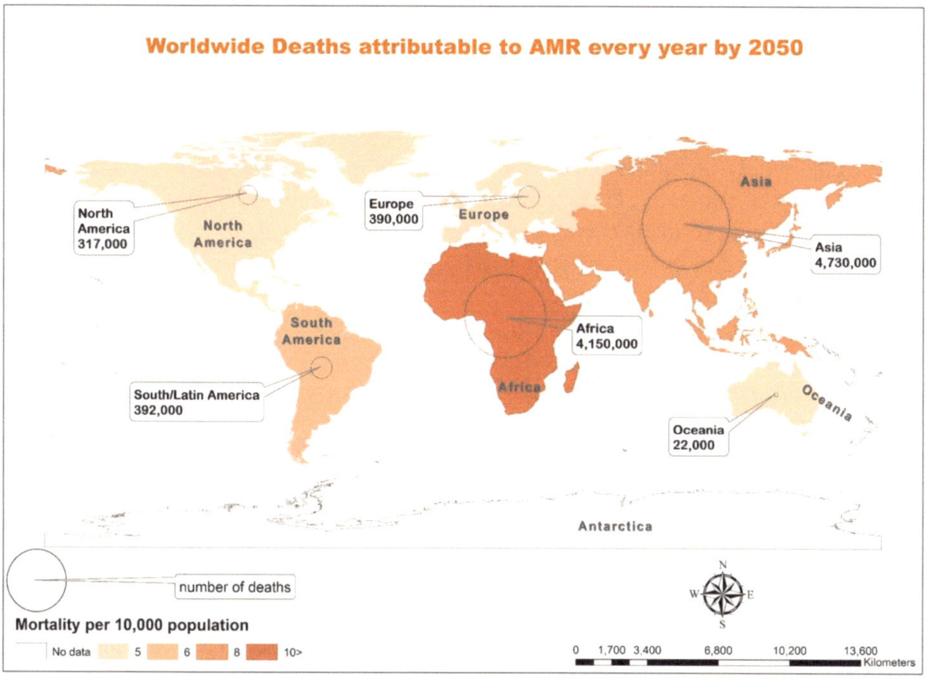

Figure 1.
An estimation of deaths caused by bacterial infection worldwide [5].

3. Types of infection

Infections can be categorized as viral, bacterial, fungal, protozoan, prion, and parasitic. Some **viral** infections are influenza, rotavirus, chicken pox, HIV, and herpes. Pneumonia, tetanus, cellulites, chlamydia, gonorrhea, etc. are the common **bacterial** infections. **Fungal** infections are ringworm, candidiasis, and athlete's foot. Malaria and African sleeping sickness are common **protozoan** infections transmitted through plasmodium and tsetse fly, respectively. **Prion** is the poisonous entities or protein infection particles which cause fatal neurodegenerative disease. Amebiasis, dysentery, and coccidiosis infections are caused by **parasites.** Antibiotics are the major agents to cope and fix these infections. There are mainly two types of antibacterial agents, i.e., synthetic antibiotics and natural antibiotics. In the following section, we will discuss antibiotics, natural antibiotics, and their mode of action.

4. Antibiotics

In the ancient times, it is believed that antibiotics were the chemicals released by microorganisms, causing prompt deleterious effect on humans. However, later this notion was reversed, i.e., these compounds were used against microbes instead of isolating from them. Antibiotics are generally of two types, **bactericidal** which kill the bacterial cell and **bacteriostatic** which inhibit the bacterial growth and may kill the bacteria. The first antibiotic was discovered by Alexander Fleming in 1928 from *Penicillium notatum*, a soil-inhabiting fungus, and the clinical trials on humans are conducted in 1940. There are five generations of different classes of antibiotics, up till now, which have been discovered and are in clinical practice.

5. Natural antioxidants as antibiotics

The increased resistance of pathogenic microorganism against antibiotic becomes a major issue around the globe from the last decade. To overcome this serious problem, it is necessary to discover a new world of antimicrobials, which are not only beneficial in bacterial infection but show long-lasting effect by boosting the immunity of the body. However, we do not skip the usage of previously practiced antibiotics as some of them show a very effective result in bacterial infection, but there is a need of advanced or may say strong antibacterials whose chemical makeup bacteria cannot be copied.

Plant synthesizes a variety of secondary metabolites (phytochemicals) which are involved in plant defense mechanism, and it is recognized that major classes of these molecules have beneficial effects on health including antioxidants and antimicrobial. The attractive antioxidant as well as antibacterial activity of phytochemicals seeks attention as it may replace the synthetic antioxidants, which cause deleterious effect on human health such as cancer. The plant kingdom is rich in various phytochemicals like phenolic acid, flavonoids, gingerol, curcumin, etc.

Phenolic acids and flavonoids are a very important class of antioxidants as it directly affects bacterial growth and causes hindrance in their pathogenic activity. The mechanism of action of antioxidants as antibacterial is still not fully understood, but some researches reveal that the attributable antibacterial activity involves three basic mechanisms: outer membrane permeability, cytoplasm leakage, and inhibition of nucleic acid formation. The interaction of polyphenols with nonspecific forces like hydrogen bonding and hydrophobic effect lipophilic forces as well as by covalent bond formation was related to microbial adhesion and enzyme and cell envelope transport protein. The antibacterial activity of polyphenols may also due to the capacity of these compounds to chelate iron, vital for the survival of almost all bacteria. Polyphenols rupture the wall, increase the permeability of cytoplasm membrane, and release lipopolysaccharides (LPS) [6].

The cell wall composition of Gram-positive and Gram-negative differs significantly as Gram-positive bacteria have thick layer of peptidoglycan along with lipoteichoic acid but lack of outer membrane. Gram-negative bacterial outer membrane consists of phospholipid, protein, and LPS and a thin layer of peptidoglycan. Both Gram-negative and Gram-positive bacterial cell walls play a very important role in osmotic protection of cell. Any damage to cell wall will decrease the tolerance of cell against osmotic pressure and ionic strength. Many researchers have demonstrated that the interaction of polyphenols with bacterial cell wall is different for Gram-negative and Gram-positive bacteria. Different interaction cites for antibacterial agents in variety of bacterial strains are shown in (**Tables 1–4**).

6. Mechanisms of action

The activity of antioxidants against bacterial inflammations is being progressively recognized. They also work synergistically with current antibacterial agents against the resistant strains of bacteria. The diversity in the structure of natural products makes it impossible for bacteria to copy its functional moieties, unlike the synthetic agents. The structure of antioxidants holds the key role in determining the antibacterial activity. Different groups of researchers investigating the relationship between flavonoid structure and their antibacterial activity generalized that active compounds share common structural features. Moreover, the unique structural

Antibacterial Action mechanism	Interaction cites	Example	References
Interaction between the bacterial cell wall	Outer membrane	Trans-anethole cause membrane integrity on *S. albus, B. subtilis, S. typhimurium, S. dysenteriae, E. coli*	[4]
		Thyme essential oils have severe effect on the listerial cell wall of L. monocytogenes leading to cell wall rupture.	[6]
		Flower essential oil of Bidens pilosa rich in monoterpene hydrocarbons and oxygenated monoterpenes which is strongly affect the membranes of gram negative bacteria	[7]
		Flavonoids (epigallocatechin, catechin, myricetin, quercetin) and aromatic phenolic compound (thymol, carvacrol, eugenol, cinnamic aldehyde)	[8]
		Obtained from dietary spice and medicinal herbs show antibacterial potential for S. aureus, E. coli, L. monocytogenes.	
	Membrane protein	Quercetin, 3-O-caffeoylquinic acid and anthocyanidins are contained within the berry leaves and branches that alter the mechanism to repair DNA thus showing antibacterial potential.	[9]
		Phenolic compound obtained from Eucalyptus globules show more activity against gram negative bacteria due to their outer lipopolysaccharide membrane.	[10]
		Quercetin obtained from yellow onion (allium cepa) has inhibitory effect on antibiotic resistant bacteria H. pylori	[11]
Interaction with cell membrane	Bilayer	Phenolic compound extracted from herbs alter the permeability of microbial cell, disrupt energy metabolism and proton motive force causing cell death.	[12]
		Essential oil of S. cumini shows activity especially for S. typhimurium.	
		Extract of Tunisian ruta chalepensis organs(leave, flower, stem) were rich in vanillic acid and coumarin which show remarkable antibacterial properties against P. aeruginosa .it is revealed that the activity was strain and origin dependent.	[13]

Table 1.
Natural antioxidants and their role in inhibiting bacterial growth in living system showing interaction between the bacterial cell wall and with cell membrane.

Antibacterial Action mechanism	Interaction cites	Example	References
Metal ion deficiency due to chelating ability	Ionic iron	Tannins from hydnora africanathunb are used for different strains of gram negative and positive bacteria.	[14]
		Spice and herbs extract rich in phenolic, flavonoids, proanthocyanidins and hydrolysable tannins show antimicrobial activity against three bacterial strains(L. monocytogenes, S. aureus, S. enterica)	
Microbial enzyme inhibition and substrate deprivation	Microbial enzymes	Quercetin cause hindrance in the production of exopolysaccharide production in K. pneumoniae, P. aeruginosa ,and Y. enterocolitica	[3]
		Ferulic acid completely inhibit colony spreading of S. aureus	
		Tannic acid along with other antioxidants inhibit B. subtilis cyclic di-AMP synthase	
Protein regulation	Repression / stimulation of the bacterial genes	Treatment of P. aeruginosa with cranberry proanthocyanidins down regulated 2 proteins implicated in ATP synthesis, a cytochrome C(PA2482 and hypothetical protein PA2481 and protein involved in DNA and RNA synthesis and acid cycle proteins(subunits of acetyl-CoA carboxylase and fumarase)	
		Treatment of P. aeruginosa with cranberry proanthocyanidins up- regulated 12 proteins related to cation transporters (such as PchD, PvdN, PhuS), 5 protein involved I amino acid synthesis (such as PA0335,PA2044, HutG) protein involved in response to stress (such as OsmC, SodM) and a hypothetical protein involved in flavonoid metabolism.	
Change in cell morphology and inhibition of nucleic acid synthesis	Formation of filamentous cells, DNA & RNA	Genistein, an isoflavone show antibacterial activity against V. harveyi and B. subtilis	[15]
Inhibition of respiratory chains of bacterial membranes	Respiratory chains	Retrochalcones from Glycyrrhiza Inflata inhibits the growth of M. luteus, S. aureus and P. aeruginosa.	[16]
Inhibition of DNA and RNA synthesis	DNA and RNA	(-)-Epigallocatechin, a flavonoid inhibits DNA and RNA synthesis in P. vulgaris and S. aureus.	[17]

Table 2.
Natural antioxidants and their role in inhibiting bacterial growth in living system showing metal ion deficiency due to chelating ability, microbial enzyme inhibition and substrate deprivation and other inhibition mechanism.

features may be essential for flavonoids to gain adjacency or uptake into the bacterial cell. Like, polyhydroxylated flavonoids show more pronounced antibacterial activity than mono-hydroxylated or non-hydroxylated flavonoids. Structural

Class	Compound	Bacteria	MIC	MBC	Mode of action
Phenolic acids	Ferulic acid	E. coli	1500	5000	Cytoplasmic membrane integrity
		P. aeruginosa	500	500	
		S. aureus	1750	5250	
		L. monocytogenes	2000	5500	
	Gallic acid	E. coli	100	2500	
		P. aeruginosa	100	500	
		S. aureus	1100	5000	
		L. monocytogenes	1250	5300	
		S. mutans	>1.2 mg/ml		
	Tannic acid	S. mutans	>0.4 mg/ml		
	Salicylic acid	S. mutans	>3.8 mg/ml		
Flavones	Flavone	Staphylococcus	50		
	7,8-	Staphylococcus	100		
	6,7-	Staphylococcus	50	–	
		S. aureus	100		
	3(OH)-flavone	S. aureus AM-176	257		
	5,7(OH)$_2$-flavone	S. aureus AM-176	103		
Flavonols	Datiscetin	P. vulgaris	100		DNA and RNA synthesis
		Staphylococcus	50		
	Morin	P. vulgaris	100		
	Quercetagetin	P. vulgaris	100		
	Robinetin	S. aureus	100		
		P. vulgaris	100		
	Myricetin	S. aureus	100		
		P. vulgaris	50		
		Staphylococcus	100		
	Galangin	Staphylococcus	6.3		
	kaempferol	Staphylococcus	50		
	fisetin	Staphylococcus	100		
	Quercetin	S. mutant	>1.5 mg/ml		
Flavanono	(+)-Dihydrorobinetin	S. aureus	200		DNA and RNA synthesis
		P. vulgaris	200		
Catechins	(-)-Epigallocatechin	S. aureus	100		DNA and RNA synthesis
		P. vulgaris	50		
		Staphylococcus	50		
vitamins	Ascorbic acid	S. mutans	>2.0		

Table 3.
Purified antioxidants extracted from plant sources and their antibacterial potential: phenolic acid, flavones, flavanonols, catechins, and vitamins.

similarity among flavonoids is too dominant that there are three probable hypotheses regarding their mechanism of action:

a. Flavonoids of same structure take same mechanism.

b. All flavonoids follow multiple mechanisms of actions.

c. All flavonoids have same sole mechanism of action.

According to a recent development, the study of mechanism of actions is not that reliable as it was assumed earlier. Like epigallocatechin gallate only induce clumping of FabG enzyme and have no such effect on other enzymes. Another such development is that flavonoids cause aggregation of bacterial cells. Clumping of bacterial cells on treatment with flavonoids causes reduction in surface area of

Class	Compound	Bacteria	MIC
Chalcones	Chalcone	AM-51 (MRSA	38.5
		AM-72 (MRSA	15.5
		AM-172 (MRSA	32.0
		AM-176 (MRSA	36.2
	2'(OH)-chalcone	AM-51 (MRSA	38.6
		AM-72 (MRSA	13.6
		AM-172 (MRSA	33.0
		AM-176 (MRSA	37.1
	2',4'$(OH)_2$-chalcone	AM-51 (MRSA	38.4
		AM-72 (MRSA	12.7
	chalcone	AM-172 (MRSA	31.0
		AM-176	34.2
	2',4'$(OH)_2$-chalcone	AM-51 (MRSA	38.7
		AM-72 (MRSA	16.3
		AM-172 (MRSA	31.6
		AM-176 (MRSA	36.6
Flavanone	Sophoraflavanone	MRSA strains	3.13-6.25
	Exiguaflavanone D	MRSA strains	3.13-6.25
	Kenusanone D	MRSA strains	3.13-12.5
	Exiguaflavanonne	MRSA strains	6.25
	Sophoraflavanone	MRSA strains	3.13-12.5
	Sophoraflavanone	MRSA strains	6.25-12.5
	Kenusanone A	MRSA strains	6.25-12.5
	Naringenin	MRSA strains	200-400
	Exiguaflavanone C	MRSA strains	12.5
	Exiguaflavannone	MRSA strains	12.5
	Leachianone G	MRSA strains	12.5

Table 4.
Purified antioxidants extracted from plant sources and their antibacterial potential: chalcone and flavanone.

bacterial population which reduce the oxygen consumption by bacteria (interruption respiratory chains). Reduction in surface area of cells decrease the nutritional uptake like uridine and thymidine (specify nucleic acid inhibition). Moreover, the prospect of baffling and the cause and effect of mechanisms of actions exist. For example, the interruption of membrane integrity by an antibacterial agent will impart negative effects on proton-motive force that directly influence the synthesis of ATP and solute transport into the bacterial cell. The deterioration of bacterial capability to produce energy and to attain nutrients results in declining capability of bacterial cell to make DNA and peptidoglycan. So, one mechanism of action may be misunderstood as multiple.

Correspondingly, if any enzyme of bacteria-like DNA gyrase is obstructed by an antibacterial agent, then this swift automated cell death and lysis. Likewise, the

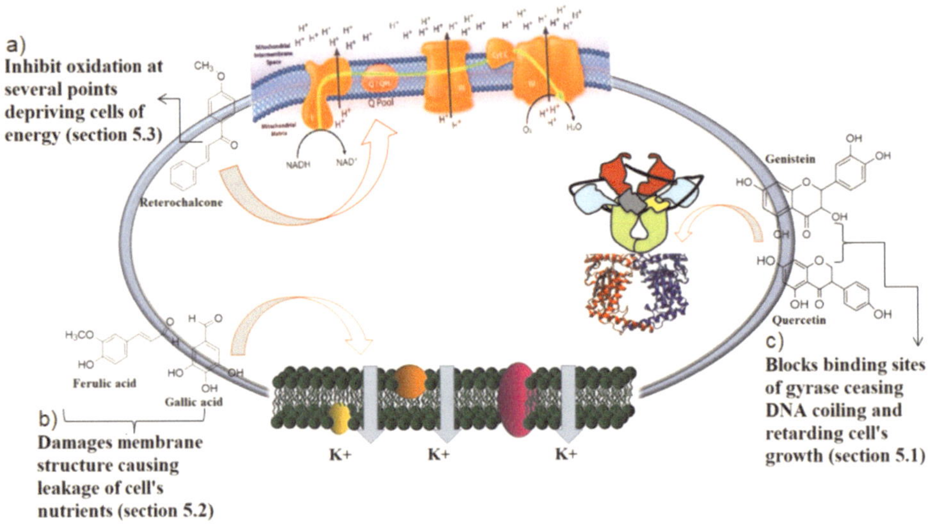

Figure 2.
The schematic layout demonstrating the natural antioxidant role as antibacterial: (a) representing inhibition of energy metabolism; (b) representing disruption of membranes; and (c) representing interruption in nucleic acid synthesis.

antibacterial agent that impedes the synthesis of nucleic acid may be misinterpreted as the agent that alters the cytoplasmic membrane functions [7].

The following mechanisms of actions are attributed to the antibacterial action of flavonoids as reported by different groups of researchers:

- Impairment of membrane functions

    a. Alteration of cytoplasmic membrane fluidity

    b. Inhibition of cell wall formation

    c. Inhibition of cell membrane formation

- Interruption of synthesis of nucleic acid

- Inhibition of respiratory metabolism

The mechanisms of action of antioxidants as an antibacterial are shown in **Figure 2**.

6.1 Inhibition of nucleic acid synthesis

Among the classes of antioxidants, flavonoids significantly show inhibitory activity against nucleic acid synthesis. Interaction of flavonoids with DNA- or with ATP-binding site of gyrase finally leads to the inhibition of nucleic acid synthesis as shown in **Figure 2**. Metabolism of DNA in bacteria comprises transcription, recombination, DNA replication, and transport of genetic information. A vital enzyme to control vigorous changes of nucleic acid is DNA gyrase. Gyrases, characteristic and crucial bacterial enzymes that change the topology of DNA, are the amiable aim to hit for the antibacterial agents. DNA gyrase, in a reaction that depends on ATP, enhances the supercoiling of DNA of bacteria, and its inactivation leads to bacterial death. Estimation of DNA supercoiling is the important parameter in assessment of flavonoids activity to inhibit DNA gyrase. It has two subunits, gyrase A that takes part in DNA breakage-resealing and gyrase B that is involved in the hydrolysis of ATP, the driving force for the DNA supercoiling. The topoisomerase (DNA gyrase) inhibitors form a cleavable complex of agent-topoisomerase-DNA or interfere with the gyrase binding to DNA (see **Table 2**).

6.1.1 Kaempferol and PMFs

Kaempferol show the strongest antibacterial activity (MIC_{50} = 25 μg/ml) against *E. coli* DNA gyrase. It inhibits the activity of gyrase enzyme that holds the key role in DNA supercoiling and bacterial growth.

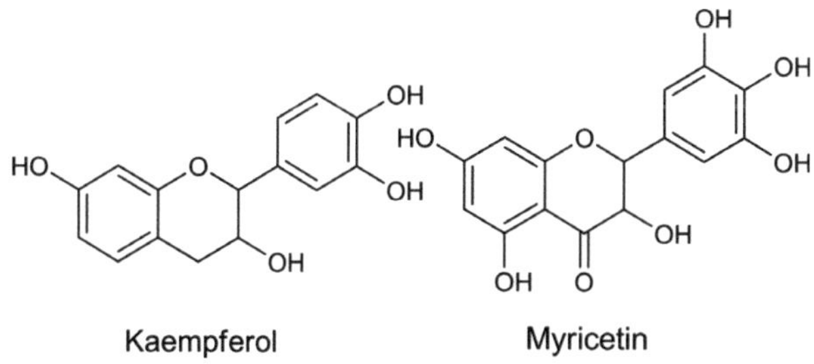

Structure of Polymethoxylated flavones

Polymethoxylated flavones (shown in structure) usually found in citrus peel possess broad spectrum antimicrobial activity. It shows antibacterial activity against *E. coli* and *S. aureus* with IC_{50} values ranging from 1.45 to 1.89 mg/ml [8] (see **Table 3** for MIC values).

6.1.2 Quercetin

Quercetin is one of the ubiquitous flavonoids, impedes the DNA supercoiling, and causes DNA to cleave. Quercetin encourages DNA scission by forming gyrase-DNA-quercetin cleavable complex. Cleavage of DNA was promoted at quercetin concentration above 80 μM in the presence of gyrase, and at 640 μM the maximum cleavage was obtained [9]. MIC values of quercetin are listed in **Table 3**. Quercetin obtained from yellow onion skin has inhibitory effect on antibiotic-resistant bacteria *H. pylori*. Sulfur and quercetin have synergistic growth inhibitory effect with beta lactam, a very functional antibiotic [10].

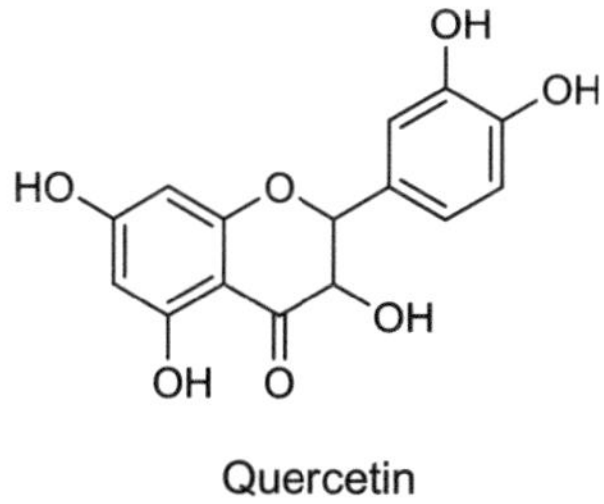

Structure of quercetin

Mode of action of quercetin inhibition includes two mechanisms:

First inhibition pathway involves rivalry at binding site of ATP at gyrase B that prevents DNA supercoiling. The second mechanism involves binding to DNA that stabilizes DNA topoisomerase II complex causing DNA to cleave [11]. MIC values for different bacterial strains are listed in **Table 3**.

6.1.3 Glycosylated flavones

Glycosylated flavones (isolated from cottonseed flour) promote topoisomerase IV-dependent cleavage of DNA in *E. coli*. Rutin is the most potent glycosylated isoflavone in exciting topoisomerase IV-dependent cleavage of DNA (CC_{50} = 1 μg/ml). It blocks the catalytic activity of type II topoisomerase in addition to alleviate the cleavable complex. At CC_{50} = 64 μg/ml, rutin inhibited the decantation action of topoisomerase IV.

6.1.4 Catechins

Catechins like epicatechin, epigallocatechin, epicatechin gallate, and epigallo-catechin gallate (structure is shown below) inhibit ATPase action because the ATP-binding site of B subunit of gyrase shares the structural similarity with these catechins. So, owing to this similarity with ATP-binding site, the catechins occupy these sites and as a result inhibits of ATPase activity. Catechins inhibit the ATPase activity in the following order, EGC < ECG < EGCG, while EC had no affect at all (for MIC values see **Table 4**) [12]. ATP hydrolysis provides vigorous force for DNA supercoiling. The inhibition of ATPase activity by catechins prevents ATP hydrolysis. In this way the DNA supercoiling is affected and so the bacterial growth.

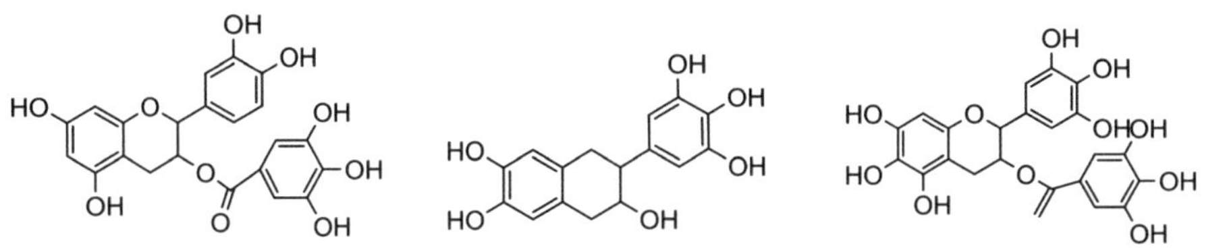

Epicatechin-3-gallate Epigallocatechin Epigallocatechin gallate

Catechin based antioxidants

6.1.5 Soybean isoflavone

SI (soybean isoflavone) could alter the supercoiling of double-stranded DNA could be altered by affecting DNA topoisomerase. By increasing the concentration of soybean isoflavone, the supercoiling activity increases and the quantity of linear and open circular DNA decreases.

At 6.4 mg/ml concentration, SI significantly inhibited the activity of both topo-isomerase I and II so stops the bacterial growth by affecting nucleic acid synthesis. Topoisomerase inhibitors form a drug-gyrase-DNA cleavable complex or disrupt the topoisomerase binding to DNA [13].

6.1.6 Genistein

Genistein is an isoflavone (shown in structure below) and characteristic of other flavonoids, apigenin, daidzein, and kaempferol for common use on the laboratory strains bacterial species like *B. subtilis*, *E. coli*, and *V. harveyi*. Addition of this flavonoid to bacterial cultures imposes drastic effects on the synthesis of DNA and RNA in almost 15 min [14].

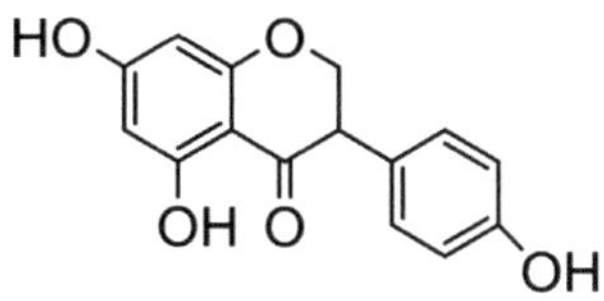

Genistein

Three hours after addition, genistein caused the bacterial cells to become elongate that cause troubled cell division and chromosome replication. MIC values are listed in **Table 3**.

Protein synthesis was also significantly inhibited by genistein but was delayed a little, suggesting that repression of translation by genistein is secondary effect.

6.2 Disruption of membranes

The outer bacterial membranes safeguard the bacterial cells from harsh environment, causing them to survive in extreme conditions. The inner membrane or the so-called cytoplasmic membrane regulates the uptake of solutes and minerals into the cell as well as the transport of proteins and other macromolecules. The alteration in membranes causes many adverse effects on functions of bacterial cells that might be very important for bacterial integrity, like uptake of mineral ions and nutrients. To study the membrane effects of antioxidants, fluorescence polarization methods using model membranes (consisting of two component: DPPC and POPC) are used. Fluorescence polarization increasingly alters in correspondence with reduction in membrane fluidity. MIC values are given in **Table 3**.

The antioxidants like polyhydroxyl flavans and catechin of green tea hinder the development of certain bacteria and affect Gram-positive and Gram-negative bacteria by damaging the structure of membranes of the bacterial cells (see **Table 1**).

6.2.1 Sophoraflavanone G

Sophoraflavanone G, a phytochemical with intensive antibacterial activity, shows very low MICs (1.56—12.5 μg/ml) against Gram-positive bacteria than Gram-negative bacteria by altering membrane functions. Increased polarization in DPPC and POPC liposomes implies that sophoraflavanone G decreases membrane fluidity (for MIC value see **Table 4**) [15].

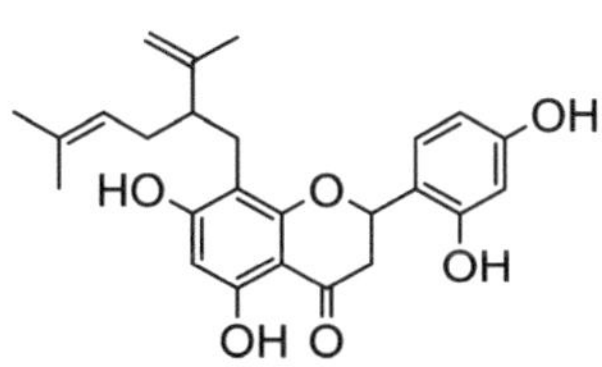

Sophoraflavanone G

6.2.2 Catechins

The pathogenicity of Gram-negative bacteria is linked to the lipopolysaccharide layer (reduce the sensitivity against antibacterial agents). That is why, the antibacterial agents demonstrate more activity for Gram-positive bacteria. Catechins intermingle and target bacterial membrane protein, fatty acid synthase, beta lactamase, and such other bacterial enzymes. Antibacterial catechins were reported to alter membrane fluidity [16]. Tea catechins impart specific agitation in the well-organized phosphatidylcholine and phosphatidylethanolamine bilayers that makeup membranes of bacteria. Epigallocatechin gallate (EGCG), a polyphenol obtained from green tea, black tea, and cocoa shows intensive activity, perturbs membranes of bacteria, and causes leakage of membranes isolated from *E. coli*. The antibacterial effects result from the interaction of catechins which interacts with oxygen, genes, and cell membranes, and these interactions produce their antibacterial effects. MIC values are given in **Table 3**.

EGCG binds straight to the peptidoglycan of *S. aureus*, affects integrity of cell and thereby decreases the acceptance of the cell to high osmotic pressure and less ionic strength. EGCG induces changes in morphology of Gram-negative bacteria depending on the acquittance of H_2O_2 and causes oxidative stress in bacteria. Flavonoids (epigallocatechin, myricetin, quercetin; structure shown below), damage membrane protein, and coagulate cytoplasm alter constituents of fatty acids and phospholipids, weaken mechanism of energy formation and metabolism, impacts the production of RNA and DNA, and abolishes translocation of proteins [17].

Epicatechin gallate (ECG) dramatically alters the physical properties of phosphatidylcholine (PC) and phosphatidylethanolamine (PE) bilayers. They cause leakage from the membranes that is known to be pronounce by the presence of PE. So, at membrane level the antibacterial properties of catechins are due to their damage to PE. So, to estimate the phospholipid specificity, in the presence and absence of PE, egg yolk model was used. The results showed that only galloylated catechins affected PE and caused prominent leakage at 6.3 mol%. Protein translocation and other such processes are to some extent related to phospholipids; so, any effect on these can significantly alter the cell metabolism of bacteria [18]. Liposome membranes are damaged by EGCG and the leakage of intraliposomal CF occurs. This damage to membranes increases the permeability of catechins for catechins to penetrate in the cell. But how catechins damage the bilayer and penetrate the cell is still unanswered [19].

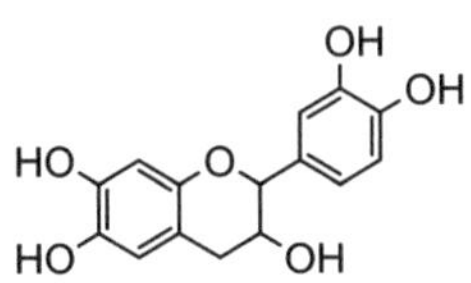

Epicatechin

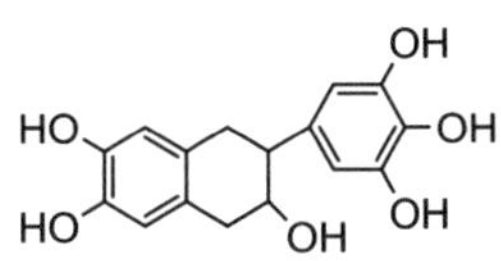

Epigallocatechin

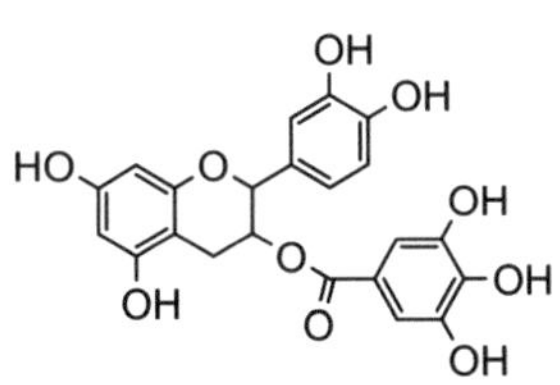

Epicatechin-3-gallate

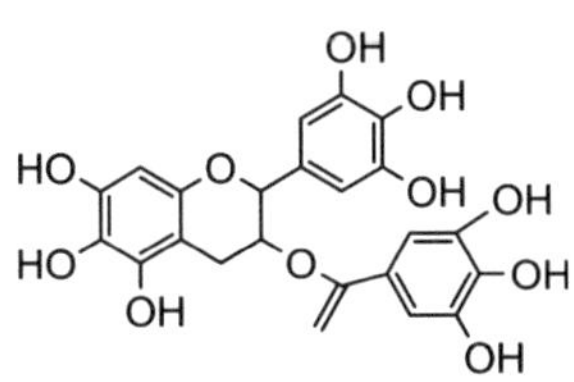

Epigallocatechin gallate

6.2.3 Ferulic and gallic acid

FA and GA cause severe and irreversible damage to the membranes causing constant leakage of the essential cell constituents. Different physiological terms are used to access the antimicrobial activities: MIC, MBC, and K^+ release in the cell. The MIC values of ferulic and gallic acids against some bacterial strains are listed in **Table 5**.

	MIC values μg/ml		
	E. coli	*P. aeruginosa*	*S. aureus*
Gallic acid	1500	500	1750
Ferulic acid	100	100	1100

Table 5.
MIC values of antioxidants against bacterial strains.

At 100 μg/ml ferulic acid and gallic acid cause 60% damage to the cytoplasmic membranes of *P. aeruginosa*. The uptake of propidium iodine (nucleic acid strain to which cell is impermeable) shows that FA and GA alter membrane integrity. In the outer membrane of Gram-positive and Gram-negative bacteria, porins (hydrophilic channels) are present that stops the hydrophobic substances from entering the cell. But some natural agents disintegrate the lipopolysaccharide layer and so damaging the permeability of the membrane causing nutrients to leak and effecting bacterial growth [20].

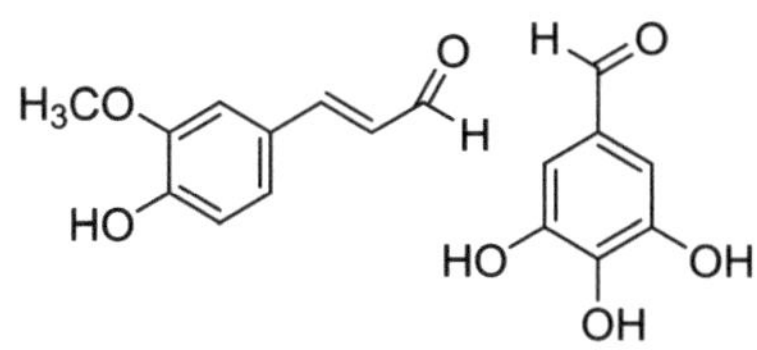

Moreover, bacterial cells have negative surface charge because of the ionic groups. The exposure to phenolic acids decreases this charge and the transport of solutes. Excess of phenolic acids cause hyper acidification that makes the cytoplasm acidic and denature the proteins present in the cytoplasm. So, the damage to membrane by acidification potentially explains the activity of phenolic acid.

Another factor that indicates the membrane damage is K^+ leakage. Because the cell's internal environment is rich in K^+, any damage to the cytoplasmic membranes causes its leakage that indicates the damage as shown in **Figure 2**.

6.3 Inhibition of energy metabolism

In bacterial cell the energy is required for the transport of solutes, uptake of metabolites, and biosynthesis of macromolecules. This energy comes from the respiratory chains like electron transport chain. Some antioxidants inhibit the respiratory chains at any step and thus depriving the cell of the energy necessary for growth (see **Table 1**).

6.3.1 Reterochalcones

Reterochalcones stops the oxygen consumption in the targeted cells and inhibits the NADH oxidation in the membranes of bacteria. The electron transport chain is inhibited in between the CoQ and cytochrome c sites as shown in **Figure 2**. The inhibition of respiratory chains stops the supply of energy to the cells thus retarding their growth [8, 21].

7. Conclusion

There is no doubt that synthetic antibiotics show quick therapeutic effect while treating bacterial infections but in parallel imposes the threat of serious gastrotoxicity, nephrotoxicity, and bacterial resistance. All these issues required special attention because we are gradually losing the game by treating bacterial infections with synthetic antibiotics—as we discussed in previous sections, natural antioxidants in its pure (isolated from raw extracts) had showed excellent potential against common infection causing bacteria, and no study has yet been reported of bacterial resistance to these compounds which firm our enthusiasm to study natural products with the aim to replace synthetic antibiotics. Finally, we can conclude that although antioxidants work slowly against bacterial growth, directly or indirectly, their action is steady and healthy—the continuous and careful evaluation in establishing antibacterial profile of isolated antioxidant can help in the utilization of natural products against bacterial infections with negligible toxicity and the fear of bacterial resistance.

Acknowledgements

The authors are very happy to pay their gratitude to Ms. Rida Siraj (MS scholar), Ms. Afshan Kanwal (PhD scholar), and the students of Dr. Ali's research group for their input in collecting and compiling the data for this chapter.

Conflict of interest

The authors declare "no conflict of interest."

Thanks declarations

The authors are highly thankful to the Higher Education Commission (HEC) Islamabad and Government College University, Faisalabad, Pakistan, for providing necessary resources to complete this project.

DOI: http://dx.doi.org/10.5772/intechopen.84864

Author details

Syed Ali Raza Naqvi[1*], Sana Nadeem[1], Sana Komal[1], Syed Ali Asad Naqvi[2], Muhammad Samee Mubarik[3], Sajid Yaqub Qureshi[3], Shahzad Ahmad[3], Ali Abbas[1], Muhammad Zahid[4], Naeem-Ul-Haq Khan[1], Syed Shujat Raza[1] and Nosheen Aslam[5]

1 Department of Chemistry, Government College University, Faisalabad, Pakistan

2 Department of Geography, Government College University, Faisalabad, Pakistan

3 Department of Wild and Fisheries, Government College University, Faisalabad, Pakistan

4 Department of Chemistry, University of Agriculture, Faisalabad, Pakistan

5 Department of Biochemistry, Government College University, Faisalabad, Pakistan

*Address all correspondence to: drarnaqvi@gmail.com

References

[1] Al-Mohanna M. Antibiotics and Chemotherapeutic Agents. 2016

[2] Moellering RC Jr. Essential characteristics of antibiotics for the treatment of seriously ill patients. Clinical Therapeutics. 1981;**4**(Suppl A):1-7

[3] Aminov RI. A brief history of the antibiotic era: Lessons learned and challenges for the future. Frontiers in Microbiology. 2010;**1**:134-134

[4] Song JH. What's new on the antimicrobial horizon? International Journal of Antimicrobial Agents. 2008; **32**(Supp. 4):S207-S213

[5] https://amr-review.org/sites/default/files/AMR%20Review%20Paper%20-%20Tackling%20a%20crisis%20for%20the%20health%20and%20wealth%20of%20nations_1.pdf

[6] Papuc C et al. Plant polyphenols as antioxidant and antibacterial agents for shelf-life extension of meat and meat products: Classification, structures, sources, and action mechanisms. Comprehensive Reviews in Food Science and Food Safety. 2017;**16**(6): 1243-1268

[7] Cushnie TPT, Lamb AJ. Recent advances in understanding the antibacterial properties of flavonoids. International Journal of Antimicrobial Agents. 2011;**38**(2):99-107

[8] Wu T et al. Structure–activity relationship of flavonoids on their anti-*Escherichia coli* activity and inhibition of DNA gyrase. Journal of Agricultural and Food Chemistry. 2013;**61**(34):8185-8190

[9] Plaper A et al. Characterization of quercetin binding site on DNA gyrase. Biochemical and Biophysical Research Communications. 2003;**306**(2):530-536

[10] Ramos FA et al. Antibacterial and antioxidant activities of quercetin oxidation products from yellow onion (*Allium cepa*) skin. Journal of Agricultural and Food Chemistry. 2006; **54**(10):3551-3557

[11] Friedman M. Overview of antibacterial, antitoxin, antiviral, and antifungal activities of tea flavonoids and teas. Molecular Nutrition & Food Research. 2006;**51**(1):116-134

[12] Gradišar H et al. Green tea catechins inhibit bacterial DNA gyrase by interaction with its ATP binding site. Journal of Medicinal Chemistry. 2007; **50**(2):264-271

[13] Wang Q, Wang H, Xie M. Antibacterial mechanism of soybean isoflavone on *Staphylococcus aureus*. Archives of Microbiology. 2010;**192**(11): 893-898

[14] Ulanowska K et al. Differential antibacterial activity of genistein arising from global inhibition of DNA, RNA and protein synthesis in some bacterial strains. Archives of Microbiology. 2006; **184**(5):271-278

[15] Tsuchiya H, Linuma M. Reduction of membrane fluidity by antibacterial sophoraflavanone G isolated from *Sophora exigua*. Phytomedicine. 2000; **7**(2):161-165

[16] Tsuchiya H et al. Comparative study on the antibacterial activity of phytochemical flavanones against methicillin-resistant *Staphylococcus aureus*. Journal of Ethnopharmacology. 1996;**50**(1):27-34

[17] Shan B et al. The in vitro antibacterial activity of dietary spice and medicinal herb extracts. International Journal of Food Microbiology. 2007;**117**(1):112-119

[18] Caturla N et al. The relationship between the antioxidant and the antibacterial properties of galloylated catechins and the structure of phospholipid model membranes. Free Radical Biology and Medicine. 2003; **34**(6):648-662

[19] Ikigai H et al. Bactericidal catechins damage the lipid bilayer. Biochimica et Biophysica Acta (BBA): Biomembranes. 1993;**1147**(1):132-136

[20] Borges A et al. Antibacterial activity and mode of action of ferulic and gallic acids against pathogenic bacteria. Microbial Drug Resistance. 2013;**19**(4): 256-265

[21] Cushnie TPT, Lamb AJ. Antimicrobial activity of flavonoids. International Journal of Antimicrobial Agents. 2005;**26**(5):343-356

Chapter 20

Diseases Related to Types of Free Radicals

Narendra Maddu

Abstract

The free radicals are reactive molecules with electron-rich groups produced during metabolic reactions occurring in the cells. These free radicals are collectively known as reactive oxygen species (ROS) and reactive nitrogen species (RNS). Lipid peroxidation products and protein carbonyls species are under the group of ROS, and nitric oxide and peroxynitrites are under the group of RNS. The malondialdehyde that reacts with LDL-C indirectly induced the risk of atherosclerosis. The protein carbonyls acts as marker of protein oxidation and exerts damage to proteins. The nitric oxide plays an important role in DNA damage, inflammation, proliferation of cancer cells, and dysfunction of apoptosis. The peroxynitrites could induce the process of lipid peroxidation, DNA damage, and may exert chronic damage to all biomolecules. The aim of the present study is that the free radicals may react with biomolecules of the cells and play an important role in the development of chronic disease conditions in the humans.

Keywords: reactive oxygen species, reactive nitrogen species, oxidative stress, pathological conditions

1. Introduction

Free radical is a molecule with an unpaired electron and capable of high reactivity [1, 2]. Free radicals are found to be involved in alteration of redox system, induced DNA damage, activation of procarcinogens, these all markers of induction of cancer [3]. Some of the radicals are the superoxide (O^{-2}), hydroxyl (OH•), alkoxy radical (RO•), and nitric oxide (NO), and nonradical species are hydrogen peroxide (H_2O_2), singlet oxygen ($^1O_2$), and peroxynitrites (ONOO—), which play an important role in the development and progression of different pathological conditions [4]. NO-induced dose-responsive DNA strand breakage and deaminations of cytosine to uracil and 5-methylcytosine to thymine account for the mutagenicity of nitric oxide toward bacteria and mammalian cells [5]. Antioxidants are proved that reduce the actions of reactive oxygen and nitrogen species, which are capable of damaging cells and tissues [6]. The proteins contain nitrotyrosine residues accumulate in cells which disrupts multiple regulatory pathways [7].

Nitroxidative stress maker species are actively engaged in the chronic disease complications, and their toxicity is reduced by antioxidants which have protective effects [8]. The enzymes of NADPH oxidases, xanthine oxidase, uncoupled nitric oxide synthase, and mitochondria act as markers of reactive oxygen species production in all metabolic cells [9]. Free radicals thus adversely alter lipids, proteins, and DNA and trigger a number of human diseases [10]. Peroxynitrites are the leading molecule of reactive nitrogen species by enhancing the process of lipid peroxidation, DNA

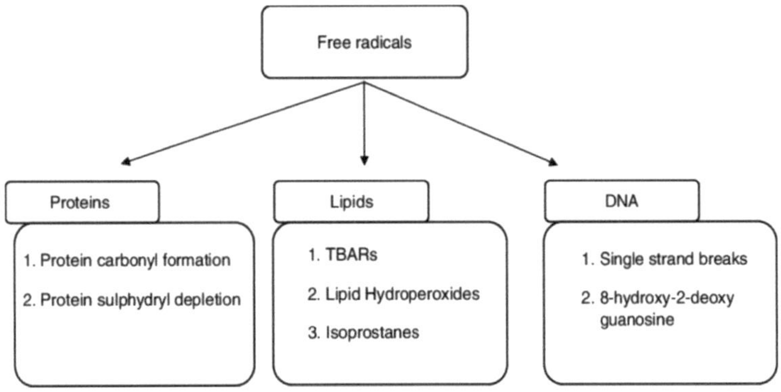

Figure 1.
Impact of free radicals on biomolecules present in cells leads to formation of adducts, markers of various diseases [19].

damage, and protein oxidation and act as molecular target for drug development for cardiovascular, inflammatory, and neurodegenerative diseases [11]. In the cells, the interaction of excess superoxides with excess nitric oxide results in the generation of peroxynitrite which specify the chronic disease conditions of stroke, myocardial infarction, chronic heart failure, diabetes, circulatory shock, chronic inflammatory diseases, cancer, and neurodegenerative disorders [12]. The reduced glutathione, glutathione disulfide, and glutathionylated proteins act as markers of redox imbalance are directly proportional to oxidative stress [13].

The ROS requires oxygen for its formation and play an important role in human health and disease [14]. The development of increased ROS production with the simultaneous dysfunction of mitochondria has been exhibited in the pathogenesis of disorders [15]. Every cell especially vascular cells are involved in the higher production of free radicals implicated in the pathogenesis of ischemic heart disease, atherosclerosis, cardiac arrhythmia, hypertension, and diabetes [16]. The scavenging role of hydrogen peroxide is performed by catalase and decreases catalase activity results in aggregation of hydrogen peroxide leads to formation of oxidative distress [17]. The aerobic metabolic reactions are faced to greater a concentration of oxygen generates and is increased oxidation it leads inflammation, mitochondrial dysfunction, and chronic kidney diseases [18]. The purpose of the present review is to investigate the role of free radicals in various physiological and pathological diseases like neuro-disorders, cancer, renal, cardiovascular, and immunological dysfunctions (**Figure 1**).

2. Oxidation and cancer

The reactive oxygen and nitrogen species (RONS) are synthesized in greater concentration by reducing antioxidant defense, and formation of redox imbalance leads to oxidative damage to the DNA and proteins in the oral squamous cell carcinoma [20]. In animals, ROS may influence cell proliferation and cell death through the activation of several signaling pathways in the development of carcinogenesis [21]. The higher level of ROS is directly proportional to the suppression of antioxidant enzymes and significant role of oxidative-induced injury in the breast cancer [22]. The prolonged exposure and intake of tobacco is strongly associated with decreased status of antioxidant enzymes, increased oxidative stress markers with the pathogenesis of oral cancer [23]. The strong correlations of ROS and RNS with lowered antioxidants are found in oral precancer and cancer [2] (**Figures 2–3**).

DOI: http://dx.doi.org/10.5772/intechopen.82879

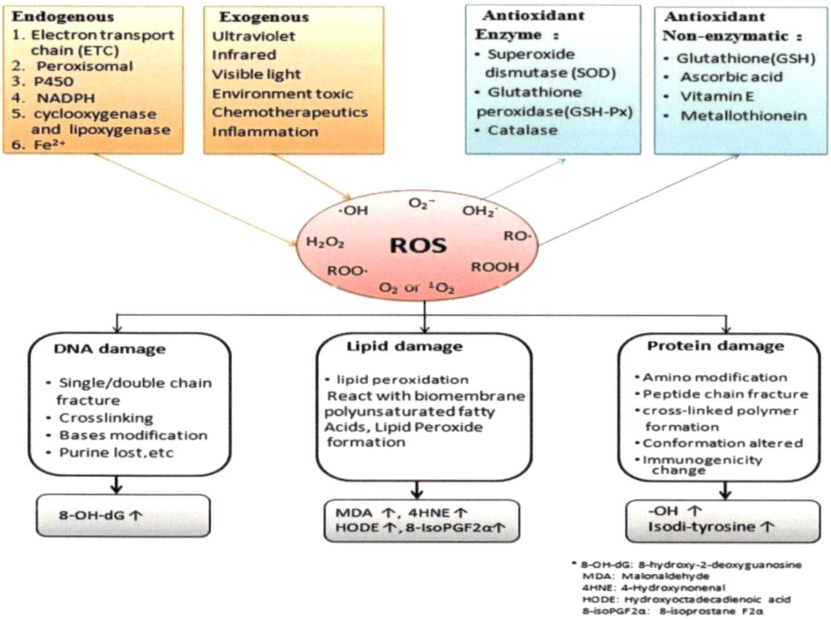

Figure 2.
The functions of free radicals on biomolecules and its consequences [24].

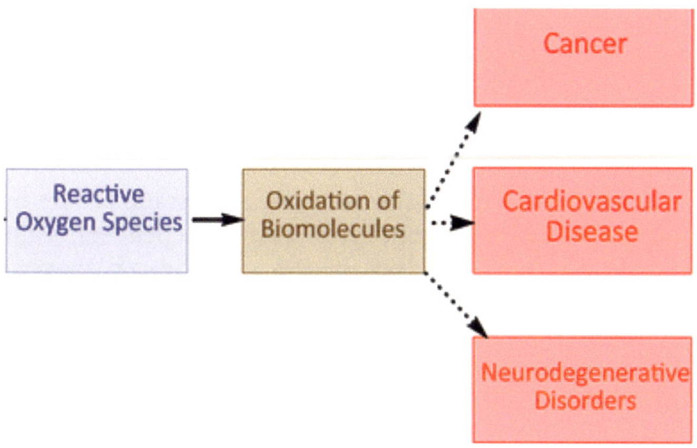

Figure 3.
Reactive oxygen species are involved in the development of various pathological disorders [38].

2.1 Free radical cause nitric oxide

The nitric oxide (NO) has dual role in health and disease and depends on its concentration. Nitric oxide is the active marker of the development of cancer by induction of angiogenesis, blood vessel formation during physiological and pathological processes [25]. NO may modulate tumor DNA repair mechanisms by upregulating p53, poly (ADP-ribose) polymerase, and DNA-dependent protein kinase (DNA-PK). The role of NO in cancer will have profound therapeutic implications for the diagnosis and treatment of disease [26]. Alterations in the NO metabolism and to increase protein nitration may contribute to the mutagenic processes and promote lung carcinogenesis [27]. NO promotes intravasation and angiogenesis to enhance cancer cell growth and increase the properties of cancer cells [28].

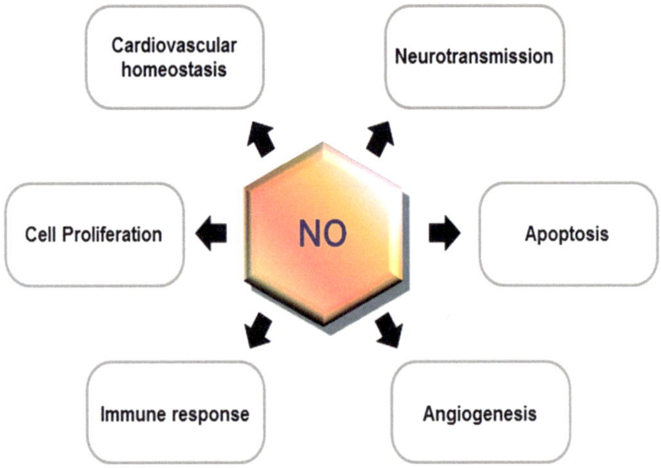

Figure 4.
The role of nitric oxide in various diseases of humans [57].

In lung cancer, a high level of NO is linked to chronic stages of cancer cells and protective role in the survival and proliferation of tumor cells by inhibiting apoptosis, increasing cell migration, and invasion [29]. NO and its role in carcinogenesis and tumor progression, as well as dietary chemopreventive agents have NO-modulating properties with safe cytotoxic profile [30]. The nitric oxide synthase 2-mediated production of NO/reactive nitrogen oxide species (RNS) is heavily involved in cancer progression and metastasis in different types of tumor (**Figure 4**) [31].

2.2 Free radical cause peroxynitrites

Peroxynitrites (ONOO—) could able to cause DNA strand breaks and oxidize cellular thiol groups in viable rat thymocytes in a dose-dependent fashion [32]. ONOO— is actively involved in the disturbances of signaling pathways of epidermal growth factors indirectly induced the process of tumorigenesis [33]. The combined effects of nitric oxide and oxidized LDL forms increase the concentrations of peroxynitrites that leads to glutathionylation of p21 ras proteins which results in aberrant activation of p21 [34]. The S-nitrosylation of PTEN, Bcl_2 enhanced DNA mutation, and inhibition of apoptosis results in cell proliferation and cell survival [35]. The peroxynitrite could modify the DNA and increase the DNA adducts which act as antigens is one of the factors for the autoantibody induction in cancer patients [36]. Levels of peroxynitrite and nitrosylhemoglobin can be used as highly informative markers of disease prognosis and therapeutic approach [37].

2.3 Free radical cause lipid peroxidation

Lipids are major structural components of the membranes and are highly addictable to oxidation by the presence of reactive double bonds [39]. The malondialdehyde (MDA), product of lipid peroxidation, reacts with low-density lipoproteins and indirectly induced the process of atherosclerosis [40]. The high level of oxidative stress is directly proportional to progression of tumor stages in lungs and pulmonary parenchyma [41]. The lipid peroxides are one of the ROS that enhance the DNA damage through mutations which results in decreased expression of tumor suppressor genes or increased expression of oncogenes [42]. ONOO— is the initiator of induction of lipid peroxidation which disrupts the membranes and lipoproteins.

These ONOO— and MDA collectively act as cytotoxic as well as mutagenic in cancer progression [43]. The formation of oxidative stress due to imbalance of redox system in the cells through increased lipid peroxidation has been associated with human health and diseases, including cancer [44]. The lower levels of cholesterol was detected in cancer cells and suspectible to attack of free radicals enabling the penetration of RONS into the interior of the cell, inducing pro-apoptotic factors [45].

3. Neurodegenerative diseases

3.1 Free radical cause peroxynitrites

The combined effects of peroxynitrite and sulfur-containing amino acids have been implicated in Parkinson's disease by performing the synergistic toxicity to a neuronal cell line [46]. The protein nitration in the form of nitrotyrosine residues is by the actions of peroxynitrite. Increased concentrations of both protein carbonyls and 3-nitrotyrosine have been reported in various neurodegenerative diseases like Alzheimer's disease (AD), Parkinson's disease (PD), and amyotrophic lateral sclerosis (ALS) [47]. The decreased activity of antioxidant enzymes with the simultaneous increase in the concentrations of peroxynitrites leads to disturbances of oxidative phosphorylation was observed in the brain mitochondria [48]. The modification of the monomers, destabilize microtubules, and major alterations in neurodegenerative diseases is performed by peroxynitrites [49]. The effects of S-nitrosylation on neuronal excitation are due to stimulation of ionotropic glutamate receptors and toxic Aβ peptides in Alzheimer's disease [50].

3.2 Free radical cause nitric oxide

In the lower doses, nitric oxide acts as a neurotransmitter of the neuronal cells, and it exerts antimicrobial activity invading microbes in macrophages [51]. Nitric oxide played an important role in the modulation of CO_2-mediated cerebral blood flow [52]. Nitric oxide is a physiological signaling molecule produced from L-arginine by enzyme of nitric oxide synthase (NOS). This enzyme occurs in three forms as neuronal (nNOS), endothelial (eNOS), and inducible nitric oxide synthase (iNOS). It increases the cGMP levels by acting as vasodilator and is involved in the neurotransmission between nervous system cells [53]. The positive association of oxidative stress and neurodegenerative conditions was observed in multiple sclerosis, stroke, and neurodegenerative disorders [54]. The ROS is actively involved in the oxidative damage to amyloid beta peptides, marker in the Alzheimer's disease [55]. The most abundant neurotransmitter in central nervous system is glutamate which acts as the initiator of NO formation, and H_2S is highly expressed in brain which is involved in the pathogenesis of various neurological disorders [56].

3.3 Free radical cause lipid peroxidation

The brain oxidative damage contributes to AD pathogenesis by the Aβ accumulation and amyloid plaque formation in the Alzheimer's disease of Tg2576 mice [58]. The imbalance of functioning endogenous antioxidant system leads to accumulation of free radicals, which not only induces the process of lipid peroxidation but also plays a central role in neurodegeneration [59]. Lipids are critical for plasticity and function of neuronal development. The abnormalities in lipid metabolism contribute to the pathogenesis of several neurodegenerative disorders like Alzheimer's disease and Parkinson's disease [60]. The relationship between lipid alterations in energy metabolism and mitochondrial dysfunction in neurodegenerative disorders [61]. Deposition of abnormal aggregated proteins and disruption of metal ion homeostasis are highly associated with oxidative stress [62]. The antioxdant and free radicals of lipid peroxidation and cognition, and cognitive response to an exercise intervention program, in adults with coronary artery disease at risk of dementia [63]. The brain is more susceptible to lipid peroxidation due to its high oxygen consumption, high level of redox metal ions, reduced antioxidant defense mechanism, and high level of polyunsaturated fatty acids [64].

4. Cardiovascular diseases

4.1 Free radical cause nitric oxide

Decreased concentrations of nitric oxide may cause constriction of coronary arteries and contribute to provocation of myocardial ischemia in coronary artery disease patients. The nitric oxide present in lower amounts exerted the vascular inflammation that could lead to oxidation of lipoproteins and foam cell formation that leads to the development of the atherosclerotic plaque [65]. These ROS actively involved in atherogenesis through their formation from enzymes of xanthine oxidase, nicotinamide adenine dinucleotide phosphate (NADPH) oxidases, and nitric oxide synthase [66]. The peroxynitrites directly increases sarco/endoplasmic reticulum calcium (Ca^{2+} ATPase) sarco/endoplasmic reticulum calcium (SERCA) activity by S-glutathiolation and irreversible oxidation of the relevant cysteine thiols in atherosclerosis [67]. An imbalance of reduced production of NO or increased production of superoxide results in the endothelial dysfunction [68].

The dual role is performed by the nitric oxide NO in the cells, and at low concentrations, it regulates normal protective functions, but at high concentration may contribute to the pathogenesis [69]. Oxidative stress, mitochondrial dysfunction, and stress-related cell death pathways (apoptosis and necrosis) are related to the improper functioning of cardiovascular system [70]. Most ROS that are generated as by-products during mitochondrial electron transport and reactive nitrogen species (RNS) are peroxynitrites and nitric oxide, contributing to the role in the development of cardiovascular disease [71]. The specific markers of ROS are altered to inflammation that enhanced the risk of atherosclerosis by diabetes [72]. The vasodilator activity of NO may be unique among therapeutic options for management of hypertension, renal disease, and left ventricular hypertrophy [73].

4.2 Free radical cause peroxynitrites

Nitric oxide is important physiological signaling molecule also known as the endothelial-derived-relaxing factor (EDRF), and can form free radicals like peroxynitrites capable of peroxidizing the LDL and proteins [74]. Formation of peroxynitrite is augmented in inflammatory-like conditions such as ischemia-reperfusion injury in the high dose manner [75]. Proinflammatory cytokines stimulate the concerted enhancement in superoxide and NO-generating activities in the heart and causes myocardial contractile failure [76]. The protein nitration and inactivation of creatine kinase during heart failure in cardiac muscles are performed by peroxynitrites [77].

Peroxynitrite depresses myocardial contractility by decreasing the ability of Ca^{2+} to trigger contraction through cGMP/cGMP-dependent protein kinase pathway [78]. The peroxynitrite exposure results in reduced sarcoplasmic reticulum (SR) Ca^{2+}-ATPase (SERCA2a isoform) activity is a major determinant of reduced contractility in heart failure [79]. Peroxynitrites that are present in higher concentrations depicts a crucial pathogenic mechanism of stroke, myocardial infarction, chronic heart failure, diabetes, circulatory shock, chronic inflammatory diseases, cancer, and neurodegenerative disorders [12]. The synergistic performance of nitric oxide, superoxides, peroxynitrites are effect on mitochondrial function and cell death [80].

4.3 Free radical cause lipid peroxidation

Abnormalities in levels of antioxidants like GSH are associated to accumulation of lipid peroxidation in chronic heart failure [81]. Increased formation of lipid peroxides and aldehydes has been observed in atherosclerosis, ischemia-reperfusion, and heart failure [82]. Atherosclerosis, the hardening of arteries under oxidative stress is related to oxidative changes of low density lipoproteins (LDL) which is an early prediction of development of cardiovascular disease [83]. The proinflammatory effects that result from the peroxidation of lipids, which provide critical structure and function in cellular membranes, are the main sites of pollutant attack in cardiovascular diseases of atherosclerosis, arrhythmia, hypertension, and stroke [84].

5. Immunological disorders

5.1 Free radical cause nitric oxide

Peroxynitrite converts low density lipoprotein to a form recognized by the macrophage scavenger receptor and that this process is associated with modification of the protein and lipid, and with the oxidation of alpha-tocopherol to alpha-tocopherol quinine [85]. The activated macrophages are involved in the production of large amounts of nitric oxide and indirectly diminish lymphocyte proliferation [86]. Tyrosine nitration is recognized as a prevalent and significant post-translational protein modification that serves as an indicator of nitric oxide-mediated oxidative inflammatory reactions [87]. Prolonged iNOS expression peroxynitrite may exacerbate inflammatory responses mediated by NF-kappaB due to prolonged inducible nitric oxide synthase [88].

NO regulates the structural and functional activity of many immune and inflammatory cells like macrophages, T lymphocytes, antigen-presenting cells, mast cells, neutrophils, and natural killer cells [89]. The proinflammatory nature of NO is actively involved in the process of inflammation only at higher concentrations [90]. The macrophages in active state are actively engaged in the production of not only NO production but also TNFα production [91]. Stimulatory effects of NO on integrin β1 expression and Talin phosphorylation were mediated by the cGMP signaling pathway, which is likely involved in wound healing [92].

5.2 Free radical cause peroxynitrites

Physiological role for ONOO— as a down-modulator of immune responses and also as key mediator in cellular and tissue injury is associated with chronic activation of the immune system [93]. In chronic inflammatory diseases, peroxynitrite formed by phagocytic cells may cause damage to DNA which acts as epitopes for the production of autoantibodies [94]. The central role of peroxynitrite is performed in the control of infections in macrophages [95]. They are produced throughout the vascular system, regulate differentiation and contractility of vascular smooth muscle cells, control vascular endothelial cell proliferation and migration, mediate platelet activation and hemostasis, and significantly contribute to the immune response [96]. Elevated reactive oxygen and nitrogen species are reduced levels of glutathione with chronic systemic inflammation with elevated levels of pro-inflammatory cytokines [97]. The ONOO— could be modified by the histone proteins that lead to formation of oxidatively nitrated histones in the initiation and progression of autoimmune inflammatory diseases [98]. Peroxynitrite represents both a pathophysiologically relevant endogenous cytotoxin and a cytotoxic effector against invading pathogens [99]. Being a mediator of protein oxidation and nitration, lipid peroxidation, mitochondrial dysfunction, and cell death, peroxynitrite represents both a pathophysiologically relevant endogenous cytotoxin and a cytotoxic effector against invading pathogens [99].

5.3 Free radical cause lipid peroxidation

Plasma malondialdehyde and glutathione levels have been used as a determinate of oxidative status in the chronic immunological disorders; systemic lupus erythematosus (SLE) is a complex [100]. 4-Oxo-2-nonenal (ONE) is a highly reactive aldehyde originating from the peroxidation of polyunsaturated fatty acids involved in the pathogenesis of autoimmune disorders [101]. The product of lipid peroxidation is 4-hydroxynonenal (HNE) that acts as specific marker of immunosenescence and aging-related disorders [102].

6. Renal diseases

6.1 Free radical cause peroxynitrites

Ischemia-reperfusion injury showed decreased levels of 3-nitrotyrosine-protein adducts. The iNOS-generated NO mediates damage in I-R injury possibly through ONOO— formation [103]. Patients with chronic renal failure (CRF) showed decreased endothelium-dependent vasodilatation to acetylcholine, have increased markers of oxidative stress, and diminished antioxidant activity [104]. ONOO— could induce entire mitochondrial protein nitration, responsible for the damage of renal mitochondria in diabetes [105]. Nitrosative stress is involved in cisplatin-induced nephrotoxicity in rats through peroxynitrite-induced nephrotoxicity and protein nitration [106]. Renal hypoxia and ischemia promotes the formation of reactive oxygen species (ROS) such as superoxide radical anions, peroxides, and hydroxyl radicals, that can oxidatively damage biomolecules and membranes, and affect organelle function and induce renal tubule cell injury, inflammation, and vascular dysfunction [107].

6.2 Free radical cause nitric oxide

The rate of whole body NO synthesis was increased in the end stage renal disease (ESRD) patients [108]. In several animal models of renal disease, the increase in NO synthesis is associated with reduced degree of glomerulosclerosis, infiltration of the kidney by invading macrophages [109]. The relations between endothelial and inducible nitric oxide synthases are perturbed in renal ischemia primarily as a result of endothelial dysfunction [110]. The nitric oxide is highly reactive and exerts its chronic effects only at high concentrations which are responsible for the complications of dialysis of patients with chronic kidney disease [111]. Patients with chronic kidney disease (CKD) have been found the decreased levels in all stages of CKD [112]. Intracellular nitric oxide (iNO) substantially increased the risk of renal dysfunction in patients with acute respiratory distress syndrome (ARDS) [113]. The process of oxidative stress affects kidney function by elevated the damage in renal vessels, glomeruli, and tubules [114]. In patients with multiple valve replacement and prolonged cardiopulmonary bypass, administration of nitric oxide decreased the incidence of acute kidney injury [115].

7. Some other type of free radicals

7.1 Hydroxyl radicals

It is the most reactive of the free radical molecules. It damages cell membranes and lipoproteins by lipid peroxidation. Damage to lipoproteins in low density lipoprotein plays an important role in atherosclerosis. •OH is formed by radiolysis of water and by reaction of H2O2 with ferrous (Fe^{2+}) ions; the latter process is termed as Fenton reaction [116, 117]. The reactive oxygen species, hydroxyl (•OH) radical is one of the potential inducers of DNA damage. A variety of adducts are formed on reaction of •OH radical with DNA. The •OH radical can attack purine and pyrimidine bases to form •OH radical adducts, which are both oxidizing and reducing in nature which in turn can induce base modifications and sometimes release of bases. Some of the important base modifications include 8-hydroxydeoxyguanosine (8-OHdG), 8 (or 4-,5-)-hydroxyadenine, thymine peroxide, thymine glycols, and 5-(hydroxymethyl) uracil [118].

7.2 Free radical cause lipid peroxidation

Lipids that contain phosphate groups (i.e., phospholipids) are essential components of the membranes that surround the cells and cell structures. Free radicals in the presence of oxygen may cause degradation (peroxidation) of lipids within plasma and organellar membranes. Oxidative damage is initiated when the double bonds in unsaturated fatty acids of membrane lipids are attacked by oxygen derived free radicals particularly by OH. The lipid free radical interactions yield peroxides, which are themselves unstable and reactive, and an autocatalytic chain reaction called propagation ensues which can result in extensive membrane, organellar, and cellular damage [116, 119]. Oxidative destruction of polyunsaturated fatty acids by lipid peroxidation is damaging because it may alter the integrity of cell membranes. [120].

7.3 Superoxide oxygen (O_2•—one electron)

It is generated by direct auto-oxidation of O2 during mitochondrial electron transport reaction. Alternatively, O2• is produced enzymatically by xanthine oxidase and cytochrome P450 in the mitochondria or cytosol [121]. O2• so formed is catabolized to produce H2O2 by superoxide dismutase (SOD), a metalloprotein. It is considered to be the least reactive type of ROS and the most commonly produced free radical in humans. Once it is produced, it triggers a rapid cascade of events that creates other free radicals.

7.4 Singlet oxygen

Singlet oxygen ($^1O_2$) is an electronically excited form of oxygen which is well known to be formed when photosensitizers such as chlorophyll or the aromatic dye rose Bengal absorb light energy and transfer some of that energy to molecular oxygen

[122, 123]. Various nonphotosensitized mechanisms for its formation have also been reported and suggested to occur in biological systems, but the importance of such endogenous singlet oxygen formation has had a controversial history [122, 124]. Ozone (O3) is best known as occurring in the stratosphere where it shields organisms on earth from ultraviolet C and much of ultraviolet B radiations, which are the most damaging UV components of solar radiations because they are readily absorbed by DNA [125, 126]. It is also known as a respiratory system-damaging pollutant in the troposphere and ironically as a therapeutic agent in alternative medicine [127]. More recently, it was shown that antibodies or amino acids catalyze the conversion of singlet oxygen ($^1O_2$) to ozone (O_3) and that this reaction occurs during the killing of bacteria by activated neutrophils [128, 129]. Since both singlet oxygen and ozone are highly reactive oxygen species, a full understanding of their mechanisms of formation and action *in vivo* is necessary. Hence, various reported mechanisms of the endogenous formation of these reactive oxygen species (ROS), the potential relevance of such pathways in human physiology, diseases and activity of these oxidants.

8. Conclusions

The free radicals are normally synthesized during metabolic reactions in the cells and disease. These free radicals are removed by various scavenging activities of cellular and noncellular antioxidants. The imbalance of excess ROS formation and diminished activity of antioxidants results in the formation of oxidative stress which is linked with various pathological chronic conditions like cardiovascular, neurodegenerative, and renal disorders.

Conflict of interest

The authors report no declarations of interest.

Author details

Narendra Maddu
Department of Biochemistry, Sri Krishnadevaraya University, Ananthapuramu, Andhra Pradesh, India

*Address all correspondence to: dr.narendramaddu@gmail.com

References

[1] Mukherji SM, Singh SP. Free radicals. In: Reaction Mechanism in Organic Chemistry. Madras: Macmillan India Press; 1984. p. 285

[2] Choudhari SK, Chaudhary M, Gadbail AR, Sharma A, Tekade S. Oxidative and antioxidative mechanisms in oral cancer and precancer: A review. Oral Oncology. 2014;**50**:10-18

[3] Sun Y. Free radicals, antioxidant enzymes, and carcinogenesis. Free Radical Biology & Medicine. 1990;**8**:583-599

[4] Halliwell B. Free radicals and other reactive species in disease. In: Encyclopedia of Life Sciences. Singapore: Nature Publishing Group; 2001. pp. 1-7

[5] Nguyen T, Brunson D, Crespi CL, Penman BW, Wishnok JS, Tannenbaum SR. DNA damage and mutation in human cells exposed to nitric oxide in vitro. Proceedings of the National Academy of Sciences. 1992;**89**:3030-3034

[6] Halliwell B. Antioxidants in human health and disease. Annual Review of Nutrition. 1996;**16**:33-50

[7] Stadtman ER, Levine RL. Protein oxidation. Annals of the New York Academy of Sciences. 2000;**899**:191-208

[8] Willcox JK, Ash SL, Catignani GL. Antioxidants and prevention of chronic disease. Critical Reviews in Food Science and Nutrition. 2004;**44**:275-295

[9] Mueller CF, Laude K, McNally JS, Harrison DG. ATVB in focus: Redox mechanisms in blood vessels. Arteriosclerosis, Thrombosis, and Vascular Biology. 2005;**25**:274-278

[10] Dalle-Donne I, Scaloni A, Giustarini D, Cavarra E, Tell G, Lungarella G, et al. Proteins as biomarkers of oxidative/nitrosative stress in diseases: The contribution of redox proteomics. Mass Spectrometry Reviews. 2005;**24**:55-99

[11] Szabo C, Ischiropoulos H, Radi R. Peroxynitrite: Biochemistry, pathophysiology and development of therapeutics. Nature Reviews. Drug Discovery. 2007;**6**:662-680

[12] Pacher P, Beckman JS, Liaudet L. Nitric oxide and peroxynitrite in health and disease. Physiological Reviews. 2007;**87**:315-424

[13] Rossi R, Dalle-Donne I, Milzani A, Giustarini D. Oxidized forms of glutathione in peripheral blood as biomarkers of oxidative stress. Clinical Chemistry. 2006;**52**:1406-1414

[14] Brieger K, Schiavone S, Miller FJ Jr, Krause KH. Reactive oxygen species: From health to disease. Swiss Medical Weekly. 2012;**142**:13659

[15] Pagano G, Talamanca AA, Castello G, Cordero MD, Dischia M, Gadaleta MN, et al. Oxidative stress and mitochondrial dysfunction across broad-ranging pathologies: Toward mitochondria-targeted clinical strategies. Oxidative Medicine and Cellular Longevity. 2014;**54**:12-30

[16] Singh R, Devi S, Gollen R. Role of free radical in atherosclerosis, diabetes and dyslipidaemia: Larger-than-life. Diabetes/Metabolism Research and Reviews. 2015;**31**:113-126

[17] Sies H. Hydrogen peroxide as central redox signalling molecule in physiological oxidative stress: Oxidative eustress. Redox Biology. 2017;**11**:613-619

[18] Lv W, Booz GW, Fan F, Wang Y, Roman RJ. Oxidative stress and

renal fibrosis: Recent insights for the development of novel therapeutic strategies. Frontiers in Physiology. 2018;**9**:105

[19] Acharya JD, Ghaskadbi SS. Islets and their antioxidant defense. Islets. 2010;**2**:225-235

[20] Bahar G, Feinmesser R, Shpitzer T, Popovtzer A, Nagler RM. Salivary analysis in oral cancer patients: DNA and protein oxidation, reactive nitrogen species, and antioxidant profile. Cancer. 2007;**109**:54-59

[21] Genestra M. Oxyl radicals, redox-sensitive signalling cascades and antioxidants. Cellular Signalling. 2007;**19**:1807-1819

[22] Kasapovic J, Pejic S, Todorovic A, Stojiljkovic V, Pajovic SB. Antioxidant status and lipid peroxidation in the blood of breast cancer patients of different ages. Cell Biochemistry and Function. 2008;**26**:723-730

[23] Patel BP, Rawal UM, Rawal RM, Shukla SN, Patel PS. Tobacco, antioxidant enzymes, oxidative stress, and genetic susceptibility in oral caner. American Journal of Clinical Oncology. 2008;**31**:454-459

[24] Zhao J, Wang S, Zhong W, Yang B, Sun L, Zheng Y. Oxidative stress in the trabecular meshwork (Review). International Journal of Molecular Medicine. 2016;**38**:995-1002

[25] Ziche M, Morbidelli L. Nitric oxide and angiogenesis. Journal of Neuro-Oncology. 2000;**50**:139-148

[26] Xu W, Liu LZ, Loizidou M, Ahmed M, Charles IG. The role of nitric oxide in cancer. Cell Research. 2002;**12**:311-320

[27] Masri FA, Comhair SA, Koeck T, Xu W, Janocha A, Ghosh S, et al. Abnormalities in nitric oxide and its derivatives in lung cancer. American Journal of Respiratory and Critical Care Medicine. 2005;**172**:597-605

[28] Cheng H, Wang L, Mollica M, Re AT, Wu S, Zuo L. Nitric oxide in cancer metastasis. Cancer Letters. 2014;**353**:1-7

[29] Luanpitpong S, Chanvorachote P. Nitric oxide and aggressive behavior of lung cancer cells. Anticancer Research. 2015;**35**:4585-4592

[30] Vahora H, Khan MA, Alalami U, Hussain A. The potential role of nitric oxide in halting cancer progression through chemoprevention. Journal of Cancer Prevention. 2016;**21**:1-12

[31] Somasundaram V, Basudhar D, Bharadwaj G, No JH, Ridnour LA, Cheng RYS, et al. Molecular mechanisms of nitric oxide in cancer progression, signal transduction, and metabolism. Antioxidants & Redox Signaling. 2018. DOI: 10.1089/ars.2018.7527

[32] Salgo MG, Bermúdez E, Squadrito GL, Pryor WA. Peroxynitrite causes DNA damage and oxidation of thiols in rat thymocytes. Archives of Biochemistry and Biophysics. 1995;**322**:500-505

[33] Vander Vliet A, Hristova M, Cross CE, Eiserich JP, Goldkorn T. Peroxynitrite induces covalent dimerization of epidermal growth factor receptors in A 431 epidermoid carcinoma cells. The Journal of Biological Chemistry. 1998;**273**:31860-31866

[34] Clavreul N, Adachi T, Pimental DR, Ido Y, Schoneich C, Cohen RA. S-glutathiolation by peroxynitrite of p21ras at cysteine 118 mediates its direct activation and downstream signaling in endothelial cells. The FASEB Journal. 2006;**20**:518-520

[35] Floyd RA, Kotake Y, Towner RA, Xing GW, Nakae D, Konishi Y. Nitric

oxide and cancer development. Journal of Toxicologic Pathology. 2007;**20**:77-92

[36] Habib S, Moinuddin Ali A, Ali R. Preferential recognition of peroxynitrite modified human DNA by circulating autoantibodies in cancer patients. Cellular Immunology. 2009;**254**:117-123

[37] Guskova E, Ivanovich Kit O, Guskova N, Goroshinskaya IA, Nerodo GA, Chernikova NV. Predictors of prognosis and assessment of effectiveness of treatment for recurrent cervical cancer. Journal of Clinical Oncology. 2017;**34**:e17024

[38] Valko M, Jomova K, Rhodes CJ, Kuca K, Musilek K. Redox- and non-redox-metal-induced formation of free radicals and their role in human disease. Archives of Toxicology. 2016;**90**:1-37

[39] Porter NA, Caldwell SE, Mills KA. Mechanisms of free radical oxidation of unsaturated lipids. Lipids. 1995;**30**:277-290

[40] Slatter DA, Bolton CH, Bailey AJ. The importance of lipid-derived malondialdehyde in diabetes mellitus. Diabetologia. 2000;**43**:550-557

[41] Zieba M, Suwalski M, Kwiatkowska S, Piasecka G, Grzelewska-Rzymowska I, Stolarek R, et al. Comparison of hydrogen peroxide generation and the content of lipid peroxidation products in lung cancer tissue and pulmonary parenchyma. Respiratory Medicine. 2000;**94**:800-805

[42] Cejas P, Casado E, Belda-Iniesta C, De Castro J, Espinosa E, Redondo A, et al. Implications of oxidative stress and cell membrane lipid peroxidation in human cancer (Spain). Cancer Causes & Control. 2004;**15**:707-719

[43] Barrera G. Oxidative stress and lipid peroxidation products in cancer progression and therapy. International Scholarly Research Notices: Oncology. 2012:137289

[44] Zhong H, Yin H. Role of lipid peroxidation derived 4-hydroxynonenal (4-HNE) in cancer: Focusing on mitochondria. Redox Biology. 2015;**4**:193-199

[45] Van der Paal J, Neyts EC, Verlackt CCW, Bogaerts A. Effect of lipid peroxidation on membrane permeability of cancer and normal cells subjected to oxidative stress. Chemical Science. 2016;**7**:489-498

[46] Marshall KA, Reist M, Jenner P, Halliwell B. The neuronal toxicity of sulfite plus peroxynitrite is enhanced by glutathione depletion: Implications for Parkinson's disease. Free Radical Biology & Medicine. 1999;**27**:515-520

[47] Beal MF. Oxidatively modified proteins in aging and disease. Free Radical Biology & Medicine. 2002;**32**:797-803

[48] Vatassery GT, Lai JC, DeMaster EG, Smith WE, Quach HT. Oxidation of vitamin E and vitamin C and inhibition of brain mitochondrial oxidative phosphorylation by peroxynitrite. Journal of Neuroscience Research. 2004;**75**:845-853

[49] Reynolds MR, Reyes JF, Fu Y, Bigio EH, Guillozet-Bongaarts AL, Berry RW, et al. Tau nitration occurs at tyrosine 29 in the fibrillar lesions of Alzheimers disease and other tautopathies. The Journal of Neuroscience. 2006;**26**:10636-10645

[50] Sun GY, He Y, Chuang DY, Lee JC, Gu Z, Simonyi A, et al. Integrating cytosolic phospholipase A_2 with oxidative/nitrosative signaling pathways in neurons: A novel therapeutic strategy for AD. Molecular Neurobiology. 2012;**46**:85-95

[51] Rosselli M, Keller PJ, Dubey RK. Role of nitric oxide in the biology, physiology and pathophysiology of reproduction. Human Reproduction Update. 1998;**4**:3-24

[52] Lavi S, Egbarya R, Lavi R, Jacob G. Role of nitric oxide in the regulation of cerebral blood flow in humans: Chemoregulation versus mechanoregulation. Circulation. 2003;**107**:1901-1905

[53] Knott AB, Bossy-Wetzel E. Nitric oxide in health and disease of the nervous system. Antioxidants & Redox Signaling. 2009;**11**:541-554

[54] Radi E, Formichi P, Battisti C, Federico A. Apoptosis and oxidative stress in neurodegenerative diseases. Journal of Alzheimer's Disease. 2014;**42**:125-152

[55] Cheignon C, Tomas M, Bonnefont-Rousselot D, Faller P, Hureau C, Collin F. Oxidative stress and the amyloid beta peptide in Alzheimer's disease. Redox Biology. 2018;**14**:450-464

[56] Panthi S, Manandhar S, Gautam K. Hydrogen sulfide, nitric oxide, and neurodegenerative disorders. Translational Neurodegeneration. 2018;7:3

[57] Kim J, Kumar GS, Choi HW, Park D, Kim WJ. A platform for nitric oxide delivery. Journal of Materials Chemistry B. 2014;**2**:341-356

[58] Pratico D, Uryu K, Leight S, Trojanoswki JQ , Lee VM. Increased lipid peroxidation precedes amyloid plaque formation in an animal model of Alzeheimer amyloidosis. The Journal of Neuroscience. 2001;**21**:4183-4187

[59] Singh RP, Sharad S, Kapur S. Free radicals and oxidative stress in neurodegenerative diseases: Relevance of dietary antioxidants. Journal, Indian Academy of Clinical Medicine. 2004;**5**:218-225

[60] Xu Q , Huang Y. Lipid metabolism in Alzheimer's and Parkinson's disease. Future Lipidology. 2006;**1**:441-453

[61] Reed TT. Lipid peroxidation and neurodegenerative disease. Free Radical Biology & Medicine. 2011;**51**:1302-1319

[62] Chen X, Guo C, Kong J. Oxidative stress in neurodegenerative diseases. Neural Regeneration Research. 2012;**7**:376-385

[63] Suridjan I, Herrmann N, Adibfar A, Saleem M, Andreazza A, Oh PI, et al. Lipid peroxidation markers in coronary artery disease patients with possible vascular mild cognitive impairment. Journal of Alzheimer's Disease. 2017;**58**:885-896

[64] Magalingam KB, Radhakrishnanm A, Ping NS, Haleagrahara N. Current concepts of neurodegenerative mechanisms in Alzheimer's disease. BioMed Research International. 2018:3740461

[65] Cannon RO. Role of nitric oxide in cardiovascular disease: Focus on the endothelium. Clinical Chemistry. 1998;**44**:1809-1819

[66] Harrison D, Griendling KK, Landmesser U, Hornig B, Drexler H. Role of oxidative stress in atherosclerosis. The American Journal of Cardiology. 2003;**91**:7-11

[67] Adachi T, Weisbrod RM, Pimentel DR, Ying J, Sharov VS, Schoneich C, et al. S-glutathiolation by peroxynitrite activates SERCA during arterial relaxation by nitric oxide. Nature Medicine. 2004;**10**:1200-1207

[68] Higashi Y, Noma K, Yoshizumi M, Kihara Y. Endothelial function and oxidative stress in cardiovascular

diseases. Circulation Journal. 2009;**73**:411-418

[69] Antosova M, Plevkova J, Strapkova A, Buday T. Nitric oxide-important messenger in human body. Open Journal of Molecular and Integrative Physiology. 2012;**2**:98-106

[70] Sack MN, Fyhrquist FY, Saijonmaa OJ, Fuster V, Kovacic JC. Basic biology of oxidative stress and the cardiovascular system: Part 1 of a 3-Part Series. Journal of the American College of Cardiology. 2017;**70**:196-211

[71] Cervantes Gracia K, Llanas-Cornejo D, Husi H. CVD and oxidative stress. Journal of Clinical Medicine. 2017;**6**:22

[72] Yuan T, Yang T, Chen H, Fu D, Hu Y, Wang J, et al. New insights into oxidative stress and inflammation during diabetes mellitus accelerated atherosclerosis. Redox Biology. 2018;**20**:247-260

[73] Ahmad A, Dempsey SK, Daneva Z, Azam M, Li N, Li PL, et al. Role of nitric oxide in the cardiovascular and renal systems. International Journal of Molecular Sciences. 2018;**19**:E2605

[74] Hogg N, Kalyanaraman B, Joseph J, Struck A, Parthasarathy S. Inhibition of low-density lipoprotein oxidation by nitric oxide. Potential role in atherogenesis. FEBS Letters. 1993;**334**:170-174

[75] Ronson RS, Nakamura M, Vinten-Johansen J. The cardiovascular effects and implications of peroxynitrite. Cardiovascular Research. 1999;**44**:47-59

[76] Ferdinandy P, Danial H, Ambrus I, Rothery RA, Schulz R. Peroxynitrite is a major contributor of cytokine-induced myocardial contractile failure. Circulation Research. 2000;**87**:241-247

[77] Mihm MJ, Coyle CM, Schanbacher BL, Weinstein DM, Bauer JA. Peroxynitrite induced nitration and inactivation of myofibrillar creatine kinase in experimental heart failure. Cardiovascular Research. 2001;**49**:798-807

[78] Brunner F, Wolkart G. Peroxynitrite-induced cardiac depression: Role of myofilament desensitization and cGMP pathway. Cardiovascular Research. 2003;**60**:355-364

[79] Lokuta AJ, Maertz NA, Meethal SV, Potter KT, Kamp TJ, Valdivia HH, et al. Increased nitration of sarcoplasmic reticulum Ca^{2+}-ATPase in human heart failure. Circulation. 2005;**111**:988-995

[80] Radi R. Peroxynitrite, a stealthy biological oxidant. The Journal of Biological Chemistry. 2013;**13**:26464-26472

[81] Campolo J, De Maria R, Caruso R, Accinni R, Turazza F, Parolini M, et al. Blood glutathione as independent marker of lipid peroxidation in heart failure. International Journal of Cardiology. 2007;**117**:45-50

[82] Ramana KV, Srivastava S, Singhal SS. Lipid peroxidation products in human health and disease. Oxidative Medicine and Cellular Longevity. 2013:583438

[83] Zhang PY, Xu X, Li XC. Cardiovascular diseases: Oxidative damage and antioxidant protection. European Review for Medical and Pharmacological Sciences. 2014;**18**:309-316

[84] Ulintz L, Sun Q. Ambient particulate matter pollution on lipid peroxidation in cardiovascular diseases. Environmental Disease. 2016;**1**:109-117

[85] Graham A, Hogg N, Kalyanaraman B, O'Leary V, Darley-Usmar V, Moncada S. Peroxynitrite modification of low-density lipoprotein leads to recognition

by the macrophage scavenger receptor. FEBS Letters. 1993;**330**:181-185

[86] Moilanen E, Vapaatalo H. Nitric oxide in inflammation and immune response. Annals of Medicine. 1995;**27**:359-367

[87] Schopfer FJ, Baker PR, Freeman BA. NO-dependent protein nitration: A cell signalingeventoran oxidative inflammatory response? Trends in Biochemical Sciences. 2003;**28**:646-654

[88] Bar-Shai M, Reznick AZ. Peroxynitrite induces an alternative NF-kappa B activation pathway in L8 rat myoblasts. Antioxidants & Redox Signaling. 2006;**8**:639-652

[89] Tripathi P, Tripathi P, Kashyap L, Singh V. The role of nitric oxide in inflammatory reactions. FEMS Immunology and Medical Microbiology. 2007;**51**:443-452

[90] Sharma JN, Al-Omran A, Parvathy SS. Role of nitric oxide in inflammatory diseases. Inflammopharmacology. 2007;**15**:252-259

[91] Kawakami T, Koike A, Amano F. Sodium bicarbonate regulates nitric oxide production in mouse macrophage cell lines stimulated with lipopolysaccharide and interferon γ. Nitric Oxide. 2018;**79**:45-50

[92] Zhan R, Wang F, Wu Y, Wang Y, Qian W, Liu M, et al. Nitric oxide induces epidermal stem cell deadhesion by targeting integrin β1 and Talin via the cGMP signalling pathway. Nitric Oxide. 2018;**78**:1-10

[93] Brito C, Naviliat M, Tiscornia AC, Vuillier F, Gualco G, Dighiero G, et al. Peroxynitrite inhibits T lymphocyte activation and proliferation by promoting impairment of tyrosine phosphorylation and peroxynitrite-driven apoptotic death. Journal of Immunology. 1999;**162**:3356-3366

[94] Ahmad R, Rasheed Z, Ahsan H. Biochemical and cellular toxicology of peroxynitrite: Implications in cell death and autoimmune phenomenon. Immunopharmacology and Immunotoxicology. 2009;**31**:388-396

[95] Prolo C, Alvarez MN, Radi R. Peroxynitrite, a potent macrophage derived oxidizing cytotoxin to combat invading pathogens. BioFactors. 2014;**40**:215-225

[96] Vara D, Pula G. Reactive oxygen species: Physiological roles in the regulation of vascular cells. Current Molecular Medicine. 2014;**14**:1103-11025

[97] Morris G, Berk M. The many roads to mitochondrial dysfunction in neuroimmune and neuropsychiatric disorders. BMC Medicine. 2015;**13**:68

[98] Khan MA, Alam K, Zafaryab M, Rizvi MMA. Peroxynitrite-modified histone as a pathophysiological biomarker in autoimmune diseases. Biochimie. 2017;**140**:1-9

[99] Radi R. Oxygen radicals, nitric oxide, and peroxynitrite: Redox pathways in molecular medicine. Proceedings of the National Academy of Sciences. 2018;**115**:5839-5848

[100] Tewthanom K, Janwityanuchit S, Totemchockchyakarn K, Panomvana D. Correlation of lipid peroxidation and glutathione levels with severity of systemic lupuserythematosus: A pilot study from single center. Journal of Pharmacy & Pharmaceutical Sciences. 2008;**11**:30-34

[101] Otaki N, Chikazawa M, Nagae R, Shimozu Y, Shibata T, Ito S, et al. Identification of a lipid peroxidation product as the source of oxidation-specific epitopesrecognized by anti-DNA autoantibodies. The Journal of Biological Chemistry. 2010;**285**:33834-33842

[102] Barrera G, Pizzimenti S, Daga M, Dianzani C, Arcaro A, Cetrangolo GP, et al. Lipid peroxidation-derived aldehydes, 4-hydroxynonenal and malondialdehyde in aging related disorders. Antioxidants. 2018;7:102

[103] Walker LM, Walker PD, Imam SZ, Ali SF, Mayeux PR. Evidence for peroxynitrite formation in renal ischemia reperfusion injury; studies with the inducible nitric oxide synthase inhibitor L-N(6)-(1-Iminoethyl) lysine. The Journal of Pharmacology and Experimental Therapeutics. 2000;**295**:417-422

[104] Modlinger PS, Wilcox CS, Aslam S. Nitric oxide, oxidative stress, and progression of chronic renal failure. Seminars in Nephrology. 2004;**24**:354-365

[105] Liang JH, Li YN, Qi JS, Jia XX. Peroxynitrite induced protein nitration is pesponsible for renal mitochondrial damage in diabetic rat. Journal of Endocrinological Investigation. 2010;**33**:140-146

[106] Chirino YI, Hernandez-Pando R, Pedraza-Chaverri J. Peroxynitrite decomposition catalyst ameliorates renal damage and protein nitration in cisplatin-induced nephtotoxicity in rats. BMC Pharmacology. 2004;**4**:20

[107] Dennis JM, Witting PK. Protective role for antioxidants in acute kidney disease. Nutrients. 2017;**9**:718

[108] Lau T, Owen W, Yu YM, Noviski N, Lyons J, Zurakowski D, et al. Arginine, citrulline, and nitric oxide metabolism in end-stage renal disease patients. The Journal of Clinical Investigation. 2000;**105**:1217-1225

[109] Klahr S. The role of nitric oxide in hypertension and renal disease progression. Nephrology, Dialysis, Transplantation. 2001;**16**:60-62

[110] Goligorrsky MS, Brodsky SV, Noiri E. Nitric oxide in acute renal failure: NOS versus NOS. Kidney International. 2002;**61**:855-861

[111] Meenakshi SR, Agarwal R. Nitric oxide levels in patients with chronic renal disease. Journal of Clinical and Diagnostic Research. 2013;7:1288-1290

[112] Reddy YS, Kiranmayi VS, Bitla AR, Krishna GS, Srinivasa Rao PVLN, Sivakumar V. Nitric oxide status in patients with chronic kidney disease. Indian Journal of Nephrology. 2015;**25**:287-291

[113] Ruan SY, Wu HY, Lin HH, Wu HD, Yu CJ, Lai MS. Inhaled nitric oxide and the risk of renal dysfunction in patients with acute respiratory distress syndrome: A propensity-matched cohort study. Critical Care. 2016;**20**:389

[114] Ratliff BB, Abdulmahdi W, Pawar R, Wolin MS. Oxidant mechanisms in renal injury and disease. Antioxidants & Redox Signaling. 2016;**25**:119-146

[115] Lei C, Berra L, Rezoagli E, Yu B, Dong H, Yu S, et al. Nitric oxide decreased acute kidney injury and stage 3 chronic kidney disease after cardiac surgery. American Journal of Respiratory and Critical Care Medicine. 2018;**198**:1279-1287

[116] Sailaja Rao P, Sireesha K, Aparna Y, Sadanandam M. Free radicals and tissue damage: Role of antioxidants. Free Radicals and Antioxidants. 2011;**1**:1-7

[117] Harsh M. Cell Injury and cellular adaptations. In: Textbook of Pathology. New Delhi: Jaypee Brothers Medical Publishers; 2010. pp. 21-34

[118] Breen AP, Murphy JA. Reactions of oxyl radicals with DNA. Free Radical Biology & Medicine. 1995;**18**:1033-1077

[119] Kumar V, Abbas AK, Fausto N. Cellular adaptations, cell injury and

cell death. In: Robbins SL, Cotran RS, editors. Pathologic Basis of Disease. Philadelphia: Saunders; 2009. pp. 15-18

[120] Agarwal HCLD, Gupta S. The role of free radicals and antioxidants in female infertility and assisted reproduction. US Genito-Urinary Disease. 2006:60-65

[121] Arnold NO. Endogenous generation of singlet oxygen and ozone in human and animal tissues: Mechanisms, biological significance, and influence of dietary components. Oxidative Medicine and Cellular Longevity. 2016:1-22

[122] Pryor WA, Houk KN, Foote CS, et al. Free radical biology and medicine: It's a gas, man! The American Journal of Physiology-Regulatory Integrative and Comparative Physiology. 2006;**291**:R491-R511

[123] Terao J, Minami Y, Bando N. Singlet molecular oxygenquenching activity of carotenoids: Relevance to protection of the skin from photoaging. Journal of Clinical Biochemistry and Nutrition. 2011;**48**(1):57-62

[124] Smith lL. Oxygen, oxysterols, ouabain, and ozone: A cautionary tale. Free Radical Biology & Medicine. 2004;**37**:318-324

[125] Balla J, Tyihak E. Direct measurement of emission of endogenous ozone from plants by GC-MS-SIM. Chromatographia. 2010;**71**:87-91

[126] Rastogi RP, Richa AK, Tyagi MB, Sinha RP. Molecular mechanisms of ultraviolet radiation-induced DNA damage and repair. Journal of Nucleic Acids. 2010:1-32

[127] Tyihak E, Oricz AMM, Ott PG. BioArena studies: Unique function of endogenous formaldehyde and ozone in the antibiotic effect—A review. Medicinal Chemistry. 2012;**8**:75-84

[128] Wentworth P Jr, McDunn JE, Wentworth AD, et al. Evidence for antibody-catalyzed ozone formation in bacterial killing and inflammation. Science. 2002;**298**:2195-2199

[129] Yamashita K, Miyoshi T, Arai T, et al. Ozone production by amino acids contributes to killing of bacteria. Proceedings of the National Academy of Sciences. 2008;**105**:16912-16917

Chapter 21

The Effect of Antioxidants on Ischemia-Reperfusion Injury in Flap Surgery

Mehmet Bozkurt, Melihcan Sezgic, Percin Karakol, Can Uslu and Tevfik Balikci

Abstract

Flap surgery has wide use in plastic surgery in the closure of tissue defects. In spite of the major advances in plastic surgery in the past years, flap surgery is still associated with significant mortality. Ischemia-reperfusion (I/R) injury, which is a complex injury associated with flap blood flow, is one of the most important causes of flap failure. The main pathophysiology underneath I/R injury is associated with reactive oxygen species, which can be prevented by certain antioxidant applications. Antioxidants have been widely used in flap surgery and I/R injury previously. There have been a lot of articles showing positive effects of antioxidants on I/R injury. In this chapter, we focus the mechanism of I/R injury and how antioxidants can able to diminish the damage, moreover demonstrating the effect of certain antioxidants on I/R injury that has been investigated previously.

Keywords: antioxidants, flap, flap failure, ischemia, reperfusion

1. Introduction

Flaps have been increasingly used in plastic and reconstructive surgery for tissue defects. Although the success rate of flap surgery reaches up to 99%, complications can occur even in the most experienced hands [1]. Vascular blood flow insufficiency is the leading cause of partial or total flap losses [2]. Ischemia-reperfusion (I/R) injury is the most important reason of vascular insufficiency to considerate. It is also the remarkable cause of flap compromise and organ dysfunction during organ transplantation and free flap surgery [3, 4].

The ischemic area of flaps is generally more distal to the region of vascular supply. Even the ischemia occurs for a short time period, it can generate reactive oxygen species (ROS). The reperfusion period, which occurs after ischemia, causes the restoration of blood flow and oxygen influx in the ischemic tissue and can finalize in cellular, inflammatory, and metabolic changes in the living cell. These changes caused by free radicals execute structural and functional alterations in the cell and may contribute to tissue necrosis [5]. This process can be prevented or decelerated with the use of antioxidant drugs that decrease the toxic metabolites responsible for tissue damage. Because postsurgical I/R injury is one of the most important causes of flap failure, in this review, we aim to show the pathophysiology of I/R injury and how the antioxidants show their beneficial effects on flap salvage.

2. Pathophysiology of I/R injury

Tissue perfusion is the most important parameter of flaps. When it is interrupted for a period of time and abruptly restored, I/R injury occurs. As long as there is timely reperfusion, ischemia results in reversible cellular damage. However, restoration of blood flow after a period of time results in an incident whereby reperfusion ends up with greater tissue injury than that which is produced by ischemia itself. I/R injury is a complex interplay between biochemical, cellular, and vascular endothelial factors. Although the clinical sequelae are organ specific, it may also involve systemic inflammatory responses [6].

The tissue damage in I/R injury is like a double-edged sword and is divided into two parts: ischemia injury and reperfusion injury. Ischemic injury may initially cause hypoxia and hyponutrition. After prolonged ischemia, the metabolic products from cells are retained and cause metabolic acidosis. When the blood supply is reestablished, local inflammation and reactive oxygen species production increase. Those lead to an activation of neutrophils and a consecutive adhesion between granulocytes and endothelial cells causing segmental vessel occlusion in postcapillary venules, transendothelial leukocyte migration, nitric oxide (NO) depletion, and the release of tissue-damaging enzymes leading to secondary injury [7] Reactive oxygen species are potent oxidizing and reducing agents that directly damage cellular membranes by lipid peroxidation [8]. The cell response is dependent on the severity of total tissue injury [9]. Cell damage induced by prolonged ischemia-reperfusion injury may lead to apoptosis, autophagy, and necrosis (**Figure 1**). Cell survival systems (control ROS generation and cell damage) are activated in short duration of I/R injury [10]. Moderate I/R injury may cause cell dysfunction by autophagy and also activate recovery systems for survival [11]. But if damage is severe, cell death may be induced via apoptotic or necrotic pathways [12].

I/R injury has effect on the microcirculation of the entire flap because of the inflammatory process and the rise in ROS in the early stages of reperfusion [13]. For this reason, insufficient microcirculation usually occurs mainly in the distal parts of the flap, which is a common cause of partial flap necrosis.

As mentioned above, total flap necrosis is most often caused by thrombosis of the pedicle causing vascular insufficiency. Immediate revision of the anastomosis is crucial to reestablish blood flow. Nevertheless, such complications can increase

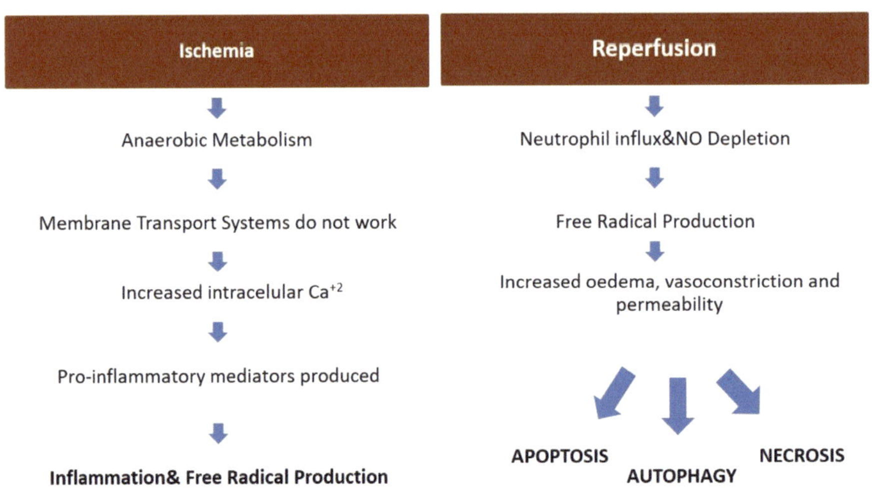

Figure 1.
Ischemia-reperfusion mechanism.

• Ischemic preconditioning
• Remote ischemic preconditioning
• Pharmaceutical preconditioning
• Thermic preconditioning
• Surgical delay
• Growth factors
• Extracorporeal shock waves
• Stem cells

Table 1.
Types of tissue conditioning.

I/R injury, which can lead to intravascular hemoconcentration, swelling of endothelium, increase in interstitial edema as well as inflammatory reactions because of the reperfusion injury. After a critical period, I/R injury can lead to a no-reflow phenomenon, which also leads to complete flap loss [14–16].

Several methods and techniques are described to protect flap from the dangerous effects of the I/R injury or minimize the stress during and after ischemia. Tissue conditioning, which is the most acceptable one, consists of preoperative, perioperative, and postoperative techniques to adapt the tissue to the ischemic stress. Multiple methods were described for tissue conditioning in **Table 1**.

Nitric oxide donation is another technique that NO administered through inhalation. NO plays a protective role via its antioxidative and anti-inflammatory functions [17], but it is not in common use in flap surgery and still remains experimental.

There are also studies aiming to prevent anti-inflammatory mediators released by leukocytes. Anti-leukocyte therapy limits leukocyte-mediated I/R injury and has focused on inhibition of inflammatory mediator release or receptor engagement, leukocyte adhesion molecule synthesis, or leukocyte-endothelial adhesion [18]. Many drugs act in this manner and have been shown to be very effective.

3. Free radical and antioxidant connection

Antioxidants that have been extensively studied in I/R injury are also found to be effective in various studies [19]. Because high amount of ROS is the primary supplement of the injury, it can neutralize the effect or prevent the mechanism from happening.

3.1 Free radical formation

Free radicals were discovered less than 50 years ago [20]. At first, they were assumed as completely harmful. Later on, advantageous biological effects of free radicals were reported. In recent studies, the role of free radicals is being researched commonly both in physiological conditions and in diseases. In molecular biology, a molecule that has an unpaired electron in its outer valence orbital that needs an extra electron to restore stability is called a free radical. They are short lived and highly reactive. The situation of instability because of the unpaired electron creates energy that has to be released instantly. In cell physiology, normal low levels of free radicals are used in autophagy, cell signaling, and antimicrobial oxidative bursts [21]. But, at higher free radical levels, the interaction with neighbor molecules such as lipids, proteins, and DNA for releasing the energy causes damage. So, free radicals are the products of normal cellular metabolism. In order to reach stability, an electron has to be stolen. The attacked molecule engages itself in a chain reaction to steal an electron from another molecule.

In aerobic organisms, oxygen free radicals launch autocatalytic reactions that finally damage the living cell. The unsaturated carbon-carbon double bonds in the exposed end groups are particularly sensitive to free radicals forming a covalent single bond at a carbon atom to form a free radical at the opposite carbon atom [22]. Free radicals interact with molecular cross-linking for increased structural organization by reducing the transport of oxygen. ROS can be produced from endogenous or exogenous sources. Endogenous ROS is produced in different cellular organs where oxygen consumption is high such as mitochondria, peroxisomes, and endoplasmic reticulum. Most of the intracellular ROS are derived from mitochondria. The amount of free radicals is determined by many factors. In periods of irregular hypoxia in mitochondrial energy synthesis, excess electron production can develop free radicals that can damage lipids, proteins, and greatly increase molecular size in increasing vicious cycles to further reduce oxygen availability for mitochondria during energy synthesis. Another major type of free radical in a living cell is reactive nitrogen species (RNS). Nitric oxide (NO) radical is formed by the enzyme nitric oxide synthase and involves in smooth muscle relaxation and various other cGMP-dependent functions [23].

Free radicals are prominent in many pathological conditions such as cancer, diabetes, cardiovascular diseases, neurodegenerative diseases, cataracts, asthma, rheumatoid arthritis, inflammation, burns, intestinal tract diseases, progerias, and ischemic and postischemic pathologies. In particular, ROS is substantial for the pathogenesis of atherosclerosis. Low density lipoprotein (LDL) accumulates within plaques and contributes to the inflammatory state when ROS concentration is high and ROS oxidizes neighbor LDLs [24]. Also, it is believed that aging is a process mediated by free radicals [25]. At the present time, each chemical step has been investigated meticulously in order to prevent cell damage and clarify free radicals.

Different reactive oxygen species are formed in biological tissue (**Table 2**). Superoxide radical (O_2^-) can be formed by adding an extra electron to the oxygen molecule. Hydroxyl radical ($\cdot OH$) can be formed in two different ways. First, it can be formed from O_2^- and H_2O_2 with a reaction catalyzed by a metal such as iron (Fe). Second, it can be formed from singlet oxygen $(^1O_2)$ reaction. Moreover, oxygen free radicals may also be formed by polymorphonuclear leukocytes in ischemic tissue.

3.2 Human body defense mechanisms

Although accumulation of this substances are harmful to cell viability, it is important to know that human body is equipped with a defense system consisting of several antioxidative enzymes, to fight with these ROS. Superoxide dismutase

Reactive oxygen species (ROS)	
Superoxide radical (O_2^-)	$O_2 + e^- \rightarrow O_2^-$
Hydroxyl radical ($\cdot OH$) 1st	$2O_2^- + 2H \rightarrow O_2 + H_2O_2/Fe^{2+} + H_2O_2 \rightarrow Fe^{3+} + OH^- + \cdot OH$
2nd	$O_2^- + H_2O_2 \rightarrow OH^- + \cdot OH + {}^1O_2$

Table 2.
Reactive oxygen species.

(SOD), glutathione peroxidase, glutathione reductase and catalase are some of these enzymes. SOD catalyzes dismutation reaction where O_2^- transforms into O_2 + H_2O_2 molecules. Catalase (heme-containing enzyme) also catalyzes the H_2O_2 reaction. H_2O_2 can also be reduced by glutathione peroxidase (GSH-P) which is selenium dependent enzyme, transforms reduced glutathione to oxidized glutathione. After that reaction oxidized glutathione is transformed into reduced for with help of nicotinamide adenine dinucleotide phosphate (NADPH). Additionally, NADPH regenerated from glucose 6-phosphate catalyzed by the enzyme glucose 6-phosphate dehydrogenase (**Table 3**).

The biochemical reaction of glutathione (GSH) is crucial. An intermolecular disulfide non-radical end product, glutathione disulfide (GSSG), is formed, which can either be exported from the cells or transformed back to glutathione by the combined action of glutathione reductase and the NADPH cofactor. Glutathione can react directly with ROS and RNS by its thiol group; also, it can aim the disulfide bridges formed inside and between proteins by the action of free radicals [26].

3.3 Antioxidants

Antioxidants are molecules against free radicals and are capable of securing or deactivating free radicals before damaging the cells. There are many antioxidant systems that work synergistically with each other to protect the body's organs and organ systems against free radical damage. There are highly complex enzymatic and non-enzymatic antioxidants: the enzymes such as SOD, glutathione peroxidase, and catalase, as well as non-enzymatic compounds such as α-tocopherol (vitamin E), β-carotene, ascorbic acid (vitamin C), and glutathione. Referred enzymes aim free radicals to delocalize their proteins into side chains and peptide bonds. Also, antioxidants may be endogenous or exogenous, such as part of a diet or dietary supplement. As we know aging is related to free radicals, nutrients rich with antioxidants contend with aging. Under oxidative stress, endogenous antioxidants may not be sufficient and dietary antioxidants may be required to maintain optimal cellular functions. According to literature, exogenous antioxidants comprise the secondary defense system against oxygen free radicals. Moreover, it is believed that ischemia-reperfusion is associated with generation of excess amounts of reactive oxygen species, the removal of which is beyond the capacity of the existing antioxidant defense system [19]. So, contribution of secondary defense system is crucial for the injury associated with ischemia-reperfusion.

Some dietary compounds that do not neutralize free radicals but increase endogenous activity can also be classified as antioxidants. An antioxidant should eliminate free radicals and be absorbed easily, and chelate redox metals at physiologically

Human body antioxidative enzymes	
Superoxide dismutase (SOD)	$2O_2^- + 2H \rightarrow O_2 + H_2O_2$
Catalase (heme-dependent enzyme)	$2H_2O_2 \rightarrow 2H_2O + O_2$
GSH-P (selenium-dependent enzyme)	$2GSH + H_2O_2 \rightarrow GSSG + H_2O$
Glutathione reductase	$GSSH + NADPH + H^+ \rightarrow 2GSH + NADP^+$
Glucose 6-phosphate dehydrogenase (G6PD)	Glucose 6-P + $NADP^+$ → gluconate 6-P + NADPH + H^+

Table 3.
Antioxidative enzymes and catalyzed reactions in human body.

relevant levels. Redox-active metals are involved in the generation of free radicals by binding strongly. It should also work in both aqueous and membrane domains and affects gene expression in a positive way.

It is a fact that all of the reactive oxygen species are formed in human body constantly but destroyed by these endogenous antioxidative mechanisms with the help of these enzymes. Endogenous antioxidants are products of the human metabolism. Except the ones that we mentioned before, human body have numerous different antioxidants. Alpha-lipoic acid (ALA), coenzyme Q, and melatonin are some of them. Alpha-lipoic acid is a disulfide derivative of octanoic acid and cysteine and a type of thiol antioxidant. ALA has significant functions such as scavenging free radicals, metal ion chelation, and antioxidant recycling. Coenzyme Q is the only lipid soluble endogenous antioxidant. It transfers electrons from complexes I and II to complex III within the mitochondria. Melatonin is produced in the pineal gland that is an indoleamine neurohormone. It has many physiopathological functions. One major function of melatonin is about oxygen metabolism to scavenge free radicals.

3.3.1 Redox homeostasis

ROS production and antioxidant capacity are in balance during the stable state of a cell and it is called "redox homeostasis" [27]. This stable state has to be reestablished in temporary derangement (**Figure 2**). When ROS concentration is detected to be high, gene expression is engaged for antioxidant activity. Signal cascades increase the amount of intracellular glutathione and other potent ROS scavengers. Thus, redox homeostasis is sustained. Another regulatory mechanism is feedback inhibition. Production of NO inactivates NO-producing enzyme, NOS. There are many physiological redox-responsive signaling pathways regulated by NO or ROS. The concentration level is modified by the balance between antioxidants and free radicals. If free radical production becomes uncontrolled, aging and diseases occur eventually.

Some major exogenous antioxidants are vitamin C, vitamin E, carotenoids, and polyphenols. Diet is the main source for exogenous antioxidants, especially fruits, vegetables, and grains [28]. Endogenous and exogenous antioxidants act in coordination in order to reach homeostasis. Vitamin C (ascorbic acid) involves in the reaction where intracellular glutathione levels raise thus protects protein thiol group against oxidation. Also, it works in cooperation with vitamin E and the carotenoids. α-Tocopherol is the most active form of vitamin E and is a membrane-bound antioxidant. The main function of it is to protect cell membrane against lipid peroxidation. Carotenoids are pigments known as the protector of plants against photooxidative processes. They contain conjugated double bonds, and in the human organism, their antioxidant activity arises due to scavenging singlet molecular oxygen and peroxyl radicals. There are many studies exhibiting that carotenoids protect the skin against photooxidative damage. Polyphenols are found in blueberry, and they facilitate increased neuronal signal transduction [29].

As previously described, the formation of high amount of ROS is the primary supplement of ischemia-reperfusion injury. Antioxidants can neutralize the effect or prevent the mechanism to develop. Considerable clinical and experimental data support the role of oxidative stress in I/R injury and emphasize the importance of antioxidant defense mechanisms in tissue protection [30]. In previous studies, it is shown that concentration of some antioxidants such as glutathione and uric acid decrease in response to ROS burst during skin flap ischemia-reperfusion [31]. So, supplementation of the antioxidants at I/R injury may help to neutralize the oxidative stress and reinforce tissue tolerance to reactive oxygen species [32].

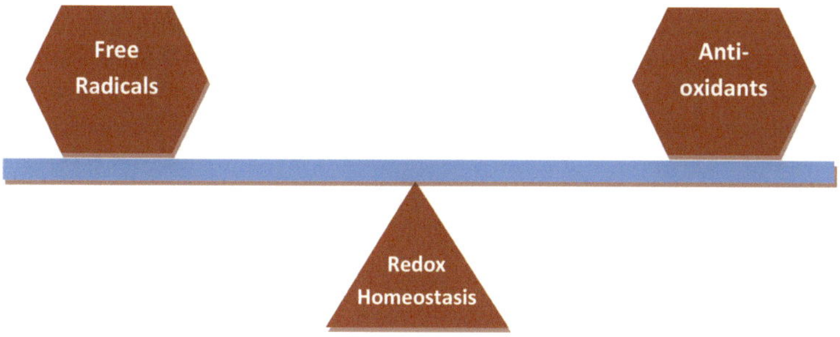

Figure 2.
Redox homeostasis.

4. Main antioxidants and effects on flap surgery

Most of the antioxidants have been proved to be beneficial versus I/R injury, with the exception of only few [19]. There are several important antioxidants that are investigated in I/R injury in previous studies as mentioned below.

5. α-Tocopherol

α-Tocopherol is the most popular one among the antioxidants; so, numerous studies were written about the positive effects of α-tocopherol in I/R injury. It can be found on foods, and also used in cosmetic and pharmaceutical industries. It is the bioavailable component of vitamin E, and appropriate consumption is considered to help to diminish risk of many chronic diseases associated to oxidative stress [33].

It is a lipid soluble antioxidant and stabilizer of membranes, has been found to decrease myocardial I/R injury and reverse contractile dysfunction by inhibition on cellular Ca^{2+} accumulation and reduce lactate dehydrogenase (LDH) release [34, 35]. Hydrophilic analog of α-tocopherol called Trolox has been studied before, and beneficial effects were shown on liver I/R injury [36].

According to Franch et al. [37], the α-tocopherol was compared with control group on rat hepatic I/R injury model. The SOD after I/R period catalases after reperfusion period, and glutathione peroxidase in all periods showed lower activities than those of control group. Erkut et al. [38] came across similar results on their study too. In rabbit skeletal muscle I/R injury model, they found out superoxide dismutase, catalase, and glutathione peroxidase levels that show the cellular injury were lower in α-tocopherol group compared with control group.

5.1 Ascorbic acid (vitamin C)

Vitamin C, one of the most popular vitamins we have heard in everyday life, has powerful antioxidant effects too. Because of the potential benefits, people pay attention to consume certain amount of fruits and vegetables these days. Ascorbic acid can protect the endothelium from direct injury by oxidants (such as H_2O_2) and prevent microvascular dysfunction. Moreover, it is proven that administration of ascorbic acid helps to decrease I/R injury [39, 40].

Because of its beneficial effects, ascorbic acid has been used in hepatic, cerebral, and renal I/R injury models in the literature [41–43] before and demonstrated positive results for end-organ protection.

There are several studies related to the effect of ascorbic acid I/R injury skin flap model. Zaccaria et al. [44] demonstrated positive effects of ascorbic acid compared with control group in rat epigastric island skin flap model. They determined higher percentage of flap survival in ascorbic acid group. On the other hand, according to Yoshida and Campos [45], vitamin c and mannitol (antioxidant group) group did not prevent or reduce the necrosis area compared with control group in rat groin flap I/R injury model.

6. β-Carotene

Carotene is called a provitamin because it can be stored in the liver and converted into vitamin A when necessary. There are two main types of carotene: alpha-carotene (α-carotene) and beta-carotene (β-carotene). β-Carotene consists of two retinyl groups and is destroyed by beta-carotene dioxygenase in the small intestinal mucosa and transformed into retinol that is a type of vitamin A.

β-Carotene is also a lipid-soluble antioxidant as α-tocopherol, interferes with lipid peroxidation by clearing away singlet oxygen, and reacts with peroxy radicals. According to Kikugawa et al. [46], β-carotene plays a preventative role in the oxidative damage process. In the literature, beneficial effects of β-carotene were shown in I/R injuries in the liver, myocardium, kidneys, and ovaries.

Karabulut et al. [47] compared vitamin A with control group in rat epigastric island skin flap venous I/R injury model in rat. By the fact in their study, after reperfusion of flaps, surviving flap area was 16% in the control group and 90% in the vitamin A group, respectively. They also combined vitamin A and vitamin E, where it was 92%.

6.1 Glutathione

Glutathione is present in all mammalian cells and has a variety of cellular functions, including amino acid transport, the maintenance of sulfhydryl groups of proteins, and the protection against oxidizing molecules and electrophilic xenobiotics. It is a tripeptide composed of glutamic acid, cysteine, and glycine. Because of strong antioxidant features, it is very popular in media in terms of healthy nutrition.

Glutathione shows its functions by clearing away O_2^- and protecting thiol groups against oxidation so that it supplies cellular integrity. In order to protect the thiol groups of proteins, a relatively high concentration of GSH is necessary. Moreover, other free radical scavengers and antioxidants (such as α-tocopherol and ascorbic acid) converted to their reduced state by GSH. Pretreatment with exogenous GSH can provide protection against gross mucosal ischemia-reperfusion injury [48]. Also, it is shown that application of intravenous GSH reduces the myocardial infarct size and decreases postischemic left ventricular dysfunction [32].

On the other hand, according to Van den Heuvel et al. [31], I/R did not significantly alter GSH concentrations in their study. They had taken biopsies from 17 DIEP flaps at the different time of surgeries but there was no immediate change in GSH concentrations compared to the concentrations at the start of surgery. They explained this finding that because the skin is less sensitive to I/R than other tissues (such as muscle, liver, and fat tissue), it may prevent antioxidant defense reactions from occurring. That could be the reason for normal levels of GSH.

6.2 Coenzyme Q_{10} (CQ10)

Coenzyme Q_{10} is an organic, natural, fat-soluble, antioxidant, endogenous vitamin-like substance (similar structure to vitamins K and E). Also called ubiquinone, it is an auxiliary factor in the intercellular electron transport chain. It has become one of the most popular nutritional supplements in recent years. It was shown in the literature as an effective antioxidant for the prevention of oxidative damage. What is more, CQ10 breaks down macromolecules to prohibit inflammatory responses [49]. Also, CQ10 is able to balance mitochondrial Ca^{2+}-dependent ion channels and prevents energy depletion in the cell [50]. In cardiovascular diseases, exogenous CQ10 has been widely applied as a dietary supplement, and it may be suggested as a therapeutic agent [51].

CQ10 has inhibitory effects for tumor necrosis factor-α (TNF-α), which may be responsible for muscle damage in I/R injury as well [52]. Moreover, it prevents the peroxidation of the cell membrane and subcellular lipids, which happens during I/R injury [53]. Hwang et al. [54] were proved that pretreatment with CQ10 had positive effects on spinal cord I/R injury and improved neurological function.

According to Ozalp et al. [55], who compared CQ10 with control group in rat inferior epigastric island flap I/R injury model, mean flap survival ratios were 88% in CQ10 group, markedly higher than the control group (51%). They also emphasized that CQ10 group had high levels of SOD and GSH compared with control group because of CQ10's antioxidant effect, which prevented lipid peroxidation during the initial phase (reduce GSH and SOD destruction).

6.3 Alpha-lipoic acid (ALA)

ALA is an antioxidant that is found in various foods and also can be synthesized in the human cells. It is also an endogenous short-chain fatty acid and a cofactor for multiple mitochondrial dehydrogenase enzymes [56]. ALA shows its antioxidant properties by the use of free radical scavenging, chelating with metals, increasing the reusability of other antioxidants, and repairing oxidative damage.

There have been a lot of articles written about ALA because of its wide range of antioxidant capabilities. The efficiency of ALA has been shown in atherosclerosis, diabetes mellitus, I/R injury, multiple sclerosis, and senile dementia [57].

In severe oxidative damage caused by I/R, levels of malondialdehyde (MDA) and nitric oxide (NO) increases [58]. ALA is capable of cleaning up MDA and NO within brain tissue [59]. Deng et al. [60] found out diminished MDA and NO levels in ALA group compared with control group in rat brain I/R injury model. They also discovered that ALA has enhanced the activities of total antioxidant capacity and SOD in rat brains. According to these findings, administration of ALA before skin flap surgery may have benefits to improve I/R injury.

6.4 Melatonin

Melatonin is a type of ethionamide that is secreted from the pineal gland, which determines the biorhythm. Moreover, it is an effective free radical scavenger and received significant attention because of its antioxidative feature. In spite of its ability to neutralize free radicals directly, also it has indirect effects, such as stimulating the activity of antioxidative enzymes (such as glutathione peroxidase and SOD) [61, 62].

Mitochondrion, which is an organelle for ATP production in the cell, has been proved to play critical roles in I/R injury. Therefore, the protection of mitochondrion can decrease I/R injury in vital organs [63]. Melatonin has been shown to restore the disturbance caused by I/R injury in mitochondria and has become a remarkable therapeutic strategy [64].

The effect of melatonin on I/R injury has been investigated in the literature for a long time. It has been shown that melatonin could be an effective neuroprotective agent for treatment of ischemic spinal cord injury [65]. Singhanat et al. [66]

explained that melatonin has cardioprotective effects against cardiac I/R injury. However, they also mentioned that the mechanism of the cardioprotective effects of melatonin were still unclear. Gurlek et al. [67] showed beneficial effects of melatonin in rat inferior epigastric flap I/R ınjury model. The determined melatonin replacement therapy causes reduction in I/R-induced flap injury.

7. Discussion

Vitamins with antioxidant properties such as vitamins A, C, and E have positive effects on I/R injury but they are not adequately effective when given alone. If they are used in combination with other vitamins and drugs with antioxidant properties, they work synergistically to decrease I/R injury. For instance, combined use of vitamin A and E in an animal model showed increase in flap survival with the help of their synergistic effect on reducing lipid peroxidation [47]. Also, vitamin E and iloprost (synthetic analog of prostacyclin PGI_2) combination demonstrated that they attenuate reperfusion injury more efficiently than their separate use, in skeletal muscle I/R injury model [68]. In addition to these, Kayiran et al. [69] showed that combined usage of vitamins C, E, acetylcysteine, and prednisolone alleviated the results of ischemia and enhanced the flap survival on free radial forearm flap. There is a wide range use of substances in the literature to prevent I/R injury, but there is no single ideal drug that can overcome this damage; so, we think that the use of combined therapy is more successful in achieving impressive results.

Because high amounts of ROS are produced in I/R injury, the amount of certain antioxidants decreases. Depletion of antioxidants does not always mean oxidative tissue damage has happened: it might simply indicate that the antioxidant system has removed the ROS and thereby consumed the present antioxidants to protect the tissues [70]. Tissue damage occurs if the ROS amount outruns the capacity of the body defense system. In other words, administration of antioxidants prior to flap surgery may help to avoid unfavorable effects of I/R injury.

Trolox equivalent antioxidant capacity (TEAC) is a measure that shows the capacity of the present hydrophilic antioxidants. In other words, it demonstrates the antioxidant level on a certain amount of tissue. According to Van den Heuvel et al. [31], TEAC concentrations was not differ 30 min later after reperfusion but there was an important decrease after 1 h of reperfusion. The TEAC concentrations were recovered in the next 1 h, showing us the body was replacing the antioxidants. These findings suggest that first hour after reperfusion is the most vulnerable period of flap to I/R injury and timing of antioxidant replacement may have an important role in preventing this injury too.

Lipids are usually primary target of free oxygen radicals in oxidative damage and lipid oxidation occurs when they exposed free radicals. Lipid oxidation is a process that generates many end products. Between these products, MDA, which is an aldehyde, is the most studied one among them [71]. Because it is the end product of the lipid oxidation pathway, measurement of MDA levels is a commonly used indicator of oxidative damage [72]. Also, MDA might help us to monitor the reaction of the body against the antioxidant support. In other words, if MDA levels are high, we can increase the antioxidant support to body in I/R injury.

Measuring MDA levels helps us to determine antioxidant therapy protocol. However, we cannot increase the dosage of antioxidants easily because they are not only antioxidant but also have prooxidant properties. Helpful effects of antioxidants are usually higher in the studies that were done in vitro comparing with the studies that were done in vivo. This fact is called "The antioxidant paradox" [73]. Many antioxidants can produce ROS at higher doses. But if they are administered at even higher doses, they can generate massive amounts of ROS that the body cannot handle. So, they can worsen oxidative stress and cause necrosis. For instance, ascorbic acid, which is widely known as a powerful antioxidant vitamin in human body, can reduce most of the ROS and other radicals. On the other hand, it has been shown that it has a prooxidant act in humans even at a dose of 500 mg/day [74]. Moreover, according to Mendes-da-Silva et al. [75], ascorbic acid was served as an antioxidant on rats at 30/mg/kg/day but they were discovered opposite effects at 60/mg/kg/day. In light of these findings, since the use of antioxidants is like a double-edged sword, careful dose adjustment is required for use in I/R injury. Further studies are necessary in order to determine completely how they act.

The effect of antioxidants on I/R injury is still under investigation. There are also substances with antioxidant properties such as flavonoids [76], thioredoxin [77], propofol [78], ebselen [79], edaravone [80], etc. which also have positive effects on I/R injury in addition to the antioxidants described previously.

8. Conclusion

I/R injury is still the most challenging problem in flap surgery. Prolonged ischemia of the flap causes irreversible infarct and flap loss, and this increases the patient morbidity. Because free radical formation is a significant step in pathophysiology of I/R injury, the help of antioxidants on I/R injury is cannot be disregarded. There have been a lot of studies proving this fact so there is a need for further studies for a better understanding of their certain effects. In this chapter, we tried to show how the antioxidants affect the I/R injury and how effective their use is. In conclusion, although the efficacy of antioxidants is not yet fully understood, we think that they will increase their medical use in the future.

Author details

Mehmet Bozkurt*, Melihcan Sezgic, Percin Karakol, Can Uslu and Tevfik Balikci
Health and Science University, Istanbul Bagcılar Hospital, Istanbul, Turkey

*Address all correspondence to: drmbozkurt@yahoo.com

References

[1] Ulusoy MG, Uysal A, Koçer U, et al. Improved flap viability site specific delivery of sildenafil citrate using fibrin glue. Annals of Plastic Surgery. 2005;**55**:292-296

[2] Smith JD, Pribaz JJ. Flaps. In: Achauer BM, Eriksson E, editors. Plastic Surgery Indications, Operations and Outcomes. St. Louis, MO: Mosby; 2000. pp. 261-290

[3] Wang WZ, Baynosa RC, Zamboni WA. Update on ischemia reperfusion injury for the plastic surgeon: 2011. Plastic and Reconstructive Surgery. 2011;**128**:685e-692e

[4] Van den Heuvel MG, Buurman WA, Bast A, van der Hulst RR. Review: ischaemia-reperfusion injury in flap surgery. Journal of Plastic, Reconstructive & Aesthetic Surgery. 2009;**62**:721-726

[5] Camargo CP, Margarido NF, Guandelini E, Vieira GA, Jacomo AL, Gemperli R. Description of a new experimental model skin flap for studying skin viability in rats. Acta Cirúrgica Brasileira. 2014;**29**(3):166-170

[6] Abela CB, Homer-Vanniasinkham S. Clinical implications of ischaemia-reperfusion injury. Pathophysiology. 2003 Sep;**9**(4):229-240

[7] Menger MD, Vollmar B. Pathomechanisms of ischemia-reperfusion injury as the basis for novel preventive strategies: Is it time for the introduction of pleiotropic compounds? Transplantation Proceedings. 2007;**39**:485-488

[8] Toyokuni S. Reactive oxygen species-induced molecular damage and its application in pathology. Pathology International. 1999;**49**:91-102

[9] Gottlieb RA. Cell death pathways in acute ischemia/reperfusion injury. Journal of Cardiovascular Pharmacology and Therapeutics. 2011;**16**:233-238

[10] McCully JD, Wakiyama H, Hsieh YJ, Jones M, Levitsky S. Differential contribution of necrosis and apoptosis in myocardial ischemia-reperfusion injury. American Journal of Physiology Heart and Circulatory Physiology. 2004;**286**:H1923-H1935

[11] Wu M-Y, Yiang G-T, Liao W-T, Tsai AP-Y, Cheng Y-L, Cheng P-W, et al. Current mechanistic concepts in ischemia and reperfusion injury. Cellular Physiology and Biochemistry. 2018;**46**:1650-1667. DOI: 10.1159/000489241

[12] Eefting F, Rensing B, Wigman J, Pannekoek WJ, Liu WM, Cramer MJ, et al. Role of apoptosis in reperfusion injury. Cardiovascular Research. 2004;**61**:414-426

[13] Im MJ, Manson PN, Bulkley GB, Hoopes JE. Effects of superoxide dismutase and allopurinol on the survival of acute island skin flaps. Annals of Surgery. 1985;**201**:357-359

[14] Harder Y, Amon M, Laschke MW, Schramm R, Rücker M, Wettstein R, et al. An old dream revitalised: Preconditioning strategies to protect surgical flaps from critical ischaemia and ischaemia-reperfusion injury. Journal of Plastic, Reconstructive & Aesthetic Surgery. 2008;**61**:503-511

[15] Menger MD, Laschke MW, Amon M, Schramm R, Thorlacius H, Rücker M, et al. Experimental models to study microcirculatory dysfunction in muscle ischemia-reperfusion and osteomyocutaneous flap transfer. Langenbeck's Archives of Surgery. 2003;**388**:281-290

[16] Menger MD, Rücker M, Vollmar B. Capillary dysfunction in striated muscle ischemia/reperfusion: On the mechanisms of capillary "no-reflow". Shock. 1997;**8**:2-7

[17] Phillips L, Toledo AH, Lopez-Neblina F, Anaya-Prado R, Toledo-Pereyra LH. Nitric oxide mechanism of protection in ischemia and reperfusion injury. Journal of Investigative Surgery. 2009;**22**:46-55

[18] Panés J, Perry M, Granger DN. Leukocyte endothelial cell adhesion: Avenues for therapeutic intervention. British Journal of Pharmacology. 1999;**126**:537-550

[19] Das DK, Maulik N. Antioxidant effectiveness in ischemia-reperfusion tissue injury. Methods in Enzymology. 1994;**233**:601-610

[20] Droge W. Free radicals in the physiological control of cell function. Physiological Reviews. 2002;**82**:47-95

[21] Navarro-Yepes J, Burns M, Anandhan A, et al. Oxidative stress, redox signaling, and autophagy: Cell death versus survival. Antioxidants & Redox Signaling. 2014;**21**(1):66-85

[22] Petersen RC, Reddy MS, Liu PR. Advancements in free-radical pathologies and an important treatment solution with a free-radical inhibitor. SF Journal of Biotechnology and Biomedical Engineering. 2018;**1**(1):1003

[23] Andrew PJ, Mayer B. Enzymatic function of nitric oxide synthases. Cardiovascular Research. 1999;**43**(3):21-531

[24] Trinity JD, Broxterman RM, Richardson RS. Regulation of exercise blood flow: Role of free radicals. Free Radical Biology & Medicine. 2016;**98**:90-102

[25] Beckman KB, Ames BN. The free radical theory of aging matures. Physiological Reviews. 1998;**78**:547-581

[26] Burk RF, Lane JM, Patel K. Relationship of oxygen and glutathione in protection against carbon tetrachloride-induced hepatic microsomal lipid peroxidation and covalent binding in the rat. Rationale for the use of hyperbaric oxygen to treat carbon tetrachloride ingestion. The Journal of Clinical Investigation. 1984;**74**(6):1996-2001

[27] Foyer CH, Noctor G. Redox homeostasis and antioxidant signaling: A metabolic interface between stress perception and physiological responses. The Plant Cell. 2005;**17**(7):1866-1875

[28] Bouayed J, Bohn T. Exogenous antioxidants-double-edged swords in cellular redox state: Health beneficial effects at physiologic doses versus deleterious effects at high doses. Oxidative Medicine and Cellular Longevity. 2010;**3**(4):228-237

[29] Lau FC, Shukitt-Hale B, Joseph JA. The beneficial effects of fruit polyphenols on brain aging. Neurobiology of Aging. 2005;**26**:128-132

[30] Collard CD, Gelman S. Pathophysiology, clinical manifestations, and prevention of ischemia–reperfusion injury. Anesthesiology. 2001;**94**:1133-1138

[31] Van den Heuvel MG, Bast A, Haenen GR, Ambergen AW, Mermans JF, van der Hulst RR. The role of antioxidants in ischaemia-reperfusion in a human DIEP flap model. Journal of Plastic, Reconstructive & Aesthetic Surgery. 2012;**65**:1706-1711

[32] Ramires PR, Ji LL. Glutathione supplementation and training increases myocardial resistance to ischemia reperfusion in vivo. American Journal of Physiology Heart and Circulatory Physiology. 2001;**281**:H679-H688

[33] Bramley PM, Elmadfa I, Kafatos A, Kelly FJ, Manios Y, Roxborough HE, et al. Vitamin E. Journal of the Science of Food and Agriculture. 2000;**80**(7):913-938

[34] Marubayashi S, Dohi K, Ochi K, Kawasaki T. Role of free radicals in ischemic rat liver cell injury: Prevention of damage by alpha-tocopherol administration. Surgery. 1986 Feb;**99**(2):184-192

[35] Massey KD, Burton KP. α-Tocopherol attenuates myocardial membrane-related alterations resulting from ischemia and reperfusion. The American Journal of Physiology. 1989;**256**:Hl192-Hl199

[36] Wu TW, Hashimoto N, Au JX, Wu J, Mickle DA, Carey D. Trolox protects rat hepatocytes against oxyradical damage and the ischemic rat liver from reperfusion injury. Hepatology. 1991 Mar;**13**(3):575-580

[37] Codoñer-Franch P, Muñiz P, Gasco E, Domingo JV, Valls-Belles V. Effect of a diet supplemented with alpha-Tocopherol and beta-carotene on ATP and antioxidant levels after hepatic ischemia-reperfusion. Journal of Clinical Biochemistry and Nutrition. 2008;**43**(1):13-18

[38] Erkut B, Özyazıcıoğlu A, Karapolat BS, Koçoğulları CU, Keles S, Ateş A, et al. Effects of ascorbic acid, alpha-tocopherol and allopurinol on ischemia-reperfusion injury in rabbit skeletal muscle: An experimental study. Drug Target Insights. 2007;**2**:249-258

[39] Kearns SR, Daly AF, Sheehan K, Murray P, Kelly C, Bouchier-Hayes D. Oral vitamin C reduces the injury to skeletal muscle caused by compartment syndrome. Journal of Bone and Joint Surgery British (London). 2004;**86**:906-911

[40] Kearns SR, Kelly CJ, Barry M, et al. Vitamin C reduces ischaemia-reperfusion induced acute lung injury. European Journal of Vascular and Endovascular Surgery. 1999;**17**:533-536

[41] Sarkar S, Mukherjee A, Swarnakar S, Das N. Nanocapsulated ascorbic acid in combating cerebral ischemia reperfusion-induced oxidative injury in rat brain. Current Alzheimer Research. 2016;**13**:1363

[42] Lee JI, Son HY, Kim MC. Attenuation of ischemia-reperfusion injury by ascorbic acid in the canine renal transplantation. Journal of Veterinary Science. 2006;7(4):375-379

[43] Hsu CC, Wang JJ. L-Ascorbic acid and alpha-tocopherol attenuates liver ischemia-reperfusion induced of cardiac function impairment. Transplantation Proceedings. 2012;**44**(4):933-936

[44] Zaccaria A, Weinzweig N, Yoshitake M, Matsuda T, Cohen M. Vitamin C reduces ischemia-reperfusion injury in a rat epigastric island skin flap model. Annals of Plastic Surgery. 1994;**33**(6):620-623

[45] Yoshida WB, Campos EBP. Ischemia and reperfusion in skin flaps: Effects of mannitol and vitamin C in reducing necrosis area in a rat experimental model. Acta Cirúrgica Brasileira. 2005;**20**(5):358-363

[46] Kikugawa K, Hiramoto K, Tomiyama S, Asano Y. Beta-carotene effectively scavenges toxic nitrogen oxides: Nitrogen dioxide and peroxynitrous acid. FEBS Letters. 1997;**404**:175-178

[47] Bilgin-Karabulut A, Ademoğlu E, Aydin I, Erer M, Gökkuşu C. Protective effects of vitamins A and E pretreatment in venous ischemia/reperfusion injury. Journal of Reconstructive Microsurgery.

2001;**17**(6):425-443. DOI: 10.1055/s-2001-16356

[48] Stein HJ, Hinder RA, Oosthuizen MJ. Gastric mucosal injury caused by hemorrhagic shock and reperfusion: Protective role of the antioxidant glutathione. Surgery. 1990;**108**:467-474

[49] Makhija N, Sendasgupta C, Kiran U, et al. The role of oral coenzyme Q10 in patients undergoing coronary artery bypass graft surgery. Journal of Cardiothoracic and Vascular Anesthesia. 2008;**22**(6):832-839

[50] Bergamini C, Moruzzi N, Sblendido A, Lenaz G, Fato R. A water soluble CoQ10 formulation improves intracellular distribution and promotes mitochondrial respiration in cultured cells. PLoS One. 2012;**7**(3):e33712

[51] Kumar A, Kaur H, Devi P, Mohan V. Role of coenzyme Q10 (CoQ10) in cardiac disease, hypertension and Meniere-like syndrome. Pharmacology & Therapeutics. 2009;**124**:259-268

[52] Boroujeni MB, Khayat ZK, Anbari K, Niapour A, Gholami M, Gharravi AM. Coenzyme Q10 protects skeletal muscle from ischemia-reperfusion through the NF-kappa B pathway. Perfusion. 2017;**32**(5):372-377

[53] Thomas SR, Neuzil J, Stocker R. Cosupplementation with coenzyme Q prevents the prooxidant effect of alpha-tocopherol and increases the resistance of LDL to transition of metal-dependent oxidation initiation. Arteriosclerosis, Thrombosis, and Vascular Biology. 1996;**16**:687-696

[54] Hwang J, Min S, Jeon Y, Hwang J, Park S, Kim J, et al. Effect of coenzyme Q10 on spinal cord ischemia-reperfusion injury. Journal of Neurosurgery: Spine SPI. 2015;**22**(4):432-438

[55] Özalp B, Elbey H, Aydın H, Tekkesin MS, Uzun H. The effect of coenzyme Q10 on venous ischemia reperfusion injury. The Journal of Surgical Research. 2016;**204**(2):304-310. DOI: 10.1016/j.jss.2016.04.075. Epub 2016 May 7

[56] Perham RN. Swinging arms and swinging domains in multifunctional enzymes: Catalytic machines for multistep reactions. Annual Review of Biochemistry. 2000;**69**:961-1004

[57] May JM, Qu Z-C, Mendiratta S. Protection and recycling of α-tocopherol in human erythrocytes by intracellular ascorbic acid. Archives of Biochemistry and Biophysics. 1998;**349**(2):281-289

[58] Wang PR, Wang JS, Zhang C, Song XF, Tian N, Kong LY. Huang-Lian-Jie-Du-Decotion induced protective autophagy against the injury of cerebral ischemia/reperfusion via MAPK-mTOR signaling pathway. Journal of Ethnopharmacology. 2013;**149**:270-280

[59] Packer L, Tritschler HJ, Wessel K. Neuroprotection by the metabolic antioxidant alpha-lipoic acid. Free Radical Biology & Medicine. 1997;**22**:359-378

[60] Deng H, Zuo X, Zhang J, Liu X, Liu L, Xu Q, et al. α-Lipoic acid protects against cerebral ischemia/reperfusion-induced injury in rats. Molecular Medicine Reports. 2015;**11**(5):3659-3665

[61] Othman AI, El-Missiry MA, Amer MA, Arafa M. Melatonin controls oxidative stress and modulates iron, ferritin, and transferrin levels in adriamycin treated rats. Life Sciences. 2008;**83**:563-568

[62] Kedziora-Kornatowska K, Szewczyk-Golec K, Czuczejko J, Pawluk H, van Marke de Lumen K, Kozakiewicz M, et al. Antioxidative effects of melatonin administration in elderly primary essential hypertension patients. Journal of Pineal Research. 2008;**45**:312-317

[63] Lesnefsky EJ, Chen Q, Tandler B, Hoppel CL. Mitochondrial dysfunction and myocardial ischemia–reperfusion: Implications for novel therapies. Annual Review of Pharmacology and Toxicology. 2017;**57**:535-565. DOI: 10.1146/annurev-pharmtox-010715-103335

[64] Reiter RJ, Mayo JC, Tan DX, Sainz RM, Alatorre-Jimenez M, Qin L. Melatonin as an antioxidant: Under promises but over delivers. Journal of Pineal Research. 2016;**61**:253-278

[65] Aydemir S, Dogan D, Kocak A, Dilsiz N. The effect of melatonin on spinal cord after ischemia in rats. Spinal Cord. 2016 May;**54**(5):360-363. DOI: 10.1038/sc.2015.204. Epub 2015 Dec 1

[66] Singhanat K, Apaijai N, Chattipakorn SC, et al. Cellular and Molecular Life Sciences. 2018;**75**:4125

[67] Gurlek A, Celik M, Parlakpinar H, Aydogan H, Bay-Karabulut A. The protective effect of melatonin on ischemia–reperfusion injury in the groin (inferior epigastric) flap model in rats. Journal of Pineal Research. 2006;**40**:312-317

[68] Bozkurt AK. Alpha-tocopherol (vitamin E) and iloprost attenuate reperfusion injury in skeletal muscle ischemia/reperfusion injury. The Journal of Cardiovascular Surgery. 2002;**43**:693

[69] Kayiran O, Uysal A, Cuzdan SS, Kocer U. Struggling with ischemia reperfusion injury. The Journal of Craniofacial Surgery. 2007 Mar;**18**(2):457-458

[70] Halliwell BGJ. Free Radicals in Biology and Medicine. 4th ed. New York: Oxford University Press Inc.; 2007

[71] Fernandez J, Perez-Alvarez JA, Fernandez-Lopez JA. Thiobarbituric acid test for monitoring lipid oxidation in meat. Food Chemistry. 1997;**59**(3):345-353

[72] Korkmaz A, Kolankaya D. The protective effects of ascorbic acid against renal ischemia-reperfusion injury in male rats. Renal Failure. 2009;**31**:36-43

[73] Siti HN, Kamisah Y, Kamsiah J. The role of oxidative stress, antioxidants and vascular inflammation in cardiovascular disease (a review). Vascular Pharmacology. 2015;**71**:40-56

[74] Carr A, Frei B. Does vitamin C act as a pro-oxidant under physiological conditions? The FASEB Journal. 1999;**13**(9):1007-1024

[75] Mendes-da-Silva RF, Lopes-de-Morais AA, Bandim-da-Silva ME, Cavalcanti GA, Rodrigues AR, Andrade-da-Costa BL, et al. Prooxidant versus antioxidant brain action of ascorbic acid in well-nourished and malnourished rats as a function of dose: A cortical spreading depression and malondialdehyde analysis. Neuropharmacology. 2014;**86**:155-160

[76] Chen G, Shen H, Zang L, Su Z, Huang J, Sun Y, et al. Protective effect of luteolin on skin ischemia-reperfusion injury through an AKT-dependent mechanism. International Journal of Molecular Medicine. 2018;**42**(6):3073-3082

[77] Yin Z, Ren H, Liu L, Chen W, Gan C, Jiao H, et al. Thioredoxin protects skin flaps from ischemia-reperfusion injury: A novel prognostic and therapeutic target. Plastic and Reconstructive Surgery. 2016;**137**(2):511-521

[78] Eroglu T, Bozkurt M, Kapi E, Selcuk CT, Kuvat SV, Tufek A, et al. A study on the effects of the use of propofol in experimental model inferior Epigastric

Island flap on ischemia-reperfusion injury. The Journal of Craniofacial Surgery. 2017;**28**(8):2193-2198. DOI: 10.1097/SCS.0000000000004049

[79] Ozyigit F, Kucuk A, Akcer S, Tosun M, Kocak FE, Kocak C, et al. Different dose-dependent effects of ebselen in sciatic nerve ischemia-reperfusion injury in rats. Bosnian Journal of Basic Medical Sciences. 2015;**15**(4):36-43. DOI: 10.17305/bjbms.2015.521

[80] Zhang DY, Kang SS, Zhang ZW, Wu R. Edaravone enhances the viability of ischemia/reperfusion flaps. Journal of Huazhong University of Science and Technology Medical Sciences. 2017;**37**(1):51-56